The Textbook of Health Psychology

This book examines the concept of health psychology following its trajectory from ancient to contemporary times. It analyses the theories, practice and research in health psychology from both Indian and Western perspectives.

The volume brings together knowledge diversified across various narrow subfields. It expounds upon physiological psychology; chronic illnesses associated with physiological systems; and biopsychosocial approaches to treatment and management with therapeutic interventions integrated throughout the book. It further discusses health promotive and health risk behaviour with reference to health policies and databases at national and global levels.

This book will be beneficial to the students, researchers and teachers of psychology, applied psychology, public health, public policy, community health, and medical and paramedical studies. It will also be indispensable to the policy-makers and NGOs working in the field of public health.

Meena Hariharan is superannuated as Professor in the Centre for Health Psychology at the University of Hyderabad, India. She is the founder-director of this centre, which was launched in 2007. She is one among the very few in India working in the area of behavioural cardiology. She has developed and validated effective intervention models for cardiac patients. Her research includes quality of doctor-patient communication and ICU trauma resilience, stress and coping. She has designed intervention packages for CABG patients and standardized scales for psychosocial assessment of cardiac patients, measurement of quality of doctor-patient communication and adolescent well-being to mention a few. She is the founder-president of the Association of Health Psychologists and the editor of the *Journal of Health Studies*.

The Textbook of Health Psychology

Meena Hariharan

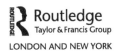
LONDON AND NEW YORK

First published 2024
by Routledge
4 Park Square, Milton Park, Abingdon, Oxon OX14 4RN

and by Routledge
605 Third Avenue, New York, NY 10158

Routledge is an imprint of the Taylor & Francis Group, an informa business

© 2024 Meena Hariharan

The right of Meena Hariharan to be identified as author of this work has been asserted in accordance with sections 77 and 78 of the Copyright, Designs and Patents Act 1988.

All rights reserved. No part of this book may be reprinted or reproduced or utilised in any form or by any electronic, mechanical, or other means, now known or hereafter invented, including photocopying and recording, or in any information storage or retrieval system, without permission in writing from the publishers.

Trademark notice: Product or corporate names may be trademarks or registered trademarks, and are used only for identification and explanation without intent to infringe.

British Library Cataloguing-in-Publication Data
A catalogue record for this book is available from the British Library

Library of Congress Cataloging-in-Publication Data
Names: Hariharan, Meena, author.
Title: The textbook of health psychology / Meena Hariharan.
Description: Abingdon, Oxon; New York, NY: Routledge, 2024. |
Includes bibliographical references and index. |
Identifiers: LCCN 2023044830 (print) | LCCN 2023044831 (ebook) |
ISBN 9781032573281 (hardback) | ISBN 9781032573304 (paperback) |
ISBN 9781003438908 (ebook)
Subjects: LCSH: Clinical health psychology—Textbooks. | Health attitudes—Textbooks. | Health behavior—Textbooks.
Classification: LCC R726.7 .H3693 2024 (print) | LCC R726.7 (ebook) |
DDC 613.01/9—dc23/eng/20240112
LC record available at https://lccn.loc.gov/2023044830
LC ebook record available at https://lccn.loc.gov/2023044831

ISBN: 978-1-032-57328-1 (hbk)
ISBN: 978-1-032-57330-4 (pbk)
ISBN: 978-1-003-43890-8 (ebk)

DOI: 10.4324/9781003438908

Typeset in Times New Roman
by codeMantra

Contents

List of figures vi
List of tables ix
List of boxes x
Foreword xii
Preface xvi
Acknowledgements xviii

1 History and Evolution of Health Psychology 1

2 Wellness, Illness, Health and Health Psychology 22

3 Positive Health Behaviour 49

4 Health Risk Behaviour 80

5 Theories of Health Behaviour 119

6 Human Physiology 186

7 Stress and Illness 240

8 Chronic Illness and Therapeutic Interventions 290

9 Psychology of the Caregiver and Careprovider 354

10 Health Resilience 402

11 Pain and Its Psychosocial Correlates 436

Index *453*

Figures

1.1	Humour and Personality Relationship	3
1.2	Body-Mind Dualism	4
1.3	Pavlov's Conditioning Experiment	5
1.4	Sigmund Freud (1856–1939)	7
1.5	Louis Pasteur (1822–1895)	7
1.6	Physiological Response to External Stimulus	9
1.7	Placebo Effect	11
1.8	Gate Theory of Pain: Psychosocial Factors	12
1.9	APA Includes Health Psychology as 38th Branch	14
1.10	Research Publications in Health Psychology	14
1.11	Indian Origin: Contributions of Ayurveda	18
2.1	Biomedical Model of Health and Illness	25
2.2	Biopsychosocial Model of Health and Illness	29
2.3	Biopsychosocial Model: Symbiotic Relationship among Factors	30
2.4	Tridoshas-Panchamahabhoota Relationship	33
2.5	Tridosha's Control over Psychophysiological Functions	34
2.6	Framework of Health Psychology	45
3.1	Illness Prevention: Primary, Secondary and Tertiary	53
3.2	Healthy Eating—Ayurveda Perspective	58
3.3	Reasons for Exercising and Not Exercising	64
3.4	Screening to Detect Disease	72
4.1	Factors Influencing Eating Behaviour	85
4.2	Body Image and Eating Behaviour	87
4.3	Smoking as Health Risk Behaviour	95
4.4	On the Road to Alcohol Addiction	100
4.5	Progression of Stages in Alcoholism and Pleasure Pain Balance Sheet	103
5.1	Health Belief Model	122
5.2	Fundamentals of Protection Motivation Theory	128
5.3	Protection Motivation Theory with Cognitive Mediation Process and Behavioural Outcome	129
5.4	Ordered Protection Motivation Schema	130
5.5	Theory of Reasoned Action	133
5.6	Theory of Planned Behaviour	137
5.7	Transtheoretical Model	139
5.8	Stages of Transtheoretical Model in Real Life	140
5.9	Stages of Precaution Adoption Process Model	149

Figures vii

5.10	Three Types of Self-Efficacy	152
5.11	Health Action Process Approach (HAPA)	155
5.12	Types of Motivation	160
5.13	Self-Determination Theory in Health Behaviour Context	165
5.14	Social Cognition Theory	169
5.15	Social Cognitive Theory & Health Behaviour	172
5.16	Self-Regulation Model	176
6.1	Structure of the Neuron	188
6.2	Neural Networking and Communication	190
6.3	Components of the Nervous System	191
6.4	Basic Concepts of Locations/Positions	192
6.5	Ventricular System of the Brain	193
6.6	Brain: Its Anatomical Divisions and Subdivisions	194
6.7	(a) Major Parts in the Brain. (b) Lobes in the Brain	195
6.8	Location of Thalamus and Hypothalamus	197
6.9	Spinal Cord: Cross-section	199
6.10	12 Pairs of Cranial Nerves	201
6.11	Structural Representation of the Peripheral Nervous System	202
6.12	Functions of the Autonomic Nervous System	203
6.13	Endocrine System	205
6.14	Structure of Human Heart	211
6.15	Respiratory System	215
6.16	Anatomy of Stomach	220
6.17	Digestive System	222
6.18	Renal System and Kidney (a and b)	225
6.19	Immune System: Functions	237
7.1	Sympathetic Adrenomedullary System (SAM)	243
7.2	Hypothalamic-Pituitary-Adrenal (HPA) Axis Response to Stress	244
7.3	General Adaptation Syndrome (GAS)	246
7.4	Cognitive Appraisal of Stress	251
7.5	Cognitive Appraisal and Coping Process in Stress	253
7.6	Sources of Stress	256
7.7	Optimum Stress Level (OSL)	262
7.8	Stress-Illness Link	267
7.9	Impact of Stress on Body Organs	268
7.10	LoC as Moderator of Perceived Stress	275
7.11	Explanatory Style of Stress	278
7.12	Stakes-Effort Balance and Stress	279
7.13	Sources of Stress for Children	281
7.14	Childhood Stress	282
8.1	Comprehensive Treatment Plan for Cystic Fibrosis	302
8.2	Aetiology of PMS (PMDD)	313
8.3	Biopsychosocial Symptoms of PMS/PMDD	314
8.4	Treatment Approaches to PMS/PMDD	314
8.5	Impact of Uncertainty on Chronic Patients	323
8.6	Cognitive Appraisal, Adaptation and Coping	328
8.7	Psychosocial Intervention to Chronic Illness: Quality of Life	333
8.8	Impact of Knowledge Intervention	341

9.1	Patient, Caregiver, Health Care Provider Triangle	355
9.2	Reciprocal Relationship between Patient and Caregiver	366
9.3	Multitasking of a Caregiver	368
9.4	Impact of Quality of Communication on Prognosis	381
9.5	Progress of Physician Burnout	391
10.1	Richardson's Resilience Model	406
10.2	Synergy Point	408
10.3	Hariharan-Rajendran Synergy Model: Pathway	409
10.4	Utilizing the 'Non-sick' Faculties for Flourishing	415
10.5	Resilience and Self-Efficacy	417
10.6	'Hope' in Chronic Patients with Resilience	419
10.7	Benefit-Finding	420
10.8	Optimizing on Abilities	423
11.1	Psychosocial Factors of Pain	443

Tables

2.1	Top ten causes of death across the globe	41
2.2	Major causes of death in the year 2020 (projections)	42
3.1	Percentage of sample in the Harris and Guten (1979) study always or almost always performing selected behaviours in order to protect their health	52
3.2	*Charaka's* 12 groups of food	56
3.3	Mental attributes associated with choice of food	56
3.4	Seasonal Considerations for healthy eating	57
3.5	Recommendation of the expert panel for age-appropriate sleep duration	65
3.6	Achievement percentage of maternity and child health activities (immunization) in India (2008–2017)	74
4.1	Top causes of death in India	81
4.2	Risk factors that cause disability and death (combined)	81
4.3	Prevalence of obesity among adults, age 18+ (%) (both sexes), 1975–2016	82
4.4	Prevalence of malnutrition in developed and developing countries (BMI < 18.5 kg/m)	84
4.5	Prevalence of HIV across the World and India (values refer to percentage)	91
5.1	Temporal details of the stages of the TTM	139
5.2	Process of change across stages of behavioural change	143
5.3	Two phases in HAPA	153
5.4	Theories of health behavioural change at a glance	179
6.1	Important glands in the endocrine system, their location, the hormones, and functions	208
6.2	Secondary sex characteristics	228
7.1	Social Readjustment Rating Scale (SRRS)	249
8.1	Prevalence of depression and anxiety among patients with chronic illness related to cardiovascular, pulmonary, gastrointestinal and dermatological diseases (prevalence per population of 1000)	319
8.2	Biopsychosocial impact of chronic illness	326

Boxes

1.1	Evaluation of Health Psychology: Time line	15
2.1	Significant Aspects of the Biomedical Model	26
2.2	Paralytic Stroke: Two Versions	27
2.3	Recovery of CABG Patient	28
2.4	Comparison between Biomedical and Biopsychosocial Models	32
2.5	Relevance of Health Psychology	46
3.1	Researcher's Box	76
3.2	Practitioner's Box	77
4.1	Synergistic Effects of Smoking and Risk Factors	94
4.2	Signs of Problem Drinking	102
4.3	Health Risks of Alcohol Consumption	109
4.4	Researcher's Box	114
4.5	Practitioners Box	115
5.1	Researcher's Box	126
5.2	Practitioner's Box	126
5.3	Researcher's Box	131
5.4	Practitioner's Box	132
5.5	Researchers' Box	134
5.6	Practitioner's Box	135
5.7	Researcher's Box	147
5.8	Practitioner's Box	147
5.9	Researcher's Box	150
5.10	Practitioner's Box	150
5.11	Researcher's Box	157
5.12	Practitioner's Box	158
5.13	Researcher's Box	168
5.14	Practitioner's Box	168
5.15	Researcher's Box	173
5.16	Practitioner's Box	174
5.17	Researcher's Box	177
5.18	Practitioner's Box	178
6.1	Summary of the Circulatory System or Cardiovascular System	214
6.2	Summary of the Digestive System	224
6.3	Summary of the Renal System	227
6.4	Researcher's Box	233
6.5	Summary of the Reproductive System	233

6.6	Summary of the Immune System	238
7.1	Summary of Stress Theories	253
7.2	Know Your OSL	262
7.3	Impact of Stress on Various Systems	274
7.4	Researcher's Box	285
7.5	Practitioner's Box	285
8.1	Chronic Illness Related to the Systems	292
8.2	Researcher's Box	349
8.3	Practitioner's Box	350
9.1	Psychosocial Intervention for the Caregiver along Patients' Phases of Disease Progression	374
9.2	Reciprocal Relationship between Doctor and Patient	378
9.3	Doctor-Patient Relationship: Impact on Health Outcome Variables	385
9.4	Factors Negatively Impacting Doctor-Patient Relationship	386
9.5	Doctor Burnout and the General Symptoms	390
9.6	Researcher's Box	395
9.7	Practitioner's Box	396
10.1	Resilience and Chronic Diseases	425
10.2	Researcher's Box	429
10.3	Practitioner's Box	430

Foreword

Notwithstanding the fact that the term 'health' has wide-ranging connotations which often vary across cultures, the concerns to ensure the quality of health and well-being are globally acknowledged. Etymologically, health signifies wholesomeness of a person. In a real-life context, health carries a strong connection with the experiences of happiness, sanity and cleanliness. The history of human civilization shows that there has been parallel existence of a range of healing systems from different epistemological positions and heterogeneous cultural contexts; the practice of biomedicine informed by scientific perspective has become the dominant one. It views human reality segmentally. Modern medical practice shows intrinsic tension due to the distancing between patients and the agents that deliver the health service. Health remains personalized while health care has become a professional matter. In essence, the North American values of egocentricity of self, mind-body dualism and marginalized role of culture constitute the basic framework for understanding health. This kind of atomization, specialization and fragmentation in matters of health is a relatively new phenomenon, and its problems are increasing. Contrarily, holistic worldviews were dominant until the past four centuries. They were located in local eco-cultural contexts, and therefore, access to them was within the reach of the common man. In most cases, the health-related processes were understood and easily comprehended by everybody. The processes of treatment and healing encompassed the personal, social, psychological and spiritual realms of life. The Indian perspectives and related thoughts and practices address the phenomenon of health and health care holistically.

It is interesting to note that the Hippocratic Oath observed that "the well-being of man is influenced by air, water, food, wind, and topography of the land. An organism is a living system". Socrates had remarked that "for us, a part can never be well unless the whole is well". Also, terms like 'health' and 'holism' are semantically very closely linked to each other. The Greek word 'hollos' stands for wholeness. In Anglo-Saxon usage, the terms whole, hale and holy stem from the same root. Thus, the holistic view has ancient roots. It is a global phenomenon. The indigenous medicine systems of India like *Ayurveda, Yoga, Siddha*, various practices of meditation, and traditional medicine in Tibet, China and Africa clearly aim at disease prevention, health promotion, managing psychosomatic and chronic conditions, and enhancing immune functioning in a holistic manner. The *Panchamahabhootas* (i.e. earth, water, fire, wind and ether/sky) are the common ingredients constituting the material existence of everything including the human body. *Ayurveda* relies on three bodily humours (i.e. *vata, pitta and kapha*) and three gunas (*Sattva*—illumination; *Rajas*—dynamism; and *Tamas*—passivity). They form a functioning unit. According to *Ayurveda*, patient, attendant, medicine and physician are the four pillars of treatment. It maintains multiple causation systems to explain the complexity of health and well-being. They are not a default concept. The dynamic state of *Samyavastha* (equanimity) is emphasized in several ways. As stated by Sushruta, the well-being of the self (*Atman*), senses and mind constitutes health (prasannatmendriyamanah, swasthamityabhidhiyate). A state of *sama* is emphasized in all aspects of bodily functioning (*Sam dosha: samagnishch sam dhatu mal kriya*). Bhagavad Gita states that evenness of mind or *samatva* is Yoga (*samatvam yoga uchyate, Gita, 2/48*). Also, there is a distinct emphasis on appropriateness. One should be *Yukta* in all aspects of life. Gita says that "*Yoga* becomes the destroyer of pain for him who is moderate in eating and recreation, who is moderate in his exertion during his actions, who is moderate in sleep and wakefulness" (Gita, 6/17). In the Yogic system (*Yoga Sutra, 2/3*), the major problems in life or *Kleshas* (afflictions) are *Avidya* (ignorance), *Asmita* (egoism), *Raga* (attachment), *Dvesha* (aversion) and *Abhinivesha* (desire to cling to life). The various systems of Yoga including *Raj yoga, Bhakti Yoga* and *Karma Yoga* are proposed. Thus, we find that biopsychosocial and spiritual factors are taken into account in diagnosis and therapy.

The indigenous systems of medicine maintain that the body has an innate capacity to heal itself and the whole is greater than the sum of its parts. It is gradually being realized that mind and matter are indistinguishable. The basic oneness of the universe with ontological holism is an emerging view. Reductionism is being replaced by a holistic paradigm. Thus, we find the emergence of disciplines like 'psychoneuroimmunology'. Malfunctioning or illness seems to take place in the context of mind, spirit and culture. Healing has religious, social and spiritual aspects. The experience of conscious involvement in the project of life and integration through self-transcendence is needed. To be a human is to be a spiritual person. In fact, traditional medicines are showing that the boundaries across systems are blurred. Indigenous is recast in a new *avatar* as herbal medicine. Also, healing is approached from a phenomenological perspective in which rituals and social relations play a key role. They hold a complementary relationship.

Holistic health care involves a person- or people-centred system of care, which optimally integrates the strategies addressing mind, body and spirit. Whole person and ongoing participation are key players in it. It implies a dynamic understanding of health and illness. The challenge is to establish a health care system to meet the criteria of equality, effectiveness, safety, ethics and cost-effectiveness, friendliness, interpersonal sensitivity, and connection with the larger social world. Health as wholeness cannot be confined to the body. This would require transcending the disciplinary boundaries and movement from compassion-based systems to people-centred approaches. Such an integrative approach is in tune with India's National Health Policy, 2017; National Education Policy, 2020; and National Digital Health Mission, 2020, and Sustainable Development Goals (SDG). It is gratifying that in 2014, the Indian government established the AYUSH ministry to cater to the needs of Ayurveda, Yoga, Unani, Siddha and Homeopathy systems, and attempts are being made to promote these systems of medicine. It promotes unconventional and alternative/complementary systems of medicine.

Holistic health care demands correct and effective prevention methods and patient-centred medical care. We also need to establish correct and dignified rehabilitation and support during illness so that the physical, mental and spiritual needs are suitably addressed. Holistic integrated care for health involves exercise, socialization, safe housing and provision for adequate means so that the restrictions that compromise health can be removed. Social care and support to assist vulnerable, socioeconomically disadvantaged and elderly people through relevant legislation and the creation of fluid organizational settings and service delivery would be required. Smooth interaction between diverse functional components for optimum survival advantage should be ensured. Unfortunately, holism is used as an attractive label to recruit customers. It may be misleading if urgent life-threatening conditions are not properly attended to. Humans are complex biological and cultural systems that require coordinated time-dependent interactions between diverse functional components for optimum survival advantage. As holistic health care is culturally acceptable, efficacious and pragmatic, sincere efforts are needed to move in this direction.

This will reduce health disparity, ensure social justice and address the health crisis, which is emerging. It's a challenge as well as an opportunity for social scientists interested in pursuing the goal of health and well-being.

The Indian tradition considers that a healthy person is autolocus (*Svastha*). As a dynamic state of harmony and balance reflecting effective mind-body functioning within the ecology, health happens to be a continuous process requiring constant monitoring and adjustment on a long-term basis. It is not a one-time or short-term affair, as it relates to the entire life span, which Indians, the Vedic seers, prayed for hundred years of an active and meaningful life: *Pashyema Sharadah Shatam*. The subdiscipline of health psychology addresses questions such as: What are the psychological influences on health? How do people stay healthy? Why do people become ill? How do they respond when they get ill? The health psychological research, therefore, engages with these and related questions and tries to evolve interventions that help people maintain health and restore it in the case of illness. In the last few decades, the field of health psychology has encompassed a wide range of issues including concerns for health promotion, illness prevention, correlates of health and illness, provisions for health care systems and development of a health policy for guiding the implementation of health measures in the society.

Unfortunately, the belief that health is primarily physical in nature still prevails in a large section of the masses. This approach misses the fact that health needs to be understood as an integration of physical, social and psychological perspectives. It is well known that psychological processes such as appraisal and social support not only shape psychological functioning on a day-to-day basis but also have long-term effects. Similarly, the roles of resilience, self-regulation, positive emotions, meaning and control of beliefs have shown that psychological processes do contribute a lot towards the promotion of health and well-being. Traditionally, the psychological aspects of health were taken into account in connection with clinical psychology and psychopathology. The gradual emergence of health psychology has shifted the attention of researchers towards the problems of stress, coping and social support as major influences on health status. In recent years, an increasingly larger number of studies were launched for delineating the factors related to health behaviour that may facilitate evolving mechanisms of health promotion, especially by introducing lifestyle changes. Since many health habits are interrelated and resist change, multiple strategies are being tried out.

It is being observed that instead of individual and group interventions, social engineering might be more effective. Critical health psychology researchers have begun to deconstruct dominant meanings of health, illness and health care. They work with participants to further understand health and illness experience and seek to achieve change and transformation in an increasing range of ways. Arenas such as health consumerism, medicalization and pharmaceuticalization have become the focus of research for critical health psychologists.

It is important for psychologists to engage with the critical emerging debates around the moral panic of the 'obesity epidemic', the construction of obesity as a disease, processes of disease mongering and the role of 'big pharma' in creating and fostering new diseases.

In some respects, legislation is also found helpful. Indeed, one needs to identify the situations, which help modification of health risk behaviours creatively. Perhaps there is no such thing as a 'health behaviour' (in the abstracted sense). Rather, social practices involving behaviours with implications for health (such as smoking) are necessarily embedded in context; they need to be studied in context to understand their meaning and the logic of their enactment. A meaningful discourse about health should be situated in a specific cultural context. This becomes more important in the Indian context where the society has been undergoing socioeconomic transformation. The concomitant processes of industrialization and urbanization have led to large-scale migration of people from villages to cities. Majority of them consist of unskilled labours working as daily wagers. The cities are experiencing unprecedented growth, leading to problems of housing, commuting to workplace, issues related to civic arrangements and provisions for health care. Especially, the lack of social security measures for a large section of the population is posing serious problems. Also, there is a visible expansion of the middle class, which is emulating the upper-middle and higher strata of the society. The result is an increase in the level of aspiration, which in turn leads to frustration and tension. In terms of health scenario, we have been witnessing a rapid rise in the incidence of cancer, cardiovascular diseases, alcohol and other substance abuse, diabetes, high blood pressure and obesity.

In this background, this book authored by Professor Meena Hariharan fulfils an important need in the field of psychology. The volume is quite comprehensive and tries to capture most of the key aspects of health psychology. It is gratifying that the author has paid attention to the Indian cultural context and documented relevant psychological contributions. They are exciting and follow different methodologies to address a wide range of issues. The volume covers most of the themes in the area and offers useful psychological perspectives.

The growing field of health psychology has uncovered many moderators and mediators of health outcomes. This field is changing the societal scenario and making a difference in the lives of people. It also has an enormous value in training, and research, as the domain of health, provides an opportunity to explore and examine psychological theories in a real-life setting. The present volume brings together wisdom from the indigenous stream and the mainstream. It attends to the foundations, processes, threats and possibilities for intervention in relation to the understanding of health and sustaining it through health protective behaviours. An interesting feature of the volume is that each chapter presents key ideas for practitioners and researchers. This furnishes a ground for building connections and pursuing interfaces across different audiences interested in the area of health. The illustrations by the artist help in easily relating the text to one's own life situations. Keeping with the contemporary health issue of chronic diseases and pain, a dedicated chapter on the pain and its psychological correlates is a value addition to the book. I take great pleasure in recommending this volume not only to the students of psychology but also to the general readers interested in delving deeper into the intricacies of health and health behaviour. I am sure that the readers from different backgrounds will enjoy reading it and researchers would venture into new and challenging areas.

Professor Girishwar Misra
Former Vice Chancellor
Mahatma Gandhi Antarrashtriya Hindi Vishwavidyalaya, Wardha, Maharashtra
Former Head, Psychology Department
University of Delhi, Delhi

Preface

As my first initiative, I along with Professor Radhanath Rath authored the book *Coping with Life Stress: The Indian Experience*, citing the Indian case studies and analyses. Many eminent psychologists of the country expressed that they expect a textbook on health psychology from me. I started going through several textbooks in the area, speaking to students, teachers, practitioners and researchers in health psychology. It gave me an insight into the needs of the people in the field and the missing links and gaps in the available textbooks. After surveying the course structure of many universities in India and abroad, the most essential chapters to constitute the textbook were identified. This book is an outcome of such elaborate background work.

The book is divided into 11 chapters. Chapter 1 'History and Evolution of Health Psychology' tracks the origin of the biopsychosocial model of health practices to ancient Ayurveda and also chronicles the development of the division of health psychology as an alternative to the biomedical model in the Western world. Chapter 2 elaborates on the concept of health and health psychology, bringing a contrast between the Western and Indian perspectives. The chapter enumerates the biopsychosocial model of health and psychosocial factors preceding, accompanying and following health and illness, and gives the broad framework of health psychology. Chapters 3 and 4 are related to health behaviour. While Chapter 3 provides an extensive account of health protective and health promotive behaviour, Chapter 4 deals with health risk behaviour. Both the chapters provide the data related to the Indian population. Besides, Chapter 3 focuses on the rich Indian practices for health promotion and protection for enhancing well-being. Chapter 5 gives extensive treatment to the theories of health behaviour. It gives a detailed account of 10 theories and their application. Chapter 6 is on the human physiology. It explains with diagrams the structure and functions of eight systems in the human body, namely the nervous system, endocrine system, cardiovascular system, respiratory system, digestive system, renal system, reproductive system and immune system. Chapter 7 is related to stress and illness. This chapter gives a broad view of the theories of stress and sources of stress. The thrust of this chapter is on the impact of stress on health related to various systems in the body. The chapter also has a section on childhood stress as a contemporary area of concern for health psychologists. Chapter 8 discusses the biopsychosocial aspects related to chronic illnesses. It can be related to the chapter on theories of health behaviour, on the one hand, and stress and illness, on the other. The chapter while giving a brief account of chronic illnesses related to the eight systems of the body places its emphasis on the psychological state, coping process of the chronic patient and psychosocial interventions such as cognitive, affective, behavioural and motivational therapies. Chapter 9 relates to caregivers and professional care providers. The contemporary research in health psychology includes the health and well-being of these two significant partners in patient care. The aspects related to their well-being and the need for systematic formal assessments and interventions are discussed extensively. Chapter 10 is on health resilience. This is a very relevant chapter that has enormous potential for future research and exploration. The purpose of this chapter is to highlight that illness experience and quality of life differ in persons with resilience. The chapter brings the issue of concept and measurement of resilience among persons with chronic and terminal illness and quality of life. It also suggests interventions for promoting resilience among people. Chapter 11 relates to psychosocial correlates of pain and pain management. Pain being a biological and emotional experience needs to be approached from biopsychosocial perspective. The chapter delineates various types of pain, various theories, and the cognitive, affective and behavioural dimensions associated with the experience of pain. The psychological interventions to pain are described.

The aspect of therapeutic interventions is integrated into the chapters to contextualize its relevance. Therefore, it is not given separate treatment in an exclusive chapter. This textbook is a modest attempt to address the needs of the students at undergraduate and postgraduate levels, researchers and practitioners in the field of health psychology. Every chapter and theory has a special box for the practising health psychologists providing the methods of assessments and interventions to the patients. Similarly, every chapter and theory has a special box for the researchers triggering innovative ideas for research in the concerned area. These suggestions, though not exhaustive, are expected to stimulate the students to think innovatively in culturally relevant lines so that the research is meaningful to the society and nation at large. The cultural relevance of this book is enhanced by citing not only the studies from the West but also the findings from Asian countries, particularly Indian studies. I hope the students, teachers, researchers and practising health psychologists find it useful for their purpose.

Acknowledgements

From the time this book was conceived until the manuscript was ready, I received support from various quarters—my gratitude to each one of them. I wish to make special mention of Dr Meera Padhy and Dr Usha Chivukula who never hesitated to invest their time in going through the parts of the manuscript and provide their inputs whenever needed. Anupam Arunachalam who added attraction to this book through illustrations deserves a special mention. The immense support, understanding and encouragement I received from my family members helped me to sustain the pressure of sticking to the schedule. My special gratitude to my sister Professor Jayashree Mohanraj for her timely support towards the end of the project. To every single person mentioned above, I express my gratitude.

1 History and Evolution of Health Psychology

Health Psychology as a distinct branch in the discipline of Psychology came into existence with the increasing need of viewing 'health' as an outcome of the symbiotic relationship between the individual's physiological and psychological functioning. Hence, the history of Health Psychology needs to be traced by following two paths—the Western and the Indian. In both, the emphasis has to be on the health practices, from ancient to contemporary times. A scrutiny of this leads to the inference that while the Western practices of medicine and progress in medical sciences significantly contributed to the evolution of Health Psychology as a distinct 38th branch of the American Psychological Association (APA), in Indian medical science and practice of medicine, it was always an integral part though not identified by the name of Health Psychology. First, we will examine the emergence of Health Psychology from the Western perspective. Then, we will identify the roots of Health Psychology in the Indian medical system.

Health Practices in the West: Emergence of Health Psychology

Health practices in different countries underwent a number of changes influenced by the nation's sociopolitical, industrial, economic and religious/spiritual needs and demands of the time on the one hand and inventions and discoveries in the field of science across the globe on the other. Though a few countries like India had a strong footing in a holistic approach to health from Vedic time, the credit for carving out the psychosocial aspects in health practices, highlighting its significance, advocating for it and christening it with a distinct name as 'Health Psychology' and establishing it as an important branch in science based on research evidence should go to the US. The emergence of Health Psychology can be tracked to about a hundred-year history of health practices in the US and Europe.

With the fall of the Roman Empire, knowledge about medical practice in the early middle age came from surviving Greek and Roman texts. Before the 4th century BC, there was a strong relationship between health beliefs and religious beliefs. Illness was believed to be the punishment of God for the sins.

4th–6th Century BCE

This period could be traced back to people's focus in the soul—rather than the physical body. As a consequence, the treatment for illness was prayers (Hajar). The patients in Greece visited temples praying to *Asclepius*, the healing God for cure. The temples, the places of healing, had a congenial environment with gardens and fountains and provided bathing and nutrition as part of the healing process. Thus, it appeared as if the common thread of Greek medicine was a combination of spirituality and patient's participation in the form of a positive diet and other healing processes such as bathing. However, the cure of illness seems to have had a strong basis on the beliefs of patients and doctors rather than any empirical evidence.

The Greeks conceived that all matter is constituted of four elements, viz. earth, water, fire and air. Later, Aristotle supported this argument and also added the fifth called 'aether'. The argument was that everything around comprised a combination of these elements in some proportion. The characteristics of the matter are determined by the proportion of these elements. Thinking along the same lines, Hippocrates (460–377 BC), regarded as the Father of Medicine, proposed the famous humoural theory. According to this theory, the human body comprises four humours or fluids, viz. blood, phlegm, black bile and yellow bile. The health and illness of human beings depended on the equilibrium of these humours. When these humours were in the right proportion, the individual enjoyed health, while disequilibrium or imbalance in their proportion caused illness. Hippocrates had concrete suggestions on the ways to maintain humoural balance through diet and exercise. This helped in shifting the role of individuals from passive to active role in sustaining wellness. Hippocrates further theorized that the dominant humour in the body determined the temperament of the individual. For example, yellow bile in excess led to a choleric temperament (short-tempered, ambitious), black bile led to a melancholic temperament (introspective, sentimental), blood as dominant humour led to a sanguine temperament (courageous, hopeful, amorous), while phlegm in excess led to a phlegmatic temperament (calm, unemotional) (Lecci & Magnavita, 2013; Clark & Watson, 2008; Arikha, 2007). Hippocrates' contributions to humoural theory can be considered significant for two reasons. First, it is the humoural theory that superseded the spiritual beliefs of illness as destiny or punishment from God, which led the church or religion to decide on health practices where the locus of control was unmistakably external. He transformed medicine into a discipline that could be taught and learned. Secondly, Hippocrates' humoural theory can be considered as the first instance of connecting physiology and psychology though not in a very scientific manner (Figure 1.1).

Further, he introduced an ethical basis to the practice of medicine, and also brought a distinct identity to the practitioners. He also set the beginning of studying the human body from the anatomical perspective and opened the thinking along the lines of the possibility of surgery. His contributions in terms of the description of diseases, and methods of preventive actions and lifestyle changes laid a strong foundation for scientific thinking for medical practice and research.

Following Hippocrates, there was a slump in scientific curiosity, exploration, discovery and invention in Europe. What was later labelled as the Big Three of Greek Philosophy had started with Socrates born in 470 BC. The philosophical discourse on the nature of the soul, its connect with intellect (mind) and dichotomy with body can be traced back to this era.

Early Period of CE

This discourse popularly known as mind-body dualism or reductionist theory of mind picked up momentum in mid-1600 with rigorous inputs from Rene Descartes who published on this in 1641.

A search for documentation on health practices revealed that after Hippocrates, there was a silence of a few centuries on any development in the area of health and biological science until 129–200 AD during which significant knowledge was added to the Science of Medicine by Claudius Galen. Galen explored the bodies of animals and humans and tracked the anatomy. His significant contributions to anatomy related to the explanation of the circulatory system, nervous system and vital organs such as brain, heart and lungs and their functions. Galen synthesized the three schools of thoughts that influenced medicine during his period, viz. the rationalists, the empiricists and Methodists (Galen, 2009). He claimed that both reason (rationalist perspective) and experience (empiricist perspective) were important for medical practice, which should also be guided by definite rules.

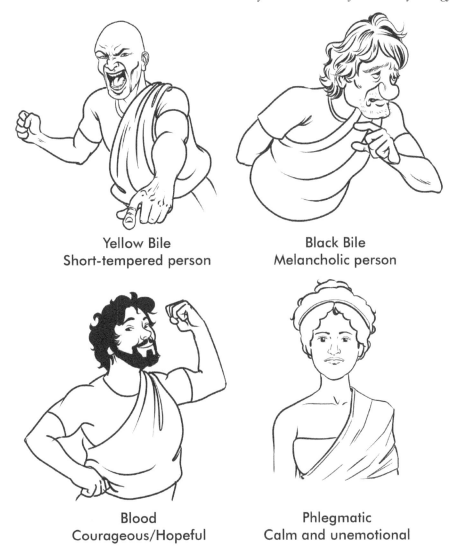

Figure 1.1 Humour and Personality Relationship.

Galen subscribed to the humoural theory of Hippocrates and endorsed the ethics evolved by him. Thus, medical science became a point of convergence for the study of science to understand the bodily process, a logic that enabled the doctor to infer the aetiology of disease that is important for correct diagnosis, prognosis and ethical principles to give a right direction in practising medicine. Galen's doctrine also was the first to trace any disease to a causative factor based on which the cause of ailments was divided into internal or external factors. He advocated that health was influenced by external factors such as air, diet and drinks and also by the individual's sleep, activity, rest and the state of mind. Here is where one can observe the argument of this great philosopher—doctor in relating body-mind balance to the sustenance of health, which is the fundamental principle in Health Psychology. Galen's contributions to medicine also extended to pharmacology as he came up with a number of recipes for preparing medical pills, powders, ointments and tinctures.

4 History and Evolution of Health Psychology

Galen's contributions can be summarized as 'the science and art of medicine' because while he advocated 'evidence-based' diagnosis and treatment, his guiding principle was also logical reasoning and ethical practices.

Galen's contributions translated into Arabic were imported into many countries like Mesopotamia, Egypt, Spain and Jerusalem where schools and universities were established that preserved the translation of Galen's work.

The Christian crusades to the Middle East in the 12th century enabled the West to recover the Roman and Greek scientific knowledge. This led to the establishment of medieval universities in Paris, Bologna and Oxford. The medical curricula in some universities taught Galen's work from the 11th century. Thus, Galen's contribution constituted a strong scientific, philosophical and ethical foundation to teaching in medical sciences.

While the contributions of Hippocrates and Galen are mentioned in helping to extricate the Science of Medicine from spirituality and religion, another name that helped in releasing the Science of Medicine from the orthodoxy of religion is Rene Descartes (1596–1650). Going by the early Greek philosophers, he strongly reasoned that the material physical body is an entity that is different from the mind that is intangible. This history of dichotomy is important to modern Health Psychology. The philosophy of the 17th and 18th century played a crucial role in determining the modern notion of human nature, social structure and the concept of being healthy (Friedman & Adler, 2011). It needs to be mentioned here that Rene Descartes emphasized body-mind dualism and their independent existence. He also referred to the fact that being independent entities, mind as a 'substantial form' is united with the human body. He suggested interaction between body and mind, though he did not elaborate on the principle on which the two distinct entities guided by different laws could make the interaction possible (Figure 1.2).

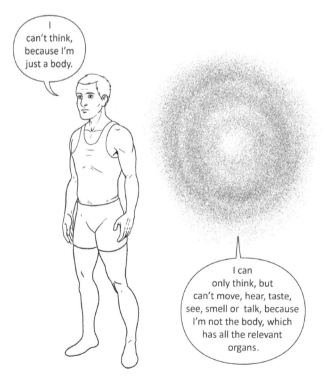

Figure 1.2 Body-Mind Dualism.

Contradicting Descartes, the famous philosopher and theologian, St. Thomas Aquinas (1225–1274) propounded that the human body considered to be 'matter' is a live human tissue. The 'mind' or 'soul' is present in every part of the human. This argument also assumes significance for Health Psychology in explaining the confluence of body and mind.

18th and 19th Century

The next significant work related to human science came from Darwin (1809–1882) who presented his Theory of Evolution. The crux of his theory was that the difference between man and animal was one of degree rather than of kind. His theory suggested similarities between humans and animals on a number of attributes.

Taking the cue of the striking resemblance between the humans and animals, the Russian physiologist turned psychologist Ivan Pavlov (1849–1936) conducted his experiments of classical conditioning on dogs, which he later extended to humans. The success of his experiments on animals and humans established the similarity of attribution between the two species. More importantly, Pavlov's work laid the strong foundation for Health Psychology by revealing the relationship between the learning behaviours and physiological responses (Figure 1.3).

The students of Psychology are well versed in the details of Pavlov's experiment. The findings proved that by artificial association, a neutral external stimulus (bell) could elicit a physiological response (salivating) in the dog. The significance of Pavlov's contribution lies in adding the knowledge that some physiological responses can be elicited, modified and controlled by way of appropriate learning or training. This has become a very powerful model for designing interventions in Health Psychology research in contemporary times.

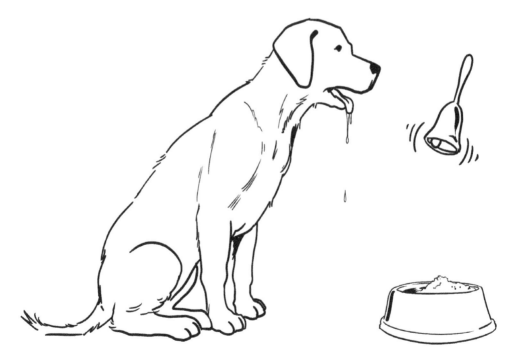

Figure 1.3 Pavlov's Conditioning Experiment.

Around the same time, the discipline of Psychology was given a boost by William James (1842–1910), known as the Father of American Psychology. A philosopher and psychologist, James' contribution to the emergence of Health Psychology may be two-fold. First, his writings based on the dual principles of pragmatism and functionalism brought an alternative to the inconclusive debate on body-mind dichotomy. Functionalism proposed that what is of significance is the individual's capacity to adapt to their environment helped by their thought and action. The principle of pragmatism assumed that it is impossible to prove an abstract absolute truth. Hence, it is of relevance to focus on the usefulness of the idea or 'truth'. These two principles in many ways helped in expansion of socially relevant research in Psychology.

In addition to the above, William James' theory of emotion, popularly known as the James-Lange theory of emotion (because he and the Danish psychologist Carl Lange independently proposed the theory), constituted the first theory that suggested a logical relationship between emotion and physiology. According to the James-Lange theory, an external stimulus triggers a physiological response. When this response is interpreted by the individual, the emotion is elicited.

It should be noted here that while Pavlov related physiological response to learning behaviour, James related it to emotions. In a way, both suggest a close association between physiology (body) and psychology (mind). Thus, the scientific knowledge moved from that of a disconnect between the physical and mental processes to that of a scientifically evident relation between the two.

The integral relationship between the body and mind was further strengthened by the focused work of Sigmund Freud (1856–1939) referred to as the Father of Psychoanalysis (Figure 1.4). Freud was practising as a physician when patients with various illnesses consulted him. Freud encouraged his patients to speak and listened to them attentively. After ten years of experience as a practitioner, he came to the conclusion that many of the illnesses with symptoms of convulsion, blindness, paralysis, amnesia or pain had no causal pathology. These somatic manifestations had underlying traumatic experiences as causal factors.

His first publication on Studies on Hysteria (1885) presented the case of Anna O who manifested multiple somatic symptoms because of traumatic events in life. His findings clearly indicated the influence of the unconscious mind on the health of the individual. Applying the theory of psychoanalysis, he explained that the emotional conflicts deeply rooted in the unconscious are converted into somatic symptoms through the voluntary nervous system. He called the condition 'conversion hysteria'. While William James' knowledge addition referred to the influence of physiological response on reaction at the mental level in the form of emotion, Freudian contribution clearly indicated that the converse is also true in the sense that the extreme emotion in the form of trauma can have its influence on the functioning of the targeted organ or system. Thus, with this suggestion of mutuality in the mind-body relationship, a future path of research in the field of Health Psychology was laid. The contemporary research in Health Psychology indicates that psychological aspects play a definite role both in the aetiology and in the treatment of illness.

When pioneering research in the field of Psychology was in progress, ground-breaking research in biological sciences also happened in the same period. Louis Pasteur (1822–1895), the French Biologist, Microbiologist and Chemist, (Figure 1.5) came with the finding of the living units called bacteria that are responsible for various diseases like cholera, typhoid, tuberculosis, pneumonia. The presence of bacteria was found in food, water and air. Subsequent research focused on preparing chemicals that could stop bacterial infections. Antiseptics and pasteurization were identified as preventive measures for bacteria. There is a need to note the involvement of bacteria in these preventive steps. Thus, while the aetiology of diseases was attributed to the

History and Evolution of Health Psychology 7

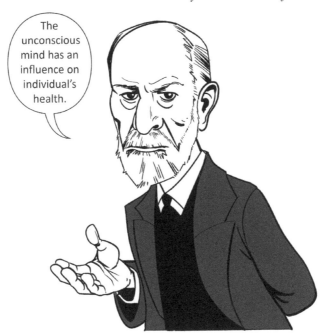

Figure 1.4 Sigmund Freud (1856–1939).

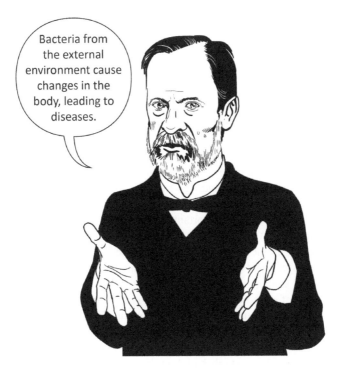

Figure 1.5 Louis Pasteur (1822–1895).

body-mind relationship in some part of the world, scientific knowledge about the environmental source of the disease was also flowing in from the same part of the world.

In the 19th century, America still had quacks and unprofessional individuals offering treatments. In a right step towards formalizing and streamlining the professional practice of medicine, the American Medical Association (AMA) was founded in the year 1847. It prescribed the minimum standards for medical education and practice. This could effectively bring regulation in medical practice enhancing the quality of patient care. However, with the physicians as regulating authority it sidelined all the other aspects not falling strictly under the realm of 'medical' denomination to peripheral levels.

In the second part of the 19th century, i.e. in 1892, the American Psychological Association (APA) was founded as an outcome of emergence of a number of academic disciplines (including psychology) in America and the progressive monument in American politics.

Following the first survey of medical schools in America at the initiative of Flexner in 1910, efforts were made to integrate psychology into the curriculum of medical training (Vevier, 1987). This proposal was further strengthened by Franz in 1911 when he attended a conference on integration of psychology and medicine organized by the American Psychological Association. He highlighted the power of psychological aspects over pharmacotherapy in the treatment and prognosis of disease (Franz, 1912). Later, as a chairperson of a committee in the APA, he surveyed the medical schools in America and came up with the recommendation for inclusion of psychology at an undergraduate level as an essential prerequisite for medical schools. This administrative move can be considered as the first step by the US for formal integration of psychology and medicine. This was further strengthened by Bott (1928) who wrote "…our conception of health must be broadened to take these mental factors fully into account" (p. 291). He recommended that psychology be a part of formal instruction in the medical curriculum. While implementing these recommendations, psychology in the medical curriculum appeared restricted to human aspects such as doctor-patient communication, patient adherence.

What made a profound impact on medical science is the discovery of penicillin by Alexander Fencing in 1928. The impact of penicillin and sulpha drugs in treating infectious diseases was electrifying. This scientific advancement was responsible for saving many lives. The high demand for these drugs for the wounded soldiers in World War II and the lives saved provided an added value to the drugs. As a consequence, the Western world saw setting up of a number of pharmaceutical companies as well as research laboratories with concerted efforts to identify chemicals for curing diseases caused by viruses and fungi. Thus, the attention of medical research shifted to microbiology and bacteriology (encyclopedia.com, 2018). Medical schools started training the students in biochemistry and microbiology, while psychology remained on the periphery. As stated by Friedman and Adler (2011) "matters of mind were increasingly left to psychiatry, newly emerging as an important specialty" (p. 6).

During the World War II, equally important to penicillin were the services of psychologists. The American Psychological Association played a crucial role in extending their services. The US government surveys availed the services of the APA in screening and recruitment into military through psychometric assessments, motivation and enhancing the morale, as well as catering to the psychiatric needs of the soldiers. William Menninger, the American psychiatrist, was appointed as the chief psychiatrist of armed forces. He played a crucial role in identifying and utilizing the services of clinical psychologists not only for the treatment of those in need of psychotherapy but also for the purposes of preventive intervention. Thus, antibiotics on the one hand and psychological interventions on the other constituted interventions for soldiers of World War II.

While Louis Pasteur's theory established the relationship between the bacteria from the external environment and disease, the decades of scientific research of Walter Cannon also referred

History and Evolution of Health Psychology 9

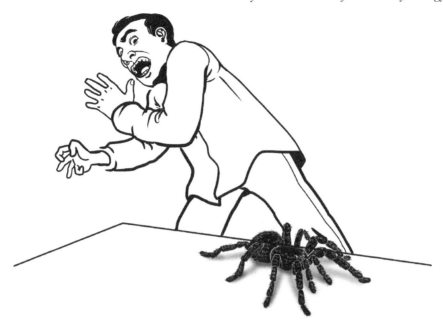

Stimuli from external environment can lead to adrenalin rush

Figure 1.6 Physiological Response to External Stimulus.

to the relationship between the external environment and its impact on physiological processes. Cannon (1932, 1942) elaborated on the physiological changes in the body in response to situations inducing emotions such as anger or fear. According to him the external stimulus has the potential to induce an emotional reaction in the human being. For example, perception of a small spider can induce the reaction of fear (Figure 1.6). He mapped the drastic changes in the functioning of vital organs resulting in increased pulse rate, respiration, rise in blood sugar level, blood pressure and more blood supply to skeletal muscles. The most significant of these is the gush of adrenaline secretion. This is called acute stress response, popularly known as fight-or-flight response. He coined the word 'homeostasis', meaning that the natural course of the body is to maintain a state of balance. In a state of severe emotions, the physiological responses bring in an imbalance of deviation in blood pressure, respiratory rate, hormonal levels and so on. This induces an observable behaviour. This chain of action subsequently leads to the restoration of balance. The theory of Cannon drove home the fact that the psychophysiological functioning of a human being has to be studied in the context of the social environment. Thus, he set the idea of a triangular relationship between body, mind and society.

20th Century

Expanding the idea of Cannon, Selye (1956) theorized the human being's natural ability to adapt to the emotional turmoil. He termed it General Adaptation Syndrome (GAS). According to him, the body's natural defence enables an individual to face the threat. However, if such defence has to be used as an adaptive measure for a prolonged period, it may cause disruption to the system. This finding that continuous exposure to stress culminates in metabolic disruption or damage perhaps can be considered a major contribution to 'Psychosomatic Medicine'.

10   History and Evolution of Health Psychology

Psychosomatic Medicine evolved from the assumption that 'soma' (the body) is influenced by the 'psyche' (the mind). The American Psychosomatic Society was founded in 1942. A number of diseases related to different systems of the body such as colitis, diabetes, arthritis, dermatitis and hypertension were also studied from this perspective.

Taking into consideration the scientific developments in the field of medicine, WHO (1948) defined health as 'A state of complete physical, mental and social well-being and not merely the absence of disease or infirmity'.

In the mid-20th century, the sociologists and anthropologists brought to the limelight the social aspects of illness. Parsons (1951, 1958) discussed the 'sick role behaviour' of the patients. The patient diagnosed with a disease is bestowed with some rights such as abstaining from work, as well as responsibilities such as seeking a treatment. Individual and cultural differences in health-seeking behaviour were highly pronounced. Some people delay in initiating treatment for even life-threatening health problems, while a few others consult doctors immediately even for very minor problems. Surfacing of these social aspects of health and illness indicates that diagnosis and treatment of illness need to consider this third dimension.

Strengthening the natural correlation between psychology and health further, in the late 1950s, Rosenman and Friedman (1981) put forth their observation that people with certain types of personality characteristics were prone to cardiac diseases. Persons with these characteristics were called type 'A' personality. Later, they established their hypothesis by their longitudinal study on a large sample. Their study specified a combination of physical, emotional, psychological and behavioural indicators.

Yet, another exciting scientific discovery of the 1950s was that of the 'placebo effect'. Though the placebo effect was known and also demonstrated from the 18th century from the time of Haygarth (1800), it was Beecher in 1955 who published a paper titled 'the Powerful Placebo' where he quantified it. The placebo effect started to gain acceptance in the medical field. This replaced the belief that it is not just the chemical pill or surgical intervention that resulted in a good prognosis, but there is a very powerful human element that contributes to the outcome of treatment. This human element could be the doctor's characteristics like what Beecher in his study termed as 'enthusiastic surgeon or the patients' belief system or faith in the doctor's treatment cure' (Figure 1.7). It could be all of them. The discovery and acceptance of the placebo effect perhaps was a significant indication to think beyond the biomedical realm for the treatment and cure of diseases.

The relationship between psychology and health was examined from a different direction by Janis (1958). He followed up the patients awaiting surgery and studied their prognosis. His findings indicated poor prognosis in patients with extremely low or high stress levels, while those with moderate stress showed the best prognosis. An examination of this opened up a new horizon of 'handling stress' or 'coping with stress'.

The contemporary psychologist Lazarus (1966) was engaged in an in-depth study on the individual's coping with stress, which continued until the 1980s. The work of Lazarus and his associate Folkman explained the significance of an individual's appraisal of a stressful situation that provided a comprehension of its manageability, its repercussions on health and the individual's choice of coping strategies. This line of research implied the shift of an individual's role from that of a passive recipient to that of an active respondent in facing any stress including the threat of illness.

In 1965, there was a major shift in conceptualizing 'pain', which until then was constructed as a physiological phenomenon. Melzack and Wall (1965) contradicted this postulate and propounded the gate control theory. They explained that the spinal cord that constitutes the first meeting point of nerves passing through different parts of the body has a series of 'gates' through which messages of pain pass. A number of psychological factors decide the opening of these

History and Evolution of Health Psychology 11

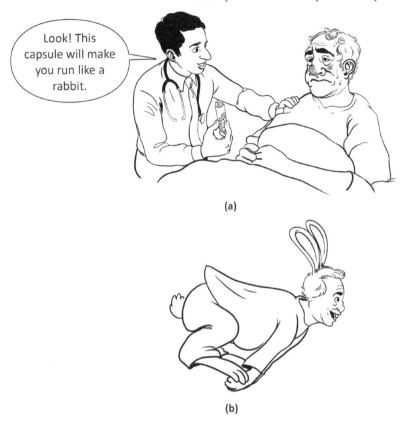

Figure 1.7 Placebo Effect.

gates allowing or delaying the pain messages to be transmitted to the brain. The pain messages are allowed by opening the gates when the individual is under stress or tension; there is a lack of activities and focus of all attention in the paining organ. Conversely, when there is a positive affect state of happiness or relaxation, or the attention is on something else that is of crucial importance and the person is engaged in an activity that demands immediate attention, the 'gates' block the travel of pain message to the brain at least temporarily. The example of the continuation of the aggressive fight by a soldier injured in the battlefield was cited to explain the absence of pain experience that would debilitate action in a life-threatening situation (Figure 1.8). This gave a new insight into the psychophysiological integral functioning.

Between 1965 and 1970, two major contributions are listed in the time line of psychology, both in the field of Clinical Psychology. Beck (1967) published the psychological model of depression. The model highlighted the role of thoughts in developing and maintaining depression.

The second milestone is a publication on behavioural therapy by Wolpe (1969). Beck expounded cognitive therapy (CT) in line with his model that thoughts, feelings and behaviour are connected. Hence, by replacing the thoughts that are unhelpful, one can change the distressing emotions and subsequent behaviours. This theory and therapeutic model had their impact in later years in evolving the Health Belief Model, and designing intervention modules for the biopsychosocial approach to health.

During the same period, there was also a landmark research that gave a strong standing for Health Psychology. Neal Miller who had been engaged in research related to learning and

12 *History and Evolution of Health Psychology*

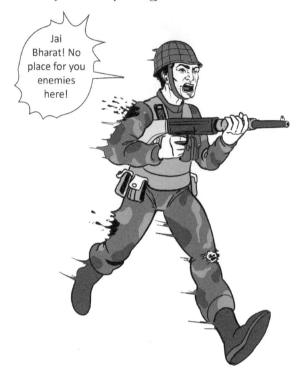

Figure 1.8 Gate Theory of Pain: Psychosocial Factors.

motivation became curious to understand the mutual influence between the brain on the one hand and learning and motivation on the other. This opened a new field of study called 'Behavioural Neuroscience'. His research demonstrated that it is possible to train the organism to control and regulate heartbeat, respiration, blood pressure and intestinal contraction, which are otherwise under the control of the autonomic nervous system. The study of Miller (1978) opened up the scope of technology-based research into the field of Psychology. Rigorous research followed in the area of biofeedback and relaxation aimed at consciously and voluntarily regulating the psychological function of the human body. This provided a very strong footing for establishing an inherent connectivity between psychological processes and health, as determined by normal physiological functioning. Biofeedback and relaxation turned out to be very important components in interventional studies of Health Psychology and are applied in different intervention modules to date.

Temporally close to this discovery was a development in the area of immunology. What in fact was an incidental observation emerged as a major contribution in evolving a special research area called psychoneuroimmunology. Ader and Cohen (1975) was studying conditioning and emotional responsiveness in rats. He along with his fellow researcher Ader and Cohen (1975) was conditioning the rats for taste aversion. The experiment required them to feed the rats with saccharin water followed by an immunosuppressant called cyclophosphamide, which induced nausea in them. Because of conditioning that associated nausea with water, the rats learned to avoid water. During the next phase of the experiment, long after the effect of immunosuppressants was washed out, when Ader and Cohen (1975) force-fed the rats with saccharin water, they began to die. The rate of death was found to be directly related to the volume of saccharin water consumed. The cause of death was contacting bacterial or viral infection. That is the consequence of weakening of the immune system. Based on this, Ader and Cohen (1975) theorized that because of the association between the saccharin water and injected immunosuppressant, the feeding of saccharin water was sufficient to induce neural signals in the brain of the rats that resulted in suppressing the immune system in the body. This gave a new insight to medical science as well as psychology that the immune system believed to be autonomous in fact is connected to the nervous system and can be influenced by it. What evolved out of it is the new insight that exposed to prolonged stress produced by life's challenges the individual's immune system is put at stake opening vulnerability to diseases caused by bacteria, virus and infection. Thus, the 19th-century knowledge that individuals were prone to diseases caused by the bacteria in the environment received added knowledge about the internal psychological state contributing to one's vulnerability. The value addition was that not everybody contacting bacteria or virus fell ill, but only those whose immune system was weak were susceptible to disease, and those under stress had a fragile immune system.

In the contemporary period, the physician George Engel investigated over six years into the sudden deaths of 170 patients. He concluded that psychological stress or trauma involving individual's self-esteem, personal threat and the humiliation or reunions following it may cause illness and even death. He postulated that the confluence of biological factors, social environmental factors like loss of a dear one and psychological factors such as inability to cope contributed to causing illness. It was Engles' efforts that advocated for replacing the biomedical approach to health that was in vogue with the biopsychosocial approach.

There was sufficient evidence to support the biopsychosocial model of Engel (1977). Evidence has been compounding from the findings of William James, Pavlov, Freud, Cannon, Selye, Janis Miller and Ader and Cohen, all of which independently suggested the important role of psychological and social environmental factors in the aetiology and treatment of illness.

After the advocacy for the biopsychosocial model of health, Health Psychology emerged as an identified branch of psychology with the American Psychological Association establishing Health Psychology as the 38th Division in the year 1978 (Figure 1.9). A few years later, in 1986 the International Association of Applied Psychology (IAAP) also established a Division of Health Psychology. Thus, America takes the credit for giving a distinct identity to Health Psychology as a specialized branch.

In the same year, i.e. 1986, the European Health Psychology Society was founded with membership from 11 countries (Schwarzer & Gutiérrez-Doña, 2000). Other countries like Canada, Australia, New Zealand, India and Japan have their own association of Health Psychology. As an initiative towards integrating the researchers in Health Psychology across the globe, in 1994, the International Society for Health Psychology Research (ISHPR) was founded, especially with a focus on bringing together researchers from developing countries.

In an effort towards consolidation of the Division of Health Psychology, the American Psychological Association, in the year 1983, organized a working conference on Education and Training in Health Psychology. The conference discussed ethical legal and cultural issues. The conference emphasized the need for a reciprocal relation between academic research and practice with an interdisciplinary orientation.

Encouraged by the distinct identity research in the field of Health Psychology picked up momentum. Concomitantly, a number of journals in the field of Health Psychology were launched. The first of them was the journal called *Health Psychology* launched in 1982 by the American Psychological Association as its official journal. Subsequent to this, the European Health Psychology Society started its journal in 1987 with a name *Psychology and Health: An International Review*. A number of other journals followed with different names such as *Journal of Health Psychology*, *British Journal of Health Psychology*, *Journal of Occupational Health Psychology*, *Journal of Health Communication*, *Japanese Health Psychology*, *Journal of Indian Health Psychology*, and *Psychology, Health and Medicine* (Figure 1.10).

14 *History and Evolution of Health Psychology*

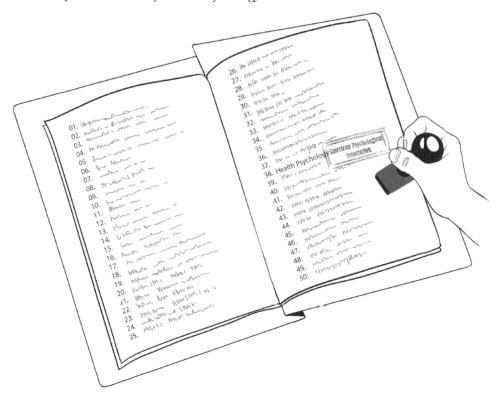

Figure 1.9 APA Includes Health Psychology as 38th Branch.

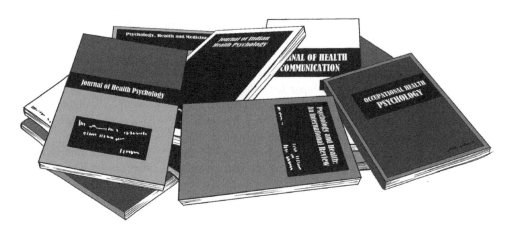

Figure 1.10 Research Publications in Health Psychology.

There is a vast scope of research in Health Psychology. The branch of Health Psychology is classified into the following sub-branches facilitating the academics and practitioners to choose their specialized field. The sub-branches that exist now are Clinical Health Psychology, Community Health Psychology, Critical Health Psychology, Public Health Psychology and Occupational Health Psychology. Several fields within Clinical Health Psychology have emerged each referring to a super-speciality. Behavioural Cardiology, Behavioural Diabetology,

Psycho-oncology, Reproductive Health are a few to name. Adequate reading material is available in each branch and sub-fields. Thus, ever since its emergence in 1978, four decades of research in the field of Health Psychology still leaves a huge unexplored area for research.

Health Psychology in India

Indian universities took some time to introduce Health Psychology in their curriculum. In the early 1990s, a few universities introduced Health Psychology as one of the subjects at the post-graduate level. The faculty teaching the subject had no formal training in the area but took the great initiative because of their keen interest and motivation.

It was in the year 2007 that the University of Hyderabad in India launched the first-ever academic unit for research and teaching Health Psychology with the author of this book as the founder Director. In the year 2008, the University of Hyderabad was the first Indian university to introduce Health Psychology as a five-year course. The Centre engaged in research in specialized branches within Health Psychology such as Behavioural Cardiology, Behavioural Diabetology, Psycho-oncology, Reproductive Health, Community Health Psychology, Geriatric Health Psychology, Pediatric Health Psychology, School Health Psychology. As the course gained popularity, the university introduced a two-year post-graduation course and a Ph.D. in Health Psychology in 2009 and 2010. Until 2019, this remains the only university in India offering a degree in Health Psychology. The chronology in the evolution of Health Psychology is projected in Box 1.1.

Box 1.1 Evaluation of Health Psychology: Time line

Time	Event
460–377 BC	Humoural theory of Hippocrates
470 BC	Socrates, Plato, Aristotle Body-mind dualism
129–200 AD	Galen's theory of causes, external and internal causal factors of illness; pharmacotherapy
1596–1650	Descartes' body-mind interaction
1809–1882	Darwin's theory of evaluation and similarities between animals and humans
1822–1895	Louis Pasteur's discovery of 'bacteria' causing acute diseases
1847	Establishment of the American Medical Association (AMA)
1849–1936	Pavlov's experiment connecting the nervous system to learning
1942–1910	William James' functionalism and significance of 'usefulness of the idea' rather than proving the absolute truth. James-Lange theory of emotion showing the relationship between the external stimulus, physiological response and brain's interpretation
1856–1939	Freud's psychoanalytic theory. Dysfunction of an organ can be caused without any pathology and because of emotional conflict
1892	Establishment of the American Psychological Association (APA)
1910	Abraham Flexner's effort to integrate psychology into the medical curriculum
1912	S. I Franz recommended that the study of psychology at the UG level is a prerequisite for medical school
1928	E. A Bott recommended psychology to be part of the medical curriculum
1928	Alexander Fleming's intervention of penicillin drug
1939–1945	World War II and active role played by psychologists in assessment, recruitment, weapon design and treatment of soldiers

(Continued)

Time	Event
1932	Walter Canon's theory of stress. External situation induces negative emotion that disturbs homeostasis in the body
1956	Hans Selye's theory; human being's natural ability to adapt to emotional turmoil unless the state is prolonged
1942	The concept of 'Psychosomatism'—bodily diseases can be caused by psychological influence
1951	Parson's emphasis on studying the disease in the sociocultural context
1958	I. L. Janis' publication of the 'placebo effect'. The prognosis is the result of factors outside the pharmacotherapy
1965	Melzack and Wall's gate control theory of pain stating pain as a psychophysiological phenomenon
1966	Lazarus' contribution to the individual's appraisal of a situation and coping with stress
1967	Beck's model of depression. The relationship between thoughts, emotions and behaviour. Cognitive therapy as an intervention for faulty thoughts
1975	Ader and Cohen's chance discovery that in response to conditioned learning, the immune system is influenced through the mediation of the brain
1976	Neal Miller's contribution to biofeedback. Response of the viral physiological system can be regulated and controlled by the training/learning process
1977	Engles' proposal for the biopsychosocial model of health
1978	APA establishes Health Psychology as the 38th Division
1982	Launching of *Health Psychology* as an official journal of the APA
1986	Establishment of the Health Psychology Division in the International Association of Applied Psychology (IAAP)

A cursory look into the time line of Health Psychology suggests that a number of factors contributed to its emergence. The first factor is the philosophical discourse on the nature of mind and the debate on its relationship with body. These discourses enabled the exploration into the abstract entity of mind. The second factor is the progressive advancement in biological sciences, be it the humoural theory anatomical mapping of the human body, discovery of bacteria or endocrinal functions. Some of the scientific progress like discovery of bacteria and the subsequent invention of penicillin and its use brought about a change in the nature of disease over a period of time. As an offshoot of this when there was a spurt in pharma industries competing with each other in manufacturing drugs, it had its impact in terms of economic viability of treatment. The third factor is efforts to institutionalize and standardize the practice and curriculum of medical sciences. This enabled to incorporate the research inputs from the field of science and accommodate relevant curriculum changes from time to time. The fourth factor is sociopolitical aspects of the world that set the stage to showcase the significant role of psychologists in the treatment process. The last, but a very important, deciding factor was the progressive development in research in the field of Psychology that consistently established the physiology-psychology connectivity, thus substituting evidence-based scientific argument that answered the age-old philosophical debate on body-mind dichotomy.

Health Psychology in the Roots of Ayurveda

While it took nearly about two millennia for the Western medical knowledge to identify the psychological principles as necessary components to be integrated into medical practice and research, Health Psychology remained an integral part of Indian medical knowledge, though not with the nomenclature of 'Health Psychology'. 'Ayurveda' is considered the root and the encyclopaedia of Indian medical science. This is more than 5000 years old, the writings of which are in Sanskrit language documented by ancient seers in India in the Vedas. Atharva Veda documents the medical knowledge in the name of Ayurveda. *Atharva Veda*, the fourth of the Vedas, was written approximately in 1500 BCE (Surendra & Prasad, 2013). The term *Ayurveda* is a combination of two words—'*Ayu*' meaning life (or that which is in constant move and hence dynamic) (Kapur, 2016) and 'Veda' meaning knowledge science. Thus, 'Ayurveda' refers to the 'Science of life' and its main focus is in the preservation of life.

The very concept of life according to Ayurveda is an amalgamation of '*Sharira*' (the body), '*Indriya*' (sense organs) and '*Satya*' (the purest form) and '*atma*' (self). Thus, the core concept of life includes the sense organs, which can be called the essential components to feed the mental processes.

The ancient Indian seers, Bharadwaja, Kashyapa and Dhanwantri, are said to be practitioners of Ayurveda. It was Agnivesh who is said to have developed the basic Ayurveda text for internal medicine. Acharya Charaka, the disciple of Agnivesh, revised the work and was responsible for handing down the knowledge to posterity. The great three classical texts of Ayurveda comprise '*Charaka Samhita*', '*Sushruta Samhita*' and '*Ashtanga Hridayam Sangraha*'. *Charaka Samhita* relates to the diagnosis, cure and prevention of disease. It documents the details of medicinal properties of 10,000 plants. *Sushruta Samhita* elaborates on 1120 health conditions, 300 operations involving 42 surgical procedures. *Ashtanga Hridayam Sangraha* refers to '*Kayachikitsa*' or internal medicine. Apart from these, the other three classics are '*Sharngdhara Samhita*', '*Bhava Prakasa*' and '*Madhava Nidanam*'.

Ayurveda conceived the human body made of '*panchamahabhootas*' or the five prime elements, viz. *Pruthvi* (Earth), *Apah* (Water), *Teja* (Fire), *Vayu* (Air) and *Akasha* (Sky). Their solitary or combinational presence in different properties is seen in various structures and functions of the body. The three main forces called '*doshas*' of the body, '*vata*', '*pitta*' and '*kapha*', have the five elements as the constituents. Depending upon the proportion of three '*doshas*' existing in the human body, the temperament or the personality or constitutional health (Prakriti) of the individual is determined. The ideal state of health and well-being is when these '*doshas*' in the right natural proportions are in perfect harmony. An increase or decrease of any creates an imbalance.

Health in Ayurveda is referred to as '*Svastha*', one who is centred in the self. Maintenance of health calls for not only a balance of the three *doshas* but also functional adequacy of body tissues ('*dhatu*'), metabolic enzymes required for digestive functioning (*agni*), proper elimination of metabolic byproducts through the excretory system (*mala*), fulfilment of needs of sensory (*indriyas*) and mental faculties (*manah*), as well as satisfaction of 'self' (*atma*).

Health in Ayurveda is defined as '*prasannatmendriyamanah*', implying a state where the physical, mental and spiritual aspects of the individual are in a state of contentment. Thus, the definition is very much inclusive and qualifies as holistic. Further, it goes on to explain 'health care' as a process that provides optimal physical and psychological state for the individual through changing seasons, by an appropriate use of sensory modalities (*artha*) and the right choice of action (karma). This in fact refers to 'stability in true self', suggesting a state of physical, mental and spiritual well-being (Sharma, Chandola, & Singh Basisht, 2007).

Ayurveda's approach to health is person-centred. The primary concern of this medical system is the prevention of disease by abiding health rather than treating the disease. In the event of failing this, the treatment efforts involve restoration of balance between the affected functions, tissues, environment and the whole person (Morandi, Tosto, Di Sarsina, & Dalla Libera, 2011). The treatment of the patient is decided on the basis of two examinations. The first is by examining the patient ('RogiPariksha') and then the disease ('RogaPariksha') (Dalal, 2016). The totality of the examination includes the physical state of the patient (disease location, symptom, digestion, metabolism, pulse, excretion matters, tongue, eyesight etc.), constitution

18 History and Evolution of Health Psychology

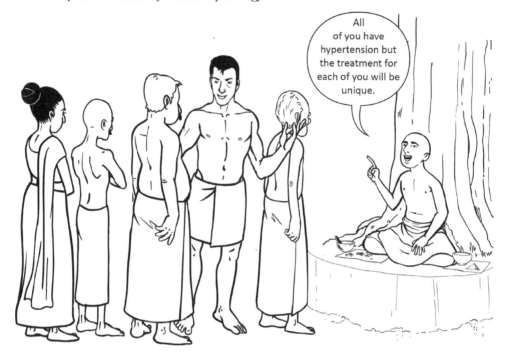

Figure 1.11 Indian Origin: Contributions of Ayurveda.

of the patient, heredity, residential location, surrounding environment and the climate or season (Figure 1.11).

The basis of Ayurveda is the assumption that each individual is unique in physical constitution and thereby the interaction between the dynamic mind and the environment also produces a unique outcome. Hence, the treatment is unique to every person. It is this characteristic of Ayurveda that did not satisfy the Western medicines' expectation of standardization and replication through clinical trials. The focus of Ayurveda is in two-fold: preventive and curative.

Ayurveda medicine pre-supposes that individual's health and well-being is determined by '*Achar*', '*Vicahr*', '*Ahar*' and '*Vihar*' meaning daily activities, thoughts and attitudes, diet and nutrition, and leisure and relaxation (Dalal, 2016).

To acquire the complex knowledge and skills involved in Ayurveda, one would have to study the discipline for 12 years to qualify as a '*Vaidya*' (doctor). With all its complexities, the system of Ayurveda also developed eight specialized branches as follows:

1   *Kayachikitsa* (Internal medicine)
2   *Balachikitsa* (Paediatric medicine)
3   *Grahachikitsa* (Psychiatry)
4   *Urdhvangachikitsa* (Issues with the upper part of the body)
5   *Shalyarogachikitsa* (Surgery)
6   *Damstrachikitsa* (Toxicology)
7   *Jarachikitsa* (Geriatrics)
8   *Vajikaranachikitsa* (Reproductive health)

The basic principles like '*dosha*' theory and person-based holistic approach are the same for all these specialized branches.

The treatment procedure in Ayurveda goes far beyond the administration of medicine or surgery. Hence, it may best suit to term it as the 'healing process'. The process of healing involves five senses, viz. sight, sound, taste, touch and smell through which the balance of '*doshas*' is achieved. Even according to contemporary psychology, sensory inputs are considered the doorways to the functioning of mind. Ayurveda's strong assumption that the mind has the power of healing the body led to therapeutic healing through the five sensations. Many problems related to the digestive system, anaemia, inflammation and burns are treated with 'colour therapy'. The discipline of psychology also assumes that colours have a direct and significant impact on health (Kurt & Osueke, 2014; Azeemi & Raza, 2005).

Healing through sound (Kumar, Badhe, & Santhiya, 2014; Lynch et al., 2018) uses music, bell, '*mantras*' and chanting. Apart from these external agents, the '*Nada Yoga*' in Ayurveda also prescribes listening to one's 'inner sound'. Of the many interventions used in Health Psychology, music therapy has proved to have a positive impact on a number of problems related to sleep, anxiety, Attention Deficit Hyperactive Disease (ADHD) and even the non-communicable diseases (NCDs). What is experimented in contemporary Health Psychology was scripted and practised in Ayurveda, the ancient Indian medicine. Researchers in the field of child development have proved the soothing effect of the sound of heartbeat on the infants.

One of the aspects of treatment in Western medicine is the prescription of diet. Ayurveda propounds six facts of taste—sweet, sour, salty, bitter, pungent and astringent. An intimate relationship is postulated between the patterns of diet and the three types of personality traits called '*trigunas*' (*Sattva, Rajas* and *Tamas*). The diet that has a good balance of these tastes is supposed to be good for health and well-being. Depending on the nature of the problem, the tastes are regulated in the prescribed diet.

Western psychology has advocated the therapeutic role of touch right from the time the child is born. Ayurveda advocated not only the sensation of touch but also appropriate pressure at various critical points through various massages. The massage therapy called '*Marna*' aims at stimulating different points for flow of energy.

What is known as 'aroma therapy' in present days was an integral part of Ayurveda. The oils made of various herbs are used as the therapeutic ingredient. Different herbs give different aromas, which when inhaled are supposed to stimulate the limbic system in the brain. The limbic system is associated with emotion. By impacting the affect of the individual, which in turn influences the disequilibrium in the body, the healing is achieved.

Thus, Health Psychology is ingrained as an integral part of Ayurveda medicine by emphasizing the body-mind integration in sustaining health, falling ill, treatment and prevention of disease. The system of Ayurveda from very ancient times is holistic in the true sense of approaching health by meticulously considering an individual's constitution, mental state, behaviour, and physical and social environment in a systematic way.

One may wonder as to why Ayurveda gave into Western medicine in India, the place of its origin. The answer lies in the political history. History has documented clearly the multiple foreign invasions suffered by India. This strongly impacted the Indian way of life. The invasions of Turkey and Afghanistan and the subsequent destruction of Indian literature and the cultural influence of the invaders resulted in departing from the lifestyle prescribed by Ayurveda and a decline in the practice of it. It also gave India a new system of medicine called 'Unani', which is a combination of Arabic medicine and Ayurveda.

Later when India came under colonial rule, the British prohibited Ayurveda. Lord McCauley decreed that Western medicine must be practised in the whole country under the governance of the East India Company. However, following India's independence, sincere attempts were made to revive Ayurveda. It is now recognized as medicine both for practice and for teaching and research. India now has a number of Ayurveda hospitals. Ayurveda is taught as an organized and recognized curriculum in colleges and universities. The Government of India now has an exclusive ministry for alternative medicine that has an acronym *Ayush* (Ayurved, Yoga, Unani, Siddha and Homeopathy).

References

Ader, R., & Cohen, N. (1975). Behaviorally conditioned immunosuppression. *Psychosomatic Medicine, 37*(4), 333–340.

Arikha, N. (2007). *Passions and tempers: A history of the humours*. Ecco/HarperCollins Publishers. https://psycnet.apa.org/record/2007-09236-000

Azeemi, S. T. Y., & Raza, M. (2005). A critical analysis of chromotherapy and its scientific evolution. *Evidence-Based Complementary and Alternative Medicine, 2*(4), 481–488.

Beck, A. T. (1967). *Depression: Clinical, experimental, and theoretical aspects*. University of Pennsylvania Press.

Beecher, H. K. (1955). The powerful placebo. *Journal of the American Medical Association, 159*(17), 1602–1606.

Bott, E. A. (1928). Teaching of psychology in the medical course. *Bulletin of the Association of American Medical Colleges, 3*, 289–304.

Cannon, W. B. (1932). *The wisdom of the body*. New York: Norton.

Cannon, W. B. (1942). Voodoo death. *American Anthropologist, 44*, 169.

Clark, L. A., & Watson, D. (2008). An organizing paradigm for trait psychology. In: O. P. John, R. W. Robins, & L. A. Pervin (Eds.), *Handbook of personality: Theory and research* (pp. 265–286). New York: Guilford Publications.

Dalal, A. K. (2016). *Cultural psychology of health in India: Well-being, medicine and traditional health care*. India: SAGE.

Engel, G. L. (1977). The need for a new medical model: A challenge for biomedicine. *Science, 196*(4286), 129–136.

Franz, S. I. (1912). The present status of psychology in medical education and practice. *Journal of the American Medical Association, 58*(13), 909–911.

Friedman, H. S., & Adler, N. E. (2011). The intellectual roots of health psychology. In: H. S. Friedman (Ed.), *The Oxford handbook of health psychology* (pp. 3–14). Oxford University Press.

Galen. (2009). Complete Dictionary of Scientific Biography. Encyclopedia.com: https://www.encyclopedia.com/science/dictionaries-thesauruses-pictures-and-press-releases/galen

Haygarth, J. (1800). *Of the Imagination: As a Cause and as a Cure of Disorders of the Body; Exemplified by Fictitious Tractors, and Epidemical Convulsions. "decipimur Specie." Hor. Read to the Literary and Philosophical Society of Bath. By John Haygarth, MDFRS Lond. and Edinb. Of the Royal Medical Society at Edinburgh, and of the American Academy of Arts and Sciences*. R. Cruttwell; and sold by Cadell and Davies, Strand, London.

Janis, I. L. (1958). *Psychosocial stress: Psychoanalytic and behavioral studies of surgical patients*. New York: Wiley.

Kapur, M. (2016). Basic principles of ayurveda. In: *Psychological perspectives on childcare in Indian indigenous health systems* (pp. 15–29). New Delhi: Springer. DOI: 10.1007/978-81-322-2428-0.

Kumar, K. D., Badhe, S., & Santhiya, S. (2014). Impact of Vedic chants intervention programme on autistic spectrum disorder. *Molecular Cytogenetics, 7*(1), P129.

Kurt, S., & Osueke, K. K. (2014). The effects of color on the moods of college students. *SAGE Open, 4*(1), 2158244014525423.

Lazarus, R. S. (1966). *Psychological stress and the coping process*. New York: McGraw-Hill.

Lecci, L. B., & Magnavita, J. J. (2013). *Personality theories: A scientific approach*. San Diego, CA: Bridgepoint.

Lynch, J., Prihodova, L., Dunne, P. J., McMahon, G., Carroll, A., Walsh, C., & White, B. (2018). Impact of mantra meditation on health and wellbeing: A systematic review protocol. *European Journal of Integrative Medicine, 18*, 30–33.

Melzack, R., & Wall, P. D. (1965). Pain mechanisms: A new theory. *Science, 150*(3699), 971–979.
Miller, N. E. (1978). Biofeedback and visceral learning. *Annual Review of Psychology, 29*(1), 373–404.
Morandi, A., Tosto, C., Di Sarsina, P. R., & Dalla Libera, D. (2011). Salutogenesis and ayurveda: Indications for public health management. *EPMA Journal, 2*(4), 459–465.
Parsons, T. (1951). Illness and the role of the physician: A sociological perspective. *American Journal of Orthopsychiatry, 21*(3), 452.
Parsons, T. (1958). Definitions of health and illness in the light of American values and social structure. In: E. G. Jaco (Ed.), *Patients, physicians and illness* (pp. 165–187). Glencoe, IL: The Free Press.
Rosenman, R. H., & Friedman, M. (1981). *Type A behavior & your heart*. New York: Fawcett Books.
Schwarzer, R., & Gutiérrez-Doña, B. (2000). Health psychology. In: K. Pawlik and M. R. Rosenzweig (Eds.), *The international handbook of psychology* (pp. 452–465). London: Sage.
Selye, H. (1956). *The stress of life*. New York: McGraw Hill.
Sharma, H., Chandola, H. M., Singh, G., & Basisht, G. (2007). Utilization of ayurveda in health care: An approach for prevention, health promotion, and treatment of disease. Part 1—Ayurveda, the science of life. *The Journal of Alternative and Complementary Medicine, 13*(9), 1011–1020.
Surendra, K., & Prasad, J. S. R. A. (2013). Concept of etiology in ayurveda and western medicine. *International Ayurvedic Medical Journal, 1*(4), 1–8.
"The Discovery and Importance of Penicillin and the Development of Sulfa Drugs." *Science_and Its Times: Understanding the Social Significance of Scientific Discovery*. Encyclopedia.com: https://www.encyclopedia.com/science/encyclopedias-almanacs-transcripts-and-maps/discovery-and-importance-penicillin-and-development-sulfa-drugs
Vevier, C. (1987). The Flexner report and change in medical education. *Flexner, 75*, 1–15.
Wolpe, J. (1969). Basic principles and practices of behavior therapy of neuroses. *American Journal of Psychiatry, 125*(9), 1242–1247.
World Health Organization. (1948). Preamble to the Constitution of the World Health Organization as adopted by the International Health Conference, New York, 19–22 June, 1946; signed on 22 July 1946 by the representatives of 61 States (Official Records of the World Health Organization, no. 2, p. 100) and entered into force on 7 April 1948. http://www.who.int/governance/eb/who_constitution_en.pdf.

2 Wellness, Illness, Health and Health Psychology

One of the often chanted *mantras* (prayers) among the Hindus is as follows:

Sarvea bhavanthu sukhinah
Sarvea santhu niramaya
Sarvea bhadrani pasyanthu
ma dukhabhaga bhaveth

The prayer is for universal wellbeing. It means "May all be happy; May all be free from illness; May all see good; May no one suffer". As referred by many sources including research papers, this prayer belongs to the Hindu scripture of Brihadaranyaka Upanishad (1.1.14). One may note here that the prayer refers to happiness, seeing good, freedom from illness and suffering—all in a single verse. Thus, it connects happiness and seeing good to freedom from illness and suffering, indicating a close connection between the physical suffering and the psychological state. This is one of the many evidences that indicates that the term 'health' has been construed as a phenomenon that encompasses more than the physical health for thousands of years. A scrutiny into the etymology of the term 'health' clearly connotes the 'wholeness' of the state. The roots of the word can be traced back to Anglo-Saxon words meaning 'whole', 'hale' and 'holy'. However, in the process of comprehending this 'wholeness', different people prioritize different aspects depending on several demographic factors and their own state of health.

'Health' as Understood by People

Researchers have studied people's understanding of the concept of health varying in the nature of their sample. Hariharan, Monteiro, Asha and Rao (2019) studied the understanding of 'health' among children from class 6 to class 10. Their survey on 667 children with a question 'what do you understand by 'being healthy?' evolved responses classified under three subthemes—the meaning of health, ways to be healthy and indices of good health. The responses referring to the meaning of health ranged from concrete aspects such as having healthy genes and the absence of disease to general abstract statements connoting the value of health such as it is 'God's gift' or 'health is greater than wealth'. It also included behavioural aspects. Their explanation in terms of indices of health matched Bennett's (2000) explanation of health in terms of 'Being', 'Having' and 'Doing'. The responses referred to 'being in peaceful state', 'having the energy and ability to work' and 'doing' in terms of play, academic performance, coping effectively—all of which reflect 'success' or accomplishment. Further, the study found that the complexity of the concept of health indicated a developmental trend as seen in the increase of complexity in their perception as they progressed in the class they studied. Children from higher classes gave a more number of responses that were multifaceted. What is to be noted here is that among children, the concept of health included not only an absence of disease and index of physical fitness, but also the state of 'wellness' indicated by their reference to 'peace' and the 'wholeness of the state' that facilitated their performance in expected fields.

A similar study conducted on Canadian children was reported by Normandeau, Wins, Jutras and Hanigan (1998). Data was collated through structured interviews and open-ended questions from 1674 children between 5 and 12 years. Children's concept of health was measured on four dimensions, viz. criteria of good health, behaviour related to 'being healthy', consequences of good health and threats to health. The results were by and large similar to the Indian study by Hariharan, Monteiro, Asha and Rao (2019). The findings revealed that children as young as five years of age included mental health in conceptualizing 'being healthy'. Three factors emerged as an index of good health. The first criteria were participation in sports and the absence of disease, both pointing to 'being functional'. The second criteria were having good mental health as indicated by 'wellbeing, feeling good about self', and having good relationships with others. The third criteria named healthy lifestyle were maintained with the practice of a healthy diet, hygiene and good sleep. The study also found differences in age, socioeconomic background and personal experience as factors influencing differences in responses. The significant inference that follows these two studies is the multidimensionality in children's concept of 'health' across cultures and time. They perceived health in a holistic way rather than a physical state.

There have been very interesting studies investigating adult's understanding of the term 'health'. Benyamini, Leventhal and Leventhal (2003) asked 500 elderly people to rate the factors important as health indices. What emerged as the most important factor was vitality or the ability to do things one is expected to do. The study also found that the ratings were affected by the current health state of the respondents. Those in good physical state mentioned things like 'the ability to exercise regularity', while those in poor health referred to their recent symptoms of poor health.

Krause and Jay (1994) conducted in-depth interviews on a sample of 158 individuals. They were asked to rate their own health status. The researchers examined the frame of reference used by the respondents. The findings indicated that the older respondents used 'health problems' while evaluating the health status, while the younger participants referred either to general physical functioning or to health behaviour. The findings also revealed differences based on race and education. Thus, the concept of 'health' is so significantly real and contemporary to the person that the explanation to a certain degree seems to be influenced by the subjective state.

Blaxter (1990) conducted a survey on the British population to examine their understanding of 'health'. She surveyed a huge sample of 9000 people who responded to a questionnaire that elicited what they thought of 'being healthy' with reference to 'identified other' and also with reference to their own self. The findings suggested that 'health' indicated the following:

1 Not being ill—no symptoms of illness and no visit to the doctor
2 Having a reserve—having a strong family, recovering fast from a surgery
3 A behaviour—taking care of one's self, regular exercise etc.
4 Vitality and physical fitness—very often, men responded with the expression of 'feeling fit', while women referred to 'feeling full of energy'. Being lively and having good social relationships were the indices of this
5 Psychosocial wellbeing—having connotation of 'mental state' such as being in harmony, feeling proud or enjoying with others
6 A function—ability to perform duties independently without experiencing any limitations

These categories suggest that people's idea of 'health' has a multidimensional characteristic rather than restricting it to the physical robustness or the absence of illness.

Herzlich (1973) conducted open interviews with middle-class professionals on their concept of health, sickness, death and their idea of relationships between individuals, society and nature. The psychosocial analysis revealed that though it was common to perceive 'health' as the absence of illness, it was not limited to this. The concept of health was constructed with all its complexity of maintaining the balance between the physical, psychological, emotional and social aspects of the individual that culminated in a state of 'wellbeing'.

One can notice that the common thread that runs across all the studies explained above is the invariable reference to disease or illness. Thus, the very concept of 'health' seems to be having an innate connection with disease or illness. The definition of World Health Organization also has a reference to disease. WHO defines health as 'A complete state of physical, mental, social and spiritual wellbeing and not merely the absence of disease or infirmity' (WHO, 1948). The fact that even WHO's definition of health has a reference of disease needs to be taken into cognizance. Though health is defined with reference to disease, the emphasis is mainly on wellbeing. Though the 'complete state of physical, mental and social wellbeing' appears to be more an ideal state, the goal of the individual should be to attain proximity to this state. The closer the one is towards this 'totality', the higher will be the wellbeing.

Models of Health

The health models were constructed depending upon whether the emphasis was on the 'Disease' or 'Wellbeing'. The biomedical model laid emphasis on the disease, while the biopsychosocial model laid emphasis on wellbeing.

Biomedical Model

The term 'biomedical' can be explained as connoting the idea that the problem of disease is biological and the solution to it is medical. The roots of the biomedical model are the reductionistic argument, which conceived body and mind as two separate and disintegrated entities. The focus of this model was the state of disease rather than the state of 'health'. The individual suffered diseases because of chemical imbalance in the body, deviation or dysfunctions of the cells or the neural network. The invention of bacteria added another scientific aetiology from an environmental source. Thus, the biomedical model propounded that disease is a manifestation of disequilibrium on a biological basis due to either internal biological dysfunction or malfunctioning or inflicted by external factors from the environment. Thus, the biological model construes the individual as a passive recipient and a 'victim' of disease.

The concept of the biomedical model perceives the human body as a mechanical mobile machine, which may go out of order due to either external intrusions or wear and tear in some specific parts. Just as the way a machine is either functional or non-functional, the medical model depicts disease and health as polar opposites. One is either healthy or unhealthy or diseased. Thus, when there is no disease, one is supposed to be healthy. When an individual is diagnosed with a disease, the treatment is administered by the doctor in the form of medicine, which 'repairs' the biomedical imbalance and cellular problem or 'removes' the external intrusions causing the diseased state.

The disease according to the biomedical model manifests in the form of symptoms either located in the specific body organ or indicated by deviation from the normal functioning of a system in the body. The diagnosis is based on these symptoms. The treatment through medication results in disappearance of these symptoms, thus shifting the position of the person from 'diseased' to 'healthy'. Thus, the concepts of health and illness are dichotomous.

This in a way promoted the idea of 'a pill for every ill'. To a certain extent, this was also evidenced when the majority of diseases were of acute nature like typhoid, tuberculosis and cholera, which were easy to cure with penicillin and sulpha drugs. Death rates due to these diseases declined remarkably.

The state of health can be labelled as a state of 'ease' and disruption to this state as 'Disease'. According to the biomedical model (Figure 2.1), the two states are mutually exclusive and dichotomous. The cause of 'Dis-ease' state could be both internal and external, with the same consequence of shifting the individual to the state of 'dis-ease' from 'ease'. However, the corrective measure in the form of treatment is necessarily external with the power of restoring the individual's state to 'ease' or 'health'. The main elements of this model are assumptions of biological functions and treatment approach based on statistical normality.

The biomedical model can be compared to the S-R model of behaviour. In both, the major common drawback was ignoring the 'Organism' as thinking, feeling and expressing entity. Hence, the criticisms of the two theories have been almost on the same ground.

The model mainly emphasizes the 'Disease pole' of the dichotomy. The conceptualization is based on 'one cause and one cure' for every disease, infirmity or dysfunction. The glaring vacuum in this model is ignoring the human being as the medium of experiencing and expressing

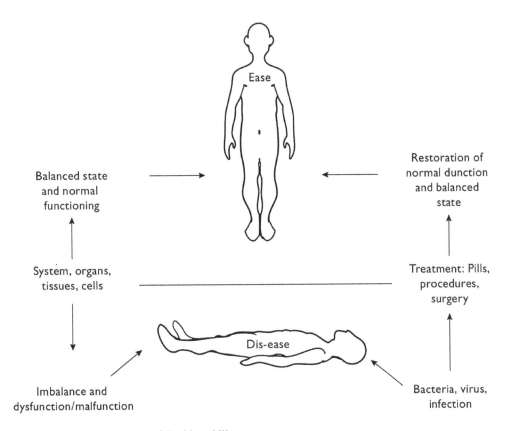

Figure 2.1 Biomedical Model of Health and Illness.

26 *Wellness, Illness, Health and Health Psychology*

Box 2.1 Significant Aspects of the Biomedical Model

1. The individual has two separate entities called 'body' and 'mind' that function independently.
2. Health and disease refer to the physical states that have no natural continuity. One is either diseased or healthy at any point.
3. Health is the absence of disease.
4. 'Disease' is a symptom physically manifested with an underlying abnormality, malfunction or dysfunction within the body.
5. The individual is a passive victim of circumstances that induce a disease in him/her.
6. The diagnosis of the disease is based on the symptoms.
7. Diseases are treated by interventions from outside by administering medication or surgery.
8. The patient is a passive recipient of treatment.
9. The cure is indicated by the absence of symptoms where the individual is assumed to have moved to the state of health.
10. Irritability, emotional turmoil or delusions are unrelated to the bodily function.

---

the symptoms of the disease. A number of syndromes with multiple underlying causes have no logical explanation in this model.

Further, the symptoms experienced and expressed by the individual have wide variations. For example, the subjectivity in experiencing pain is scientifically endorsed by the gate theory.

The formula of cause and effect is not satisfactory considering the absence of universality in its operation. For example, the biomedical theory has no satisfactory explanation as to the process by which, exposed to the same environment and bacteria, only some individuals prove vulnerable, while others do not get the disease.

The definition of health as polar opposites fails to explain the phenomenon where despite the disease or injury, the individual functions at an optimal level. Similarly, it also has no explanation when there is dysfunction of the organ with no underlying pathology. Hence, Radley (1994) stated that explaining health and disease in dichotomy is just a linguistic artefact. As observed by Siegel (1986), the biomedical model assumes that 'disease catches individual rather than the individual catching the disease', thus reducing the role of an individual to an 'absorbing agent'.

The lacunae of the model can be best understood from the example in Box 2.2. The example presents two versions of the diagnosis, impairment and prognosis of the disease.

A 50-year-old IT executive suffered a paralytic stroke of his left part of the body six months ago. His left leg still has a drag, and his left hand has not achieved perfect coordination. The IT executive, though permitted by the doctor to resume normal routine, has not returned to work.

In box 2.2 both the versions are true in terms of diagnosis, impairment and prognosis. The doctor's version is based on the objective assessment, while the patient's version is based on his subjective experience. Both are based on 'Perception'. The doctor's perception is grounded in his medical knowledge, professional experience and skills, while the patient's perception is based on his beliefs, attitudes, expectations and values. The doctor's version is that of disease, while the patient's is that of illness.

Box 2.2 Paralytic Stroke: Two Versions

Dimensions	Doctor's version	Patient's version
Diagnosis	Mild stroke, with a history of hypertension	Severe stroke
Impairment	Slight weakness of the left leg and mild coordination dysfunction in the left arms. Language and cognition intact	Left leg doesn't work. Left hand is useless
Prognosis	Good. Able to do almost all activities Is fit to return to work	Have become handicapped Unable to play tennis or cycle Still feel very sick Cannot go back to office

Kleinman (1980) brings a clear distinction between the two. 'Disease' according to Kleinman refers to the bodily condition, the presence of pathology that is for the doctor to diagnose and treat. 'Illness' refers to the experience of that disease by the patient, the way the person understands the disease. This happens in the backdrop of a number of factors such as the individual's knowledge about the disease, belief about its impact, past experience, expectations and the values related to a number of factors such as autonomy, dependence. Dalal (2016) observes, "clearly, disease is a medical term; illness refers to psychological side…" (p. 10). By reducing the role of the patient into a passive recipient of the disease and treatment, the biomedical model turned a blind eye to the psychological factors of the patient that makes the prognosis a reality. All the personal psychological characteristics of the patient operate in a social context but not in isolation. For example, the patients' knowledge and experience about the disease originates from the social source. Similarly, the expectations and values also have a social context and relevance. The biomedical model is totally silent on this dimension.

The example in Box 2.3 clarifies this aspect.

An examination of the case described in Box 2.3 clearly reveals the social influence (family being the first social agent) on the individual's recovery from surgery. While the medical assessment and advice are for resuming the normal social roles, the indulgence of the social support system (which, in middle-class Indian society, is overwhelming, particularly in the event of illness) prolongs one's return to the state of 'health' from that of 'disease'. In the words of one Indian Cardiac Interventionist, "the actual problem for the Cardiologist is not the patient who is advised bypass surgery, but it is the so called friends and acquaintances of the patient who narrate the cases they 'know' and induce a set of beliefs and attitudes in the patient". A patient who has narrated two cases of deaths following surgery by two independent 'friends/relatives' suffers high anxiety induced by internalization of consequences and negative thoughts.

The social aspect of the disease encompasses the capacity of the patient to fulfil the responsibilities in a social role to the expectations of society. The level of expectations influences his continuation of ceasing the role of the patient. Thus, while 'disease' is a doctor's assessment and 'illness' is a patient's experience, 'sickness' is the social role of the person determined by society. The biomedical model has no single reference to this aspect.

The biopsychosocial model of health evolved out of the inadequacies inherent in the biomedical model.

Box 2.3   Recovery of CABG Patient

The 58-year-old man has been discharged from hospital after Coronary Artery Bypass Grafting (CABG). The box presents the doctor's advice, inputs from the social support system and patients' reaction/response in three separate columns. This presentation relates to six weeks after the surgery.

Dimensions	Doctor's advice	Social support (family)	Patients' reaction/response
Diet	Low on oil and carbohydrate Low salt High fibre	Food served has no oil and no carbohydrate No salt Boiled vegetables and fruits	Food is tasteless. I have not regained my appetite
Activities	Can gradually resume normal activities. Can resume all his roles. Should walk regularly	Assistance and support extended in every activity. Patient's family roles are transferred to other members. Walking can wait for some more time because it was 'heart surgery' that you have undergone	It is taking very long for my recovery. I don't know when I will be 'normal' again
Work	Can return to work	You have accumulated a lot of leave. Use them now and take a complete rest	My professional responsibilities are now on my counterpart. I cannot take so much stress now
Prognosis	Recovery is good	Take your own time. You are sick. You have our support	I am still sick

Biopsychosocial Model

The biopsychosocial model of health evolved from the criticisms of the biomedical model. Engel (1977), a strong critique of the biomedical model for its excessive focus on biological aspects for aetiology and medical aspects for cure, proposed the biopsychosocial model. As the name suggests, the biopsychosocial model gives prominence to psychological and social factors as significant contributors to health and illness in addition to the biological factors.

At the very outset, the biopsychosocial model rejects the two assumptions of dichotomy as conjectured in the biomedical model. The first is the dichotomy of health and disease as two opposite poles. To explain it further, the biopsychosocial model, which construes body and mind as two separate entities, rejects their independent functioning. It conceives a close and continuous interaction between the body and mind contributing to the state of health or illness. Its challenge to the dichotomy of health and illness is on the ground that there is a possibility of positioning oneself between these two poles. First of all, recovery from certain illness could be a slow and gradual process where there is a scope for the person to move gradually from illness to wellness. Secondly, illness may vary in severity and consequences. While some may be a temporary indisposition, some may be severe causing permanent infirmity (e.g. amputation of a limb) while some other may be terminal. Thirdly, while the polar opposite position may be somewhat true in case of acute illnesses, in case of chronic diseases like hypertension, arthritis, diabetes, one may find the BP 'slightly high', 'very high' or normal; and the same with the sugar levels in the blood. Finally, even when the BP is high one may not label oneself as 'sick'. Thus, the biopsychosocial model postulates health (wellness) and illness not as two separate and independent concepts but as two ends of the continuum varying in degree.

As indicated in Figure 2.2, it is possible for an individual to position oneself at any point of the continuum depending upon one's own judgement that includes the medical diagnosis and label, as well as one's own subjective perception of 'illness'. The optimum state of health or wellness is a conceptual position when the individual feels highly energetic and happy and shows an optimum level of performance. By envisaging the position of the individual on any point of the continuum, the model places equal importance to both health/wellness and illness, both of which are states that come out of a symbiotic relationship between biological, psychological and social factors.

This model, in fact, can be viewed as an extension of the biomedical model. While the biomedical model emphasizes one cause and one treatment, the biopsychosocial model propounds that multiple factors interplay as determinants of health and illness. One may wonder about the possibility of interaction between the three factors named in the model. It may sound improbable, but the macro-level factors of psychological and social processes interact with biological factors at the micro level. This is explained using the system theory. According to the system theory, all levels of organization in an entity are hierarchically connected to each other. A change in any one level impacts all the other levels bringing changes therein. Adopting it in the biopsychosocial model of health, it can be explained that the biological factors involving the micro-level process are nested within the psychosocial aspects that involve the macro-level process. Any changes in the micro level (e.g. biochemical imbalance) bring about a concomitant change in the macro level (e.g. mood changes and social response to the affective disposition). The vice versa is also accepted. The multidimensionality of 'biopsychosocial' factors is explained in the model as constant operating forces starting from aetiology, symptom manifestation to the treatment process.

The crux of the biopsychosocial model lies in answering the question 'when does a person feel he/she is sick?' Engel (1977) explains that some individuals express a somatic condition or an emotional upheaval as 'problem of living', while others perceive it as 'illness'. The reason

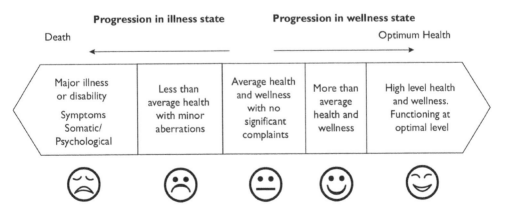

Figure 2.2 Biopsychosocial Model of Health and Illness.

lies in whether or not the person is willing to live the 'sick role' and seek health care. Again, the surfacing of symptoms experienced in the form of pain has several expressions varying in form and degree as a function of demographic and cultural factors (Mohan, 2010). Engel further explains the concept of being sick with 'grief' in people experiencing grief reporting 'ill' with both somatic and psychological symptoms. Given such complexity, the practising physician should have knowledge in the field of psychology and understand the social processes in the context of the patient in addition to his knowledge and skill in medicine. Alternatively, the diagnosis and treatment process must involve a teamwork that includes expertise from all the three fields concerned.

Viewed from the prism of the biopsychosocial model, one realizes as to how the aetiology, symptoms/syndromes, treatment and prognosis of illness or the state of wellness can be explained from a wide spectrum of possible forces operating in combination. Figure 2.3 summarizes the complex confluence.

The health and illness status of the individual is determined by the curious interplay between the three forces. For example, the mere genetic predisposition of the individual does not result in the illness (e.g. cancer) in the person. Only when the lifestyle behaviour of the person (smoking) subscribes substantially to place him/her in the 'at-risk' category does the person get cancer. Similarly, though the environment is full of staphylococcus infection, not everyone exposed to the infection is affected, but a person who has been exposed to severe stress such as bereavement in the family contacts the infection because the stressful experience would have weakened the immune system. This is about the aetiology of illness or health. A more complex situation of all the forces interplaying with each other is explained in the following case.

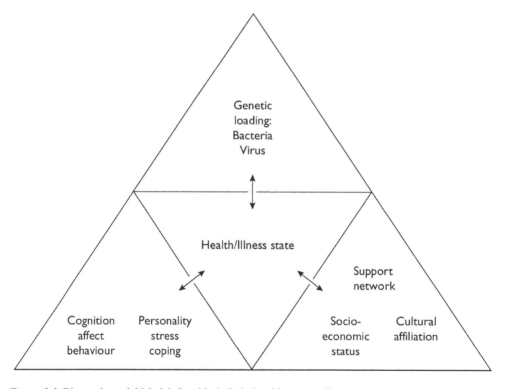

Figure 2.3 Biopsychosocial Model: Symbiotic Relationship among Factors.

Venkat, a small-scale carpenter, has a six-year-old son diagnosed with a congenital cardiac condition that could be cured with a major surgery costing few lakh rupees. This was informed to Venkat by the doctors when the child was four years old. The economic status of Venkat made such expensive treatment non-viable. The illiterate parents resigned to 'destiny' as the condition of the boy worsened limiting his physical functioning and giving rise to several medical emergencies, which were attended to by the family. The condition of the child was casually mentioned to a client where he was doing the interiors. The client took the initiative in mobilizing funds from philanthropists for the treatment of the child. Now, it is the economic condition that led to worsening of the condition of the child and the social support network that restored the 'wellness' in the child. The child who was physically weak due to the progressive cardiac problem was inattentive, cranky and crying frequently, gradually turned alert, active and happy following surgery. This shows the impact of the social status on the physical and psychological state.

The biopsychosocial model focuses on the individual rather than the disease. The model places partial responsibility for the status of health on the person in terms of health-inducing behaviour (e.g. regular exercise or nutrition's diet) or health risk behaviour (e.g. smoking, consumption of alcohol or eating junk food). Similarly, the treatment process is not confined to the administration of medication. It includes inculcating required functional knowledge about the illness (laying the cognitive foundation) introducing therapeutic intervention to bring desirable change in the affect state when the patient is found to have high levels of anxiety or depression (restoring desirable affect state) and bringing about a change in the behaviour that is not conducive for sustaining a positive state of health (initiating behavioural change). Thus, the biopsychosocial model of health addresses all the factors mentioned in the WHO definition of health in 'totality' and upholds the holistic perspective of health. The model shifted the concept of 'health' from a 'state' determined by internal and external factors to that of a 'status' achieved by the individual by playing an active role in practising behaviour that helps in the endeavour and creating a social network that supports and promotes such desirable behaviour. The status of health and illness is dynamic and susceptible to changes due to the interplay of the biological, psychological and social forces. The goal of the individual is to reach the ideal state of the optimum health, and the efforts ideally should be moved towards this end in the continuum.

Thus, the biopsychosocial model of health could overcome a number of criticisms that the biomedical model faced. In order to drive home the advantages of the biopsychosocial model, the two models are contrasted in Box 2.4.

Ayurveda and Biopsychosocial Model

The Western idea of the biopsychosocial model of health evolved over several millennia of advancement in the field of health. But Ayurveda, the ancient medical practice in India, had the biopsychosocial model as an integral part of knowledge, practice and skill in the science of medicine. Conceptualization of 'health' in Ayurveda is very rich in its inclusiveness. Dalal (2016) writes about Ayurveda, "This system of medicine offers a different perspective on life and health, in which wholeness, integration, freedom, connectivity, creativity and enjoyment figure as central concerns" (p. 15). This ancient science is one that construes 'health' with no reference to illness. In Sanskrit (the language in which Ayurveda is documented), health is expressed as *'swastha'*, broken into two parts—*'swa'* meaning 'self' and *'stha'* meaning placed or situated. Thus, the term *'swastha'* refers to 'Being in one's own natural state'.

According to Vedic scriptures (from where Ayurveda originated), the natural state of the human being is that of *'Ananda'* or 'bliss'. The concept of *Ananda* or bliss supersedes the concept of 'happiness', which is mostly related to mundane achievements. This inner state of *'Ananda'*

Box 2.4 Comparison between Biomedical and Biopsychosocial Models

Grounds of comparison	Biomedical	Biopsychosocial
Basic assumption	Body-mind dichotomy	Close interaction between body and mind though they are separate entities
Cause of illness	Internal factors such as chemical imbalance, genetic factors or external factors like bacteria, virus invading the body	Biological factors as described in the biomedical model, psychological factors involving cognition, affect and behaviour or social factors like SES, pressure for social conformity
Role of the patient	Passive victim	Active participant
Treatment (a) Target (b) Process (c) Outcome (d) Assessment (e) Responsibility	(a) Disease (physical state) (b) Medication, surgery, radiation (c) Absence of symptoms (physical) (d) Objective (e) Doctor	(a) The person as a whole (b) Medication, surgery, radiation and interventions to bring changes in emotion and behaviour (c) Absence of physical symptoms, change in behaviour with higher adherence and positive change in emotions (d) Objective and subjective (e) Doctor and patient
Health-illness relationship	Mutually exclusive, opposite poles	One and the same concept. Two poles of the same continuum
Relationship with psychology	Psychological state may be a consequence of illness but not the cause	Psychological factors can be both the cause or consequence of wellness and illness

is the natural existential condition of the human being. Thus, the state of 'health' is possible only with the convergence of the positive state of physical, mental, social and spiritual factors in life.

For the purpose of understanding, the state of *'Ananda'* may be translated to 'General state of wellbeing'. Verma and Verma (1989) defined the General state of wellbeing as "Subjective feeling of contentment, happiness, satisfaction with life experiences and one's role in the world of work, sense of achievement, utility, belongingness and no distress, dissatisfaction or worry".

Physical Body, Bioenergy and Constituents: Panchabhootas and Tridoshas

The Ayurveda model postulates a human body is made of *'panchamahabhootas'*, viz. *'Pruthvi'* (Earth), *'Apah'* (Water), *'Tejas/Agni'* (Fire), *'Vayu'* (Air) and *'Akasha'* (Sky). This conglomeration of five elements consists of the bioenergy called *'tridoshas'*—*'vata'*, *'pitta'* and *'kapha'*. The relationship between the 'panchabhootas' and 'tridoshas' is explained in Figure 2.4. As can be seen, vata is the outcome of *'pruthvi'* and *'vayu'*, i.e. Earth and Air. *'Pitta'* is related to *'Tejas/Agni'*, i.e. Fire, while *'kapha'* is the manifestation of 'Apah', i.e. Water. Thus, the human being is a microcosm of the macrocosm (Surendra & Prasad, 2013).

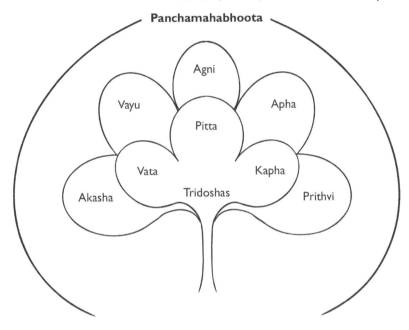

Figure 2.4 Tridoshas-Panchamahabhoota Relationship.

'*Tridoshas*' are the three forces susceptible to being vitiated (Dosha = Vicious). In Ayurveda, a human being is not conceptualized as a system of organs but as a system of relationship of functions. The '*tridoshas*' refer to biological functions like movement, transformation, support and growth (Jayasundar, 2010).

Ayurveda assumes that the human being's physical constitution and personality make-up are influenced by the *tridoshas* or the three humours in the body. All the physiological and psychological functions are controlled, moderated and balanced by the '*tridoshas*'. Further, there is a sound integration among the three. The psychophysiological functions of the '*tridoshas*' are explained in Figure 2.5.

Relationship between Tridoshas and Trigunas

As explained in the figure, the main functions of the *tridoshas* are movements, coordination, action, transformation, sustenance, stability and control of not only the physiological functioning but also the psychological functioning. Each of the *doshas* is connected with functioning at the physical and mental level. Just as the way the body is identified with the *tridoshas,* the mental faculties are also classified into three characteristics, viz. '*Sattva*', '*Rajas*' and '*Tamas*'. All the three are referred to as '*trigunas*'. Sattva refers to the truth or reality. It is qualified with clarity, divinity, and head and heart (thought and feeling) integration. '*Rajas*' translated as 'royal' is characterized by agitation, desire, anger, wilfulness and pursuit of power, stimulation and entertainment. Thus, it is full of vitality and action. '*Tamas*' has the qualities of inertia, inactivity, insensitivity and resistance. For both '*tridoshas*' and '*trigunas*', the building blocks are *panchamahabhootas*. In every individual, one or the other *dosha* and one or the other *guna* are dominant.

34 *Wellness, Illness, Health and Health Psychology*

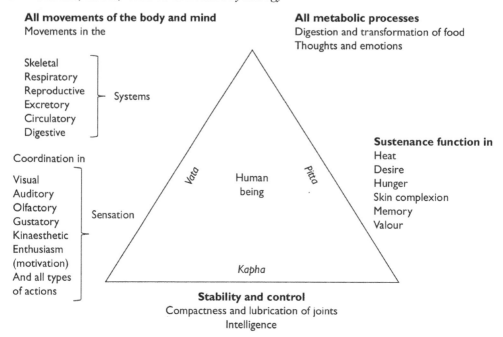

Figure 2.5 Tridosha's Control over Psychophysiological Functions.

While the model ascribes separate identity to body and mind, there is a strong integrated functional relationship between them. The *'tridoshas'* and *'trigunas'* are not mutually exclusive in their functional characteristics. Each of the three *'gunas'* has one dominant *'dosha'* in it. *'Sattva'* guna has *'pitta'* as the dominant *'dosha'*, while it also carries traces of *'vata'* and *'kapha'*. *'Rajas'* has *'vata'* as dominant *'dosha'* with *'pitta'* also present in the subdued level. *'Tamas'* has *'kapha'* as the only *'dosha'* present in it. It is possible that an individual's body is dominated by one *'dosha'*, while mind *(guna)* is dominated by another. The equilibrium *(sama)* between these three forces summarily responsible for the functioning of human beings indicates *'swastha'* or health. Disequilibrium at any level has an impact on disequilibrium at other levels causing illness or *'aswasthata'*. A person who enjoys a healthy status is the one who is fully functional to fulfil the four *purusharthas*, viz. achieve *'Dharma'* (social responsibilities), gain *'Artha'* (monitory returns), have *'Kama'* (sensual enjoyments) and attain *'Moksha'* (liberation) (Rastogi, 2009).

The concept of mind in Ayurveda is identified with three separate functional expressions, viz. *'Manas'* (thoughts), *'Buddhi'* (Intelligence) and *'Ahankara'* (Ego). These three, while functionally independent, work in good coordination, which is governed by consciousness (Shroff, 2017).

Sources of Vulnerabilities

According to the Ayurveda model, disease or 'Aswasthata' can be caused due to imbalance between the three *'doshas'* in the physical body or mind whose vulnerability originates from three sources (Surendra & Prasad, 2013):

1 *'Asatmendriyartha Samyoga'*. This refers to the overuse or underuse of the sense organs. This is what is expressed as understimulation or overstimulation in the parlance of psychology.

Exposure to extreme light, or darkness for prolonged periods, being in an environment of noise pollution, exposure to extreme heat or cold, indulgence in eating or inhalation of polluted air can result in illness. The modern psychology has proved the stressful consequences of overexposure to each of these sensations, and also, the devastating effects of prolonged deprivation may manifest at the physical plane in the form of headache, nausea, digestive disorders, fever and cold or at the mental plane in the form of strain, anxiety depression or a manifestation as mild as irritability.

2 *'Prajnaparadha'*. This translates to intellectual blasphemy. This has a behavioural loading. The source of disease is mainly due to the behavioural deviation. Ayurveda characterizes it with 'intellectual error'. This can be elaborated with the example of initiating and sustaining smoking behaviour despite the full knowledge that it has a potential health risk. This also refers to the impulsive behaviour that results because of the lack of control over 'mind'. Violation of hygiene in sexual practices, substance abuse, violation of traffic rules, and entertaining negative thoughts leading to unacceptable behaviour come under this classification. Each of these actions in combination leads to the loss of health and causes illness.

3 *'Kala'*. This third influencing factor refers to seasonal variations. Seasonal variations will cause an imbalance in the *tridoshas*. In addition, the consumption of food not suited to the external environment (season) also is considered as improper for health. The prescription of Ayurveda is living in harmony with the environment. *'Kala'* also refers to *'Kala parinama'* or transformations related to time. This connotes variation in body's susceptibility to diseases due to changes brought by progression in age. It also includes the impact of variation in day and night on the body. Thus, the 'human being' is the epicentre of the Ayurveda.

Ayurveda Approach and Biopsychosocial Characteristics

Thus, the Ayurveda model traces the aetiology of disease to multiple causes related to the biological factors, psychological factors and the environmental sources. Apart from body and mind, the Ayurvedic concept of health also includes aspects indicating true balance with society. It involves maintaining harmony with family, friends and work by following customs and traditions and pursuit of spiritual life. Inclusion of the spiritual dimension to the model helped to bring vitality to other three aspects. While spirituality has been an important integral part in the Ayurveda model, it was proposed to be added only in the year 1998 by WHO in their Executive Board, which has not yet accepted and adopted by their general membership body (Dalal, 2016).

Ayurveda, so deeply rooted in the biopsychosocial model, advocates diagnosis and treatment of the disease not based on uniformity or standardization but based on the unique *'Prakruti'* or constitution of the individual. The system with the *'tridoshas'* impacting body and mind independently results in such complexity that standardizing is not possible.

The emphasis of Ayurveda, true to its nomenclature (The Science of Life), is more on the prevention of disease through following a healthy lifestyle. The Ayurvedic 'way of life' practised in daily living prescribes food preference, leisure activities and other preventive and promotive health measures that ensure quality of life and longevity. However, should there be a disequilibrium resulting in illness, the model does have provision for the treatment process, which is unique for every person. The treatment assumes the interconnectivity between body and mind and treats the whole person but not the diseased part. Hence, it may be appropriate to term the treatment of Ayurveda as 'healing' rather than curing. The healing involves medicines, diet and lifestyle activities to restore the functional imbalance of *'doshas'* (Jayasundar, 2010). The treatment regimen includes intervention at the sensory level such as exposure to colours, tastes, sounds, touch and aroma, body massages, medication for purging and practice of Yoga (which includes meditation).

Prescribed Lifestyle in Ayurveda

In Ayurveda, Yoga is prescribed as both part of treatment and health promotion or 'way of life'. The term 'Yoga' originates from 'Yug' meaning 'uniting' (Shroff, 2017) mind, body and universal spirit. The *Ashtanga Yoga* prescribed by *Ayurveda* includes *Yama, Niyama, Asana, Pranayama, Pratyahara, Dharana, Dhyana* and *Samadhi*. They refer to moral code, self-purification, posture, control over breath, control over thoughts, concentration, meditation and attaining oneness or integration. The holistic approach is very evident from the spectrum of aspects brought under regulation. Yoga includes the practice of *'asanas'* (set postures of the physical body), *'pranayama'* (breathing exercises) and *dhyana* (meditation), all of which have proved to heal physical ailments related to cardiovascular, pulmonary, digestive, reproductive and other physiological systems, restore and sustain emotional balance, and inculcate stability in physical and mental health. Control over senses, thoughts, enhancing concentration and practice of meditation speak about the significance given to cognitive and social aspects of health behaviour. The Yogic practices help the individual recondition the neuromuscular and neuroglandular systems. This prepares the individual to encounter and cope successfully with stress and strain of life.

Thus, Yoga helps develop resistance in body and mind and promote vitality. The other preventive measures are *'Dinacharya'* (daily routine), *'Ritucharya'* (seasonal diet) and *'Sadvritta'* (social behaviour). *Dinacharya* refers to adherence to personal hygiene that starts from brushing the teeth in the morning to following sleep hygiene. *Ritucharya* prescribes the diet regimen that should suit seasonal variations. *Sadvritta* elaborates on the desirable social behaviour based on religions as ritual practices, relationship with family, friends and other significant social agents. *Sadvritta* demands that emotions and behaviour are maintained in balance as a partial requirement of good health. Thus, the onus of good health is majorly on the individual, rather than on society or doctor.

The biopsychosocial model of Ayurveda places a great emphasis on the individual and 'self-awareness', which includes physical, mental, social and spiritual dimensions of self. This awareness also implies that the individual perceives 'self' as part of the system with all its complexity.

"The social health model of Ayurveda is directed bottom up from individual to population" (Morandi, Tosto, Di Sarsina, & Dalla Libera, 2011). The personal, social, cultural, motivational and spiritual life of individuals in the society constitutes the social health.

Thus, the Ayurveda model is biopsychosocial in nature. It is a holistic approach to health that gives a comprehensive picture of health with a functional integration between body, mind, behaviour and environment, each of which is significant from the aetiological, healing, preventive and promotive perspective of health.

Health Psychology

Having explained the biopsychosocial model in detail, it becomes simple to define and easy to understand what 'Health Psychology' is. Health Psychology, the 38th branch of the American Psychological Association, is an applied branch of psychology where all the principles of psychology are applied in the context of health. The definition that was widely accepted goes like this:

> Health Psychology is the aggregate of the specific educational, scientific and professional contributions of the discipline of Psychology to the promotion and maintenance of health, the prevention and treatment of illness, the identification of etiologic and diagnostic correlates of health, illness and related dysfunctions and improvement of health care system and health policy formation.
>
> (Matarazzo, 1980, p. 815)

To elaborate on the definition, Health Psychology refers to the application of all the principles of psychology evolved out of theoretical knowledge from education, from scientific research and experience of professional practice in the field of health. These principles equally applied to different dimensions of health and health care aim for health promotion and maintenance, illness prevention, tracing the aetiology and treatment of illness. It is also applied in the field of diagnosis of illness and their symptoms and syndromes. Thus, the overall goal of Health Psychology is to strengthen the structure and function of the health care system and then influence the health policies at national and global levels.

The theory and practice of Health Psychology revolve around answering a few basic questions:

1 Who are the people who become sick? Who are the ones who stay healthy and why?
2 Who among the sick recover? How and why?
3 How to promote recovery from illness?
4 How to prevent illness?

Postulating theories, parameters investigated in research and interventions introduced in practice related to the questions posed above focus on the cognitive, affective, motivational, behavioural and personality domains of the human being. Thus, the inquiry is into the dynamics of cognition and motivation related to the disease, affective state preceding, during and following illness, behavioural practices labelled as health risk or health promoting as part of the lifestyle that might have contributed to becoming ill, staying sick or recovery. Apart from these, Health Psychology also examines the contributing factors from social environments such as the social support, cultural practices, health values, health literacy and health communication in the context of the individual and the sociocultural environment.

Psychological Factors as Antecedents of Disease

Tracing the aetiology of the disease to psychological antecedents, Friedman and Rosenman (1974) found a significant relationship between type 'A' personality and coronary heart disease (CHD). Type A personality was found to be characterized by a behavioural pattern comprising three components, viz. a sense of time urgency, competitive spirit and striving for achievement and easily aroused hostility. With these components, it can be easily imagined that type 'A' people lead a life with a fast pace, work longer hours, are constantly under stress to achieve targets, show impatience with team members who work at a slower pace, are highly competitive and push themselves towards the goal. The physiological functioning (particularly the cardiovascular system) of these people is likely to take the brunt of the lifestyle, thus making them vulnerable to coronary heart diseases. This has been proved in a number of studies across the globe. In a study on 2750 men who were tested on type 'A' behaviour, it was found that the high scorers had twice the incidence of coronary heart disease compared to low scorers (Jenkins, Rosenman, & Zyzanski, 1974). Decades later, a group of Australian researchers (Bunker et al., 2003) in their study attempted to identify psychosocial risk factors of coronary heart disease (CHD), development and progression. They found that depression, social isolation and lack of quality social support were independently and consistently related not only as the cause of coronary heart disease but also in the prognosis of the treatment. They did not find any evidence of a relationship with type 'A' behavioural pattern. They strongly recommended that these constitute the risk factors and hence need to be included in the assessment package of CHD risk assessment, as well as CHD management. Further, they argued that this research evidence needs to be taken seriously while framing the public health policies.

Psychosocial Aspects of Illness Experience and Treatment Package

Apart from identifying the psychosocial antecedents to illness, Health Psychology also investigates into the relationship between illness experience and psychosocial factors. It was found by Chivukula, Hariharan, Rana, Thomas and Andrew (2017) that psychosocial care in the ICU also made a difference in wellbeing levels of patients during their post-CABG stay in the ICU. These studies are elaborated in a later chapter related to chronic illness. These findings clearly indicate that the illness experience of the patients can be decreased by including psychosocial care as an integral part of the treatment regimen for patients. As indicated by the biopsychosocial model, when the individual falls ill, it is not just the physical body that experiences the pain, but the cognitive and affective domains also undergo an upheaval. Emotional blaming through psychosocial care ensures that the 'healing' is to the individual and not just the diseased organ. When the target of treatment is the individual as a whole, the perceived support provides a cushioning effect in lowering the illness experience.

While psychosocial care was found to impact the illness experience, the latter also has its influence on recovery and post-illness health status. If the treatment regimen excludes the focus on the cognitive and affective state of the patient and treats only the impaired part of the organ, its impact may show on the recovery and prognosis. Mossey, Mutran, Knott and Craik (1989) followed up on 219 female patients who had fractured their hip while in community-dwelling. The findings indicated that high levels of depression following the surgery had an association with poor recovery in physical and psychosocial functioning. This is a clear pointer that the patients' affective state during illness cannot be kept outside the realm of the treatment regimen. The affective state of the patient has a significant influence on the recovery from illness. A follow-up study on Indian patients who underwent CABG surgery (Thomas, Hariharan, & Rana, 2016) found that those patients whose psychosocial intervention addressed the distress levels in the post-surgery phase showed a faster pace of recovery and a higher level of functioning at physical and psychological levels. The study found that the prognosis was closely related to the level of post-surgical distress. This study is discussed in detail in a later chapter.

Thus, the scope of Health Psychology covers the trajectory from the state of wellness, to the state of illness, and the return to the state of wellbeing, thus following the full circles in individual's health status.

Aims and Scope of Health Psychology

It may be easy to infer from the above discussion the aims and goals of Health Psychology. The aims of Health Psychology as an established branch can be broadly classified into two:

1. Theorizing the biopsychosocial processes in health
2. Applying the biopsychosocial module in promotion, prevention, diagnosis, care and healing covering the entire spectrum from wellness to illness and back

Continuous inputs from research in the field cater to both.

1. **Theorizing:** The academic endeavours of Health Psychology rest in its continuous attempts to understand and explain the theories in vogue and developing and testing the new theories. For example, evaluating the role of certain personality disposition or behavioural pattern in causing a specific future illness is part of theorizing. Similarly, it may be theorized that patients with low levels of motivation will have low adherence levels to medical advice and thus have a slower pace of recovery. All the theories are validated by testing with empirical

studies. Theoretical orientations of Health Psychology assume equal value as the application because they supplement each other. The aim of understanding, explaining, developing and testing theory may include relating behavioural antecedents to an illness, predicting unhealthy behaviour based on health beliefs (smoking behaviours based on health beliefs), assessing the connectivity between psychology and physiology (e.g. cortisol secretion under stress), explanation of the psychological factors in illness experience (e.g. depressive state magnifying the pain experience) or highlighting the significance of psychological factors in treatment regimen (e.g. relaxation therapy in the pre-surgery phase to enhance pace of recovery from surgical wound).

2 **Application:** Health Psychology as a professional branch aims to apply the theoretical postulates into practice. This is possible in the following four contexts:

  a **Patient Care:** Having understood the relationship between the psychological inputs in illness perception and experience, the onus of developing modules of psychosocial care for the patients and including them as part of treatment intervention is on the policy-makers and health psychologists. For example, reassuring a patient in the ICU that the family members are present in the attenders' lounge goes a long way in enhancing perceived social support in the patient. Similarly, explaining to the patient about the procedure of lumber puncture to draw fluid from bone marrow in terms of the purpose, the degree of pain and the cooperation from the patient help in laying a cognitive base in the patient, thereby pre-empting the anxiety that would be induced when the patient is involved as a passive participant. Ensuring a free flow of communication from the health providers expressing empathy, providing information, explaining discomfort or revealing expectations constitutes an important segment of care.

  b **Illness Cure:** Health Psychology presumes that 'cure' is achieved when the individual returns to the status of 'health' on biopsychosocial criteria. In other words, the parameter of cure is not only the absence of physical symptoms like pain, indigestion or giddiness, but also a stable emotional state, well-functioning cognition and ability to discharge social responsibilities without any hitch. For example, a patient, eight weeks after the CABG, may be assessed by the cardiac surgeon and certified 'fit' by him on his cardiac functions. However, the patient still feels depressed and perceives himself as not yet fit to return to his work or engage in routine activities. He may complain of sleep disturbances with flashes of experiences he had during his ICU stay. In such instances, the patient is not classified as 'cured' and 'fit' by a health psychologist.

  c **Health Promotion:** Health Psychology focuses on the behaviours that impact health. Understanding the dynamics of health risk behaviour such as smoking, substance abuse, violation of sleep hygiene, indulgence in unprotected and unsafe sexual practices or violation of traffic rules thereby enhancing one's vulnerability to accidents helps in targeting such behaviour and developing methods and modules to change them. Secondly by examining the belief system in an individual, culture or society, Health Psychology can predict the upcoming health behaviour. Applying the principles of learning, motivation and cognition, Health Psychology targets the beliefs to bring a change in concomitant behaviour or by bringing a change in the behaviour, thereby enhancing the belief system. The final goal of both is to replace the faulty health beliefs with the right ones and substitute the health-compromising behaviour with health-promoting behaviour. Minimizing the health risk behaviour and optimizing health-promoting behaviour is done at the individual level of patients and also at the mass level as public health measures. For example, designing school health programmes to inculcate personal hygiene through hand-wash training in children promotes healthy behaviour and also prevents some bacteria-based gastrointestinal problems in children. Similarly, the patient's maintenance of smoking behaviour is understood as a habit reinforced by oral stimulation. As a remedy, harmless edible and chewable oral stimulant herbal chewing gums are invented to substitute the health-compromising behaviour of smoking. Thus, understanding the cognitive-behavioural basis and consequences of health opens up a wide spectrum of designs and modules to change the behaviour and promote health.

d **Illness Prevention:** Prevention of illness can be at two levels, viz. prevention of onset of illness and prevention of relapse or progression of illness. For both, health education is the right intervention. Health Psychology offers effective intervention for creating awareness about the preventive steps for certain acute illness and management practices for certain chronic illness. The health education modules include individual interventions like counselling, public health awareness measures through media, and group interventions like focused training programmes and support group meetings. The interventions involve changing lifestyle for patients diagnosed with chronic illness. For example, a patient diagnosed with primary hypertension can be educated on changing lifestyle with a regulated diet, regular exercise and ritualistic adherence to medication so as to prevent any cardiovascular disease. An effective awareness programme for rural adolescents is designed to create awareness about the HIV/AIDS as a consequence of unsafe sexual practices. Both the modules are termed as preventive intervention. One prevents the progression of a potential cardiac condition, while the other works as a non-initiator of a health risk behaviour in a potential population.

When the theories of Health Psychology are thus tested and validated through application, the results of the research studies constitute a strong basis for translating the practices as recommendation for formulating health policies. The health care system thus evolved is more likely to be foolproof, robust and patient-friendly.

Need for Health Psychology

A number of factors at micro and macro levels were combined to enhance the relevance of Health Psychology in the contemporary period.

Change in Lifestyle

Major technological advancements and economic programmes have brought drastic changes in human behaviour. The use of devices has become an integral part of life, determining the postures and restricting the physical mobility of the individual. The two examples are the use of mobile phones and computers, which have turned into essential devices for information inflow and communication channels. As a result of this, the motor activities of the middle-class educated population are governed by the computers and mobile phones hooking up their visual attention and postures to the position of the devices. The use of mobile phones has reached even the remotest rural parts of India where a homemaker, farmer, high school student, and small-scale vendor and people of all ages and all walks of lives constitute the consumer group. The mobile phone use has reached a stage of addiction with people getting glued to the device for communication, information, entertainment or relaxation. As a consequence, the posture and gait of the persons are gradually dictated by the devices. This has become a major threat to natural physical mobility and activities contributing to physical fitness. The second major change at the micro level is due to the disturbance in the biological clock, particularly among the youth in developing countries. Employment opportunities based on global connectivity demand the youth to adjust their biological clock to the requirement of the countries they are linked to. Sometimes, when the job requirement involves multinational coordination, the individual may not have a definite biological clock. While this is the case with the middle- and upper-class youth, the youth of developing countries from the lower socioeconomic group are adapting to similar demands following their enrolment in organizations such as security agencies, driving or construction companies (to name of few), where they work on the shift system. Such lifestyles result in low or no sleep hygiene, and untimely diet habits. Sweeping changes and disturbances in these two dimensions that assume great significance for maintaining sound health leaves a society where a portion of population do not adhere to a specific routine. The third gross shift at the micro level is seen in the diet preference. In a country like India, there used to be huge diversity in the ethnic food that varied from region to region mainly suiting the climatic conditions, food cultivation and availability as a natural process of synchronizing the physical body to the seasonal changes. However, due to the development in transporting modes, the availability of food and preference for it have broken the regional boundaries, thus collapsing the nature's contribution to physical fitness of the individuals.

This indicates a major shift in lifestyle. Alongside these and because of these, the stress levels in general have shot up. Faulty coping strategies to encounter the stress involve indulgence in health risk behaviour such as smoking, overconsumption of alcohol, use of tranquillizers.

Lifestyle Diseases and Demand for Behavioural Change

The sedentary lifestyle, disturbed biorhythm, irregular diet, high stress levels and health risk behaviour place the individual at high risk for non-communicable diseases (NCDs). This is reflected in the increased prevalence of NCDs at the global level and in India. There is a shift in the major causes of death in the past two decades; Alzheimer's disease and diabetes mellitus, which were not in the top ten causes of global morality in the year 2000, have occupied the 5th and 7th rank in the year 2016. Table 2.1 shows the change in the percentage of deaths for the top ten causes between the years 2000 and 2016. The projection for the year 2020 is also shown in Table 2.2.

The comparison of figures in the years 2000 and 2016 and of projections for the year 2020 suggests that the NCDs and diseases caused due to lifestyle are shifting up in their rank order as a major cause of death.

The nature of NCDs is chronic and demands 'self-care' through efficient management of the disease. This prerequisites behavioural change. Behavioural change can happen through

Table 2.1 Top ten causes of death across the globe

Year 2000	Rank	Year 2016
Ischaemic heart disease (13.4)	1	Ischaemic heart disease (16.6)
Stroke (9.9)	2	Stroke (10.2)
Lower respiratory infection (6.4)	3	Chronic Obstructive Pulmonary Disease (5.3)
Chronic Obstructive Pulmonary Disease (5.7)	4	Lower respiratory infection (5.2)
Diarrhoeal disease (4.3)	5	Alzheimer's disease (3.5)
Tuberculosis (3.2)	6	Trachea, bronchus, lung cancer (3)
HIV/AIDS (2.8)	7	Diabetes mellitus (2.8)
Preterm birth complication (2.6)	8	Road injury (2.5)
Trachea, bronchus, lung cancer (2.4)	9	Diarrhoeal disease (2.9)
Road injury (2.2)	10	Tuberculosis (2.3)

Source: Shelley E. Taylor (2006).

Table 2.2 Major causes of death in the year 2020 (projections)

Rank	Disease or injury
1	Ischaemic heart disease
2	Unipolar major depression
3	Road traffic accidents
4	Cerebrovascular disease
5	Chronic Obstructive Pulmonary Disease
6	Lower respiratory infection
7	Tuberculosis
8	War
9	Diarrhoeal disease
10	HIV

Source: WHO (2018); figures in bracket indicate percentage.

appropriate knowledge transmission followed by motivational counselling, continuous guidance and monitoring. Health care professionals have a major role to play here. In a country like India, the doctor is considered to be a supreme health care provider. However, the doctor-patient ratio in the country is dismally poor with 1:1800 (Deo, 2013). In observation by the author and her research team, the average consultation time of a cardiologist with a patient was found to be seven minutes (Thomas, Hariharan, Rana, Swain, & Andrew, 2014). This is because of the work overload of the doctors trying to manage the health care system.

Through the biomedical model, the patient's condition clearly demands an appraisal and communication about the seriousness of the disease and its slow progression, the need for changes in lifestyle, its advantage, creating alertness about any emergency signals, and delineating a caution against the adversities of non-adherence or low adherence or inefficient management of the disease. However, the doctor is neither adequately trained to adopt such health communication to the varying intellectual, educational and age levels of the patients nor do they have time to discharge this responsibility. Under such circumstances, the approach of diagnosis and treatment remains limited to the biomedical model with suboptimal prognosis. It is in this context that Health Psychology and health psychologists play a pivotal role in designing and administering disease-specific interventions to optimize the outcome of treatment or management of the disease.

Significance of Considering Comorbid Psychological Condition

With advancements in medical sciences, the medical profession branched into specialization and super-specialization. The consequence of this shifted the focus of professionals from the individual as a whole to the specific parts of the body organs concerned. As an outcome, the advocacy of the biopsychosocial approach to health lost its strength and the biomedical approach is embraced. Treatment of the disease in isolation of the psychological status of the patient, especially when the illness is non-communicable disease, remains incomplete, because adherence behaviour is closely related to the psychological morbidity. For example, a patient being treated for a cardiac-related disease needs to have high adherence to medical prescription in order to have effective management. Medical prescription in this case includes, besides being regular with medication, regular exercise and a strict diet regimen. In case the patient suffers from moderate to severe depression that is not diagnosed, the adherence level is likely to be low. This is because depression is known to be associated with a lack of motivation, lowered attention, memory, inertia and sluggish disposition. These characteristics lower the motivation for action in terms of being regular in taking medication, or initiating regular exercise or following a special diet.

Thus, the low adherence is more a consequence of the comorbid condition of depression than any economic or adverse effect of medication. A number of studies proved a strong relationship between adherence and prognosis. Thus, ironically, progress in non-communicable disease, resulting in irreversible serious adverse conditions, is more due to super-specialization and micro-specialization in the field of medicine that failed to adopt a holistic treatment approach.

Up until the 1980s, the physicians in India had quality interactions with patients. They used to spend interacting with patients in the process of eliciting information related to symptoms and syndromes. This has gradually reduced as the diagnosis is mostly dependent on technology and is 'evidence-based'. The role of the doctor in the initial consultation is to identify the relevant investigations in the form of pathological tests, ECG, echocardiogram, treadmill test etc. Once completed, the doctor relies more on the piece of paper carrying the results of the tests than on the patient. Thus, the erstwhile 'human touch' in the process of care and cure is now replaced with invasion by biotechnology though with a very well-intended goal of 'better precision and objectivity'. However, as a natural consequence the patients feel the absence of 'healing'. In affiliation-oriented cultures like India where social support is valued high for its role in healing, the absence of quality communication between the doctor and the patient certainly creates a vacuum in health care.

Lifestyle Risk: Concern for All Economic Classes

Yet, another change in the macro level is related to the global economy resulting in paradoxical coexistence of unaffordability of quality health care and neglect of health care due to high affordability. The divide in affordability has been becoming sharper between the poor and the rich. The poor find it difficult to spend on any medical emergency or major medical intervention due to highly technology-driven practices in corporate hospitals and the lack of facilities in government hospitals. On the contrary, high affordability of the rich tends to drive them to a lifestyle not contributing to sustaining health. For example, longer work hours, confining oneself to air-conditioned rooms, the use of automobiles for saving time, and handling high levels of stress in a competitive world negatively contribute to 'naturally being healthy'. Among the middle class, the unnatural working hours, unusual load of work, not able to see and enjoy the concrete output, and shifts in work timings reduce the time for any meaningful social interaction with family and friends. This adversely affects the 'general wellbeing' of individuals.

As a consequence of these changes, the third layer in the macro level (the environment) also changed. Instead of the natural physical environment, one gradually adapts to the artificial environment with artificial lighting, air conditioners, room fresheners, synthetic food and consciously created silence in workplaces. On the contrary, the poor continue to live in unhygienic physical environments with subnormal living conditions, low levels of literacy, unhealthy and health-compromising behavioural practices.

Population belonging to all the three socioeconomic classes need to be understood in their typical context. All the three groups are in dire need of health education for better health promotion and illness prevention. While this is the scenario in India, the health care system even in the US seems to be no better "…health care systems are often perceived to be inefficient, ineffective and unfit for purpose. This is especially the case in the US where the largest per capita expenditure is producing some unimpressive outcomes" (Mark, Murray, Evans, & Estacio, 2011, p. 15).

Though medicine tries to appropriate the credit for decline in acute diseases and improved longevity, the other version from critics attributes it to factors like education and poverty reduction (McKeown, 1979).

It is difficult to state if the enhanced need and relevance of Health Psychology are 'because of' or 'in spite of' advancement in the field of biotechnology.

The Framework of Health Psychology

Health Psychology functions in a framework. The elaborate explanation of the need and relevance of Health Psychology in the contemporary context referred to a number of factors at micro (individual) and macro (economic/social/political) levels. It can be inferred from the discussion that the framework of Health Psychology expands from micro to macro levels. It can be conceptualized as four interconnected levels at which Health Psychology functions. This is explained in Figure 2.6. The goal of Health Psychology is to optimize the individual's health status. In order to attain this goal, the framework has to expand to the sociocultural level, as well as political, economic levels.

The individual is positioned with certain static factors like gender and genetic predisposition, as well as dynamic factors like age. These factors have their influence on the health of the person directly and independently, as well as in combination. The individual opts for a certain lifestyle that is determined by individual factors such as age, gender and personality while being influenced by the environment (physical and sociocultural). The choice of one's lifestyle and the social-cultural environment are mutually complementary. Similarly, the existing systems of education, organization and employment, health care, agriculture, food production and the opportunities for inculcating, maintaining and sustaining health and wellbeing within the systems impact the social structures and opportunities for social networking. Even here, there is mutuality in the factors at these two levels influencing each other.

At the micro level, Health Psychology functions at the individual level of patients and doctors. The main concern is health care with its spectrum of all dimensions. It includes working with patients and doctors with a goal of enhancing patient participation in the treatment process, enhancing adherence behaviour, working on behavioural lifestyle changes in patients as a measure of preventive practice, and working towards optimizing health communication between the doctor and the patient for enhancing prognosis. There are specialists among health psychologists functioning at different levels.

Scope of Health Psychology in Specialized Branches

A clinical health psychologist is the person who engages at the micro-level functioning. A clinical health psychologist can be a practitioner or researcher in this field. There are two steps at the macro level. The physical environment in which the individual lives has a significant bearing on the individual health. In addition, the local cultural influences in terms of health beliefs, healing practices and health values contribute to individual lifestyle and vice versa. A close network in the community constitutes a healthy and sound social support for the patient. Utilizing the support through formal and informal methods is enhanced through training. Some of the best interventions have communities as partners in promoting health and prevention of illness. Communities are taken for the level of analysis. Interventions that are planned by taking community inputs have been found to be very effective since the feeling of alienation is avoided. Community health psychologists work at this macro level of framework. The most effective methods are action plans at this level.

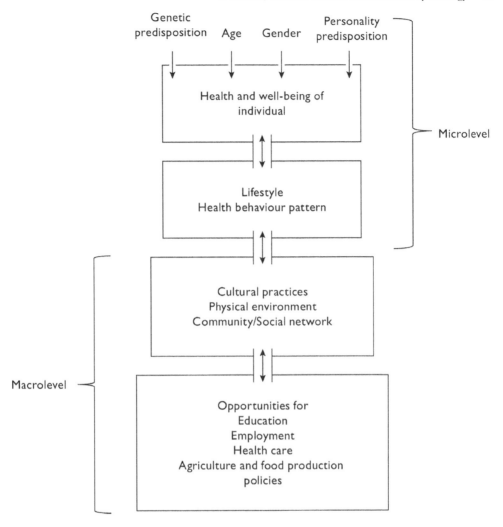

Figure 2.6 Framework of Health Psychology.

The larger horizon is the last level, where Health Psychology takes into consideration the larger national or global set-up in which the individual is placed. This takes into account the way systems work. The systems of education, health, employment and agriculture in a nation are governed by national policies. Each of them has an influencing role in determining health and wellness. For example, the curriculum of science in the existing system and opportunities to gain entry into the system are closely related to the health literacy and awareness of the individuals in society. Similarly, employment opportunities and the type of employment in the health care system and its quality, agricultural and food production in a country contribute largely to the individual health. All these are the outcome of policies at the national level. The role of Health Psychology is to create public awareness about issues related to health, enhance health literacy at a large scale, and inculcate hygiene in the physical environment in a campaign mode by choosing the contents carefully and presenting in a form through the powerful models/agents that triggers the motivation. Public health psychologists work in this area, which helps feeding the policies based on population behaviour and bring change in people's behaviour to enhance the acceptability of natural policies on health and implement them successfully. For this, the public health psychologist works on the cognition and behaviour of the larger population.

Yet, another function of Health Psychology concerns the unequal distribution of power across the population and the impact of it on health experience and behaviour. The divide in health experience and behaviour is mainly due to differences in opportunities resulting in a wide economic gap. Health Psychology also works on the measures to narrow down the gap in health inequality, by working on the methods to prioritize social justice and universal rights to health irrespective of gender, age, education, race and socioeconomic background. People who work towards it at the wider macro level are called critical health psychologists. Again, this is closely related to national health policies. The significance of Health Psychology in the contemporary period is summarized in Box 2.5.

As an epilogue, it is necessary to point out that despite the dire need, the specialized branch of Health Psychology has not yet given its due prominence in the Indian health care system. The replacement of the biomedical approach with the biopsychosocial approach will have to be driven by a health policy with a meticulous implementation plan. This requires unstinted research feedback from Health Psychology to policy levels. Innovative research and groundbreaking findings, and reinvention of the Indian health system are the expected efforts from the experts in the field.

Box 2.5 Relevance of Health Psychology

1 Progressive increase in prevalence of non-communicable diseases related to lifestyle
2 Treatment of non-communicable diseases calls for efficient management through lifestyle changes
3 Growing popularity of technology-driven, evidence-based approach to treatment minimizing the 'healing touch'
4 High doctor-patient ratio resulting in decreased time and communication during consultation
5 Need for quality communication to enhance cognition and bring behavioural change necessary for disease management
6 Behavioural change and lifestyle management require interventions to enhance health literacy
7 Increase in the number of surgical interventions calls for psychosocial interventions to minimize pre- and post-surgical psychological distress for enhancing the pace of recovery
8 Chronic pain needs psychosocial intervention and behavioural change for effective management
9 Public health measures to increase health awareness to popularize preventive measures need interventions suited to the cognitive levels of target groups
10 Treatment of the disease ignoring the negative affect state as a comorbid condition will get only suboptimal outcome

References

Bennett, P. (2000). *Introduction to clinical health psychology*. Oxford: Oxford University Press.

Benyamini, Y., Leventhal, E. A., & Leventhal, H. (2003). Elderly people's ratings of the importance of health-related factors to their self-assessments of health. *Social Science & Medicine, 56*(8), 1661–1667.

Blaxter, M. (1990). *Health and lifestyles*. London: Routledge.

Bunker, S. J., Colquhoun, D. M., Esler, M. D., Hickie, I. B., Hunt, D., Jelinek, V. M., ... & Tonkin, A. M. (2003). "Stress" and coronary heart disease: Psychosocial risk factors. *Medical Journal of Australia, 178*(6), 272–276.

Chivukula, U., Hariharan, M., Rana, S., Thomas, M., & Andrew, A. (2017). Enhancing hospital well-being and minimizing intensive care unit trauma: Cushioning effects of psychosocial care. *Indian Journal of Critical Care Medicine: Peer-Reviewed, Official Publication of Indian Society of Critical Care Medicine, 21*(10), 640.

Dalal. A. K. (2016). *Cultural psychology of health in India: Well-being, medicine and traditional health care*. New Delhi: Sage.

Deo, M. G. (2013). Doctor population ratio for India-The reality. *The Indian Journal of Medical Research, 137*(4), 632.

Engel, G. L. (1977). The need for a new medical model: A challenge for biomedicine. *Science, 196*(4286), 129–136.

Friedman, M., & Rosenman, R. H. (1974). *Type A behaviour and your heart*. Greenwich, CT: Fawcett.

Hariharan, M., Monteiro, S. R., Asha, D., & Rao, C. R. (2019). Perceptions of health: A developmental trend in Indian school children. *Child Indicators Research, 12*(4), 1351–1368.

Herzlich, C. (1973). *Health and illness: A social psychological analysis* (Vol. 5). New York: Academic Press.

Jayasundar, R. (2010). Ayurveda: A distinctive approach to health and disease. *Current Science, 98*(7), 908–914.

Jenkins, C. D., Rosenman, R. H., & Zyzanski, S. J. (1974). Prediction of clinical coronary heart disease by a test for the coronary-prone behaviour pattern. *New England Journal of Medicine, 290*(23), 1271–1275.

Kleinman, A. (1980). *Patients and healers in the context of culture: An exploration of the borderland between anthropology, medicine, and psychiatry* (Vol. 3). University of California Press, Berkeley

Krause, N. M., & Jay, G. M. (1994). What do global self-rated health items measure? *Medical Care, 32*, 930–942.

Matarazzo, J. D. (1980). Behavioural health and behavioural medicine: Frontiers for a new health psychology. *American Psychologist*, 35(9), 807.

McKeown, T. (1979). *The role of medicine: Dream*. Oxford: Blackwell.

Mohan, H., (2010). Cultural Markers in expression of pain and Trauma. In Hariharan, M., Padmaja, G., and Padhy, M. (eds.), *Trauma and Pain management: Biopsychosocial Perspectives* (pp. 71–78). New Delhi: Global Vision Publishing House.

Morandi, A., Tosto, C., Di Sarsina, P. R., & Dalla Libera, D. (2011). Salutogenesis and ayurveda: Indications for public health management. *EPMA Journal, 2*(4), 459–465.

Mossey, J. M., Mutran, E., Knott, K., & Craik, R. (1989). Determinants of recovery 12 months after hip fracture: The importance of psychosocial factors. *American Journal of Public Health, 79*(3), 279–286.

Normandeau, S., Wins, I., Jutras, S., & Hanigan, D. (1998). A description of 5-to 12-year old children's conception of health within the context of their daily life. *Psychology and Health, 13*(5), 883–896.

Radley, A. (1994). *Making sense of illness: The social psychology of health and disease*. Sage.

Rastogi, S. (2009). Ayurveda for comprehensive healthcare. *Indicators, 3*(4), 5.

Shroff, F. M. (2017). What is ayurvedic health care and how is it applicable to the Modern Day. *Journal of Nutrition and Human Health, 1*(2), 17–29.

Siegel, B. S. (1986). *Love, medicine and miracles*. London: Arrow Books.

Surendra, K., and Prasad, J. S. R. A. (2013). Concept of etiology in ayurveda and western medicine. *International Ayurvedic Medical Journal*, *1*(4), 1–8.

Taylor, S. E. (2006). *Health psychology*. New Delhi: Tata McGraw-Hill Education.

Thomas, M., Hariharan, M., Rana, S., Swain, S., & Andrew, A. (2014). Medical jargons as hindrance in doctor–patient communication. *Psychological Studies*, *59*, 394–400.

Verma, S. K & Verma, A. (1989). *Manual for PGI general wellbeing Measure*. Ankur Psychological Agency.

WHO. (1948). Definition of Health. http://www.who.int/suggestions/faq/zh/index.html

World Health Organization (2018). *Top ten causes of death*. https://www.who.int/news-room/fact-sheets/detail/the-top-10-causes-of-death

3 Positive Health Behaviour

Srinivas, a 52-year-old professor in a Central University, wakes up at 5 in the morning and goes for his walk from 5:30 am to 6:30 am. He does his Yoga exercises from 7 am to 7:45 am, has boiled vegetables and curd for his breakfast and goes for work by 9 in the morning. He usually has his lunch at 1 pm. He eats one cup of rice, dal and vegetables for lunch. He sips green tea two to three times between 9 am and 6 pm. About three evenings a week, he plays tennis with his students. Evenings during the weekend are spent with his family. He returns to bed between 10.30 pm and 11 pm every night.

Rajesh is a 48-year-old neighbour of Srinivas. He works in an IT company. His office timings are not fixed. Sometimes, he leaves for office at 7 am, while there are days when he goes to office around 2 pm. He returns home very late past midnight. He wakes up at different timings depending upon the time he has to leave for office. As a result, he skips his breakfast when he wakes up late. He often states that his job demands are such that he has to work in the time zones of various countries. As a result, it is almost impossible for him to set a daily routine to maintain timings of his meals or sleep. He claims that he accommodates his meals and sleep to when he 'gets time'. He endorses that he is under a lot of stress. According to him, the only way to get over stress is to come out of the chamber in the office and smoke a cigarette. He also says that the weekends are spent 'drowning himself' in good drinks—the only way to relax.

Madhavi, a 35-year-old woman running her boutique, has been suffering from neck pain. She has been speaking to her clients about her pain. She called her brother on phone and explained to him about her pain and the occasional dizziness she has been experiencing. One of her clients suggested that she must see a neurologist. Her brother told her that it could be spondylitis. Her husband asked her to appoint a manager to look after the boutique for some time and take rest. Madhavi was planning to visit the doctor. However, she continued to speak to her clients about her pain.

Srinivas, Rajesh and Madhavi, all of them can be analysed on their 'health behaviour'. While the narrative of Srinivas predominantly focused on health-promoting behaviour, Rajesh's lifestyle helps us identify 'health risk behaviour'. Madhavi's can be described as 'illness behaviour'.

What Is Behaviour?

Before engaging in explanation of health behaviour, it may be of help to recapitulate the concept of 'behaviour'. In simplest terms, it refers to any action or response (e.g. eating behaviour) to a stimulus that can originate from within (hunger, thirst) or from the external environment (e.g. snacks served in a platter and offered by a guest). The goal of a behaviour is to reach a state of equilibrium from disequilibrium. The disequilibrium state can be physiological (e.g. reduced blood sugar level or hypoglycaemia) or psychological (e.g. experience of fear on sighting a terrorist). They indicate simple affect states like fear. It may be a complex disequilibrium at the cognitive level involving indecisiveness about the correct treatment line for the newly diagnosed illness. Only when the disequilibrium is slightly pronounced, it acquires the strength to create unrest in the person to drive him/her to action leading to the restoration of equilibrium. Secondly, if the behaviour has a positive value associated with intrinsic or extrinsic reward, it would be easier for behaviour to get strengthened.

What Is Health Behaviour?

Having explained the concept of behaviour, it is easy to understand 'health behaviour' by extending the same explanation in the context of health. Health behaviour is an action or response to any stimulus originating from within or from an external environment with a goal of maintaining equilibrium in terms of health and wellbeing. It could be a proactive behaviour with a goal of sustaining equilibrium or a remedial behaviour with the goal of restoring equilibrium. In other words, it refers to any behaviour that protects the status quo, prevents the probable illness or promotes the existing state of health. Summing up all the above, Gochman (1997) defined health behaviour as "Behaviour patterns, actions and habits that relate to health maintenance, to health restoration, and to health improvement" (Vol. 1, page 3).

Behaviour in the context of health refers to something that one does or refrains from doing, which may not always be consciously or voluntarily undertaken. A number of personal factors such as beliefs, values, perceptions, motivations, emotions, personality make-up may contribute to the health behaviours. Thus, between the stimulus and the response the 'organism' factor plays a crucial mediating role.

Taylor (2006) has defined the health behaviour as "Behaviours undertaken by people to enhance or maintain their health" (p. 47). Whether it is health enhancement or maintenance of the existing health status, there is a necessary reference to the baseline assessment so that the outcome in terms of improvement is ascertained. Thus, it calls for a definite objective assessment process.

The goal of health behaviour is maintenance, restoration and improvement. The three types of health behaviour denominated by Kasl and Cobb (1966) fit into the framework of the individual goal. They are as follows:

1. Health behaviours with an aim to prevent diseases (e.g. eating a balanced diet, exercising daily)
2. Illness behaviours with an aim to seek remedy (e.g. complaining about symptoms and seeking advice from family, friends, relatives)
3. Sick role behaviours with an aim to get well (e.g. taking the prescribed medication, taking leave from work to rest)

While the behaviours under points 2 and 3 relate to short-term behaviours until restoration of health, the preventive behaviours delineated under point 1 refer to long-term behaviours with the goal of sustaining the existing state of health or preventing illness. These behaviours are something that get integrated into a lifestyle. Lifestyle refers to the individual's way of living that includes one's interests, attitudes, opinions, values, behavioural orientation and behaviour. The behaviour related to lifestyle manifests in the way one interacts with the physical, psychological, social and economic environment on a day-to-day basis. The lifestyle of an individual is primarily guided by the needs, motivation and priorities set by the individual. It has the influence of a number of factors such as family, socioeconomic background, cultural norms, peer group and personality factors. Some aspects of lifestyle like the options in type of food, clothes, leisure activities and entertainment are consciously chosen by the individual, while the others are determined by external factors, particularly in the Indian context. For example, the job one is engaged in, the working hours and the traffic one has to drive in daily are to a large extent beyond one's control. For example, a daily wage labourer engaged in a construction company has no control over the type of labour or the timings of the work. Further, many a time one is not left with an option of choosing an alternative given the limitations in the options that suits one's skill, qualifications and personal and family needs.

Lifestyle and health behaviours are closely related. Any change in any aspect of lifestyle is likely to bring a concomitant change in health behaviour and vice versa. For example, upward mobility in job bringing with it an elevated economic status may also increase the family's frequency of eating out, holiday trips or mode of transport. Similarly, a change in health behaviours may result in the change of lifestyle. For example, an individual keen on reducing the weight may decide to increase the number of kilometres he/she walks every day. As part of this newly inculcated health behaviour, he/she may decide to walk the five kilometres to the workplace instead of using the car. Thus, lifestyle has had a tremendous impact on the individual's health particularly since the beginning of the new millennium in India because of the fact that the majority of the diseases suffered by a human kind have a close link with the health behaviours.

One might integrate into the lifestyle either health protective behaviour or health risk behaviour based on the influencing factors that compete among themselves. In this context, it is relevant to explain the concepts of health protective behaviour and health risk behaviour.

Health Protective Behaviour

The phrase 'health protective behaviour' appears rather self-explanatory. At the outset, we may say it refers to any activity that an individual undertakes to 'protect' one's own health. This raises several questions such as does it include the behaviours of an ill person seeking treatment? Does it include those behaviours undertaken for a specific result but the outcome is either absent, suboptimal or counterproductive? Does it assume that the individual involved in health protective behaviour is aware of his/her present health status and the health protective behaviour is an endeavour to either improve the status or sustain the status quo? The definition addresses all these issues. They defined health protective behaviour as "Any behaviour performed by a person regardless of his or her perceived or actual health status, in order to protect, promote or maintain his or her health, whether or not such behaviour is objectively effective toward that end" (Harris & Guten, 1979). An examination of this definition clearly indicates that a behaviour undertaken with a 'positive intent' of maintaining or improving one's health status qualifies to be called health protective behaviour. It does not concern if the end result is fruitful in realizing the objective. Secondly, the behaviour need not have the stamp of approval from health care professionals as 'beneficial to health'. Thirdly, the behaviour may be undertaken by any individual irrespective of the current health status.

In their classical study, Harris and Guten (1979) surveyed 842 subjects and found out from them the three most important things that they do to 'protect' their health. The results revealed that the top response in terms of the percentage of the sample endorsing it referred to nutrition, food and eating conditions, sleep, rest, relaxation physical activity or physical recreation.

Major items in the list relate to physical fitness. Table 3.1 presents all the 30 items in the list.

Matarazzo (1984) made a reference to health protective and health risk behaviour with two unique appropriate terms. He named the following two sets of health behaviour:

1 Behavioural immunogens (behaviour that protects health)
2 Behavioural pathogens (behaviour that puts health at risk)

52 Positive Health Behaviour

Table 3.1 Percentage of sample in the Harris and Guten (1979) study always or almost always performing selected behaviours in order to protect their health

Behaviour	Percentage
Eat sensibly	66.0
Get enough sleep	66.0
Keep emergency phone numbers near the phone	65.0
Get enough relaxation	56.4
Have a first aid kit at home	53.1
Destroy old or unused medicines	52.3
See a doctor for a regular check-up	51.1
Pray or live by the principles of religion	47.5
Avoid getting chilled	47.4
Watch one's weight	47.0
Do things in moderation	46.4
Get enough exercise	46.0
Avoid parts of the city with a lot of crime	41.2
Don't smoke	41.1
Check the condition of electrical appliances, the car etc.	40.0
Don't let things 'get me down'	39.3
Fix broken things around home right away	39.2
See a dentist for a regular check-up	36.6
Avoid contact with doctors when feeling okay	35.3
Spend free time outdoors	33.7
Avoid overworking	33.0
Limit foods like sugar, coffee, fats	31.9
Avoid over-the-counter (OTC) medicines	30.2
Ignore health advice from lay friends, neighbours, relatives	29.0
Take vitamins	24.1
Don't drink	24.0
Wear a seat belt when in a car	22.8
Avoid parts of the city with a lot of pollution	21.5
Discuss health with lay friends, neighbours, relatives	17.1
Uses dental floss	15.9

Source: Harris and Gluten (1979) Page 20, table 2.

Just as the way the immune system prevents any antigens from invading the body to cause illness, the set of positive health behaviours is useful in preventing illness. For example, exercising regularly or eating nutritious food high in fibre and protein and low in carbohydrates and fat helps in preventing cardiovascular diseases. Similarly, an individual with a family history of cardiovascular disease indulging in heavy smoking behaviour in fact is placing oneself vulnerable to cardiovascular diseases just as allowing the pathogens into the body. Thus, the two terminologies related to behaviours are very appropriate.

Illness Prevention

With increasing awareness and intervention measures in the field of both medicine and behavioural sciences, illness prevention assumed a major role at multiple levels. Sarafino (2016) explains three predominant influences on illness prevention, viz. behavioural, environmental and preventive medical efforts. Out of these, the behavioural influence explains measures undertaken at an individual level to protect one's own health. The environmental measures indicate steps taken at the macro level in the interest of public health. Both these measures can be grouped under 'preventive behaviour'.

Positive Health Behaviour 53

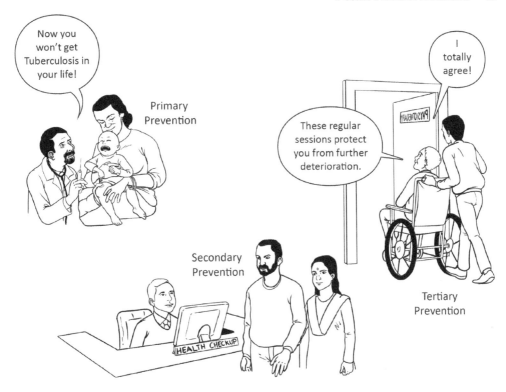

Figure 3.1 Illness Prevention: Primary, Secondary and Tertiary.

'Preventive behaviour' normally suggests a proactive behaviour before the invasion of illness. This seems to be a misnomer. According to Herndon and Wandersman (2004) and Runyan and Gould (1985), there are three levels of prevention out of which only one relates to the action before the illness or injury. They are primary prevention, secondary prevention and tertiary prevention (Figure 3.1).

Primary Prevention

This refers to the proactive measures one takes in anticipation of the probability of the illness or injury. Examples of primary prevention go to the extreme farsightedness of examining the blood groups of the man and woman before the decision to get married so that they avoid the hazard of the offspring being born with certain diseases. The medical technology also provides scope for genetic screening. Availing such facilities is part of preventive behaviour. Getting the infants and children vaccinated against certain illnesses like tuberculosis, diphtheria, polio, smallpox is part of primary prevention.

Positive health habits such as brushing twice, flossing the teeth, washing hands before meals, washing feet after an outing, setting time for meals and sleep are basic health behaviours that can be inculcated in children.

Behaviours such as wearing the helmet while riding a two-wheeler or the seat belt while in car are the preventive behaviours practised by adults. A physician or a health psychologist in a hospital setting can play a significant role in promoting primary prevention.

The health policy of different nations takes care of primary prevention in the form of vaccination programmes. A number of diseases are eradicated through primary prevention as national policy. For example, smallpox has been eradicated from India through large-scale vaccination. Polio is by and large prevented through the pulse polio programme. What is significant from the point of health behaviour is that despite the fact that immunization is widely advertised and carried out as a national welfare measure, not all people avail the facility.

Secondary Prevention

It may be appropriate to describe secondary prevention as an action of 'nip it at the bud'. Sarafino (2016) defines secondary prevention as 'actions taken to identify and treat an illness or injury early with an aim of stopping or reversing the problem'. Routine annual health check-ups come in aid when problems are identified at an early stage for timely intervention and to protect the quality of life. There are a number of cases where serious arterial blocks are identified during routine health check-ups. Interventions with procedures of angioplasty or Coronary Artery Bypass Grafting (CABG) surgery also popularly known as bypass surgery could avert cardiac emergencies.

For example, women with a family history of breast cancer are recommended regular mammograms and this is emphasized for the women whose mother had a history of breast cancer. Similarly, men after a particular age are advised screening for prostate cancer.

Another type of secondary prevention relates to responding immediately to the symptoms of illness. For example, irritation and discomfort in the throat indicates the onset of common cold. Immediate response with vitamin C supplementation helps in arresting the full-blown cold.

Secondary prevention behaviour will be initiated only when the person has the basic understanding of the consequences of aggravation of the situation. For example, a person who knows that the symptoms of appendicitis include pain in the stomach will seek medical consultation. Further, those with internal health locus of control and high self-efficacy are likely to believe that averting the situation or arresting the aggravation is something that can be done by oneself.

Tertiary Prevention

Tertiary prevention refers to the action or behaviour after the individual suffers illness or injury. It relates to the action initiated with an intention of softening the impact of the injury or illness that has long-lasting consequences. Action taken to prevent recurrence, minimize the damage or prevent further progression is grouped under this. The examples are artificial limb rehabilitation programme for a limb amputee, physiotherapy programme for a patient diagnosed with chronic arthritis.

Tertiary prevention in certain health problems is included in the treatment package. For example, forming the support groups for patients with chronic illnesses facilitates sharing of strategies by patients in managing the disease. Vocational rehabilitation programmes help the patients. Through the training programmes, the patients learn new skills after their optimal recovery. A cancer patient where the doctors say that no further treatment will be of help is looked after to keep the patient comfortable to the maximum extent. Thus, it can be inferred that the goal of tertiary prevention behaviour is to optimize the quality of life given the fact that the patient is already a victim of the disease or injury.

We can sum up the three types of prevention by stating that primary prevention is a behaviour with a goal of stopping the disease from affecting the person. Secondary prevention is the behaviour that is initiated to check and verify if everything is fine with health and in case not to identify and prevent the disease at the very early stage itself. Tertiary prevention is the behaviour that is initiated to handle the disease or injury already impacting the person in a way to optimize quality of life.

Of all the behaviours constituting one's lifestyle, eating, sleep and exercise are the ones that form the repetitive everyday activities. Let us examine how these activities can be converted into health-promoting or health risk behaviour.

Diet

Eating behaviour is something that has the influence of family, culture, region, climate and values. The schedule of eating, the options of food, the company while eating, method of food preparation, serving and eating are majorly influenced by the family and child-rearing process. Later in adolescence, it has a peer influence. Further, after marriage it is also likely to be influenced by the choices of the spouse and his or her habits. Thus, the food habits formed in early life are susceptible to changes at different stages of life owing to various factors.

What we eat, to a large extent, decides the state of our physical health as per the Western medical sciences. However, Ayurveda goes a little further and states that what we eat determines not only our physical health but also our temperamental disposition or personality disposition. The influence of the type of diet on our health and wellbeing is well documented. A diet rich in protein, fibre and minerals is recommended as a good diet. However, this cannot be a universal principle for all age groups across developmental span. An adequate amount of proteins, carbohydrates and fat apart from minerals and fibres help the children in their growth and development. The recommended ingredients and the quality of food vary with age. However, what goes as a universal principle is the consumption of good quantity of fresh fruits and vegetables irrespective of the age. The reason for this is the presence of fibre, vitamins and antioxidants in fruits and vegetables. Fibre is essential for good digestion and excretion, while minerals are considered healthy for the body. Antioxidants function as protection from diseases like cancer. In a meta-analysis of 170 studies, Block, Patterson and Subar (1992) found that 132 studies indicated that fruits and vegetables function as protection against cancer. Key et al. (1998) in their meta-analysis involving data on 76,000 adults found that vegetarianism helped in reducing the risk of ischaemic heart disease. A vegetarianism diet seems to have health promotional advantages over the non-vegetarian diets. Misra, Balagopal, Raj and Patel (2018) studied 1038 randomly selected Asian Indians in the US, to find out the association between this group and patients with diabetes, obesity and metabolic syndrome. The findings suggested that the vegetarian diet has a protective factor against diabetes but not obesity or metabolic syndrome. Thus, while we can say the vegetarian diet as an eating behaviour constitutes a shield against certain lifestyle diseases, one cannot claim to be protected from all illnesses by just following the vegetarian diet.

Despite the awareness about the benefits of including vegetables and fruits as a major part of the meal, it is also observed that they do not top the list of food preference, particularly among the young population. The reasons could be many. It could be because of the association of unpleasantness. Particularly for those children who were force-fed these items when they were children, these items are somewhat aversive. For those from lower socioeconomic groups, the problem could be affordability. For many others, it could even be the fact that other 'tasty' and 'crunchy' items have a preference over the fruits and vegetables. In a study by Haste (2004), the majority of children's food preference was found to be guided by taste rather than the nutritional value.

Food preferences for an individual depend on a number of factors such as the cooking method, product, components, taste, texture, smell and appearance. The orientation they get as a child goes a long way in setting the habit.

Schools play a significant role in motivating children on healthy dietary behaviour. In some schools in India, every child has to get one fruit as part of his/her lunch every day. This helps in inculcating the behaviour, which over a period of years spent in the schools settles as a dietary habit.

Healthy Eating: *Ayurveda* Perspective

Eating healthy constitutes a significant part of *Ayurveda*. It is *Ayurveda* that has talked in great detail about the diet and healthy eating behaviour that included not only a prescribed diet, but also the preparation, eating environment, mental state while eating and constitution of the body. *Ayurveda* includes five types of food in the diet, variation within that is prescribed for the three types of body constitution, viz. '*vata*', '*pitta*' and '*kapha*'. The five types of food are cereal and pulses, vegetables and fruits, spices, nuts, seed and oil, and dairy products (Sarkar, Kumar, Dhumal, Panigrahi, & Choudhary, 2015). According to *Ayurveda*, food or '*Ahara*' is one of the three pillars of life. The other two pillars are sleep and sexual behaviour. Thus, '*Ayurveda*' included the three important daily life activities as three pillars of a healthy life.

First of all, according to *Ayurveda*, eating the right quantity of food helps maintain positive health. The quantity is decided by one's age and seasonal variations. This is because *Ayurveda* believes that the digestive power of an individual varies with age and season. With reference to quantity of food, the universal principle of *Ayurveda* is to fill only two thirds of the stomach with solid and liquid. The one third left empty helps the easy movement of gastric that aids in the digestion process. According to *Charaka*, the stalwart of *Ayurveda*, the right quantity of food, promotes life span (Nishteswar, 2016). *Charaka* also prescribed 12 groups of food as mentioned in Table 3.2.

The type of food consumed has a close association with mental attributes called 'trigunas'. Table 3.3 presents the types of food associated with the three mental attributes.

According to '*Ayurveda*', the six psychological expressions, viz. *Kama, Krodha, Lobha, Moha, Mada* and *Matsarya* (Lust, Anger, Greed, Desire, Attachment and Ego), are closely linked to the type of food one eats (Payyappallimana & Venkatasubramanian, 2016). The Ayurvedic facts presented in Table 3.3 clearly suggest that healthy eating behaviour can include

Table 3.2 *Charaka's* 12 groups of food

S.No.	Sanskrit expression	English equivalent
1	Sukadhanya	Corns with bristles
2	Samidhanya	Pulses
3	Mamsa	Meat
4	Saka	Vegetables
5	Phala	Fruits
6	Harita	Raw vegetables/salads
7	Madya	Wine
8	Ambu	Water
9	Gorasa	Milk
10	Ikshuvikara	Products of sugarcane
11	Kritanna	Prepared food
12	Aharayogi	Food accessories, e.g. oil, spices, salt

Table 3.3 Mental attributes associated with choice of food

Trigunas (mental attributes)	Type of food consumption
Sattva guna (purity/wisdom/contended state)	Fresh fruits, vegetables, fresh juice, grains, nuts, seeds, water, cow's milk, honey and herbal tea
Rajas guna (action/excited state)	Spicy food, deep fries and baked food, pungent things like onion, garlic, chillies, sweets, pulses
Tamas guna (inertia/ignorance/lethargic state)	Food that is not fresh, e.g. stale food, frozen food, junk food, large quantities of garlic, meat and alcohol

Table 3.4 Seasonal Considerations for healthy eating

Season	Guidelines for eating
Winter (Hemanta and Shishira)	Can have heavy food as digestive power is increased due to contact with cold wind
Spring (Vasanta)	Light, easily digestible food to be taken. Heavy food and sweets to be avoided
Summer (Greeshma)	Sweets, cold, liquids to be consumed. Food that is pungent, hot, sour or salty to be avoided
Rainy (Varsha)	Wheat, barley, vegetable soup, rice with meat are recommended. This helps maintain normal digestive power
Autumn (Sarat)	Sweet, light, bitter and cold food and drinks are recommended

Sattvic and *Rajasic* food in good balance while avoiding the *Tamasic* food for providing wisdom and agility that connote wellness.

Healthy eating according to '*Ayurveda*' should take into consideration the seasonal variations, because the digestive power of the body varies with the outside atmosphere. Table 3.4 gives general guidelines for eating as per the season.

Ayurvedic concept of nutrition and diet is not generic in nature. It is worked out and tailor-made depending upon the '*Prakriti*' or constitution of the individual. Designed this way, the prescribed diet ensures preserving health in all individuals. Even in the West, some nutritionists have adopted Ayurvedic principles in inventing individual constitution-based recipes (Satyavati, 2008).

As a universal guideline, *Ayurveda* recommends beverages at room temperature, neither hot nor cold. It also suggests the timings for eating. It is recommended to have lunch as the large meal. The rationale is that between 12 noon and 2 pm, when the sun's heat is the strongest, the digestive 'fire' is also strongest. The dinner that is suggested to be light is recommended before 8 pm. Apart from setting timings for eating, the other suggestion of *Ayurveda* for healthy eating behaviour refers to the posture and medium. It recommends that sitting on the floor cross-legged is the right posture for eating. Sitting in a chair when the legs hang down, the blood flow is more to the lower extremity. Further sitting cross-legged on the floor keeps the digestive organs in a right position. It is said that when one eats in this posture, the brain receives the message when to stop eating. *Ayurveda* advocates using one's own fingers for eating instead of a spoon. The argument is that the sensory neurons in the fingertips feel the temperature and texture of food and communicate to the brain so that the system gets ready for the exact type of food even before it touches the tongue. Further, it claims that certain types of microorganisms get filtered out in the skin of the fingertips (Figure 3.2).

With reference to eating behaviour, *Ayurveda* recommends the ambience for healthy eating. It says that eating in an environment that is pleasant, with good settings that appeal to the other sense organs, helps in healthy metabolism. Hence, we see that the place of dining at home is normally done with appealing visuals, light music, good ventilation and indoor plants. The same trend is observed in good restaurants.

One of the very important aspects related to healthy eating is one's affect state while consuming the food. *Charaka* categorically mentioned that even the right type of food in the right quantity fails to be digested well if the individual's affect state is negative with emotions of grief, fear, anger or sorrow while partaking of food (Nishteswar, 2016).

Thus, we find *Ayurveda* has a holistic perspective on eating behaviour for health promotion. Despite such elaborate guidelines, the large chunk of Indian population is not found to be aware of this and adhering to these guidelines.

58 *Positive Health Behaviour*

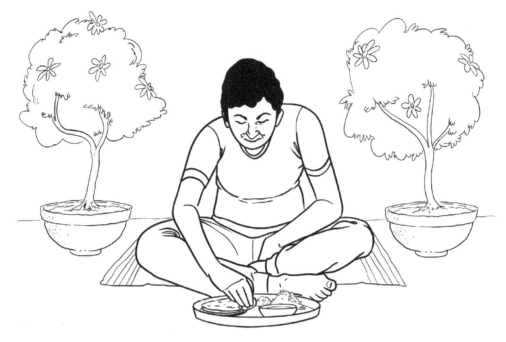

Figure 3.2 Healthy Eating—Ayurveda Perspective.

Physical Exercise

Physical exercise is a health protective behaviour. According to World Health Organization (2004),

> Physical activity is defined as any bodily movement produced by skeletal muscles that require energy expenditure. Exercise is a subcategory of physical activity that is planned, structured, repetitive and purposeful in the sense that the improvement or maintenance of one or more components of physical fitness in the objective.

Physical exercise involves the skeletal and muscular system. The positive benefits of exercise are directly reaped by these two. The bones and all the muscles including the soft muscles like heart, stomach and lungs become healthy and stronger. We see the positive impact of the exercise on circulatory, respiratory and gastrointestinal systems. The relationship between physical exercise and health is indicated by the fact that physical inactivity is found to be the fourth major risk factor for mortality at the global level accounting for 6% of deaths. Further, it is estimated that about 21%–25% of cancer in breast and colon, 27% of diabetes mellitus and 30% of ischaemic heart problems can be traced back to lack of physical exercise.

Exercise Inadequacy: Impact on NCDs

A longitudinal study on Harvard graduates by Paffenbarger, Hyde, Wing and Hsieh (1986) followed up 16,936 alumni of Harvard University for 12–16 years. During this follow-up, a total of 1413 subjects had died. It was found that those who died of cardiovascular or respiratory causes were found to have less engagement in physical exercise or sports. The risk of premature death was found to be positively related to lower levels or the absence of exercise. The risk was found to be higher for those engaged in sedentary work.

There is a flood of research that proved the benefits of physical exercise and fitness with a lowered risk of a number of non-communicable diseases (NCDs). One can inculcate the habit of physical exercise at any point in life and reap the prospective benefit of the same. Blair et al. (1995) in their prospective study found that people who transited from the state of 'unfit' to the fitness state over a five-year period showed a 44% reduction in the relative risk of death compared to those who continued to remain unfit.

Exercise as a habit is considered a strong health protective step. This helps staying fit, which means sustenance of good health and wellbeing. In a study by Erikssen et al. (1998), the participants whose fitness was highest at the baseline, which was either maintained or improved over a prolonged period, had the lowest risk of premature death.

Physical exercise as a habit is found to be a very good preventive behaviour in reducing the risk of the lifestyle diseases, as well as arresting the progression of the same. Reiner, Niermann, Jekauc, and Woll (2013) carried out a review and meta-analysis of 15 longitudinal studies with a minimum of five years of follow-up to examine the relationship between physical activity and lifestyle disorders such as obesity, coronary heart disease (CHD), type 2 diabetes, Alzheimer's disease and dementia. The results indicated a long-term association between physical activity and each of these diseases.

Exercise and Impact on the Immune System

Exercise is not only helpful for chronic lifestyle diseases but is also found to have a positive impact in preventing minor short-term illnesses such as common cold, viral infection and bacterial infections. This happens because exercise helps enhancing the function of the immune system and prevents multiplications of antibodies in the body.

There are several theories that attempt to explain the logic of the way exercise enhances the efficiency of the immune system. However, none of these theories are supported by empirical studies. Nevertheless, these theories can be summed up into the following points:

1. Physical activity enhances the function of lungs during the exercise. This may result in the flushing out the antibodies from the respiratory system. Thus, those engaged in moderate regular exercise are less likely to suffer from upper respiratory problems like cold, cough or throat infection.
2. Exercise results in the release of adrenaline, noradrenaline and cortisol. The cortisol has the characteristic of destroying the T and B cells (white blood cells). When the proportion of these cells decrease in the body, the message goes to the brain and more of these are produced by bone marrow. However, unlike the situation of stress, the cortisol secretion stops very soon and the state of equilibrium in cortisol levels is reached. When this process is repeated daily with exercise, the WBC levels in the blood always remain high. Thus, the efficiency of the immune system is enhanced and sustained.
3. Exercise enhances the blood circulation. Consequently, the WBCs in the blood get circulated rapidly. This enables them to detect the virus, bacteria or infection faster and put a defence against them, thus preventing illness.
4. During exercise, the body temperature rises. The bacteria do not grow fast in the higher temperature.
5. The release of endorphins during exercise contributes to enhance immune functioning.

The above arguments of exercise refer to moderate exercise. As long as there is moderate physical exercise, the impact is positive. The relationship between the exercise and health outcome is like an inverted bell. Once it crosses the moderate level, the impact may be negative in terms of health benefits.

Impact of Exercise on Mental Health

Health includes not only physical health and fitness, but also the mental health component constitutes a significant part of it. Exercise is called a health-promoting behaviour because of its positive impact on overall wellbeing that includes the mental health of the individual. The process can be explained theoretically. It is summed up into the following points:

1 Endorphin results in the feeling of euphoria, a 'feel-good' factor. This directly results in a positive affect state. This natural peptide chemical in the body released during physical exercise interacts with the receptors in the brain that impacts the mental state. As a result, the individual is helped to stay focused in positive affect and is less impacted by pain. It has a lot of commonality with the prescribed anti-anxiety drug. Thus, with the release of endorphins regular exercise helps in reducing stress, depression and ward off anxiety.
2 Regular exercise increases the blood supply to the brain. The brain receives adequate oxygen and nutrients. This helps the neuronal health—manifested in neuron growth and signalling.
3 Exercise is found to help in neurogenesis, i.e. creation of new neurons in the hippocampus. The hippocampus is the part of the brain associated with memory, emotional regulation and learning. New neurons in the hippocampus are used in storing new memories by keeping the old ones separated. Thus, through exercise, processing and storing of new information is facilitated by its impact on the hippocampus.

The positive psychological impact of exercise need not be accompanied or explained by any physiological evidence. There may be a number of psychological benefits with no measurable or observable changes at the physiological level. Rajeski (1994) was categorical when he stated "it is misguided to theorize that explanations for psychosocial outcomes will ultimately be reduced to some physiological system (e.g. cardiac related cortical activity) or neurochemical activity" (p. 1053). Exercise has to be prescribed, trained and accepted as a therapeutic intervention for mental illnesses. Martinsen (1990) in his review of literature found that the non-aerobic exercises had equivalent results to effects of anti-depressants. There are a number of studies that found the positive impact of exercise even on patients with schizophrenia in terms of perceived energy, endurance and positive affect state.

In general, physical exercise has a stimulating effect on almost all physiological systems in the body. As a result, the skeletal and muscular systems are toned up, and circulatory and respiratory systems being activated also influence the other systems like renal system whose functions are clearly associated with them. Sharma, Madaan and Petty (2006) identified a number of benefits of exercise on general mental health that can be summarized into the following points:

1 The quality of sleep is enhanced
2 There is an increased interest in sex
3 Improvement in endurance
4 Experience of relief from stress
5 Experience of positive affect state

6 Perceived increase in energy levels
7 Improvement in mental awareness

Apart from all the other aspects discussed until now, exercise if carried out as a part of daily activity in a group setting has an indirect impact on positive mental health. This is derived because of its facilitating expansion of the social network and social support that contributes to wellbeing.

Exercise: *Ayurveda* Perspective

Exercise in Sanskrit is called '*vyayama*'. *Ayurveda* advocates '*vyayama*' as part of '*Dinacharya*' meaning daily activities. The master of *Ayurveda*, *Charaka*, defined *vyayama* as 'any physical activity which is desirable and is capable of bringing about the stability in body and increases the strength of body'. *Sushruta* defined it as 'anything which brings about tiredness or exhaustion in the body' (Singh, 2017).

Enumerating the health benefits of *vyayama, Charaka* and *Sushruta* identified a few that included both physical and mental health aspects. This is understandable because the very concept of health according to *Ayurveda* is holistic. First, this health protective behaviour enhances the digestive fire that results in pacifying the '*doshas*'. It is found to mellow down the '*Kapha*' and burn up the excessive weight or obesity so that the body maintains good shape and 7contours. According to *Ayurveda*, '*vyayama*' enhances the digestive power to the extent of processing even the incompatible diet. The increased blood flow into the body parts and the sweating as a consequence of *vyayama* bring good lustre to the body. It not only makes the body strong but also enhances the person's endurance for fatigue, thirst, heat and cold, and optimizes the immune system. In other words, *Ayurveda* identified the positive impact of *vyayama* in terms of body strength, stamina and immunity. Thus, the reasons cited by Western medicine have been identified and propagated by *Ayurveda* thousands of years ago.

Ayurveda recommends variations in the intensity of *vyayama* based on the individual's age, stamina of body, region of living, time and type of diet. Thus, in line with its fundamental principle of 'one size does not fit all', the recommendation of v*yayama* follows the guideline of suiting to the individual and environmental characteristics. Winter and autumn seasons are said to be the best for intensive vyayama. This also matches with the Western advocacy of lowered intensity of exercise during summer. Similarly, while Western Science recommends morning time for exercise to optimize the results because the Basal Metabolic Rate (BMR) is low at this time, Ayurveda also recommends mornings as the best time for the reason that after the whole night's fast, the *Kapha dosha* is pacified by exercise. In other words, what it suggests is that in the morning, the fats in the body would get burnt because of the absence of carbohydrates.

Ayurveda is very clear about individual limits in *vyayama*. It has no ambiguity in stating that too much of exercising is counterproductive. The body constitution that is '*vata*'-dominant needs less exercise. Hence, limiting to activities like walking suffices the need. '*Pitta*'-dominant body constitution requires a moderate amount of exercise such as swimming, while '*Kapha*'-dominant bodies demand intense exercise like aerobics.

Ayurveda helps in identifying what is right and what is excess exercise. Sign of adequate exercise includes appearance of sweat, enhanced respiration and feeling of lightness of the whole body (Bagde, Sawant, Sawai, Dhimdhime, & Swami, 2015). It says that one should stop the activity if one experiences difficulty breathing through the nose and automatically open the mouth to breathe. The second indication to stop exercising is when one starts sweating in the forehead and sweat drops start dripping from the tip of the nose. One should stop the activity on noticing any one of the two indications.

Yoga

Yoga asana is a unique form of exercise. Having its roots in Indian philosophy, *Yoga* has been in practice for millennia, though it is gaining popularity across the globe in the last few decades. Broadly, it connotes 'way of life', while '*Yoga asanas*' refer to exercise. '*Yoga asana*' majorly includes various physical postures, regulation of breath, meditation and deep relaxation. Each of the above has a positive effect on physical and mental wellbeing. Life force, which is called *Prana Shakti*, refers to the vital energy. The practice of *Yoga* is found to contribute to enhancing the same (Satish, 2012).

Specific *asanas* are prescribed based on the need for risk prevention. *Yoga* exercise includes not only the asanas or body postures but also procedures to relieve one of stress, anxiety and tension. They have a calming effect on the person. Pranayama, a breathing exercise, involves inhalation of air through the right nostril and exhalation of air through the left. This is followed by inhalation by the left nostril and exhalation from the right. This process completes one cycle. By doing so, the lungs expand and contract optimally. The regulation of breathing is a slow and deep rhythm contrary to what happens when one is under stress. Thus, the message sent to the brain is one of the 'non-stress' situations resulting in a positive mental state. This exercise helps in reducing anxiety state of mind. According to Satish (2012), *Yogasanas* ensure *Sthiram* (stability) and *Sukham* (comfort) connoting the tranquillity of mind.

The calming and relaxing effects of *Yoga* are studied by a number of researchers in a scientific way. Sohani et al. (2018) in a quasi-experimental study exposed 52 women to 12 *hathayoga* training sessions spread across four weeks (three sessions per week each for a duration of 60–70 minutes). At the end of the training, a comparison of baseline and post-Yoga training, stress, anxiety and depression revealed a significant decrease in the levels of all the three. This indicates the positive impact of *Yoga* on negative mental states.

Yoga asanas have been in practice for both cure and prevention of a number of non-communicable diseases. Those who practise it as a preventive measure include both normal and at-risk populations. Sharma and Knowlden (2012) reviewed 17 studies related to the practice of *Yoga* either as a prevention or as an effective management measure for type 2 diabetes mellitus. The studies reported using various *Yogic* practices such as *Yoga asanas* (body postures), *pranayama* (breath regulating), *shatkriyas* (cleansing exercises) or *Yoga nidra* (Indian version of relaxation exercise). The subjects included were healthy volunteers and diabetic patients. The outcome measure was blood glucose levels. They found that out of the 17 studies, reviewed 9 studies showed a significant decrease in blood glucose levels following intervention of practising *Yoga*.

The practice of *Yoga* is normally adopted for general fitness and wellbeing, which constitute a major prevention against illnesses. If this practice has to be set in as a habit, it needs to be inculcated from childhood. The unique feature of *Yoga* is that it suits all age groups and benefits the practitioners significantly. Training in *Yoga asana* is being formalized in many schools in India, Europe and America. The practice of *Yoga* by schoolchildren not only keeps them physically fit but also helps them in prevention of negative emotions. Velasquez, Lopez, Quinonez and Paba (2015) conducted a study on 125 Colombian schoolchildren of lower socioeconomic status from classes 5, 8 and 9. Children's anxiety, aggression, depression and socioemotional competencies were assessed before and after the intervention. The intervention on *Yoga* was given for 12 weeks at the rate of twice a week. The results revealed that the *Yoga* intervention had the potential to reduce children's problems of anxiety.

Yoga can be the best preventive measure if adopted by those in the high-risk group for any disease or complications. Practised systematically under supervision, *Yoga asanas* reduce the risk levels.

In an interesting study, Rakshani et al. (2012) found evidence of the beneficial effects of *Yoga* among the high-risk pregnant women. Their sample included 68 high-risk pregnant women. They randomly assigned them into intervention and control groups. The 30 participants in the intervention group received one-hour *Yoga* session thrice a week in addition to their standard care. The 38 participants in the control group received standard care and conventional antenatal exercise like walking during the same time. Thus, both the groups received exercise under supervision. The intervention was given from the 12th to 28th week of pregnancy. Their health was monitored throughout pregnancy, and the health of the baby after delivery. It was observed that the participants in the intervention group who were given Yoga practice had significantly fewer pregnancy-induced hypertension, gestational diabetes or intra-uterine growth retardation compared to the control group. Further, the babies born to these women were significantly fewer compared to the control group in complications such as 'small for gestational age', and low Apgar scores.

Thus, exercise, in any form like daily walks or aerobics, *vyayama* or *Yoga asana*, if integrated into lifestyle forms a good preventive shield against many illnesses and also helps one stay physically fit and psychologically sound.

Exercising and Not Exercising: Major Reasons

What motivates some people to follow a strict exercise regime? The factors that motivate a person could be highly varied. Very few go for exercise for its intrinsic value, and say that they exercise because the very activity is highly pleasurable. Those who are guided by such intrinsic motivation are less likely to drop out anywhere in the midway. They are likely to adopt it as a very natural activity of their daily routine. The others are guided by extrinsic motivation. Some may adopt exercise regimes to maintain physical fitness. The reward for them lies in the outcome. As long as the outcome is maintenance of fitness, they are likely to continue the behaviour. Physical appearance that includes body weight and body shape is associated with one's self-esteem. Protection of one's self-esteem is a strong motivating factor. Any indication that the weight control or body shape has deviated from the expected limits motivates them to intensify their endeavour. A few individuals may discover that exercise as a routine activity sustains a positive mood. They may even create time for additional slots of exercise when experiencing a negative affect state. Yet, others follow the exercise regimen to adhere to medical advice, because they are diagnosed with hypertension, obesity or coronary heart disease or diabetes mellitus. The motivation for them is likely to be external pressure, obligation or a positive social support from a family member or a peer who encourages, accompanies or monitors their adherence. People whose exercise behaviour is not guided by self are more likely to experience frequent lapses that may even convert into dropouts. The reason cited by them often is external, like lack of time, inadequate facilities, the absence of social support, suboptimal or no outcome. Studies have proved that people who are regular in exercising perceive more positive outcomes (Dzeewaltowski, 1989), less obstacles (Marcus, Rakowski, & Rossi, 1992) and internal control (Norman & Smith, 1995) (Figure 3.3).

In a study by WHO (2004) on a sample of 1,62,000 children and adolescents between the group of 11 and 15 years from European and North American countries, it was found that a very small percentage of the sample engaged in moderate exercise. The results revealed that on average, 35% of boys and 22% of girls practised moderate exercise of a minimum one hour for five days a week. The highest percentage of subjects were from the US (57.1% boys and 41.8% girls), while the lowest percentage of girls were from France (11.7%) and the lowest percentage of boys were from Italy (22.6%) (Morrison & Bennett, 2006).

64 *Positive Health Behaviour*

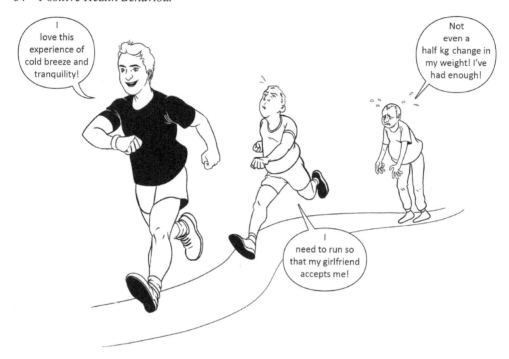

Figure 3.3 Reasons for Exercising and Not Exercising.

Sleep Behaviour and Its Significance

Prabhas, a 45-year-old senior executive of an overseas company in Mumbai, India, shocked everyone when he collapsed and died when he was getting ready for office. The medical report identified the cause of death as a massive cardiac arrest. It was shocking to everyone because Prabhas was known to be a fitness freak. He had the right diet that was by all standards considered 'healthy' in terms of quality, quantity, frequency and timing. He never missed his daily exercise (in fact the day before he died, he had participated in the marathon run). He had no health risk behaviour like smoking or alcohol consumption. He created for himself a very strong social support network that included his family. He was not found to be under stress. He was not obese nor was he ever told by doctors in any of health check-ups that he was at risk for coronary heart diseases. The physician friend of Prabhas solved the mystery by revealing that Prabhas used to sleep for not more than four hours every night. He also added that he had cautioned Prabhas that the cumulative inadequate sleep was a potential threat to his health. Prabhas never took that seriously and believed that he could make the best and productive use of life by working longer hours. Thus, following all the other important doctrines of the healthy lifestyle could not prevent premature death for Prabhas just because he violated the one important doctrine called adequate and healthy sleep.

Sleep is one of the vital requirements of good health and wellbeing. By no parameter, it can be placed second to either a healthy diet or an adequate physical exercise. It is a different matter that sleep is not often discussed, analysed or inquired as a part of health assessment. Until recent years, not many therapeutic interventions were designed or tested for enhancing the sleep quality and quantity, except the prescription of a pill to induce sleep. The increasing research in the area of sleep and their repeated findings reiterating the need for quality sleep and the negative consequences of sleep deprivation contributed to the emergence of sleep as one of the health behaviour.

Table 3.5 Recommendation of the expert panel for age-appropriate sleep duration

Age	Recommended (hours)	May be appropriate (hours)	Not recommended (hours)
0–3 months (newborns)	14–17	11–13 / 18–19	<11 / >19
4–11 months (infants)	12–15	10–11 / 16–18	<10 / >18
1–2 years (toddlers)	11–14	9–10 / 15–16	>9 / <16
3–5 years (pre-schoolers)	10–13	8–9 / 14	<8 / >14
6–13 years (school-aged)	9–11	7–8 / 12	<7 / >12
14–17 years (teenagers)	8–10	7 / 11	<7 / >11
18–25 years (young adults)	7–9	6 / 10–11	<6 / >11
26–64 years (adults)	7–9	6 / 10	<6 / >10
≥ 65 years (old adults)	7–8	5–6 / 9	<5 / >9

Source: Hirshkowitz et al. (2015).

A rough estimation reveals that we spend about one third of our lives sleeping. However, this is not to be considered 'waste of life time'. A number of regeneration activities take place in our physiological system during our sleep. Regeneration is a very essential cause for our rejuvenation in the morning. Thus, sleep constitutes a very significant aspect of maintaining our health and fitness. There is so much of variation in perception and practice of sleep behaviour that the need for standardization was felt by experts and practitioners in the field of health. The National Sleep Foundation of America constituted a panel of experts from various disciplines to come up with recommendations for duration of sleep for various age groups. The experts were from the discipline of sleep, gynaecology, paediatrics and gerontology. The 18-member committee came up with their recommendations for duration of sleep for age groups starting from newborns to old adults. Their recommendations included three categories, viz. 'Recommended hours', 'May be appropriate' and 'Not recommended'. They published their recommendations in the Journal of National Sleep Foundation 'Sleep Health' in 2015. Their recommendations are presented in Table 3.5.

The adequacy of sleep seems to have an association with a number of factors related to physical health.

Sleep Duration and Body Weight

Obesity or overweight is undoubtedly endorsed as a health risk and associated with a number of diseases. In a study by Taheri, Lin, Austin, Young and Mignot (2004), the authors included 1024 volunteers identified with a sleep disorder in the sample. They took night-time polysomnography (an instrument that measures the quality and quantity of sleep). The fasting blood samples were collected, and the levels of serum leptin and ghrelin (hormones that regulated appetite) and many other chemicals and hormone levels in the blood were measured. Analysis was carried out to find the relationship between these measures in the blood, BMI and sleep duration.

The results clearly showed a 'U'-shaped graph, indicating a curvilinear relationship between the sleep duration and Body Mass Index (BMI). Lower duration of sleep was associated with higher BMI. Secondly, shorter sleep duration was also found to be related to low leptin and high ghrelin. Such difference in these hormone levels results in increased appetite. One can logically infer the higher BMI with lowered sleep hours and increased appetite. Contrary to short sleepers, good sleepers tend to consume lower calories.

Sleep and Immune Function

When a person suffers sleep deprivation for a prolonged duration, the vulnerability to illness is found to be higher. This is observed in day-to-day life. When students study the whole night and attend their academic activities in the daytime, and continue their routine for a long time, some of them fall sick forcing them to rest and thus make up for the lost sleep. However, even when such sleep deprivation is temporary and short, the impact is seen in one's immune system functioning. Irwin, McClintick, Costlow, Fortner, White and Gillin (1996) conducted a study on 42 healthy male volunteers. The participants were deprived of one night's sleep between 10 pm and 3 am, and their blood samples were collected following the sleep deprivation. The results found a fall in the natural immune responses manifested by NK (Natural Killer) cell activity. The immune response resumed to the baseline level after a night's recovery sleep. This study indicates the immediate adverse impact of loss of sleep on the immune system. This, in fact, justifies the expert committee recommendation that sleeping for shorter duration is not advisable.

There have been a number of studies that established the association between sleep and immune function and inflammation. Inadequate sleep and its association with Inflammatory Bowel Syndrome have been noticed in a large number of patients (Kinnucan, Rubin, & Ali, 2013). It is possible to improve their disease condition by introducing sleep intervention.

Sleep and Non-communicable Diseases

The example cited at the beginning of the section on sleep speaks about the significant close association between sleep and cardiac health. Prabhas, despite adopting all other health behaviour, suffered the fatal cardiac arrest because of cumulative sleep deprivation. A review of studies that measured sleep and cardiac health was done by Cappuccio, Cooper, D'Elia, Strazzullo and Miller (2011). They received a total of 15 studies that had a sample of 4,74,684 men and women. Some studies indicated the positive relationship between short duration of sleep and a greater risk of dying of coronary heart diseases (CHDs) or stroke. Long duration of sleep was also found to be associated with a higher risk of CHD, stroke and cardiovascular diseases (CVDs). Thus, the meta-analyses indicated that both shorter and longer duration of sleep were predictors of cardiac illness.

Next to cardiovascular disease is diabetes, the incidence of which is on the progressive rise. Adequate sleep is found to be an important factor in levels of blood sugar and insulin secretion. Inadequate sleep negatively impacts this equilibrium. Spiegel, Heprault and Cauter (1999) conducted an interesting experiment on a sample of 11 men. These participants were restricted to just four hours of sleep per night for six nights. This was called 'sleep-debt condition'. Later on, this sleep deprivation was compensated with 12-hour sleep per night for six nights. This phase was called 'sleep-recovery period'. They were tested for glucose tolerance, thyrotrophin concentrations, cortisol concentrations and sympathetic system activities in both the conditions. The results indicated lower glucose tolerance and thyrotrophin concentration and an increase in cortisol concentration and sympathetic nervous system activities during the sleep-debt condition. This is good evidence of harmful consequences on metabolism of carbohydrates and endocrinal functions due to inadequate sleep. This is compared to the process during ageing. Hence, it can be inferred that chronic sleep deprivation may culminate in severe age-related chronic disorders.

Sleep and Mental Health

Sleep, an everyday routine behaviour of the individual, not only affects the various physiological system–related physical health, but has its influence on the mental wellbeing too. The individual's cognitive and emotional states are deeply influenced by sleep. Many of us must have experienced that if we were busy working until very late at night completing an assignment or attending an emergency, the efficiency in our work dropped the following day. Our attention and perceptual process work at the suboptimal level, and concentration on work dilutes, and we find ourselves unable to solve some 'not-so-difficult' type of problems. Further, our affect state is not very positive. We find ourselves irritable, disinterested and sensitive. While these could be the temporary mental states of short deprivation of sleep for a night or so, the cumulative sleep deprivation or prolonged inadequacy of sleep can be more devastating to the individual's mental health. Depression is found to have a close association with poor quality of sleep.

The affect state normally has a spillover effect on one's social interactions. People become less perceptive about other's feelings and hence may respond inappropriately. This, leading to an action-reaction chain, may leave the person socially less responsive. Experiments on emotional facial recognition confirmed this fact (Leech, 2018). There are studies that proved the impact of sleep loss in processing emotional information. In a social context, processing of emotional information, as well as responding with emotional empathy, is important. Only when there is a combination of these two, there will be a good social interaction, which is one of the dimensions of health and wellbeing.

Guadagni, Burles, Ferrara and Lavia (2014) found that sleep deprivation adversely affects emotional empathy. They assigned 37 healthy volunteers into three groups. One group was deprived of sleep for one full night. The second group was allowed normal sleep for the night at house. The third group was not manipulated on night's sleep. The sleep-deprived group and the normal sleep group were tested on emotional empathy before and after the night. The third group that was not manipulated on sleep was tested on emotional empathy twice during the day. The results showed a significant difference in the post-test only in case of the sleep-deprived group. The scores in the post-test were lower for this group. This indicates that healthy individuals with poor sleep habits may score low on their 'social health', which constitutes an important dimension of overall health and wellbeing.

The sleep duration and quality that constitute important components of health and wellbeing have been neglected in the diagnosis and treatment process of medical science for a significantly long period when this science was engrossed in its new inventions. The one method adopted by the medical science for problems of insomnia or inadequate sleep was pharmacotherapy.

Healthy Sleep: *Ayurveda* Perspective

Ayurveda considered sleep as an important constituent of health. Hence, the sleep habits, significance of sleep and guidelines for healthy sleep are discussed in detail. '*Nidra*' (sleep) in *Ayurveda* is considered one of the '*trayopastambhas*' (three subpillars), which balances the individual's health. It is one of the three biological needs of the individual, the other two being eating/drinking and sexual satisfaction. It describes sleep as exhaustion of mind and soul, and as a state of inactivity of mind, and sensory and motor organs that become stationary. There is inertia in consciousness, when the intellect, affect and the body are in deep rest (Shukla, Prashant, Shukla, Baghel, Vyas, & Vellela, 2014).

The contribution of good sleep to health is enumerated from various dimensions. First, it helps in recuperation of cells and the nervous system in the body. It is during sleep that the growth process is on. The cell regeneration improves the physical strength, vigour and glow in the skin. Further, it is assumed to improve digestion, and other metabolic functions and restoration of body tissues.

From the point of mental health, *Ayurveda* feels that sleep enhances neural plasticity. This in turn helps in consolidation of new information input and the earlier memories that had not yet stabilized. Thus, sleep is an essential health behaviour that strengthens the cognitive functioning. It also helps in the creation and sustenance of a positive affect state, i.e. happiness.

Ayurveda refers to two types of sleep, viz. natural sleep (*swabhavika*) and abnormal sleep (*aswabhavika*). According to *Charaka*, there are seven causes of sleep, each one of which is different in its type:

1 '*Tamas*'—this characterizes inertia
2 '*Kapha dosha*'—dominance of phlegm
3 Mental exertion
4 Physical exhaustion
5 '*Agantuka*' that indicates progression of disease leading to imminent death
6 Outcome of complication of other diseases
7 The very time of night (natural physiological sleep)

The natural sleep during night-time is considered to be normal, while the rest are grouped under abnormal. Ayurveda has specific views on the timings of sleep for health and wellbeing. According to its doctrines, the best time to go to sleep is six hours after sunset and waking up before the sunrise. It prohibits sleep in the first and last parts of night (Tripathy & Tripathy, 2011).

A person who follows the guidelines is likely to follow a definite routine and pattern for sleep, which is considered a healthy habit. Improper or erratic sleep timings lead to a number of negative health outcomes. This includes generalized weakness, body rigidity and heaviness of the body, giddiness, fever, skin-related problems like eruption of rashes, itching, pain, respiratory problems like cough, dyspepsia or problems in the throat, nausea and digestive problems. It also casts a negative impact on mental functioning such as negative affect state like sorrow and lowering of happiness, apart from the lowered cognitive functioning mentioned earlier.

It strongly recommends against resisting sleep. According to *Ayurveda*, resisting sleep leads to a number of symptoms that range from body pain, drowsiness, excessive yawing, headache and heaviness in eyes. All these can be managed by good sleep.

Ayurveda prescribes specific guidelines to enhance the quality of sleep and optimize the health benefits. This includes the environment, posture, bed type.

The Physical Ambience

The room where one sleeps should be calm, clean and uncrowded. The bed should be comfortable with clean bed linen. The height of the cot is recommended at the knee joint level. The surface of the bed has to be even soft and comfortable.

Sleep Posture

The sleep posture should be easy. Lying down in an easy posture helps mitigate fatigue and soothes the '*dosha*' of '*vata*'. It also helps in the healthy growth of the physical body. *Ayurveda* prohibits the prone posture while sleeping. Many people have a habit of sleeping on their tummy. This induces back aches and interferes with digestion.

Mental State

It is desirable to engage in virtuous thoughts before sleeping and waking up. This helps sustain the positivity. Indulging the negative thoughts is avoidable at the time of going to bed or rising in the morning. Divine thoughts and saying one's prayers at bedtime and waking up are prescribed in *Ayurveda* for better health and wellbeing. A mild massage before sleep is recommended to remove fatigue and induce a pleasant sense of relaxation that promotes good sleep. *Ayurveda* recommends massage prior to sleep for removal of '*kapha*' and '*vata*' *doshas*.

Finally, Ayurveda believes in flowing with nature, but not deviating from it. Hence, it strongly advocates against staying awake during night or sleeping during the daytime. Sleeping during daytime is not prohibited for infants, the elderly, sick persons and everyone during summer. Unfortunately, those working from India for other countries with different time zones have no option but to deviate from this recommendation of *Ayurveda*. Studies to understand the health problems of such employees may provide us with sound statistics to substantiate the argument. The *Ayurveda* system argues that violating the rule and staying awake at night results in a number of symptoms such as giddiness, body stiffness, headache, restlessness, lowered levels of concentration. This occurs because of '*vata dosha*', '*pitta dosha*' and '*kapha dosha*' getting vitiated. Shukla et al. (2014) identified the diseases associated with different sleep patterns. For example, they linked daytime sleep with obesity, a typical skin disease named as '*Visarpa*' and gouty arthritis, untimely sleep patterns with indigestion etc.

Health Screening Behaviour

Apart from following the healthy diet, regular exercise and having adequate sleep, health protection includes health screening behaviours. Health screening refers to 'a programme designed to evaluate the health status and potential of an individual'. The outcome of screening may be a diagnosis of a particular disease or a finding that the person neither has a particular disease nor is at risk. The screening may involve documenting the family health history, physical examinations, radiological examinations, laboratory tests, health counselling or psychoeducation following the tests. Health screening behaviour is normally voluntary and periodical.

Screening behaviour helps in two ways:

1 It serves the purpose of identifying the risk factors for illness, particularly chronic illness so that it can be either checked or delayed through behavioural change.
2 It helps in detecting certain diseases, which have not yet manifested because of their asymptomatic characteristics.

Screening for Health Risk

Screening for health risk basically relates to assessment of future health status. In case the screening identifies risk for any illness in future, it leaves good scope for taking immediate steps to encounter it successfully so that the possibility of illness is blocked, minimized or delayed. In certain cases, the initial screening may warrant further investigations for an accurate pointer. Screening for risk factors includes investigation, physical examination or biochemical assessments for the following:

1. Cardiovascular risks
2. Diabetes risks
3. Genetic screening for adults (e.g. Huntington's disease, muscular dystrophy) and foetus (e.g. Down's syndrome)
4. Antenatal screening
5. Eye check-up for cataract, glaucoma etc.

Periodic assessment of blood pressure, blood cholesterol levels, treadmill test etc. helps in identifying if there is any cardiovascular risk in the person. Testing of blood glucose levels in fasting, as well as random checks, places one either in the normal, diabetic or borderline category. Such scheduled screening is of significance to educate the person placed in the 'at-risk' category. For example, a person whose blood pressure readings place one in the pre-hypertension group has to be educated on the adverse impact of smoking for hypertensive patients that puts one under a high risk for cardiac illnesses. In case the person is overweight, the risk of cardiac disease is higher with a pre-hypertension state. Weight reduction, cessation of smoking and change in diet may be of great help in preventing a pre-hypertensive person from transiting to a hypertension state. Similarly, a person who tests 'borderline' on blood sugar level can follow a moderate exercise regime and cut down on carbohydrates in the diet as a precautionary step. In India, frequent free medical camps are organized for specific screening assessments such as cardiac illness, diabetes, problems related to eye both in urban and in rural areas. However, enrolling for such screening calls for motivation in the individuals concerned.

Yet, another screening that the physicians are advising the adults is for testing the levels of vitamins D_3 and B_{12} in the blood. They are tested by taking the blood sample. It is believed that the majority of the Indian middle-class population suffer from low vitamin D that is a major contributor to many diseases related to bones, cancer, depression, general fatigue to mention a few. Deficiency in vitamin B12 places one at a risk for Alzheimer's disease as per the physicians. Detecting the deficiency in these two at the right time and putting the individual on supplements for an adequate period, or educating them to have exposure to sunlight or change in diet to enhance the intake of B_{12}-rich food also is highly beneficial. Creating a cognitive base about the benefits of early interventions rather than cautioning about serious repercussions after one is diagnosed with the disease enables a person to give serious consideration to go for intervention and change the health behaviour.

The first-ever screening test that one faces is soon after birth. It is called 'Apgar test', developed by an anaesthesiologist named Virginia Apgar. 'Apgar' also is used as an acronym for what it tests. The parameters taken into consideration for scoring are Appearance, Pulse, Grimace, Activity and Resistance. This is a very important assessment that the doctor makes on a newborn baby to ensure normalcy based on the skin colour or appearance of skin, heart rate, reflex, muscle or motor skill, and respiration. This helps the doctor in evaluating the present health status of the newborn and if the baby is likely to require any treatment in future.

While all the screening tests mentioned above are relatively common, what is uncommon but is sometimes very useful is the genetic screening. It is particularly useful in case the person is the carrier of a genetic disorder. For example, in case of the muscular dystrophy, the females in the families could be carriers. However, the ethical issue here is how does the outcome of such screening help? Would it be ethical to educate the woman to forego having children? Treatment options may be very expensive for any genetic problems. How ethical is it to advise for diagnosis when the treatment is not affordable or remote?

The World Health Organization (WHO) has come up with a following set of criteria for population-wide screening tests:

1. For ensuring potential benefits to the health of people, screening has to be done only for diseases that may have serious consequences.
2. The test administered should have no harmful effects, and it should have passed the reliability check.
3. Only those diseases where early detection is beneficial for effective treatment should be screened for. Further, there should be clear scientific proof that treatment prior to the manifestation of symptoms is more effective.
4. Public should be given an opportunity to make informed decisions. For this, neutral information has to be made available to them. For self-screening, particularly for diseases like breast cancer apart from these, individual training and education is also given.

Studies on screening behaviour and mortality rates caused by specific diseases are inconclusive about the outcome of screening in terms of early detection and treatment. Hence, the medical advice is very cautious in this regard.

People's decision to adopt screening behaviour or avoid it is determined by a number of psychosocial factors:

1. Absence or inadequate knowledge about the condition and benefits of screening. This may even be associated with the level of education and economic status
2. Generalized fear of pain, discomfort or the bad outcome
3. Embarrassment regarding the procedure one has to go through as part of screening (e.g. physical examination)
4. Age and gender. Younger people, however, have a tendency to avoid screening behaviour
5. Lack of knowledge or faith in the outcome
6. Distrust in the system
7. Lethargy or inertia or complacence
8. Lack of or low self-efficacy when it comes to self-screening
9. Not associating any seriousness with the purpose
10. Not perceiving oneself as possible or probable victims of the disease

Screening for Detecting Disease

People not having any manifestations or symptoms of a disease go for testing for the specific disease. The purpose of this is either to rule out the presence of the disease or to detect it at the very early stage to treat it most effectively. For example, women with a family history are advised to go for screening for breast cancer and cancer of cervix. This benefits by initiating early treatment and good prognosis in case cancer is detected in the screening. This basically constitutes secondary prevention (Figure 3.4).

72 Positive Health Behaviour

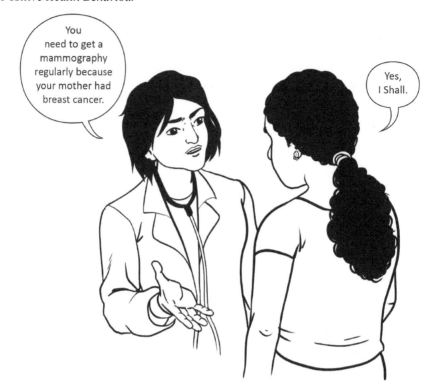

Figure 3.4 Screening to Detect Disease.

Some of the screenings may place an outcome that involves serious decision-making by the affected person and family. For example, for a pregnant woman at her middle age, a screening detects if the foetus has the possibility of mental retardation like Down's syndrome. In case there is detection of it, there is no treatment for it. Hence, the prospective parents will have to decide on continuing or terminating the pregnancy. Such decisions have multidimensional factors influencing and complicating the process of decision-making. There are multiple emotions involved, such as fear, anger, guilt, religious considerations, ethics and values, social and cultural influences—all these making the decision-making process very difficult. Hence, in such a screening procedure it is desirable to involve a health psychologist in the team.

Immunization Behaviour

Immunization constitutes the first major health protective behaviour for any individual. The first immunization for a person (during infancy) depends on the immunization behaviour of the parents since the child is a passive recipient. Immunization involves challenging the human immune system with a vaccine composed of modified pathogens. Apart from protecting the individual, it also reduces the circulation of the infecting agent among the population. The modified pathogen injected into the human system by way of vaccination has sufficient characteristics of the original pathogen. Thus, they activate the immune system and create a long-term

Positive Health Behaviour 73

immunity in the recipient. Vaccinations occasionally induce allergic responses, fever etc., which are mild and short-term illnesses. Sometimes, this emerges as one of the causes of avoidance of immunization.

The WHO's purpose of the proposal of universal immunization is because some diseases that need to be eradicated require every individual to be protected. For example, certain illnesses like smallpox could be eradicated through the process. The same is being done with polio for the past three decades. As part of such efforts, infants before the completion of the first year are targeted so that they are caught much before the risk of infection. In case of certain other vaccines, the recipients of the vaccine may not be the target. For example, rubella vaccination to the women of child-bearing age is to protect the foetus but not the recipient herself.

While it is assumed that vaccination is mainly for children, it is also required for adults in special circumstances. For example, adults travelling to different parts of the world need to protect themselves against some of the region-specific diseases. Adults engaged in occupations that place them vulnerable are recommended to take appropriate vaccines. For example, nurses are normally advised to get themselves vaccinated for hepatitis B in view of their coming in contact with patients on a daily basis. Pregnant women are given the tetanus toxin (TT) vaccination.

Though immunization is known as a major health protection measure, there is still a failure of receiving immunization. The causes are many, though the major cause is ignorance or lack of knowledge. Many people go for vaccination because the local hospital or health centre or the health worker reminds them and do a follow-up and get the infants vaccinated, but not with the full knowledge or the serious repercussions of not getting vaccinated. While this is the situation in a developing country like India, even in the US, the knowledge levels were found to be very low. Kimmel et al. (1996) reported the knowledge level regarding the importance of vaccination in parents of children under five years of age. They found that 47% of parents were unaware of the contagious nature of polio. About 36% were ignorant about the fact measles could be fatal, while 44% of parents did not know that H. influenza could lead to meningitis in childhood. Such ignorance is the main cause of non-adherence to immunization.

Immunization rates are found to vary with the socioeconomic status of the families. While one of the influences may be knowledge-deficit, the equally important cause is the lack of access, or prioritization of activities related to their survival need.

Families with a more number of children tend to neglect immunizing younger children. This is because with the expansion of family, their responsibilities for older children increase, and in the process, the priority of immunizing children born later takes a back seat.

Because of the nature of occupation, certain families move from place to place depending on the availability of employment. For example, those employed in construction work do not stay in one location continuously. It is difficult for the primary health care workers to keep track of them and follow up on immunization of children.

A very important factor that contributes to the individual's immunization behaviour is the attitude of the staff in the health care centre. A sense of commitment on the part of the health care staff, a convincing communication and the attitude of going the extra step to help the family adhere to the schedule go a long way in immunization compliance in a community.

While the national initiative for immunization is one of the priorities of the Ministry of Health, the achievement of 100% target rests on a number of factors discussed above. Table 3.6 presents the achievement in terms of the percentage immunized for various vaccines from the years 2008 to 2017.

Table 3.6 Achievement percentage of maternity and child health activities (immunization) in India (2008–2017)

Year	TT (pregnant women)	DPT (3rd dose)/ pentavalent (3rd dose)	DT (5 years)/ DPTS	Polio (3rd dose)	BCG	Measles
2008–2009	85.9	96.3	58.2	99.4	108.0	96.8
2009–2010	83.7	99	72.7	98.5	101.1	94.8
2010–2011	80.7	91	40.7	90.1	95.4	88.5
2011–2012	80.6	89.6	41.5	85.4	93.4	88.9
2012–2013	78.0	84.2	43.9	87.8	93.2	89.6
2013–2014	80.3	75	47.1	90.2	93.6	89.2
2014–2015	78.9	89.43	52.29	87.12	92.4	87.27
2015–2016	78.95	89.8	54.7	87.98	93.7	89.14
2016–2017	77.32	88.23	67.76	86.67	90.44	88.11

Source: HMIS portal (Status as on 10 Jan 2018); https://cdn.downtoearth.org.in/pdf/NHP-2018/pdf

DPT vaccine is a combination of immunization against three diseases, viz. diphtheria, pertussis and tetanus. Diphtheria is a bacterial infection transmitted through close physical and respiratory contact. Pertussis also known as whooping cough is also a bacterial respiratory infection. It causes severe cough with a typical whoop often causing vomiting. It lasts for a duration of several weeks. Tetanus is not a disease that is transmitted. It is caused by a potent neurotoxin that grows in tissues such as dirty wounds or umbilical cord if the delivery has not been in hygienic conditions.

BCG vaccine is against tuberculosis. It is the cause of more than two and half billion deaths across the globe by 1990. Tuberculosis bacteria have been a great challenge as the bacteria have been found to become multi-drug-resistant. This happens when the patients drop out of the treatment before it is cured.

Polio is known as poliomyelitis. It is an acute viral infection. It spreads through the faecal-oral route. The probability of its transmission is high in places with poor sanitation. Poliovirus infection is asymptomatic. There is a high probability of paralysis because of the virus.

Measles is an acute viral infection. It is transmitted through respiratory contact. It may even lead to secondary infections in the respiratory tract or gastrointestinal tract, which could be fatal.

Going by the characteristics of these diseases, it is certainly cost-effective to get oneself immunized rather than going for the treatment of the infected. Given the fact that the major reasons for non-compliance are knowledge-deficit, problems of prioritization and logistics, efforts need to be invested in effective health communication, reaching out and psychoeducation to the parents and drive to enhance health literacy in the community.

Immunization Drive in Rural India

The introduction of Accredited Social Health Activists (ASHA) under the National Rural Health Mission by the Government of India brought in knowledge dissemination about immunization. The ASHA volunteers who are necessarily a member of the community successfully created awareness about the benefits of immunization and took the mothers to the health centres for getting their children vaccinated. For this, they were paid a monetary incentive of a token amount (Rao, 2014).

Immunization Behaviour through Patient Education

Effective patient education, particularly in rural Indian set-up, depends on quantity, quality and clarity of information packed in communication. Further, an authentic source of communication, and the agent who communicates have their own value. In case of immunization behaviour, it is desirable to expand patient education to cover the family and community at large. Mass media campaigns with sharp and crisp messages were found to be helpful in increasing the percentage of immunization. Awareness programmes in the campaign mode involving national public figures, local authorities and popular community representatives are found to have a positive impact and enhance the immunization behaviour in communities.

The patient or community education programmes will have to be so designed in order to address various apprehensions and dissipate the myths about the immunization, particularly among the uneducated and from socioeconomic backgrounds. When the benefits of immunization are highlighted, alongside the focus on the probability of negative outcomes of failure to immunize presents the complete picture. That enables them to reflect and make an informed choice by prioritizing immunization.

Factors Influencing Positive Health Behaviour

Positive health behaviour, like any behaviour, is guided by the principles of learning behaviour and consolidating it. We can identify two major principles contributing to health behaviour:

1 Operant conditioning—the basic principle of operant conditioning is reinforcement. According to this, any behaviour when performed gives pleasure and satisfaction, or satisfies any need is likely to be repeated. For example, a person joining a weight reduction programme who targets a weight loss of three kilograms in a month undergoes rigorous exercise and consumes a restricted diet. Both the activities call for 'foregoing' something like physical comfort and food of one's choice. However, at the end of the month if the weight loss is found to have hit the set target, that is considered a reward. Now, it is more likely that the person continues the programme.

Just as the way reinforcement strengthens a health protective behaviour, it also works the same way in strengthening a health risk behaviour. Let us explain this by taking smoking behaviour as an example. An adolescent boy hardly had any peer group of his own on entering the new college. He tried to associate himself with a group that was very prominent in the college. There was not much acceptance shown by them. After a fortnight, he passes by the group with a cigarette in his hand and finds few members of the group calling him to the college canteen for having tea together. This peer acceptance satisfying his need for affiliation is for his smoking behaviour. Hence, this smoking behaviour, which is a health risk, is likely to strengthen and continue.

Taking another health risk behaviour as an example, we can explain the way reinforcement works in strengthening a health risk behaviour. A young adult faces the stress of breaking up a relationship with his girlfriend. He is unable to cope with the situation of rejection. His emotions of sorrow, anger, guilt and revengefulness, as well as love, are in conflict. This impacts his eating and sleeping negatively. In such a state, on the insistence of a friend he sits down to consume alcohol. He experiences a sense of relaxation. He can eat a meal and can have long hours of sleep. He finds that alcohol could help him to come out of his stress (though temporarily). Now, he is more likely to consume alcohol for getting rid of his present stress and perhaps even in future.

The second important principle related to operant conditioning is extinction. When the consequence of the behaviour that helped in strengthening it is removed, the behaviour gets weakened. For example, when the loss of weight in the subsequent month is not substantial, the person may not adhere to the strict exercise and diet regimen. Similarly, when smoking behaviour fails to meet with peer acceptance, it may get weakened unless there is some pleasure sensation derived from it.

Another example of extinction is in relation to healthy eating. If a child being inculcated into healthy eating behaviour is given one rupee every day for finishing vegetables and fruits served in meal, he/she is likely to eat them every day even if he does not particularly enjoy them. But when this one-rupee reward is stopped, he/she is more likely to stop this healthy eating behaviour.

The third principle of operant conditioning relevant in the context of health behaviour is punishment. When a behaviour brings a consequence that is painful or unpleasant, it is not likely to be repeated. For example, initiating physical exercise in the morning as part of the weight reduction programme may be undertaken by an individual. Suppose, on the second or third day of his jogging early in the morning, he is chased by the street dogs and trips and falls in the park, he is less likely to persevere with the activity of jogging. Similarly, the first-time smoker, when experiences an asthma attack within one hour of smoking, is less likely to continue the behaviour. Thus, an unpleasant consequence of a health behaviour, be it a health protective or health risk behaviour, is likely to stop the behaviour than to continue it.

2. Social Learning or Modelling—many of our behaviours are learned through observational learning. When a person of significance behaves in a particular way and is rewarded for the behaviour through admiration, acceptance, bestowing of power, fame or any desirable manner, the observed behaviour is more likely to be emulated by us. In the context of health behaviour, if the parents, siblings, teachers, peers or any significant person in the life of a child indulges in good health practices such as healthy diet, following sleep hygiene, practising Yoga and the child observes societal acceptance and acclaiming such behaviour, it is more likely for the child to adopt the same. The same principle follows in case of health risk behaviour. If the child finds the father an authority figure smoking or drinking, and the father is highly respected both within the family and in society, the child is likely to take to smoking and drinking when he grows into adolescent or adult.

Be it health-promoting behaviour or health risk behaviour, a number of factors have their influence on its continuation or cessation.

Box 3.1 Researcher's Box

- There is a need to compile scientific Indian data on healthy eating. This can be done for different age groups. Along with the diet patterns, psychological parameters such as goal setting behaviour, perseverance, health beliefs, self-efficacy can be tested and correlated with diet.
- The impact of psychoeducation on a healthy diet can be studied through pre-test/post-test designs. This can be combined with a qualitative study where the adherence to a healthy diet can be combined with interviews on the factors contributing to adherence and non-adherence.

- Studies with a correlational design can be planned to find out the psychological correlates of different types of diet and disciplined and undisciplined eating habits. Personality variables, physical agility aspects, wellbeing, stress levels, affect states, quality of life and happiness index can be correlated with diet.
- Studies can be planned to examine the impact of certain interventions such as music therapy, *Yoga*, meditation and other relaxation exercise on the quality of sleep. These interventions can be compared with other practices like watching television shows before sleep, working on computers, internet or using mobile phones preceding sleep time.

Box 3.2 Practitioner's Box

- Patients reporting difficulty in compliance with eating behaviour (irresistible binge eating) can be educated on stimulus control by storing just adequate food and only healthy or prescribed food.
- Procrastination or frequent lapses in adhering to an exercise regimen can be handled well by introducing social support intervention. Either a family member or a good friend can be tagged to the exercise as a companion.
- Support groups for *Yoga* and exercise work as a good motivator.
- Clients with sleep problems have to be screened on their pre-sleep activities. Any activity that disrupts the secretion of melatonin will have to be handled with care.
- Psychoeducation and counselling on sleep hygiene are very significant because the majority of lay persons have no cognition of it.
- There is a need to educate all clients on the age-specific sleep requirement and the need for quality sleep to maintain wellbeing.

References

Bagde, A. B., Sawant, R. S., Sawai, R. V., Dhimdhime, S. R., & Swami, N. B. (2015). Preventive aspect of vyayama (physical exercise). *International Journal, 3*(1).

Blair, S. N., Kohl, H. W., Barlow, C. E., Paffenbarger, R. S., Gibbons, L. W., & Macera, C. A. (1995). Changes in physical fitness and all-cause mortality: A prospective study of healthy and unhealthy men. *Jama, 273*(14), 1093–1098.

Block, G., Patterson, B., & Subar, A. (1992). Fruit, vegetables, and cancer prevention: A review of the epidemiological evidence. *Nutrition and Cancer, 18*(1), 1–29.

Cappuccio, F. P., Cooper, D., D'elia, L., Strazzullo, P., & Miller, M. A. (2011). Sleep duration predicts cardiovascular outcomes: A systematic review and meta-analysis of prospective studies. *European Heart Journal, 32*(12), 1484–1492.

Dzeewaltowski, D. A. (1989). Toward a model of exercise motivation. *Journal of Sport and Exercise Psychology, 11*(3), 251–269.

Erikssen, G., Liestøl, K., Bjørnholt, J., Thaulow, E., Sandvik, L., & Erikssen, J. (1998). Changes in physical fitness and changes in mortality. *The Lancet, 352*(9130), 759–762.

Gochman, D. S. (1997). Provider determinants of health behaviour. In: David S. Gochman (Ed.), *Handbook of health behaviour research II* (pp. 397–417). Boston, MA: Springer.

Guadagni, V., Burles, F., Ferrara, M., & Iaria, G. (2014). The effects of sleep deprivation on emotional empathy. *Journal of Sleep Research, 23*(6), 657–663.

Harris, D. M., & Guten, S. (1979). Health-protective behaviour: An exploratory study. *Journal of Health and Social Behaviour, 20*(1), 17–29.

Haste, H. (2004). *My body, my self: Young people's values and motives about healthy living*. London: Nestlé Social Research Programme.

Herndon, J. E, Wandersman, A. (2004). Prevention. In Christensen, J. A., Martin, R., & Smyth, M. J. (Eds.), *Encyclopedia of Health Psychology* (pp. 220–221). Kluwer Academic/Plenum Publishers.

Hirshkowitz, M., Whiton, K., Albert, S. M., Alessi, C., Bruni, O., DonCarlos, L., ... & Neubauer, D. N. (2015). National Sleep Foundation's sleep time duration recommendations: Methodology and results summary. *Sleep Health, 1*(1), 40–43.

Irwin, M., McClintick, J., Costlow, C., Fortner, M., White, J., & Gillin, J. C. (1996). Partial night sleep deprivation reduces natural killer and cellular immune responses in humans. *The FASEB Journal, 10*(5), 643–653.

Kasl, S. V., & Cobb, S. (1966). Health behaviour, illness behaviour and sick role behaviour: I. Health and illness behaviour. *Archives of Environmental Health: An International Journal, 12*(2), 246–266.

Key, T. J., Fraser, G. E., Thorogood, M., Appleby, P. N., Beral, V., Reeves, G., ... & Mann, J. (1998). Mortality in vegetarians and non-vegetarians: A collaborative analysis of 8300 deaths among 76,000 men and women in five prospective studies. *Public Health Nutrition, 1*(1), 33–41.

Kimmel, S. R., Madlon-Kay, D., Burns, I. T., & Admire, J. B. (1996). Breaking the barriers to childhood immunization. *American Family Physician, 53*(5), 1648–1666.

Kinnucan, J. A., Rubin, D. T., & Ali, T. (2013). Sleep and inflammatory bowel disease: Exploring the relationship between sleep disturbances and inflammation. *Gastroenterology & Hepatology, 9*(11), 718.

Leech, J. (2018). 10 Reasons why good sleep is important. Retrieved on July 13, 2019 from www.healthline.com/10-reasons-why-good-sleep-is-important

Marcus, B. H., Rakowski, W., & Rossi, J. S. (1992). Assessing motivational readiness and decision making for exercise. *Health Psychology, 11*(4), 257.

Martinsen, E. W. (1990). Benefits of exercise for the treatment of depression. *Sports Medicine, 9*(6), 380–389.

Matarazzo, J. D. (1983). Behavioral health: A 1990 challenge for the health sciences professions. In J. D. Matarazzo, N. E. Miller, S. M. Weiss, & J. A. Herd (Eds.), Behavioral health: A handbook of health enhancement and disease prevention. New York: Wiley.

Misra, R., Balagopal, P., Raj, S., & Patel, T. G. (2018). Vegetarian diet and cardiometabolic risk among Asian Indians in the United States. *Journal of Diabetes Research*. doi: 10.1155/2018/1675369

Morrison, V., & Bennett, P. (2006). *Health psychology: An introduction*. England: Prentice-Hall International.

Nishteswar, K. (2016). Ayurvedic concept of food and nutrition. *Journal of Nutrition & Food Sciences, 6*(4), 1–8.

Norman, P., & Smith, L. (1995). The theory of planned behaviour and exercise: An investigation into the role of prior behaviour, behavioural intentions and attitude variability. *European Journal of Social Psychology, 25*(4), 403–415.

Paffenbarger Jr, R. S., Hyde, R., Wing, A. L., & Hsieh, C. C. (1986). Physical activity, all-cause mortality, and longevity of college alumni. *New England Journal of Medicine, 314*(10), 605–613.

Payyappallimana, U., & Venkatasubramanian, P. (2016). Exploring ayurvedic knowledge on food and health for providing innovative solutions to contemporary healthcare. *Frontiers in Public Health, 4*, 57.

Rajeski, W. J. (1994). Dose-response issues from a psychosocial perspective. In: C. Bauchard, R. J. Shephard, and T. Stephens (Eds.), *Physical activity, fitness and health* (pp. 1040–1055). Champaign II. Human Kinetics Publishers.

Rakhshani, A., Nagarathna, R., Mhaskar, R., Mhaskar, A., Thomas, A., & Gunasheela, S. (2012). The effects of yoga in prevention of pregnancy complications in high-risk pregnancies: A randomized controlled trial. *Preventive Medicine, 55*(4), 333–340.

Rao, T. (2014). The Impact of a Community Health Worker Program on Childhood Immunization: Evidence from India's' ASHA' Workers. Available at SSRN 2444391.

Reiner, M., Niermann, C., Jekauc, D., & Woll, A. (2013). Long-term health benefits of physical activity–A systematic review of longitudinal studies. *BMC Public Health*, *13*(1), 813.

Runyan, D. K., & Gould, C. L. (1985). Foster care for child maltreatment: Impact on delinquent behaviour. *Pediatrics*, *75*(3), 562–568.

Sarafino, E. P. (2016). Context and perspectives in health psychology. In: S. Sutton, A. Baum, and M. Johnston (Eds.), *The Sage handbook of health psychology*. doi: 10.4135/9781848608153

Sarkar, P., Lohith Kumar, D. H., Dhumal, C., Panigrahi, S. S., & Choudhary, R. (2015). Traditional and ayurvedic foods of Indian origin. *Journal of Ethnic Foods*, *2*(3), 97–109.

Satish, L. (2012). Yoga as positive psyhcological intervention strategy. In: A. Yadava, D. Hooda, and N. R. Sharma (Eds.), *Biopsychosocial issues in positive health* (pp. 153–158). New Delhi, India: Global Vision Publishing House.

Satyavati, G. (2008). *Ayurvedic concepts of nutrition and dietary guidelines for promoting/preserving health and longevity* (pp. 210–228). New Delhi, India: Nutrition Foundation of India.

Sharma, M., & Knowlden, A. P. (2012). Role of yoga in preventing and controlling type 2 diabetes mellitus. *Journal of Evidence-Based Complementary & Alternative Medicine*, *17*(2), 88–95.

Sharma, A., Madaan, V., & Petty, F. D. (2006). Exercise for mental health. *Primary Care Companion to the Journal of Clinical Psychiatry*, *8*(2), 106.

Shohani, M., Badfar, G., Nasirkandy, M. P., Kaikhavani, S., Rahmati, S., Modmeli, Y., & Azami, M. (2018). The effect of yoga on stress, anxiety, and depression in women. *International Journal of Preventive Medicine*, *9*(1), 21.

Shukla, A., Prashant, D., Shukla, A., Baghel, A. S., Vyas, M. K., & Vellela, J. (2014). Relevance of sleep for healthy living: An Ayurvedic perspective. *Ayurveda Journal of Health*, *XII*(3), 27–34.

Singh, D. (2017). Physical exercise: Perspective in Ayurveda. *Journal of Advanced Research in Ayurveda, Yoga, Unani, Sidha and Homeopathy*, *4*(1–2), 33–36.

Spiegel, K., Leproult, R., & Van Cauter, E. (1999). Impact of sleep debt on metabolic and endocrine function. *The Lancet*, *354*(9188), 1435–1439.

Taheri, S., Lin, L., Austin, D., Young, T., & Mignot, E. (2004). Short sleep duration is associated with reduced leptin, elevated ghrelin, and increased body mass index. *PLoS Medicine*, *1*(3), e62.

Taylor, S. E. (2006). *Health Psychology*. New Delhi: Tata McGraw-Hill Education.

Tripathy, I., & Tripathy, D. S. (2011). *Yogaratnakava, Nityapravrittiprakara, Sootra*, 259 (p. 66). India: Chaukambha Krishnadas Academy.

Velásquez, A. M., López, M. A., Quiñonez, N., and Paba, D. P. (2015). Yoga for the prevention of depression, anxiety, and aggression and the promotion of socio-emotional competencies in schoolaged children. *Educational Research and Evaluation*, *21*(5–6), 407–421.

WHO. (2004). Global strategy on diet, physical activity and health. https://journals.sagepub.com/doi/pdf/10.1177/156482650402500310#:~:text=The%20overall%20goal%20of%20the,reduced%20disease%20and%20death%20rates

WHO. (2004). Young people's health in context: Health behaviour in school-aged children (HBSC) study (International report from the 2001/2002 survey). Edited by C. Currie, C. Roberts, & A. Morgan. Retrieved from www.euro.who.int

4 Health Risk Behaviour

Health risk behaviour refers to any behaviour adopted by an individual, voluntarily or imposed with or without knowledge of its implications that increases the individual's susceptibility to a disease, either by precipitating a predisposed potential or by creating a new vulnerability. Just like the positive health behaviour, the health risk behaviour is also closely associated with the lifestyle of the individual. The individual, in an attempt to satisfy the needs organized in hierarchy, initiates certain behaviour. There are a number of materials and methods to satisfy these needs. Exercising the options in choice of these materials and methods demands application of discretion in terms of the health outcomes. When the discretion is not used due to ignorance or deliberately ignored for any reason, there is a possibility of adopting health risk behaviour for the sake of immediate need satisfaction. Health risk behaviour associated with everyday life relates to diet, sleep, physical activities and sexual behaviour. We have discussed positive health behaviour related to these areas. Now, we will examine health risk behaviours related to the same.

As a very small and interesting exercise, choose about ten adults in your family, neighbourhood or the academic institution you are studying. Ask them two questions: (1) If they have any long-term health problems And (2) apart from medication has their doctor advised them of any changes in their daily life?

If you consolidate your responses, you may have under the 'do's' of doctor's advice aspects related to diet, exercise and sleep, and under 'don'ts' aspects related to smoking and alcohol consumption. The behaviour that is classified under the category of the doctor's advice of 'don'ts' is health risk behaviour.

By examining the top ten causes of death in India in the years 2007 and 2017, changes in the ranking of few causes are observed. Table 4.1 presents the rank change in a period of one decade.

The risk factors for disability and deaths are combinedly listed for both the years. Table 4.2 presents the risk factors. It may be observed that out of the 12 risk factors, four are related to behavioural risk; two classified under metabolic risk are closely related to diet and exercise.

About 36% of diseases and deaths have contribution from behavioural risk factors, suggesting that the probability of disease and death in these cases is enhanced by health risk behaviour. Hence, we will discuss these three health risk behaviours under this section. In addition, we will also discuss the health risk in the context of sexual behaviour.

DOI: 10.4324/9781003438908-4

Table 4.1 Top causes of death in India

S. No.	Diseases	Ranking in 2007	Ranking in 2017
1	Ischaemic heart disease	1	1
2	Diarrhoeal diseases	2	4
3	Chronic Obstructive Pulmonary Diseases	3	2
4	Neonatal disorders	4	7
5	Lower respiratory infection	5	5
6	Stroke	6	3
7	Tuberculosis	7	6
8	Asthma	8	8
9	Road injuries	9	12
10	Self-harm	10	14
11	Diabetes	13	9
12	Chronic kidney disease	14	10

Source: www.healthdata.org/India

Table 4.2 Risk factors that cause disability and death (combined)

Metabolic risks	Environmental/occupational risks	Behavioural risks
High blood pressure	Air pollution Water, Sanitation and Hygiene (WASH)	Malnutrition, dietary risks, tobacco consumption Alcohol consumption
High fasting blood glucose High LDL High Body Mass Index (BMI)	Occupation risks	

Source: www.healthdata.org/India

The health risk behaviour can be grouped into the following three broad categories:

1 Deviation and unhealthy practices introduced into the everyday natural behaviour that is universal, e.g. eating behaviour, sleep and sexual behaviour that are very natural and essential biological requirements for survival. When these behaviours are practised in a manner that poses risk to health, they are identified as unhealthy / health risk behaviour.
2 Acquiring a new unhealthy behaviour that is not natural or required for survival, e.g. smoking, alcohol consumption.
3 Behaviour that is in violation of rules, set for one's own safety and thereby positioning oneself vulnerable to risk, e.g. violating driving speed limits, not wearing a helmet or fastening seat belts, speaking on mobile phone while driving.

Behavioural Deviation from Healthy Practices

Very often, one tends to give in to the biological and social pressures and engage in behaviour that is known to cause a minor or temporary harm to health and sometimes a major and long-term harm to health. While ignorance is sometimes the cause, impulse and feeling obligated are also the reasons when one deviates with complete cognizance about the consequences.

Unhealthy Diet

Healthy diet recommendations include consumption of adequate quantities of vegetables, fruits, legumes, nuts and grains. Not following these recommendations is unhealthy. Further, substituting this with a diet rich in fat, sugar and salt is further unhealthy. Deviating from dietary guidelines contributes to a number of diseases like coronary heart diseases, cancer and gastrointestinal diseases to name a few. Also, inadequate fruit and vegetable consumption contributed to 6.7 million deaths across the globe (Lim et al., 2012). Further, adequate consumption of fruits and vegetables is found to lower the risk of cardiovascular diseases, and cancer in the stomach and colorectal region.

How does unhealthy food impact your health? It is a misnomer that a stomach full of meal takes care of nutritional needs. It is highly possible that a person is over-fed and yet suffers nutritional deficiency. Thus, 'what' is consumed is more important than 'how much' is consumed. Higher nutritional values are found in whole foods like cereals, lentils, vegetables and fruits. Thus, one of the repercussions of unhealthy food is nutritional deficiency.

An increase in consumption of processed food high in saturated fat, sugar and salt is one of the causes of weight gain and obesity. The added weight places pressure on every part of the body and enhances the risk for a number of metabolic diseases like hypertension, diabetes and cardiovascular diseases, sleep apnoea, liver diseases, infertility and stroke. High consumption of a sugar-rich diet results in erratic glucose levels that spike up and fall repeatedly. This may cause insulin resistance, meaning decreased sensitivity to insulin. When this condition is uncorrelated and prevails, it may lead to type II diabetes. A diet high in fat, sugar and salt contributes to placing one at high risk for hypertension, cardiovascular diseases and stroke.

When this awareness is present, and despite such messages being continuously transmitted through social media, why do people deviate from healthy eating and indulge in an unhealthy diet?

Obesity is found to be one of the consequences of improper choice of diet. Irrespective of the economic status, there is a progressive increase in the prevalence of obesity across nations. Table 4.3 presents the percentage of population above 18 years suffering obesity.

A comparison is made across eight countries that included developed and developing countries from the American, European and Asian continents. It is observed that in the past 45 years, the increase in prevalence of obesity across these countries is somewhere between three-fold to about 17-fold. What is more alarming is that in the Asian countries where the problem of obesity was almost non-existent with below 1% prevalence, the increase is multifold by the year 2016. One of the reasons for this progressive trend could be the gradual change in dietary habit, particularly among the children and the youth over a period of two decades. The availability of a

Table 4.3 Prevalence of obesity among adults, age 18+ (%) (both sexes), 1975–2016

Year	US	Canada	UK	Indonesia	China	Japan	Sri Lanka	India
1975	11.9	9.8	9.4	0.4	0.5	1	0.6	0.3
1980	13.7	11.3	10.7	0.6	0.6	1.2	0.7	0.5
1985	16	13.1	12.3	0.8	0.9	1.4	0.9	0.7
1990	18.7	15.2	14	1.2	1.2	1.5	1.2	0.9
1995	21.9	17.6	16.2	1.8	1.7	1.8	1.6	1.2
2000	25.5	20.5	18.6	2.6	2.4	2.1	2.1	1.6
2005	29	23.3	21.4	3.6	3.2	2.6	2.8	2.1
2010	32.3	26	24.2	4.9	4.4	3.3	3.7	2.8
2015	35.6	28.8	27.2	6.5	5.9	4.1	4.9	3.7
2016	36.2	29.4	27.8	6.9	6.2	4.3	5.2	3.9

Source: https://www.who.int/gho/ncd/risk_factors/overweight_obesity/obesity_adults/en/

global variety of food in every country, the exposure to aggressive marketing and the attractive schemes attached to the processed food are the main causes of obesity. This is particularly true in case of India. If there has been continuous innovation in the variety of food in any country, it has to be India. With wide variations in geographical location, seasons and suitability for age groups, India has been very enterprising in its culinary skills utilizing the locally grown cultivation. Hence, food in any region has always been very healthy and suitable for all age groups. However, with globalization, processed food with high levels of carbohydrate, fat, salt and sugar has started attracting the appetite of a new generation. Combined with a rise in purchasing power and paucity of time for elaborate cooking, the frequency of eating the processed food has been on the rise progressively. In addition to that, the job demands of the new generation have interfered sufficiently with the discipline of the 'the family meal-time'. As a result, eating behaviour among Indian children and youth has violated the principles of 'what', 'when' and 'how'. What is appetizing and attractive has replaced what is nutritious and recommended; the specific timings for breakfast, lunch and dinner are increasingly being replaced with whenever one gets time or whenever one is awake. The norm of eating and sitting relaxedly with family at the dining table is now a rare phenomenon in middle-class Indian families. It is substituted with eating while travelling, watching television or working. Thus, it may not be an exaggeration to state that 'healthy eating' has violated all rules of quantity, quality, timings, method and manner. All these aspects are discussed in detail under health protective behaviour.

While obesity is one extreme of consequence of unhappy eating behaviour, the other extreme is the prevalence of malnutrition. Table 4.4 presents the decadal data on prevalence of malnutrition in eight countries. While India saw a phenomenal increase in the prevalence of obesity between the years 1975 (0.3%) and 2016 (3.9%), there is a noticeable fall in the prevalence of malnutrition (BMI < 18.5) in men and women in India between the years 1975 (men, 36.14%; and women, 18.8%) and 2014 (men, 24.5%; and women, 24.9%). However, the fact remains that about 25% of Indian men and women are still malnourished.

The table clearly shows the contrast between the developed and developing countries in terms of percentage of prevalence. While the developed countries have less than 2% of population suffering from malnutrition, it is a two-digit percentage in developing countries. India has the largest percentage of prevalence.

The two tables are clear indicators of the unhealthy status of about 29% of Indian adult population suffering the consequence of an unhealthy diet (obesity 3.9 + about 25% malnourished = circa 29%).

What is malnutrition and what is obesity? Both malnutrition and obesity can be determined by measuring Body Mass Index (BMI). The logic is based on the healthy or accepted norm for the weight for height. The formula for calculating BMI is

$$\text{BMI} = \frac{\text{Weight(kilogram)}}{(\text{Height(meters)})^2}.$$

The BMI between 18.5 and 24.9 is normal, between 25 and 29.9 is overweight, while more than 30 is obese. Similarly, BMI less than 18.5 is considered underweight. Underweight is taken as an index of malnutrition.

Pooja, Yadava and Sharma (2012) enumerated the multiple risk factors associated with high BMI. It is found to be related not only to physical illness but also to psychological wellbeing and cognitive function.

Now, let us try to understand obesity, whose prevalence is found to be on the increase across the globe. In terms of BMI, obesity is defined as a condition where the BMI of the person is

Table 4.4 Prevalence of malnutrition in developed and developing countries (BMI < 18.5 kg/m)

Year	US Men	US Women	Canada Men	Canada Women	UK Men	UK Women	Indonesia Men	Indonesia Women	China Men	China Women	Japan Men	Japan Women	Sri Lanka Men	Sri Lanka Women	India Men	India Women
1975	2.1	4.1	1.5	4.3	2.2	4.6	23.3	26.2	11.4	14.6	9.2	10.8	22.0	24.3	36.4	37.4
1985	1.3	3.5	0.9	3.0	1.5	3.4	22.7	23.6	10.8	12.7	7.3	9.9	21.4	21.4	34.0	34.9
1995	0.9	2.6	0.7	2.2	1.2	2.0	21.3	20.2	9.3	10.7	5.9	9.4	20.3	18.6	31.6	32.2
2005	0.7	2.1	0.5	1.7	0.9	2.1	18.5	16.8	6.0	8.1	5.0	9.4	18.2	15.1	28.2	28.7
2014	0.6	1.9	0.4	1.4	0.6	1.8	14.9	13.6	3.4	6.0	4.5	10.0	15.9	11.9	24.5	24.9

Source: Ezzati et al. (2016).

more than 30. There are degrees of obesity. A BMI between 30 and 39.9 is called moderate or clinical obesity, while a BMI above 40 qualifies one as severely obese.

The problem of obesity in many cases is traced to genetic predisposition, lower metabolic rates or hormonal imbalance. Nevertheless, eating behaviour is one of the associated factors. It is just not the eating behaviour (in terms of option for high fat, high carbohydrate food) but also in combination with a disproportionately low physical activity that results in obesity. A high-calorie diet and preference for a sedentary lifestyle end up in failure to burn the calories consumed. They tend to get deposited as adipose in the body. A number of studies stated overconsumption of fast food (normally high in fat content) and less intake of recommended healthy food as health risk behaviour among the adolescents (Singh et al., 2006). Sunitha and Gururaj (2014) stated that India is encountered with the challenge of nutritional transition as there is a shift in choice from traditional diets that are high in cereals and fibres to the Western food high in sugar, fat and animal source of food that is identified to be associated with non-communicable diseases in later years of life.

An obese person seems to be trapped into a vicious circle of high food consumption and low physical activity. Sometimes, the appetite of obese persons is high because of the imbalance of the hormones leptin (associated with appetite) and serotonin (associated with satiation). High levels of leptin enhance the appetite, while high levels of serotonin induce satiation. When these two levels are not in right balance, there is a heightened appetite leading to eating more. When the body weight increases further due to eating more, the individual finds it difficult to engage in physical activities.

Prevalence of obesity among Indian children is a matter of concern for the health care professionals, nutritionists and schools. Sunitha and Gururaj (2014) mentioned a meta-analysis, which indicated that 12.6% of Indian children are overweight, while 3.3% are obese. Among children between 10 and 19 years of age, the prevalence of overweight was found to be between 9.9% and 19.9%. This indicated the potential for early onset of obesity.

Despite high awareness about healthy eating and wide information dissemination on the adverse impact of unhealthy processed food, fast food or junk food, why do people indulge in such unhealthy behaviour?

Eating behaviour is influenced by multiple factors. The individual with his/her personality factor, family, culture, society and environment has a major role in setting a basic eating behaviour, as well as bringing about a change in the pattern that is almost set. Figure 4.1 depicts the various factors influencing the eating behaviour.

Various factors play a dominant role of deviation from healthy eating at different stages of life.

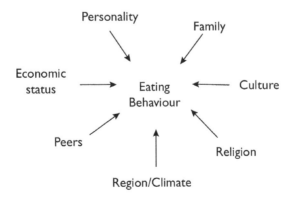

Figure 4.1 Factors Influencing Eating Behaviour.

Childhood

The diet preferences develop in the early stage of life. In fact, it is well integrated into the child-rearing process. Parental influence on the choice of food plays a major role in prioritizing the nutritional value over the other factors such as appearance, texture, smell, colour and taste of food.

Adolescence

Even though the family trains the children in healthy food habits, the adolescent age has a high probability of having peer influence in food preferences. Peer groups' influence on food is so high that one may deviate from the quality, quantity, timing and environment of eating. It is in the adolescent age that children shift their food preferences to junk food. They tend to eat at odd times, miss their meal, choose the food based on media and marketing influence, and experiment with food prohibited by one's religion or family because of the value system. A striking example of experimenting with meat-eating behaviour by Mahatma Gandhi sends a powerful message about the peer influence on shifting food preferences at adolescent age. Yet, another factor that attracts the adolescent eating behaviour is the prestige tag that a food item carries. Eating expensive food and visiting expensive restaurants are the outcome of both attractive commercial advertisements and peer pressure. In short, it can be stated that eating behaviour in adolescent age is not just to satisfy the hunger but also to satisfy the need for affiliation and self-esteem. Very often, in need satisfaction, factors higher in hierarchy get the better of the basic physiological need. Every time such needs are satisfied, the behaviour of 'wrong eating' gets strengthened. Kinard and Webster (2012) explored into the causes that abet unhealthy eating among adolescents in the US. They identified three factors, viz. influence of parents, peers and self-efficacy contributing to unhealthy eating.

Of these, they found self-efficacy as the strongest influence. The hope that this study provides to the intervention research is that the influence of marketing and advertisement can be neutralized by parental influence and self-efficacy. In other words, an adolescent with a high self-efficacy and strong parental support for healthy eating behaviour is less likely to sacrifice healthy eating (Figure 4.2).

Yet, another factor that plays a role in eating behaviour is body image, closely associated with the self-esteem of the person. During adolescence, there is a growth of skeletal and muscular structure. As a result, particularly in girls, the body shape is rounded. This might prompt the girls to cut down on the unhealthy diet, fast or miss meals to gain the appearance of slim, delicate—all leading to undernourishment or malnutrition. The reverse may happen in case of boys whose body image requires strong muscular structures and gain in height. This may lead them to prefer food high in calories and fat. In addition to this, the appetite of the adolescent is negatively impacting if there is an onset of smoking behaviour or alcohol consumption. These two habits are known for lowering their appetite for food, thus contributing to nutritional deficiencies.

Adulthood

For the adults, the professional responsibilities may overpower the need for timely meals. As a result, those hard-pressed for time may tend to miss their meals, and substitute a meal with aerated drinks or bakery products easy to consume while taking little time off from the working table. Further, the majority of the Indian youth, both men and women, are engaged in jobs that demand a different country's time zone. The consequence of this is not only on one's own

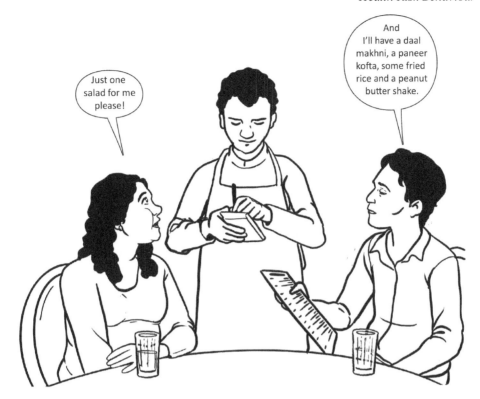

Figure 4.2 Body Image and Eating Behaviour.

eating, but also on the compromise of healthy family meals, both in terms of regularity, punctuality and quality. This is because everything is guided by the video calls after office timings that may overlap with family meal-time.

Elderly

The elderly people deviate from healthy eating for a totally different set of reasons. Their taste buds are not active. As a result, their engagement in eating good food decreases. The lowered olfactory sense fails to stimulate them with good aroma of food. The impaired hearing interferes with sustaining a good meal-time conversation. Thus, meal-time gradually ceases to be a social interaction time. Problems with dentition make chewing an effort; as a result, some may even perceive eating as a 'job' without much incentive. This makes it difficult for them to chew vegetables and fruits. Weak gastrointestinal functioning and problems with digestion prompt them to avoid certain types of food though they are rich in nutrients. Though the prescribed diet for them demands inclusion of fruits, vegetables, grains, protein food, dairy products and oils, they may prefer liquid or semi-solid food for the various reasons discussed above.

Thus, the reason for preference for unhealthy food varies with age.

Unhealthy Sleep Behaviour

We have already discussed under health protective behaviour the definition of healthy sleep, the impact of sleep deprivation on physical and mental health and the age-specific recommended duration of sleep. In this section, we will discuss about what is unhealthy sleep and sleep hygiene. This section is not to discuss sleep disorders but to focus on sleep behaviour that is unhealthy.

Sleeping behaviour is part of daily life and is as much significant as eating behaviour. During sleep, the brain and body get replenished, which is essential for sustaining health and wellbeing.

Stages of Sleep

Before we go on to discuss unhealthy sleep, it is relevant to briefly explain how sleep is induced and the stages it goes through. As the daylight turns into dark after sunset, the body secretes a hormone called melatonin. This hormone is secreted by the pineal gland. The stimulus for it is the lowering of light or setting in darkness. As the level of melatonin released into the blood goes up, the alertness of the individual goes down, and sleep is induced. The melatonin level in the blood is high for about 12 hours. The body clock gets set to induce sleep at night. It is not just the clock, but the bright light or the absence of it plays a crucial role in release of melatonin.

From the time of falling asleep at night to waking up the next morning, the sleep passes through five stages. It takes about 90 minutes to go through these five stages. Every night's sleep sees about four to six cycles of these stages.

Stage 1 of sleep is a transitional phase when one is in and out of consciousness. The muscles that start relaxing may also give a jerk sometimes jolting one off the sleep.

Stage 2 sleep is light sleep. During this stage, the heart rate begins to slow down and the body temperature drops. The brain waves also start slowing down. About 50% of our sleep compromises stage 2.

For the purpose of explaining, stages 3 and 4 are normally combined as they consist of deep sleep. It is difficult to wake up someone from this stage of sleep. These two stages are characterized by slow waves hence known as slow wave sleep (SWS). The EEG records show delta waves in this stage. The characteristics of these stages are drop in the heart rate and blood pressure, and slower and rhythmic breathing. The body is paralysed and immobile. This is the phase of sleep that is known to be highly rejuvenating. Hormones promoting growth (by replenishing muscles and tissues) and appetite control are released. The blood circulation to the muscles increases. By this, the nutrient and oxygen supply to muscles increases, thus aiding in their restoration.

Stage 5 sleep is known as Rapid Eye Movement (REM) sleep. The rest of the stages are Non-Rapid Eye Movement (NREM) sleep. About 20% of our sleep is spent in REM sleep. During this stage, the eyeballs move rapidly, the breathing is shallow and irregular, and heart rate and blood pressure that were low in previous stages start rising. This is the stage an individual dream. This stage of sleep helps in revitalizing the brain and readies it for the activation for the following day.

A healthy sleep consists of four to six cycles of these stages in a night. Any activity that disrupts induction of sleep or the sleep cycles can be labelled as an unhealthy sleep habit.

Habits That Interfere with Sleep

Exposure to technological gadgets like T.V., mobile phone, computer, tablet or any electronic screen, including e-book, gives the stimulus of bright light. This in turn interferes with melatonin secretion. Thus, working on any of these gadgets before bedtime may wade away the sleep because they interrupt secretion of melatonin.

Many people do not undergo the five stages of sleep. As a result, though they sleep for adequate duration they do not feel 'rested' when they wake up in the morning. People who do not reach stages 3 and 4 of sleep do not have the advantage of tissue and muscle replenishment and revitalization of brain functioning. As a result, they feel tired and mentally less alert the following morning. The outcome of this is compromising efficiency in the daytime activities and discharge of responsibilities. Some people experience difficulty in falling asleep. Some others have problem staying asleep, while others experience difficulties waking up after sleep. All the above indicate problems, and there could be a number of causes for the same. We will concentrate here only on behavioural causes.

Many people have the habit of having their dinner just before sleep. It is possible that the late meal disrupts the peaceful sleep. As soon as one eats, the gastric juices start secreting. In a lying-down position, they may flow towards the throat. Further, the digestive activity in the body also has the potential to interfere with sleep.

Some people have the habit of consuming coffee, tea, alcohol or chocolates, or smoking a cigarette in the evening. They function as good stimulants, particularly if consumed within three hours of sleep time. The caffeine, alcohol or nicotine functions as effective stimulants and prevents one from falling asleep.

Watching an emotional T.V. serial, engaging in active telephonic conversation or indulging in emotional arguments before bedtime results in secretion of adrenaline that activates the sympathetic nervous system, and keeps the person in an arousal state, which is counterproductive for sleep.

Sleeping behaviour can be trained as a good conditioned response, which can be elicited by conditioning with a time, place and ambience that includes darkness. This calls for a 'sleep discipline'. Failure in sleep discipline is also a failure in sleep conditioning.

Unhealthy sleep behaviour leads to a number of health repercussions that include cardiovascular diseases, obesity, lowered cognitive function, negative affect state and also increase in the accident proneness. In view of all these, measures to improve sleep hygiene are strongly recommended.

Sleep Hygiene

Sleep hygiene is recommended so that the unhealthy sleep habits that are clear health risk behaviour are substituted with positive sleep behaviour. The following are a few guidelines to enhance sleep quality:

1. Dinner is recommended at least two hours before sleep time.
2. It is healthy to inculcate the habit of setting a specific sleep time. This facilitates the secretion of melatonin as a conditioned response.
3. Avoidance of caffeine, nicotine products and alcohol prior to sleep insulates one from being subjected to stimulants. Burke et al. (2015) conducted a double-blind, placebo-controlled study for 49 days. The results revealed that consumption of coffee to the magnitude of a double espresso, three hours prior to the routine sleep time, resulted in about a 40-minute phase delay in melatonin circadian rhythm in subjects. This was equal to about half the magnitude of phase delay caused by three-hour exposure to evening bright light.
4. Avoidance of any electronic screen devices prior to sleep facilitates melatonin secretion.
5. The bedroom with proper ambience of dim light/darkness, temperature between 18 and 24 degrees, soothing bed linen, pleasant and wild wall paintings, soft and clean bed induces relaxation.
6. A warm bath or a mild massage before sleep, and consumption of warm milk or light liquid high in minerals help in inducing sleep.

7   People working for long hours may find it useful to have short naps of 60 minutes that boost their physical and mental energy. Sometimes, one may have all the five stages of sleep within the short nap. Thus, it is not so much about the duration of sleep, but the quality of it that determines whether the sleep is healthy or unhealthy. In a study by Goldschmied, Cheng, Kemp, Caccamo, Roberts and Deldin (2015), 40 subjects were divided into two groups, viz. nappers and no-nappers condition. The nappers were allowed a brief mid-day nap, while the no-nappers were not allowed to nap. They were measured on emotional control and frustration tolerance. Results indicated a higher degree of emotional control (measured by impulsivity) and frustration tolerance among the nappers, while no-nappers showed a contrasting result. Thus, when the long shifts have become imperative for certain professions, forcing them to violate healthy sleep behaviour, compensation through short daytime naps may prove effective in shielding away the adverse impact on the affect states. A certain type of physical exercise or yoga during the day may facilitate good sleep. In a Pennsylvanian study, Chheda, Baritta and Gallagher (2015) used the data of 4, 29 and 110 adults surveyed in 2013 in Behavioural Risk Factor Surveillance System. They examined whether the identified ten types of activities showed any association with typical duration of sleep in comparison with no activity or walking. They found that those who adopted walking for exercise were found to have better sleeping habits. However, the impact was much better in those who adopted activities like running, yoga, gardening or playing golf.
8   Meditation promotes healthy sleep. Meditation brings the same effect of total relaxation to the body and mind. A number of studies proved the slowing of heart rate and blood pressure, regulated breathing, and drop in skin temperature and muscle tone during meditation. Such experiences bring the effects of calming the physiological and the psychological states, which is highly conducive to sleep.
9   Finally, sleep hygiene guidelines recommend against oversleeping. Sleeping for longer hours than what is recommended for the age may prove counterproductive to health. A study established a close association between longer hours of sleep and the susceptibility to stroke (Leng et al., 2015). Their prospective study on 9692 subjects between 42 and 81 years with 9.5 years of follow-up identified 346 cases of stroke. The results found a strong association between long sleep and increased risk of stroke. Those who reported persistently long hours of sleep or a remarkable increase in sleep duration over a period of time had a higher risk of stroke.

Unhealthy Sexual Behaviour

Sexual behaviour originates from a biological need, just as eating behaviour originates from the biological need for food when one is in the state of hunger. Similar to the exercise of discretion in eating healthy or unhealthy, even in sexual behaviour, it is the discretion of the individual that enables one to have healthy sexual behaviour. The absence of it leads one to indulge in unhealthy sexual behaviour. What is risky or unhealthy sexual behaviour? It refers to engaging in that sexual behaviour with another person that increases the probability of either one of them transmitting the infection to the other, becoming or making the partner pregnant when it is unwanted. Unlike the other health risk behaviour that involves only the person concerned, the sexual risk behaviour involves the second person who is the partner. Thus, the concept of risk behaviour is determined by two persons. In case one of the two is infected with sexually transmitted diseases, has multiple partners that in fact enhance the probability of being infected, or insists and indulges in unprotected sex, the risk for the other person is high.

The most vulnerable group for unhealthy sexual behaviour is the adolescent and young adult group. Stimulated by the new experience induced by hormonal secretion, unable to handle the pressing physical need that is majorly precipitated by exposure to the media, challenged by the peers, in their new search for identity and acceptance, driven by curiosity and need for new experience the adolescents, particularly those with no proper family guidance are found to engage in unhealthy sexual behaviour. In an Indian study, Singh and Misra (2012) found the indulgence in sexual intercourse among adolescents in India. The incidence was, however, found to be significantly higher among boys than girls, and among adolescent boys in metropolitan cities compared to the urban- and rural-dwelling boys. Among the girls, the incidence was found to be significantly higher among girls in metropolitan cities than those from urban or rural area. Two significant factors related to risk behaviour are the incidence of unprotected sex and sexual victimization. Boys and particularly those from metropolitan cities were found to have a protective sex compared to girls in general and compared to boys from urban and rural dwellings. Metro boys reported a higher incidence of sexual victimization than those from urban and rural backgrounds. Contrarily, a larger incidence of sexual victimization was reported by girls from urban background.

The above study throws insight into few facts. Irrespective of the geographical background, the Indian adolescents are found to indulge in sexual behaviour, including unprotected sexual practice. Secondly, the incidence of sexual victimization suggests that sustained relationship with partners is not a universal phenomenon. Either due to immaturity or manipulative, exploitative tendencies or because of other reasons, some partners feel victimized. Thus, there is a physical and psychological dimension to the unhealthy sexual behaviour.

One of the glaring and often quoted consequences of unprotected sexual intercourse is contacting Human Immunodeficiency Virus (HIV) and Acquired Deficiency Syndrome (AIDS). Table 4.5 presents the prevalence of HIV in population at the global level and in India.

The table enables to infer two facts. First, compared to the scenario at the global level, the prevalence of HIV in India at any time point is much lower. Second, between 1991 and 2002 there has been a progressive increase in the percentage of prevalence of HIV in India. Thereafter until the year 2017, there has been a declining trend. This suggests the effectiveness of awareness programmes as a public health measure. What used to be considered a stigma in society and taboo to discuss about is no more considered so presently. In a study by Nagpal, Rajendran, Hariharan, Seema and Rao (2017), the awareness about HIV/AIDS among schoolchildren studying in class 6th to 12th, results revealed a progressive increase in the knowledge levels on multidimensional levels about HIV/AIDS. Multidimensionality of knowledge refers to various aspects of knowledge such as the causes, symptoms, risks, duration, outcomes. Results also showed a progressive decrease in the misconception about HIV/AIDS.

Table 4.5 Prevalence of HIV across the World and India (values refer to percentage)

Global		India	
Year	Percentage	Year	Percentage
1990–1991	0.3	1991–1992	0.1
1992	0.4	1993	0.2
1993–1994	0.5	1994	0.3
1995–1996	0.6	1995–1996	0.4
1997–1999	0.7	1997–2002	0.5
2000–2006	0.8	2003–2006	0.4
2007–2011	0.7	2007–2011	0.3
2012–2018	0.8	2014–2017	0.2

Source: https://ourworldindata.org/hiv-aids

Trigger to Unhealthy Sexual Behaviour

Indulgence in unhealthy sexual behaviour poses a great threat of contacting sexually transmitted diseases that include HIV/AIDS. What are the factors responsible for driving the people to unhealthy sexual behaviour. The assumption is that it is the adolescent population who are found to adopt unhealthy sexual behaviour. However, studies on adults infected with HIV also suggest the practice of unhealthy sex. Some of the possible reasons for this are mentioned under the following points:

1. High impulsive behaviour on the part of either of the sexual partner may leave no time for protective measures.
2. Ignorance or knowledge deficit about the repercussions drives one towards the unsafe behaviour.
3. The misnomer of enhanced pleasure without protection, on the part of either of the partners, may coax or convince the other to yield.
4. Absence of perception of severity of the consequences drives one for the unhealthy behaviour. Perception of pleasurable outcome in such cases is likely to overpower the negative consequences perceived as low in severity.
5. Normally, even with the awareness of the consequences, there may be complacence and tendency to undermine one's own susceptibility to adverse consequences. This may result in risk behaviour.
6. High affiliation need and the fear of losing the partner may drive a person to the risk behaviour.
7. Low self-efficacy and hesitation in speaking and persuading the partner or lack of communication skills in convincing the partner about the consequence of the risk behaviour could also be a reason.
8. Peer pressure and acceptance, particularly among adolescents, may result in the risk behaviour.

A few studies have identified the causes behind unprotected sexual behaviour. Fauk et al. (2017) in their study on Indonesian homosexual men identified psychosocial factors contributing to unsafe sexual behaviour. They grouped them into behavioural, cognitive and environmental factors. Behavioural determinants identified factors such as having multiple sexual partners, indulgence in group and transactional sex practices as contributing to unprotected sex. Cognitive causes included knowledge deficiency about HIV/AIDS and condoms, expectation of pleasurable experience and low self-efficacy to discuss with the partner the use of condoms or HIV status.

Knowledge deficiency has been found as one of the contributing factors. In a Chinese study, Li, Huang, Cai, Xu, Huang and Shen (2009) explored to identify the determinants of sexual behaviour among the adolescent children of migrant workers. Their sample included 2821 adolescents around 14 years of age studying in schools. They measured knowledge, attitude and behaviour in relation to the risk of HIV and other sexually transmitted infections (STI). The results identified that the factors that contributed to sexual behaviour among adolescents of migrant workers are lower family income, first sexual intercourse experience at a younger age, deficient knowledge about HIV/AIDS and scarce communication on issues related to HIV/AIDS. Thus, limited information on reproductive health is found to emerge as one of the main reasons for health risk behaviour related to sex.

Lack of knowledge about HIV and other sexually transmitted diseases places a normal adolescent or adult at high risk if one adapts unprotected sexual practice and more so if one indulges in having casual partner or multiple partners. This is because there would be no way to know if the partner is infected with HIV, since those infected are also found to participate in unprotected sex.

In a study on the HIV-infected sample in Ethiopia, Engedasket, Worku and Tasfaye (2014) found that 22.2% of the sample practised unprotected sex. Women, being single and long association with the partner were some of the factors associated with unprotected sex. Apart from this, restricted communication with the partners on the issue of safe sex and use of condom was also found to be a significant cause for practising unhealthy sexual behaviour.

Studies in India reported that 15%–22% of men and 1%–6% of women between the age group of 15–24 years engage in premarital sex (Mehra, Savithri, & Coutinho, 2002). Another study in the state of Gujarat, India, reported that 40% of males and 7.4% of females between 15 and 24 years have multiple partners, while 32% of males and 3.2% of females have sex in exchange for money (Sujay, 2009). In yet another study by Kumar et al. (2011) among 2475 unmarried boys and girls, only 22.3% of boys and 6.3% of girls were found to have protected premarital sex.

In view of the emergence of knowledge deficit and low self-efficacy as factors contributing to unhealthy sexual behaviour among various populations, the intervention measures related to reproductive health need to focus on efforts towards enhancing the knowledge base about the consequences of unhealthy sex and the high possibility of susceptibility for anyone who gives in to it even once.

Health Risk Behaviour as Acquired Habits

Two major health risk behaviours that are acquired during the course of life are smoking and alcohol consumption. Both these behaviours are initiated and gradually stabilized and mostly lead to addiction. Both have a number of health hazards. We will discuss these two health risk behaviours under this group.

Smoking Behaviour

Smoking or tobacco smoking refers to that behaviour that consists of drawing into the mouth, and usually, the lungs smoke from burning tobacco (West & Shiffman, 2016). When one inhales the tobacco smoke, one takes in the concentration of a number of carcinogens and a number of toxic chemicals. It contains carbon monoxide and gas. Carbon monoxide has the potential to displace oxygen from haemoglobin. As a reaction, the body produces more red blood corpuscles to compensate for the loss.

When one inhales the tobacco smoke, one takes in the concentration of a number of carcinogens and a number of toxic chemicals. It contains carbon monoxide and gas. Carbon has the potential to displace oxygen from haemoglobin. As a reaction, the body produces more red blood corpuscles to compensate for the loss.

According to the report by the World Health Organization (2013), about six million premature deaths per year worldwide can be attributed to smoking behaviour. Premature death refers to death from a smoking-related disease in a person who would otherwise have died later because of other reasons. Further, the smokers suffer diseases of old age 10 years earlier than the non-smokers (Jha & Peto, 2014).

When one inhales the chemicals and gas from the tobacco, they interact with a number of factors to cause damaging effects. It is just not the nicotine that harms the health. But there seems to be a synergistic impact. Taylor (2006) brought to light the synergistic effects of smoking. Box 4.1 describes this in brief.

Smoking is found to be associated with a number of diseases that impact cardiovascular, respiratory, reproductive, immune, gastrointestinal and nervous systems. In fact, it appears to have an adverse effect on all the systems of the body. Smoking has been found to be associated with an array of diseases such as coronary heart disease, stroke, cancer of lungs and upper airways

> **Box 4.1 Synergistic Effects of Smoking and Risk Factors**
>
> 1 The effect of smoking and cholesterol in combination is a high rate of morbidity and mortality due to cardiovascular diseases. The magnitude of risk is much higher than adding up the risk for the two. The interaction happens because nicotine in tobacco stimulates the release of free fatty acids. This result is the synthesis of triglycerides, which in turn decreases the HDL production.
> 2 For reasons unknown, smokers who are underweight have a greater risk of mortality compared to those whose weight is within the normal range.
> 3 Smoking is found to interact with stress. Male smokers experience an increased heart rate as reaction to stress, while for female smokers, the heart rate decreases as a reaction to stress, while the blood pressure shoots up. Both the reactions pose a risk to cardiac health and may even cause a cardiac emergency.
> 4 Female smokers, who have the genetic disposition of inability to break certain chemicals, have those chemicals (from smoking) in their blood. This increases their risk for breast cancer.
> 5 Smoking is found to be related to anxiety. In a way, the relationship between smoking and anxiety is one of conditioning. When one encounters an anxiety-provoking situation, and smokes a cigarette, the nicotine in tobacco changes the level of neuroregulators like acetylcholine, noradrenaline, dopamine, vasopressin and endogenous opioids. Acetylcholine and endorphin help in reducing the anxiety. Thus, a higher level of nicotine becomes conditioned to removal of anxiety. But when the nicotine level drops, one may experience anxiety until the level is restored by smoking. Similarly, any encounter with anxiety-inducing situation may trigger the need for smoking a cigarette (Figure 4.3).

and Chronic Obstructive Pulmonary Disease (COPD) (West, 2017). As per estimations, smoking increases the risk of coronary heart disease and stroke by two to four times (US Department of Health and Human Services, 2014). The same report also estimated the smoking increases the risk of lung cancer in men by 25 times, and developing lung cancer in women by 25.7 times.

How does smoking impact the circulatory system? Because of smoking, the blood vessels get damaged. The vessels become thick and narrow the path for blood flow. This results in heightened blood pressure, enhanced heartbeat and sometimes formation of blood clots. When a clot blocks blood flow to part of the brain or rupture in and around the brain, the consequence is a stroke. These clots can also cause blockage or reduced blood flow to the legs.

When the blood circulation is impacted, there is the possibility of its negative effects on all parts of the body. Skin is present all over the body. The impact of poor blood circulation can be seen on the skin. Because of the impaired blood flow, the oxygen supply to the skin takes the toll. This causes damage to the collagen and epithelial tissues. As a result, wound healing will be delayed, making surgeries a risky option even in emergencies. Because of impaired flow to the legs, walking becomes strained and painful.

How does smoking impact the respiratory system and cause respiratory diseases? The behaviour of smoking is one where the smoke is directly into the respiratory system and the smoke reaches the lungs. The smoke of cigarettes has a number of chemicals that directly impact the respiratory pathway and the lungs. Young adolescents, initiating the smoking behaviour, run the risk of preventing the growth of their lungs. The chemicals in the smoke have the potential to slow down the growth of lungs. The various chemicals also damage the airway, which narrows down gradually. The narrowed airway restricts and obstructs the flow of air resulting in a limited

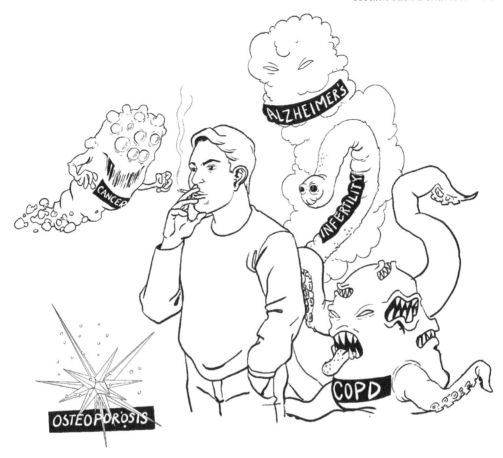

Figure 4.3 Smoking as Health Risk Behaviour.

inflow of oxygen to the lungs. The injury to lungs and airway causes Chronic Obstructive Pulmonary Disease. The narrowing down of the airway and blockage therein may lead to asthma.

How does smoking result in cancer? According to the report of the US Department of the Health and Human Services (2014), the cigarette smoking is responsible for 30% of all cancer deaths. Though the nicotine in tobacco per se does not cause cancer, the 69 chemicals present in tobacco are found to be carcinogenic. As a result of high carcinogenic content, smoking behaviour increases the risk of cancer to all the parts of the respiratory system, such as nose, sinuses, voice box, throat, pharynx and larynx. In addition, it also contributes to cancer in other parts of the body such as oesophagus, stomach, pancreas, kidneys, bladder and colon. It also causes myeloid leukaemia.

Apart from cardiovascular disease, cancer and respiratory diseases, which have been reiterated by a number of research findings, smoking is also found to pose a risk factor for a number of health hazards. According to a report of the US Department of Health and Human Services (2014), smoking is considered a risk factor for blindness, deafness, back pain, osteoporosis and serious peripheral vascular disease that may lead to amputation.

Mouth, the first contact of cigarettes, also takes the negative consequences of it. The teeth get discoloured because of nicotine stain. Tobacco reduces the flow of saliva in the mouth. Saliva is a natural cleansing agent for the teeth. Deprived of this, the teeth become vulnerable to decay.

According to the report of US Office of the Surgeon General's Report (1988), smoking can cause osteoporosis and degenerative disc diseases. Since the bone density is affected, one may suffer from spine and hip fractures. The impact of smoking can also be observed in reproductive health. It reduces the sperm count in men and causes impaired ovulation and egg function in female smokers (Gometz, 2011).

A UK report on Action on Smoking and Health (2013) states that smoking results in reduced fertility in both genders. Women who smoke during pregnancy have the risk of miscarriage, underdeveloped foetus, neonatal death, respiratory disease or mental health problems in the child.

The health hazards are not limited to active smokers, but it extends to other family members who by virtue of their presence in the immediate environment constitute passive smokers and have all the risk that smokers carry with them.

In addition to the physical health risk hazards, smoking also poses a risk to mental health in cognitive functioning and affect state. Smoking poses one to the risk of Alzheimer's disease and vascular dementia (de Toledo Ferraz Alves et al., 2011). Smoking, though may enhance the mental alertness and memory as an immediate result, in fact has the risk of addiction for it whenever one faces the challenge of any cognitive-related risk. Knowing that smoking, an acquired health risk behaviour, is proved to play such havoc with the health of the people, why do people smoke? Why do they relapse after quitting? The answers to these questions can be provided from a pure psychosocial perspective.

Antecedents to Smoking

Smoking behaviour is one that an individual learns and sustains at some point in life. It does not satisfy any of the basic biological needs (unlike eating, and sleeping that a human being inherits from birth). It is of interest to explore and identify the factors that drive an individual first to initiate the behaviour, then sustain it and then be unable to quit the same.

The studies worldwide endorse the fact that the majority of tobacco users get inducted into the habit during adolescence. Sunitha and Gururaj (2014) in their article referred to a WHO report that stated that more than 150 million adolescents were tobacco users. Parasuraman, Kishor, Singh and Vaidehi (2009) in their National Family Health Survey 3 mentioned that 40% of Indian men and 5% of women between the age groups of 15 and 24 years involved in consuming tobacco. Global Youth Tobacco Survey (GYTS) in the years 2006 and 2009 surveyed 180 schools. It found that cigarette smoking among 13- to 15-year-olds increased from 3.8% in the year 2006 to 4.4% in the year 2009 in India. Thus, there is enough evidence across the globe and in India that one gets inducted into the behaviour at a very early age of adolescence.

This can be examined from the perspective of learning (what reinforces), motivation (what needs are satisfied), cognition (what belief systems give rise to the behaviour) and emotions (what emotional states are associated with the behaviour). Let us first examine the factors that contribute to initiating the behaviour.

Smoking Behaviour: Contributing Factors

The major factors attracting the adolescents to initiate smoking behaviour include models in family disputes or peers.

Family: Adolescents who have at least one parent who smokes are likely to be smokers. This is because of observational learning. When the children see the parents an authority figure adopting the behaviour, and particularly if they find that the smoking behaviour is being rewarded and accepted by others, they are likely to internalize the behaviour in the process of imitation and modelling.

Secondly, if the family is in some major crisis like a member of the family being caught and booked under some criminal case, the main bread earner losing the job, parents undergoing marital problems or separating the child, they are likely to take to smoking behaviour as one of the deviant escape mechanisms.

Peers: In the majority of cases, the first cigarette is smoked in the presence of someone, which is very often a peer or a group of peers. Starting to smoke normally starts when one is in the company of those who are trying to smoke or have already started smoking. It may start in an adolescent either for peer acceptance or as a curiosity and experimentation or because of proving one's own 'toughness'. Those who have a high need for affiliation are more likely to take on to smoking for gaining acceptance in the group. When the affiliation need is not satisfied by the family, one is more likely to seek this affiliation in peer groups.

The initial 'starters' are likely to transit into regular smokers if the peer group has already transited to regular smoking, if their academic orientation is weak, and if they are influenced by pro-smoking attitude, cannot depend on parental or family support or have already been initiated into consumption of alcohol.

Smoking and Self-Image

Very often, the smokers are projected as 'strong, tough, straight' protagonists in media. Dinh, Sarason, Peterson and Onstad (1995) found that early adolescence onwards, the image of a smoker is conceptualized as a rebellious, mature, tough individual. Thus, these characteristics get associated with the smoking behaviour. Those adolescents experiencing feelings of inadequacies or insecurity may try to take umbrage under smoking behaviour that provides them such image. This serves as a good compensation for them. Low self-esteem, external locus of control, dependency, feeling of powerlessness and social isolation have the potential to adopt smoking behaviour (Taylor, 2006).

Adolescents who have an aggressive tendency are attracted to smoking. Those under severe stress and depressive state, or experiencing distress or trauma are likely to get initiated into smoking. For them, the temporary relief from the negative state is highly reinforcing. Hence, the behaviour is likely to get strengthened.

In an article, West (2017) propounds that the smoking behaviour gets maintained mainly because of positive and negative reinforcing properties of nicotine itself. For a smoker, according to him the negative health repercussions are far and remote. Naturally while weighing the same, immediate rewards against the remote and uncertain negative impacts, the rewards emerge more attractive.

In an attempt to identify the determinants of smoking, Karadoğan, Önal and Kanbay (2018) conducted a survey on 2505 college students, pursuing two- or four-year degree programme. The findings in a way seemed to be in confirmation of the fact that people with a smoking parent are likely to be a smoker. The results revealed that 36.1% students who smoked had father as a smoker and 10.3% had mother as a smoker; and 15.3% had a sibling who smoked. Five factors emerged as closely related to the existing smoking behaviour. They are the gender (being a man), enrolment in a two-year programme in the college, having at least one smoker in the family, having all close friends as smokers and consumption of alcohol. The findings are in consonance with the factors we already discussed. While the presence of smoking member in the family and peer group as smokers needs no further explanation, the fact that the smokers were also alcohol consumers confirms that health risk behaviours are likely to be present in multiples. The findings that enrolment in a two-year degree course was associated with smoking suggest a lower academic orientation among the smokers.

The study by Cronk and Piasecki (2010) reiterated the presence of other smokers as an influencing factor. In addition to it, their study found that the strongest predictor was their living outside their original location. Further, when their place of living had no restriction on smoking, the students were found to be more likely to take to smoking. Very often, the peer influence casts a significant impact when there is no counterinfluence of family. Hence, it is very common to find students starting to live in hostels who yield to this health risk behaviour due to peer influence and unhealthy models.

Tobacco Consumption

In an Indian context, apart from cigarette smoking, tobacco is consumed in various other forms, the most popular being *paan* (betel leaves) with *zarda* (tobacco), *gutkha, khaini* and *hookah*. Even in consumption of these, the first window is the stage of adolescence. The impact of tobacco on health is the same in any of its forms. The prevalence of these is high in South Asian countries. *Paan* chewing is highly common in countries like India, Bangladesh, Pakistan, Sri Lanka, Thailand, Cambodia, Malaysia, Indonesia, China and many other Asian countries (Mukherjea, Modayil,Tong (2014)).

However, the smokeless tobacco consumption has some unique additional consequences. Chewing of these products results in oral mucosal lesions, seen as white plaque and periodontal disease. Smokeless tobacco is found to cause submucous fibrosis, a chronic devastating condition that has the potential for oral cancer (Niaz et al., 2017). According to these authors, smokeless tobacco consumption produces carcinogenic (potential to cause cancer) and genotoxic (a toxic agent that damages DNA molecules in genes causing mutations, tumours etc.) compounds on oral epithelium cells.

Paan masala is a mixture of areca nut commonly referred to as betel nut, slaked lime, catechu and other agents for flavour. It is available in many forms in India. Enumerating the harmful effects of it, Garg, Chaturvedi, Mishra and Datta (2015) identified its potential to damage almost all systems in the human body. Apart from causing the oral submucous fibrosis that may progress to cancer, it is known to have toxic effects on liver, kidneys and testes. It may even cause increased creatinine and deformities in sperm.

Very often, because of its taste and flavour, children get curious and get initiated into it. Like any other tobacco consumption habit, chewing *paan* or *gutkha* also leads to an addiction. In a study on schoolchildren between 10 and 15 years of age, Metgud, Murugesh, Kumar, Priya and Rashmi, Naik and Tak (2018) found that 28% of schoolchildren chewed *gutkha*. Of this, 25% were girls, while 75% were boys. While 70% of children believed that it is a bad habit, 30% did not label it as a bad habit. About half of the children in the sample were unaware of its harmful effects on health.

In view of various research findings, consumption of smokeless tobacco calls for equal attention, particularly in South Asian nations.

Alcohol Consumption

Consumption of alcohol is a health risk behaviour at an individual level. Just like tobacco consumption, this is an acquired behaviour that is likely to turn into a habit and later an addiction. When any addiction turns endemic in any society or nation, it becomes a social or national concern. Thus, consumption of alcohol and alcohol-related morbidity, mortality, crime and accidents have become a global concern.

World Health Organization gives an alarming picture related to the consequences of alcohol consumption. According to the WHO (2018) source, about three million deaths amounting to 5.3% of all deaths every year across the world are attributed to harmful consumption of alcohol. About 13.5% of deaths in the age group of 20–39 years are traced to be related to alcohol. A harmful use of alcohol is associated with more than 200 diseases, injuries and health conditions. Alcohol is causally related to a number of NCDs, injuries, and mental and behavioural disorders.

As per the fact sheet of the National Family Health Survey (NFHS-4) (2015–2016), 28.7% of urban men and 29.5% of rural men consume alcohol. A total of 29.2% of Indian men consume alcohol. Among women, 0.7% of urban women and 1.5% of rural women consume alcohol. However, there seems to be a declining trend in overall consumption of alcohol. When we compare with NFHS-3 (2005–2006), the consumption of alcohol was higher among both men and women. It declined from 31.9% to 29.2% among men and 2.2% to 2.1% among women.

The usual defence of people who consume alcohol is that they are 'within limits' and are 'moderate drinkers'. The standard drink according to the US criteria is 14 g or 1.2 ounces of beer, 8 ounces of malt liquor, 5 ounces of wine, or 1.5 ounces of distilled spirit like gin, rum, vodka or whisky. According to them, the prescription of standard has a gender difference. Binge and excessive drinking is defined for men and women differently. Women who have more than four drinks and men having more than five drinks on a single occasion are considered binge drinkers. For women, eight or more drinks per week and for men 15 or more drinks per week are considered 'excessive' drinks (Division of Population Health, 2018).

The standard prescribed by the US cannot be universal. In an article published in The Lancet, Wood et al. (2018) broke the myth of the 'standards' prescribed. Their study was on a huge sample of 5,99,912 current drinkers. Alcohol consumption was found to be linearly associated with stroke and coronary diseases. With regard to the amount of consumption, the results stated that, compared to those who reported consumption between 0 and less than 100 g of alcohol per week, those whose consumption was between 100 and 200 g per week, 200 and 350 g per week or more than 350 g per week had a lower life expectancy of six months, one to two years or four to five years respectively at the age of 40 years. The fact that the results did not mention any gender differences in risk or life expectancy questions the differential prescription of 'standard' based on gender. Further, based on the association between the quantity of alcohol and the health risk, as indicated by their study, the safe limits for alcohol consumption appear to be much lower than the standards recommended by the US government. The data did not suggest the absence of health risk among 'moderate drinkers' but indicated 'lower risk of' non-fatal heart attacks, and other cardiovascular problems.

Thus, setting a 'one-size-fit-all' standard threshold seems to have problems, because the threshold seems to be influenced by a number of other factors such as body weight, gender, rate of consumption of alcohol, present state of health, medication being taken. Hence, it may not be logical to claim that everybody below a set threshold of consumption is in a health safe zone (Achenback, 2018).

In view of the above, we shall discuss broadly the alcohol consumption as a health risk behaviour and impact of alcohol consumption on health.

Onset and Progression of Drinking Behaviour

A curious question that strikes many minds is how does one acquire the behaviour of alcohol consumption? How does this drinking progress into a habit and then an addiction? (Figure 4.4)

100 *Health Risk Behaviour*

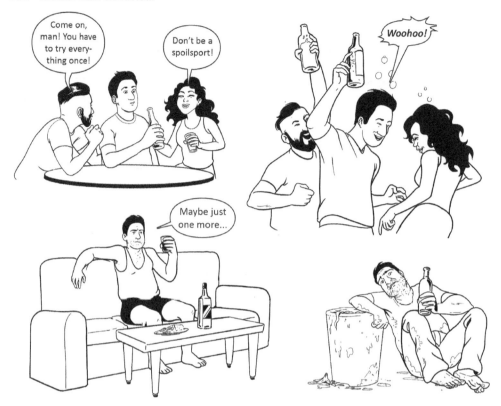

Figure 4.4 On the Road to Alcohol Addiction.

Like many acquired behaviour, it is likely to begin as a one-time curiosity or experimentation behaviour. From there, either because of the rewarding experience or due to peer pressure it continues. Further, it is found to repeat because of its immediate positive reinforcement value. Before one realizes, it has turned into a habit and then an addiction where he/she has already become dependent on this substance. Studies have identified genetic and socioeconomic factors contributing to the consumption of alcohol. However, the prominent influencing factors have emerged as psychological-behavioural and sociocultural factors contributing to alcohol-consuming behaviour, from the time of onset to progression to problem behaviour.

Onset of Alcohol Consumption

Very typically, the first incident of consuming alcohol happens in the presence of others. The reasons cited are either curiosity and experimentation or a social behaviour for deriving pleasure. Over time, the frequency of this 'social behaviour' increases. The instance of drinking in company of the peer group, social circles or colleagues gradually increases in frequency. The purpose of consumption of alcohol then smoothly transits from 'social reasons' to other reasons. There is a high possibility of peer pressure and peer acceptance as the reasons for initial drinking.

Drinking alcohol as a social behaviour with a purpose of deriving pleasure gradually shifts to one that helps one to relieve pain or fatigue. Mackinnon, Bhatia and Nadkarni (2017) in their qualitative study found the participants citing fatigue, pain, boredom as causes of drinking. They grouped them under 'functional use' of alcohol. A person who starts using it for relief from fatigue is likely to turn to it when he/she is too tired to wait and drink in company. Thus, the probability of drinking alone picks up.

Apart from physical fatigue and pain, the purpose is likely to expand to psychological stress. In such instances, any situation of life stress such as job demands, financial crisis, family interpersonal conflicts, any major life events or minor daily hassles, instead of triggering an active coping behaviour, may elicit the alcohol consumption behaviour, which can qualify as escape-avoidance coping strategy that focuses on temporarily reducing the emotional reaction in the face of stress.

Boredom stress is yet another reason for people taking to drinks, particularly those who already have had the first few drinks. Having no specific long- or short-term goals to pursue, unemployment or underemployment leaves a lot of free time at hand. Such boredom itself causes stress and may lead one to 'switch off' by adopting drinking behaviour.

Progression in Drinking

According to Mackinnon, Bhatia and Nadkarni (2017), "the progression from casual to problematic drinking is characterized by drinking alone". This has further characteristics of drinking behaviour associated with the availability of money and phases alternating between abstinence and heavy drinking. The period of the absence of drinking is used for rationalizing that one is not addicted and that one is capable of quitting at one's own will.

The availability of money poses an attraction to spend it on alcohol. Thus, gradually the individual progresses from spending available money to buy necessary quantity of alcohol to buying lower quality of alcohol if available funds are inadequate for a quality alcohol.

Problem Drinking & Alcoholism

The health risk behaviour of alcohol consumption may place one at the level of a casual drinking problem or alcoholic drinking behaviour.

Problem drinking refers to that behaviour where the consumption of alcohol results in substantial social, psychological and medical problems. However, the body of the consumer of alcohol is not physically dependent on alcohol. On the contrary, 'alcoholism' necessarily includes physical dependence on alcohol in addition to problems to health and life. A problem drinker may have alcohol, and interrupt the routine life as a result of which one may miss work, important social obligation and school/college/university, because of drinking. However, the person can go for days, weeks and even months without consuming alcohol. This is not possible for an alcoholic, because he/she is physically dependent on it. As soon as the alcohol level in the blood goes down, the person experiences a craving for it and has to consume alcohol. Without that, he/she may manifest withdrawal symptoms. This physiological dependence is manifested in certain fixed patterns in the drinking behaviour that requires a specific type of alcohol in specific quantity at specific time of the day. Alcoholics develop tolerance for alcohol. Unless the blood maintains a certain level of alcohol, they find it difficult to function and crave for a drink. While this is the significant feature of an alcoholic's behaviour, the problem drinker has a number of signs. Alcoholism and problem drinking may coexist. Box 4.2 presents the signs of a problem drinker.

> **Box 4.2 Signs of Problem Drinking**
>
> 1. Missing regular job/school/college or responsibilities
> 2. Avoidance of company of family and friends and preference to be alone
> 3. Depression, anger and violence manifested
> 4. Financial problems because of spending beyond one's capacity
> 5. Conflicts with family and friends and problems in the interpersonal relationship
> 6. Unsafe decisions in areas of crucial importance, e.g. unsafe sexual behaviour, financial hardships
> 7. Prone to get involved in illegal activities
> 8. Driving under the influence of alcohol
> 9. Experience of blackouts
> 10. Loss of memory when intoxicated

An individual who starts as a casual drinker may gradually progress to the stage of a problem drinker or alcoholic. The progression is also described in terms of stages. Jellinek (2018) described the following five stages of alcoholism.

Stage 1: Pre-alcoholism

At this stage, drinking begins as a social activity. However, the tendency to progress to advanced stages has certain warning signals. If someone is drinking because the social context is appropriate where everyone is drinking—only to be part of the social group—it may not be a cause for concern. However, if the purpose of drinking in the social environment is to get the experience of 'feeling better', it needs to be taken as a signal of being in the pre-alcoholic stage. Further, when the purpose of drinking is to handle stress, fatigue, pain, bothering thoughts or anxiety, probably one is in the pre-alcoholic stage and needs intervention.

Stage 2: Early Alcoholic

This stage is characterized by an ambivalence that has a combination of growing discomfort with drinking and difficulty to resist it. One may be found compromising on certain values by lying to family and friends about the drinking, hiding the alcohol or spiking one's soft drinks with alcohol. Between the irresistibility and shielding from the others, one may get obsessed with the thoughts about drinks.

Stage 3: Mild Alcoholic

This is a crucial stage that marks one transit ahead to addiction or retracts from the habit of drinking. This is the stage when the changes in physical appearance and behaviour usually make the fact obvious to those in close relation like family and friends. Physical symptoms of weight gain or loss, developing bloated stomach, flushy face may be the first signs to be observed by others. In addition, irritability, drinking during odd hours, missing work, or social functions for reasons of drinking or coping with the hangover during those times also reveal to others that the person is in an unhealthy phase of alcoholism. What is unique about the stage is that the person has cognition about getting trapped in addiction. One may also make attempts to resist and quit the habit. But the urge to drink is often successfully met with the help of external help. However, there may be some rare instances where the individual retracts from this health risk behaviour with one's own efforts.

Stage 4: Late Alcoholic

In this stage, the impact of long-term alcohol use becomes inevitable. The impact is shown on both physical and mental health. One may develop alcohol-associated physical illness like cirrhosis of liver, ulcer or cancer in the digestive organs or cardiovascular diseases to name a few. In addition, it may not be unusual to see people in this stage developing dementia, paranoid ideas etc. In this stage, some are found to manifest fearfulness that is inexplicable. Certainly, all these physical and mental health problems that are highly uncomfortable if not painful prompt one to stop drinking. But any attempt to discontinue may result in withdrawal symptoms that range from tremors to epileptic attack, anxiety, irritability and hallucinations. Hence, in order to overcome it, one may continue the habit.

Thus, it is an irony that as shown in Figure 4.5, the drinking behaviour that initiates because it gives a 'feel-good' factor or pleasure progresses for escape from stress, pain and fatigue transits to one of discomfort and then settles down to a behaviour, which despite negative impacts if stopped results in unpleasant physical and mental states. Thus, what starts as a pleasure-seeking behaviour reaches a stage where one has to sustain it in order to avoid pain.

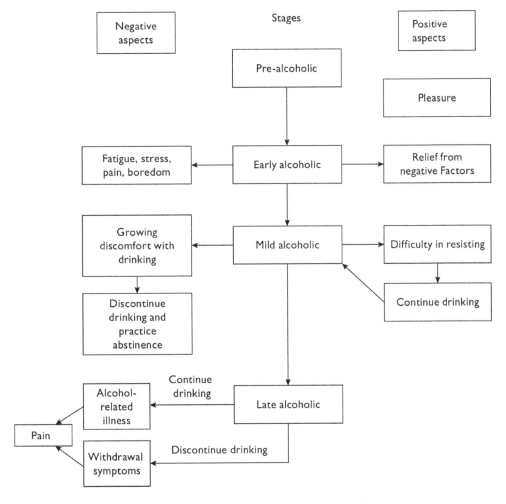

Figure 4.5 Progression of Stages in Alcoholism and Pleasure Pain Balance Sheet.

The progression along stages depends on a number of factors. Jackson (2010) studied the progression in 3331 youth between 12 and 18 years for treatment. He studied the age at which the first drink was consumed, first monthly drinking, first time one had more than five drinks, on a weekly basis, then daily basis. The results revealed that the participants reached the milestones at relatively young age and the transition between stages was swift. The transition was impacted by ethnicity and gender. Girls and Whites transited swiftly. Those who started at very early age of 10 years or earlier progressed relatively slow.

Alcohol Consumption and Consequences

Alcohol is an intoxicant. It consists of a number of chemicals that may interact with the biochemicals and produce certain reactions both at physical and at mental levels. These impacts can be immediate and sustained for short term or long term. Irrespective of the purpose for which one drinks, the impact of alcohol on physical and mental health occurs depending upon the volume of alcohol consumed, frequency and duration of drinking. Let us discuss the short-term and long-term consequences of alcohol consumption.

Short-Term Effects

One need not be a habitual drinker to have short-term effects of alcohol. To a certain extent, the short-term effect is determined by the body's tolerance to alcohol and the speed with which it is consumed. Keller and Vaillant (2018) state that liver has the capacity to metabolize roughly not more than one standard drink per hour, which varies with the individual's weight, age, gender and liver functioning. If the speed of drinking is high, and one consumes more than a standard drink in an hour, the blood alcohol level rises with every drink and the person gets intoxicated. Alcohol affects the central nervous system. As a part of its impact, there is likely to be a lowered communication between the body and mind, resulting in difficulties in coordination. As a result of this, the reflexes may take longer, and the body's reaction time may be higher than normal. Very often, one may observe a person under the influence of alcohol unable to maintain the physical balance. It slows down the information processing. Consequently, there is a change slowing down between the sensory inputs like visual, auditory, olfactory, gustation or kinaesthetic. The outcome of this is seen in a time gap between these inputs and the feeling experienced about these sensations. This culminates in a response delay. When blood alcohol levels rise very high, it may result in medical emergency due to alcohol poisoning. Drinking may give rise to a spectrum of temporary health problems that range from flushed skin, vomiting or passing out.

The cerebral cortex has a type of neurotransmitters called gamma-aminobutyric acid (GABA). This is the main inhibitory neurotransmitter in the brain. This facilitates communication among the brain cells. GABA plays a role in reducing the activity of neurons in the brain and central nervous system. This in turn impacts the body and mind by enhancing the relaxation and calmness, reducing the stress experience, bringing in balanced mood, alleviating pain and aiding in good sleep. Alcohol increases the level of GABA. This results in a drop in body temperature and lowered heartbeat.

Alcohol lowers the behavioural inhibitory centres in the brain by acting on moods, emotion and reactions. As a result, a person low in inhibition and high in relaxation tends to do so, say act and react in a way without any restraint, which under normal circumstances, one would not do because of the use of wisdom, discretion and restraint. It may start with becoming more talkative, pleasant and energetic. But with additional intake of alcohol, one may gradually manifest slurred speech, physical imbalance and aggressive act too. One tends to manifest exaggerated expressions of emotions under the influence of alcohol. This has a scientific explanation from the neuropsychological perspective. The prefrontal lobe of the brain is responsible for emotional control, aggressive thoughts and actions. It can precipitate the emotion already experienced. The emotional control is lost because the impact of alcohol on the prefrontal lobe is such that one loses the discretion of the limit. As a result, the expression of emotions goes out of hand.

One of the temporary effects of intoxication due to alcohol is blurred vision or double vision. This is temporary and gets back to normal with the impact of alcohol coming down during the day or the following morning. Blurry vision is usually the impact of binge drinking that amounts to about four drinks within two hours. The other impact seen in the eyes is the bloodshot eyes. This is the outcome of changes in blood pressure or dehydration.

Behavioural Risk of Alcohol and Repercussions

Because of lowered inhibition and less control on emotional expressions under the influence of alcohol, the way one behaves has potential risks for its impact on health. There is a possibility of risky sexual behaviour that includes unprotected sex, or having multiple partners resulting in unwanted pregnancies and sexually transmitted diseases (Naimi, Lipscomb, Brewer, & Colley, 2003). A number of studies have found miscarriage, stillbirth or foetal alcohol spectrum disorder (FASD) among women who are pregnant (WHO, 2014; Naimi et al., 2003).

A series of studies proved that while under the influence of alcohol, one experiences warm friendly sensations associated with enhanced socialization. This triggers a tendency to flirt with those who are 'perceived attractive' because of the influence of alcohol, but leads to feelings of regret the following day on finding the partner unattractive. This phenomenon of perceiving people more attractive under the influence of alcohol is called 'beer goggles'.

Consumption of alcohol in combination with cigarette smoking was found to have a higher impact on 'beer goggles' effect.

The impact of alcohol in lowering the inhibition has a higher possibility of leading a person to criminal behaviour. This is because the individual's emotional control is lowered and logical thought is temporarily suspended or inhibited. A person under the influence of alcohol is more prone to try other drugs, which are highly injurious to health. Because of the uncontrolled emotions under the influence of alcohol, persons are found to get aggressive and engage in fights that they would not do in normal conditions.

Long-Term Effects

The long-term negative effect of alcohol is almost on every system of the body. It impacts the nervous system, and endocrine, cardiovascular, digestive, reproductive and immune systems of the body. Let us examine each one of them.

Impact on Nervous System

Chronic drinking behaviour may cause a permanent damage to the brain resulting in impaired memory and related problems. Chronic alcohol consumption can even lead to a brain disorder called the Wernicke-Korsakoff Syndrome. This is caused by thiamine or vitamin B1 deficiency. They refer to two separate conditions that may coexist. Wernicke's disease (WD) is developed due to alcohol misuse or malnourishment. Very often, chronic drinkers miss their meals or under-eat due to the influence of alcohol. Hence, their chances of being affected by WD are high. The symptoms include double vision, drooping upper eyelid, loss of muscle coordination. Wernicke's disease may lead to Korsakoff's syndrome. A combination of these two manifests a confused mental state, amnesia, difficulty in comprehension, putting words into context and hallucination. Yet, another sign is the tendency of exaggerated storytelling (Krause & Roth, 2015).

Drinking alcohol over a long period of time may result in shrinking of the frontal lobe. This results in functional impairments in emotional control, short-term memory, reasoning and judgement. The brain finds it difficult to create long-term memories, making rational choice and many other vital functions. The damage that alcohol causes to the central nervous system results in numbness or tingling sensations in the hands and feet.

Thus, the nervous system suffers both structural and functional impairments as a result of long-term alcohol-consuming behaviour.

Impact on Cardiovascular System

People who consume alcohol have a higher risk of cardiac health problems compared to those who do not drink. Monico (2019) states that drinking alcohol has complicated impacts on cardiovascular health. As per WHO (2018) report, the global estimated deaths due to alcohol-related cardiovascular diseases in the year 2016 were 5.93 lakhs. The complications related to cardiovascular health include hypertension, irregular heartbeats, problems in the pumping power of the heart, formation of blood clots and strokes. Heart attacks and a condition called cardiomyopathy due to sagging of heart muscle are also common among alcohol consumers (Piano, 2017). Excessive drinking also results in anaemia.

Impact on Digestive System

In the long course, alcohol damages the digestive system. The impact on the digestive system may not be envisaged at the beginning stage, but one would come to know of it only after the damage is caused. The alcohol content may result in damaging the tissues of the digestive tract, and prevent the intestines from assimilation of nutrients. As a result, one may suffer from malnutrition.

When the digestive tract comes in contact with alcohol repeatedly, the walls may get damaged resulting in ulcers and haemorrhoids. This is caused due to dehydration because of heavy drinking. Further, there is a risk of cancers in the entire path of the digestive system, starting from mouth, throat, oesophagus, stomach, duodenum, intestine and colon.

Alcohol consumption also causes acidity, bloating of stomach, diarrhoea and painful stools in the people.

Damage to the Liver and Pancreas

Liver is a supportive digestive organ. The job of the liver is to flush the toxic matter out of the system. Alcohol is toxin. Thus, when alcohol is consumed the liver has to be active to screen out the toxic contents. This is done efficiently when the quantity and speed of consumption is within the reasonable limits so that the liver is put to its optimal activity. However, when the consumption crosses the capacity of liver's efficiency, the liver is put to overuse. Further, the alcohol has the potential to damage the tissues of the liver. This leads to scarring, which is called cirrhosis of liver. The long-term use of alcohol also results in alcoholic fatty liver disease. This indicates that the functional efficiency of the liver is suboptimal. With increasing damage to the liver, removal of toxins from the system becomes harder. Building up of toxic waste in the body is life-threatening.

Pancreas is considered a supportive part of the digestive system, as well as a part of the endocrine system. It is critical in producing insulin and glucagon, which are essential in regulating the blood glucose levels. A damaged pancreas may result either in low insulin production for utilizing the sugar or in excess of it leading to hypoglycaemia or hyperglycaemia. Excessive alcohol consumption triggers abnormal activation of these enzymes leading to a condition called pancreatitis. Pancreatitis is inflammation of pancreas that adversely affects digestion. If the insulin production is impaired, one may have diabetes and its side effects. Long-term abuse of alcohol places one at a risk of having pancreatic cancer, which spreads very fast and may turn fatal.

Impact on Reproductive System

We have discussed the risks of sexual behaviour as a short-term consequence, when the person is under the influence of alcohol. Now, we discuss the impact of consumption of alcohol excessively or regularly over a period of time on the reproductive system as a long-term impact, and it may lead to problems related to reproductive health. In men, it is one of the causes of erectile dysfunction, and in women, irregularity in the menstrual cycle. Alcohol consumption disrupts production of sex hormones and libidinal deficiency. Alcohol abusers from both genders have low fertility as a consequence of long-term use.

Impact on Kidneys

The kidneys have the delegated function of filtering harmful substances from the blood. Alcohol has toxic matter to be filtered. Both binge drinking and regular heavy drinking have the potential to damage the kidneys, because the more the alcohol in the blood, the more the demand on the function of kidneys. Binge drinking may lead to a condition called 'acute kidney failure'. Though this is a temporary condition and is curable, occasionally it leads to a permanent kidney damage. Heavy drinking is found to increase the risk of kidney disease by two-fold. It is worse when drinking is combined with smoking. This combination is found to increase the chance of chronic kidney disease (CKD) by five-fold.

Consuming alcohol is found to increase the chance of hypertension. Chronic hypertension that is not managed efficiently increases the risk of kidney damage. When alcohol damages the liver, its major functioning of filtering the blood of toxic matter is impaired. Because of this, the demand on the kidney is enhanced. The overfunctioning results in damage of the organ.

Impact on Skeletal System

Alcohol interferes with the production of vitamin D. Absorption of calcium in the body is aided by vitamin D. When the vitamin D level goes low in the body, it disrupts absorption of calcium. The resultant condition is deficiency in calcium. Calcium deficiency in turn leads to weak bones, osteoporosis, associated with pain and disability.

Impact on Immune System

There has been evidence to suggest the association between alcohol consumption and adverse effects related to immune system functioning. Alcohol adversely affects the innate immunity and adaptive immunity. This weakens the body's defences against infections, placing a chronic drinker vulnerable to a wide range of diseases caused by viruses, bacteria and infections. The behavioural risk factors of many of the people suffering from tuberculosis and pneumonia have identified alcohol abuse.

The first contact point of alcohol is the gastrointestinal tract. It adversely impacts the structure and integrity of the gastrointestinal tract. Consumption of alcohol results in damage to the epithelial cells, T cells and neutrophils in the GI system. This causes damage to the barrier and leaves a scope for the microbes to leak into the circulation.

Respiratory infections are also caused by alcohol. Alcohol disrupts the ciliary function in the upper respiratory path, damages the neutrophils and macrophages, and by impairing the epithelia of lower airways leaves the system vulnerable to infection.

Alcohol is found to be the culprit in people's recovery from physical trauma like burn, haemorrhage, shock and brain injury (Sarkar, Jung, & Wang, 2015). By impacting the immune system, alcohol leaves the abuser at risk for frequent illnesses.

Impact on Vision

When a person consumes more alcohol than what can be processed by the liver, the toxic substance enters into the bloodstream reaches various organs causing immense damage. The optic nerve is one such organ vulnerable to the damage. Alcohol changes the breathing pattern resulting in reduced oxygen intake. When the oxygen level in the blood is low, many sensitive tissues get damaged. Tissues in the optic nerve are once again the target. As a result of this, optic nerve suffers from macular degeneration. Macular degeneration affects the vision by making colours less vibrant and shapes fuzzy.

Some studies have found an association between alcohol abuse and development of cataract at younger age.

Impact on Mental Health

The short-term impact on cognition, affect and behaviour was already discussed earlier. What we will discuss here is the long-term impact of alcohol on mental health. An excessive use of alcohol may result in certain mental disorders such as depressive disorder, sleep disorder, bipolar disorder or psychotic disorder—all induced by alcohol. They are possibly associated with intoxication or withdrawal. Hence, they can be considered temporary (APA, 2013).

Alcohol abuse also may cause certain mental illnesses that either develop from the disorder or precede it. Illnesses such as major depression, anxiety, schizophrenia and bipolar disorder may have alcohol abuse as antecedence (Shivani, Goldsmith, & Anthenelli, 2002).

Psychosocial Repercussions

The impact of alcohol abuse is not limited to one's own physical and mental health. It impacts the family significantly, and the individual's relationship with the members of family, as well as others in the social circle that includes friends, colleagues, neighbours and relatives. Thus, the social dimensions of health take a toll.

An alcohol abuser is more likely to indulge in domestic violence than a person who does not abuse alcohol. Domestic violence creates trauma not only in the victim but also in all the family members, more so in children. Late-night episodes of violence create not only the trauma, but also sleep disturbances and its negative impact. Children's image of the parent involved in violence, and the victim of it in their impressionable age influences their perception of the social agents, trust and relationship with adults. Overall, it impacts their personality and personal values.

Binge drinking and alcohol dependence tend to move the person away from peers and normal social contacts, and either isolate oneself or form a group of people with the same tendency. As a result of this, the person and the family experience a type of social isolation that is more or less self-imposed. Sometimes, the family undergoes financial crisis because the alcohol abuser diverts money to the drinks bypassing other priority expenditure, and sometimes because major part of the expenditure goes into the treatment of frequent illnesses, the person suffers. Thus, the impact is not just on the wellbeing of the abuser but on the health and wellbeing of the entire family.

Box 4.3 gives a summary of the harmful health impacts of alcohol consumption.

Box 4.3   Health Risks of Alcohol Consumption

I   Impact on brain and mental health
1. Shrinking of the frontal lobe
2. Amnesia
3. Problems with attention, perception, concentration, learning, transfer of memory from short term to long term.
4. Lack of control on emotions, aggressive behaviour
5. Depression, anxiety
6. Schizophrenia, bipolar disorder
7. Hallucinations
8. Wernicke-Korsakoff Syndrome

II   Impact on cardiovascular health
1. Hypertension
2. Irregular heartbeats
3. Decreased pumping power of heart
4. Formation of blood clots
5. Stroke
6. Heart attack
7. Cardiomyopathy
8. Anaemia

III   Impact on digestive system
1. Malnutrition
2. Ulcers and haemorrhoids
3. Cancer in any part of the digestive tract
4. Diarrhoea
5. Acidity and bloating of stomach
6. Painful stools
7. Liver cirrhosis
8. Fatty liver
9. Pancreatitis
10. Cancer in pancreas/liver
11. Acute kidney failure
12. Chronic kidney disease

IV Impact on skeletal system
1. Vitamin D and calcium deficiency
2. Osteoporosis

V Impact on immune system
1. Pneumonia
2. Tuberculosis
3. Infection to any part of the body

VI Impact on vision
1. Blurred vision
2. Double vision
3. Early development of cataract
4. Macular degeneration
5. Optic nerve damage

VII Impact on reproductive health
1. Infertility in both genders
2. Unprotected sex/multiple partners leading to STD
3. Unwanted pregnancy

VIII Impact on renal system
1. Acute kidney failure
2. Chronic kidney disease

IX Impact on psychosocial life
1. Lowered inhibition and socially unacceptable behaviour
2. Domestic violence and strained interpersonal relationship
3. Self-imposed social isolation
4. Financial difficulties

Internet and Social Media Addiction

Internet addiction is characterized by excessive use, which is indicated by loss of sense of time and neglect of other basic needs, withdrawal syndrome manifested in anger, tension and depression in the face of computer inaccessibility. One of the highly prevalent health risk behaviours of 21st century is addiction to internet, social networking sites, such as Facebook, Twitter, WhatsApp, Instagram and any other form of social media. Addiction refers to a compulsive behaviour where people feel the compulsion to do certain activities repeatedly and so often that it turns to be a harmful habit because it interferes with the productive life of the individual such as academic work, professional responsibilities or family and social responsibilities. There is a difference between other addictions and this. For example, alcohol or cigarette is such whose use can be totally abstained, but the use of internet and social network has become an integral part of life in the 21st century. Hence, total abstinence cannot be advocated. However, when someone uses the media in excess checking the status and messages and twittering continuously that they consider the other productive and obligatory activities a hindrance to this, or prioritize the networking activities over the others, then it is a health risk behaviour or an addiction.

The impact of this addiction on health is two-fold: first, the effect of radiation on the nervous system; and second, the impact on family and social relationships and overall effect on decreased productivity.

Cell phones emit radiofrequency radiation, which is feared to be absorbed by the parts nearest to the device. There has been a series of studies to examine if this non-ionizing radiation causes cancer to the brain or casts other harmful effects on health. The findings were conflicting. Though few studies suggested an association between the use of cell phone and the malignant or non-malignant tumours, they failed to establish any cause-effect relationship (Grell et al., 2016; Schoemaker et al., 2005; Larjavaara et al., 2011, Cardis et al., 2011). Based on the mixed epidemiological findings that are inconclusive on the association between radiofrequency radiation and cancer, the International Agency for Research on Cancer classified radiofrequency fields as 'possibly carcinogenic to humans (group 2B)'. Research in this case is still continuing. In the absence of evidence of 'no risk', restricted use of mobile phones is advisable.

One conclusive evidence against the use of mobile phone is its use while driving. Because of distraction of attention, the risk of an accident is high. The accident risk increases with age because of delay in reaction time to brake. The risk is said to be equal to 0.05% of the blood alcohol level (Maier, Blakemore, & Koivisto, 2000).

While the hazardous effects of mobile phone on physical health are still under investigation for establishing cause-effect relationship, the addiction certainly is found to impact the mental health.

Alhassan et al. (2018) conducted a study to find out university student's addiction to mobile phone use and its association with depression. Their study on 935 students indicated a positive linear relationship between mobile phone addiction and depression. Qualification of school education and higher smartphone addiction were significant predictors of depression.

The use of mobile phones or internet itself is not related to mental health problem. It is the addiction to its use that may pose problems. The compulsion to check the messages, or the negative affect generated in the absence of an immediate response to a post or a message sent to someone is some of the indications of addiction. Panova and Lleras (2016) in their study on university students brought some clarity to the association between internet use and stress and anxiety. They studied a sample of 300 students' internet and mobile phone use, the motivation for the use and their mental health. The findings clearly showed that those who in their response described an addictive style of behaviour scored higher on depression and anxiety. Further, the motivating factor for use of the devices played a significant role. Those who used internet or mobile to fight their boredom did not show depression or anxiety. Thus, only when it was a compulsive behaviour, there was an association between anxiety and depression. The follow-up experimental study contributed in yet another way. It was found that during a stressful experimental situation, those having a cell phone but not using it were found to be less likely to be affected by the stress compared to those who were not having the cell phone. Thus, having a cell phone is found to provide a sense of severity.

The technology and electronic devices like laptop, notebook, tablet or mobile phone have occupied an important space in modern life. Their use has come to be an integral part of daily life. However, the discretion between judicious use and misuse decides the fine line between wellness and health risk.

What Maintains Health Risk Behaviour?

Most of the health behaviours are inculcated by parents as part of child-rearing, e.g. eating healthy diet, setting a fixed bedtime, getting good physical exercise, wearing seat belt and other habits of hygiene like brushing teeth, having a bath and maintaining hygiene in clothing. When there is consistency in training children in these aspects, they are likely to get integrated as values in children. However, inconsistent parenting on these issues leaves the children confused and to switch between compliance and deviation. Later on depending upon stronger influence by the peer group, media and exposure to knowledge, one may tend to cultivate a belief system of his/her own. This belief system plays a crucial role in guiding the health behaviour of the individual.

Of the major factors that play a role in sustenance of health risk behaviour are the cognition, motivation, need satisfaction, affect state, social support and self-efficacy. Let us discuss them in brief.

Cognitive Factors

Individual's knowledge level plays a significant role in the behaviour. The absence of knowledge, wrong knowledge or knowledge deficiency about the outcome of the health risk behaviour plays a great role in the individual's continuation of behaviour. For example, when the individual is unaware of the adipose deposit in the body with consumption of each meal of fat-rich food, the ignorance of the impact of alcohol on the GABA levels or being blind to the fact that about 60 different chemicals are puffed in with each cigarette, he/she is ignorant about the magnitude of damage it causes to health. Further, there also seems to be a conscious blinder drawn by oneself to absorb such information. There is normally a tendency for selective information absorption where one counts on the number of persons not having any health issues despite the health risk behaviour rather than seeing the other side of the coin.

Most of the health risk behaviours are initiated during adolescence when one is energetic, healthy and active. The negative impacts of the health risk behaviour are not shown on oneself immediately, and hence do not form part of 'experiential knowledge accumulation'. The cumulative negative impact event what constitutes part of knowledge appears remote and theoretical. Cognition formed through experience is more overpowering than the cognition gained through hearing or reading.

As a result of this, one's belief system is not likely to attach high value to the information on the seriousness of the implications of health risk behaviour or the probability that one may be vulnerable to the implications spelt out.

Yet, another factor associated with the continuation of health risk behaviour is the pace of progression of health risk behaviour. The progression is normally gradual, and sometimes, the marginal increments are not even taken into cognizance by the person. Hence, it is likely that the person may not even endorse it as a serious health risk behaviour, warranting any concern for change.

The people indulging in health risk behaviour normally keep company of those who also do the same. This opens the scope for mutual endorsement of selective information that reinforces their behaviour and refutes or ridicules those that contradict their behaviour. This happens as a part of avoidance of cognitive dissonance.

Motivational Factors

In case the person prefers to continue the health risk behaviour despite the knowledge about their negative impact, the health risk behaviour must be satisfying some need. If the health risk behaviour such as binge eating, binge drinking or smoking is resulting in the immediate experience of pleasure, it constitutes immediate reward or immediate goal satisfaction. On the contrary, the potential harmful effect manifests sometime in future. When these two are compared, the probability for gratification of need is higher than giving up the pleasure-providing behaviour in view of a punishment that appears remote in time.

An individual with a definite long-term goal in life pursues it. Anything that comes in the way of blocking the goal is not attractive to him/her. Thus, an adolescent or young person whose life goal is associated with health and fitness is less likely to yield to the immediate goal satisfaction of health risk behaviour compared to one who either has no definite life goal or has a goal that is not associated with health and fitness.

Factors Related to Affect State

The negative affect state is painful. No one wishes to be in the negative affect state for long. Any behaviour that helps one to get out of the negative affect state is considered desirable and rewarding.

The chemical components in tobacco and alcohol have the characteristic of creating a sense of relaxation in the consumer. Thus, a person under stress or negative mood experiences a sense of relief from that state. Thus, the conditioning between the health risk behaviour and relief from the stress establishes and the behaviour gets strengthened because of reinforcement value.

Social Support

Social support of people who constitute 'significant others' in a person's life is valued highly, particularly in the Indian context because Indian culture associates great value with affiliation need satisfaction. When the social group that also indulges in health risk behaviour constitutes the valued support network, the individual is likely to continue the behaviour. On the contrary, if the family and friends who disapprove of one's health risk behaviour constitute a significant social network, then one is likely to make efforts to withdraw from the behaviour.

Self-Efficacy

Self-efficacy is the individual's assessment of one's own ability to do things. A person with low self-efficacy is likely to maintain the status quo and not found successful in changing the behaviour. A number of personal factors as one's self-esteem, self-confidence and locus of control also contribute to continuing or ceasing the health risk behaviour.

Family Support and Involvement

The understanding, empathy, support, guidance and involvement of family are very essential at two stages, viz. as a preventive measure and once the behaviour is set in, to help the person out of it (in case of addiction) and into the health-promoting behaviour (in case of the absence of compliance in case of diet, exercise or sleep).

The parental support and modelling help not only the adolescents, but even for adult, the family plays a significant role in introducing and sustaining health-promoting behaviour and weaning someone off the health risk behaviour. The reluctant spouse when accompanied by life partner is more likely to comply with daily exercise than when nagged about non-compliance. Bringing creativity into kitchen may help a fussy eater to comply with the nutritive food.

Treating an adult addicted to tobacco or alcohol with empathy is very important. This needs to be treated as a health problem rather than a deliberate deviant behaviour. Support, empathy and mild challenge to the individual's self-efficacy work in a positive direction rather than playing a passive helpless recipient role in the context of domestic violence, or inappropriate behaviour under the influence of alcohol or being a willing passive smoker when the adult takes to tobacco smoking. Empathy in combination with disapproval of health risk behaviour helps in convincing the adult to seek professional help to change the health risk behaviour. Efforts at changing the person's health risk behaviour with no alternative positive behaviour may not be successful compared to a situation where a positive substitute is offered to occupy the time, energy and pleasure sought in the health risk behaviour.

Box 4.4 Researcher's Box

- Cognitive intervention on healthy diet and its impact on schoolchildren can be studied with following steps:

    1. Make a diet survey and identify children practising unhealthy diet
    2. Measure and record their BMI
    3. Provide them a 30-minute cognitive intervention on risk involved in unhealthy diet
    4. Provide them daily diary to record the details about every meal and in between munches
    5. Test them on relevant psychological and social parameters
    6. Correlate the psychosocial parameters with the adherence recorded in daily diary

- Impact of cognitive intervention on sleep hygiene can be measured. This calls for a pre- and post-intervention test of sleep hygiene practised by the sample. Other psychological, environmental and social parameters can also be tested in addition to sleep hygiene in order to find the influence of these associated variables.
- Survey designs can be planned to find out the prevalence of any of the health risk behaviour across ages. This helps in compiling scientific data on Indian population.
- Studies can be planned to compare the relative effectiveness of cognitive intervention, motivational interviewing and affective intervention in relinquishing a health risk behaviour and sustaining the same.
- Longitudinal studies can be designed to measure the impact of cognitive intervention against smoking and alcohol consumption on schoolchildren of different ages and socioeconomic status, and geographical locations.
- Knowledge, attitude and practice of various health risk behaviour can be studied in children and adolescents to predict their future health risk behaviour. Follow-up on them can validate the predictability.

Box 4.5 Practitioners Box

Patients diagnosed with diseases related to health risk behaviour require weaning them off the behaviour. The health psychologists can adopt appropriate behaviour therapy depending upon the other psychosocial parameters of the client. A few of them are suggested below:

1. Aversion therapy for the people wishing to give up smoking or alcohol consumption. The use of mild negative stimuli conditioned with the behaviour in laboratory setting followed by natural setting may be of help.
2. Cognitive and affective intervention through short video clippings or effective PowerPoint presentation produce good results.
3. Using successful case studies of person who stopped specific health risk behaviour like tobacco smoking or alcohol consumption may work as a good motivator.
4. Similarly, video clippings projecting the cases where the continuation of health risk behaviour resulted in adverse effects in progression of disease also may bring in a realistic perception of severity and susceptibility of health risk behaviour.
5. Counselling the client, family counselling and building social support groups for giving up the health risk behaviour are some of the best practices worth their trial.

References

Achenback, J. (2018). Moderate drinking guidelines are too loose study says, Health & Science, *The Washington Post* (WP company LLC, US). Retrieved from http://www.washingtonpost.com/national/health-science/moderate-drinking-guidelines-are-too-loose-study-says Retrieved on 01 June, 2019.

Action on Smoking and Health. (2013). *Smoking and reproduction*. London. Retrieval from http://www.ash.org.uk/files/documents/ASH_112.pdf

Alhassan, A. A., Alqadhib, E. M., Taha, N. W., Alahmari, R. A., Salam, M., & Almutairi, A. F. (2018). The relationship between addiction to smartphone usage and depression among adults: A cross sectional study. *BMC Psychiatry, 18*(1), 148.

American Psychiatric Association. (2013). *Diagnostic and statistical manual of mental disorders* (5th ed.). Washington, DC: American Psychiatric Association.

Burke, T. M., Markwald, R. R., McHill, A. W., Chinoy, E. D., Snider, J. A., Bessman, S. C., ... & Wright, K. P. (2015). Effects of caffeine on the human circadian clock in vivo and in vitro. *Science Translational Medicine, 7*(305), 305ra146–305ra146. doi: 10.1126/scitranslmed.aac5125

Cardis, E., Armstrong, B. K., Bowman, J. D., Giles, G. G., Hours, M., Krewski, D., ... & Brown, J. (2011). Risk of brain tumours in relation to estimated RF dose from mobile phones: Results from five Interphone countries. *Occupational and Environmental Medicine, 68*(9), 631–640.

Chheda, J., Baritta, H., & Gallagher, R. (2015). Yoga, running, weight lifting and gardening: Penn study maps the types of physical activity associated with better sleep habits. *Penn Medicine News,* June 4, 2015.

Cronk, N. J., & Piasecki, T. M. (2010). Contextual and subjective antecedents of smoking in a college student sample. *Nicotine & Tobacco Research, 12*(10), 997–1004.

de Toledo Ferraz Alves, T. C., Scazufca, M., Squarzoni, P., de Souza Duran, F. L., Tamashiro-Duran, J. H., Vallada, H. P., ... & Busatto, G. F. (2011). Subtle gray matter changes in temporo-parietal cortex associated with cardiovascular risk factors. *Journal of Alzheimer's Disease, 27*(3), 575–589.

Dinh, K. T., Sarason, I. G., Peterson, A. V., & Onstad, L. E. (1995). Children's perceptions of smokers and nonsmokers: A longitudinal study. *Health Psychology, 14*, 32–40.

Division of Population Health. (2018). National Centre for Chronic Disease Prevention and Health Promotion, U.S. Department of Health and Human Service. Retrieved from http://www.ccc.gov/alcohol/fact-sheets/alcohol-use.html. Retrieved on May 31, 2019.

Engedashet, E., Worku, A., & Tesfaye, G. (2014). Unprotected sexual practice and associated factors among people living with HIV at ante retroviral therapy clinics in Debrezeit Town, Ethiopia: A cross sectional study. *Reproductive Health, 11*(1), 56. doi: 10.1186/1742-4755-11-56

Ezzati, M. et al (2016). Trends in adult body-mass index in 200 countries from 1975 to 2014: A pooled analysis of 1698 population-based measurement studies with 19·2 million participants. Lancet, 387, 1377–1396.

Fauk, N. K., Crutzen, R., Merry, M. S., Putra, S., Sigilipoe, M. A., & Mwanri, L. (2017). Exploring determinants of unprotected sexual behavioursfavouring HIV transmission among men who have sex with men in Yogyakarta Indonesia. *Global Journal of Health Science, 9*(8), 158–164. doi: 10.5539/gjhs.v9n8p47

Garg, A., Chaturvedi, P., Mishra, A., & Datta, S. (2015). A review on harmful effects of pan masala. *Indian Journal of Cancer, 52*(4), 663.

Goldschmied, J. R., Cheng, P., Kemp, K., Caccamo, L., Roberts, J., & Deldin, P. J. (2015). Napping to modulate frustration and impulsivity: A pilot study. *Personality and Individual Differences, 86*, 164–167.

Gometz, E. D. (2011). Health effects of smoking and the benefits of quitting. *AMA Journal of Ethics, 13*(1), 31–35.

Grell, K., Frederiksen, K., Schüz, J., Cardis, E., Armstrong, B., Siemiatycki, J., ... & Hours, M. (2016). The intracranial distribution of gliomas in relation to exposure from mobile phones: Analyses from the INTERPHONE study. *American Journal of Epidemiology, 184*(11), 818–828.

Jackson, K. M. (2010). Progression through early drinking milestones in an adolescent treatment sample. *Addiction, 105*(3), 438–449.

Jellinek, E. M. (2018). The four stages of alcoholism, Alcohol.org, an American Addiction Centre's Resource. Retrieved from http://www.alcohol.org/alcoholism-types/stages Retrieval on June 3, 2019.

Jha, P., & Peto, R. (2014). Global effects of smoking, of quitting, and of taxing tobacco. *New England Journal of Medicine, 370*(1), 60–68.

Karadoğan, D., Önal, Ö., & Kanbay, Y. (2018). Prevalence and determinants of smoking status among university students: ArtvinÇoruh University sample. *PloS One, 13*(12), e0200671.

Keller, M., & Vaillant, G. E. (2018). Alcohol consumption. *Encyclopaedia Britannica in, 30*, 437–450.

Kinard, B. R., & Webster, C. (2012). Factors influencing unhealthy eating behaviour in US adolescents. *International Journal of Consumer Studies, 36*(1), 23–29.

Krause, L., & Roth, E. (2015, December 10). Wernicke-Korsakoff Syndrome. Retrieved January 4, 2017, from http://www.healthline.com/health/wernicke-korsakoff-syndrome

Kumar, G. A., Dandona, R., Kumar, S. P., & Dandona, L. (2011). Behavioral surveillance of premarital sex among never married young adults in a high HIV prevalence district in India. *AIDS and Behavior, 15*(1), 228–235.

Larjavaara, S., Schüz, J., Swerdlow, A., Feychting, M., Johansen, C., Lagorio, S., ... & Berg-Beckhoff, G. (2011). Location of gliomas in relation to mobile telephone use: A case-case and case-specular analysis. *American Journal of Epidemiology, 174*(1), 2–11.

Leng, Y., Cappuccio, F. P., Wainwright, N. W., Surtees, P. G., Luben, R., Brayne, C., & Khaw, K. T. (2015). Sleep duration and risk of fatal and nonfatal stroke: A prospective study and meta-analysis. *Neurology, 84*(11), 1072–1079. doi: 10.1212/WNL.0000000000001371

Li, S., Huang, H., Cai, Y., Xu, G., Huang, F., & Shen, X. (2009). Characteristics and determinants of sexual behavior among adolescents of migrant workers in Shangai (China). *BMC Public Health, 9*(1), 195.

Lim, S. S., Vos, T., Flaxman, A. D., Danaei, G., Shibuya, K., Adair-Rohani, H., ... & Aryee, M. (2012). A comparative risk assessment of burden of disease and injury attributable to 67 risk factors and risk factor clusters in 21 regions, 1990–2010: A systematic analysis for the Global Burden of Disease Study 2010. *The Lancet, 380*(9859), 2224–2260.

Mackinnon, N., Bhatia, U., & Nadkarni, A. (2017). The onset and progression of alcohol use disorders: A qualitative study from Goa, India. *Journal of Ethnicity in Substance Abuse, 18*(1), 89–102.

Maier, M., Blakemore, C., & Koivisto, M. (2000). The health hazards of mobile phones: The only established risk is of using one while driving. *British Medical Journal, 320*, 1288–1289.

Mehra, S., Savithri, R., & Coutinho, L. (2002). Sexual Behaviour among Adolescents and Young People in India, Some Emerging Trends. *M AMT A, Working Paper* (3).

Metgud, R., Murugesh, C. J., Kumar, B. S., Priya, N. K., Rashmi, P., Naik, S., & Tak, A. (2018). Prevalence, knowledge, and attitude of gutkha chewing among school children of Arsikere, India. *Journal of Cancer Research and Therapeutics, 14*(2), 368.

Monico, N. (2019). The Physical & Psychological Effects of Alcohol. Alcohol.org, An American Addiction Centre's Resource. Retrieved from http://www.alcohol.org/effects Retrieved on June 5, 2019.

Mukherjea A, Modayil MV, Tong EK (2014) Paan (pan) and paan (pan) masala should be considered tobacco products. *Tobacco Control*, Published Online First: 21 October 2014. doi: 10.1136/tobaccocontrol-2014-051700

Nagpal, A., Rajendran, A., Hariharan, M., Seema N. D. S. N., & Rao, C. R. (2017). Conceptualizing HIV/AIDS: Developmental trend in school children. *IOSR Journal of Nursing and Health Sciences, 6*(6), 74–81.

Naimi, T. S., Lipscomb, L. E., Brewer, R. D., & Gilbert, B. C. (2003). Binge drinking in the preconception period and the risk of unintended pregnancy: Implications for women and their children. *Pediatrics, 111*(Supplement 1), 1136–1141.

NFHS-3 (2005–2006). National Family Health Survey-3, Volume 1, *Ministry of Health and Family Welfare, Govt. of India.*

NFHS-4 (2015–2016). India Fact Sheet, National Family Health Survey-4, 2015–16, *Ministry of Health and Family Welfare, Govt. of India.*

Niaz, K., Maqbool, F., Khan, F., Bahadar, H., Hassan, F. I., & Abdollahi, M. (2017). Smokeless tobacco (paan and gutkha) consumption, prevalence, and contribution to oral cancer. *Epidemiology and Health, 39*, e2017009.

Office of the Surgeon General of the United States. (1988). *The health consequences of smoking-nicotine addiction*. U.S. Department of Health and Human Services [USDHHS] 1988, p. 9.

Panova, T., & Lleras, A. (2016). Avoidance or boredom: Negative mental health outcomes associated with use of Information and Communication Technologies depend on users' motivations. *Computers in Human Behavior, 58*, 249–258. doi: 10.1016/j.chb.2015.12.062

Parasuraman, S., Kishor, S., Singh, S. K., &Vaidehi, Y. (2009). A profile of youth in India. National Family Health Survey (NFHS-3) India 2005–06.

Piano, M. R. (2017). Alcohol's effects on the cardiovascular system. *Alcohol Research: Current Reviews, 38*(2), 219.

Pooja, Yadava, A., & Sharma, N. R. (2012). Body mass index: A vital marker of health. In: A. Yadava, D. Hooda, and N. R. Sharma (Eds.), *Biopsychosocial issues in positive health* (pp. 63–74). New Delhi: Global Vision Publishing House.

Sarkar, D., Jung, M. K., & Wang, H. J. (2015). Alcohol and the immune system. *Alcohol Research: Current Reviews, 37*(2), 153.

Schoemaker, M. J., Swerdlow, A. J., Ahlbom, A., Auvinen, A., Blaasaas, K. G., Cardis, E., ... & Klaeboe, L. (2005). Mobile phone use and risk of acoustic neuroma: Results of the Interphone case–control study in five North European countries. *British Journal of Cancer, 93*(7), 842–848.

Shivani, R., Goldsmith, R. J., & Anthenelli, R. M. (2002). Alcoholism and psychiatric disorders: Diagnostic challenges. *Alcohol Research and Health, 26*(2), 90–98.

Singh, A. K., Maheswari, A., Sharma, N., & Anand, K. (2006). Lifestyle associated risk factors in adolescents. *Indian Journal of Pediatrics, 73*, 55–60.

Singh, A. P., & Misra, G. (2012). Adolescent lifestyle in India: Prevalence of risk and promotive factors of health. *Psychology and Developing Societies, 24*(2), 145–160.

Sujay, R. (2009). Premarital Sexual Behaviour among Unmarried College Students of Gujarat, India Health and Population Innovation Fellowship Programme Working Paper, 2009; No 9. New Delhi: Population Council.

Sunitha, S., & Gururaj, G. (2014). Health behaviours& problems among young people in India: Cause for concern & call for action. *The Indian Journal of Medical Research, 140*(2), 185.

Taylor, S. E. (2006). *Health Psychology.* New Delhi: Tata McGraw-Hill Education.

US Department of Health and Human Services. (2014). *The health consequences of smoking—50 years of progress: A report of the Surgeon General.* Atlanta, GA: US Department of Health and Human Services.

West, R. (2017). Tobacco smoking: Health impact, prevalence, correlates and interventions. *Psychology & Health, 32*(8), 1018–1036. doi: 10.1080/08870446.2017.1325890

West, R., & Shiffman, S. (2016). *Smoking cessation* (3rd ed.). Abingdon: Health Press.

Wood, A. M., Kaptoge, S., Butterworth, A. S., Willeit, P., Warnakula, S., Bolton, T., … & Bell, S. (2018). Risk thresholds for alcohol consumption: combined analysis of individual-participant data for 599 912 current drinkers in 83 prospective studies. *The Lancet, 391*(10129), 1513–1523.

World Health Organization. (2013). *WHO report on the global tobacco epidemic, 2013: Enforcing bans on tobacco advertising, promotion and sponsorship.* Geneva: World Health Organization.

World Health Organization. (2014). *Protecting unborn babies from alcohol-related harm.* Geneva: World Health Organization.

World Health Organization. (2018). *Global status report on alcohol and health 2018* (pp. 73–74). Geneva: World Health Organization.

5 Theories of Health Behaviour

Health behaviour is explained from various theoretical perspectives. Theorists have explained the phenomenon from the angle of perception, cognition, motivation, social influence, incentives and personality factors such as self-efficacy. Every theory has its own merits and loopholes. The subsequent theories evolved with a purpose of plugging the deficits in the previous theory. Thus, it is a process of evolution. In the end, the researchers may choose the most appropriate theory in order to explain the health behaviour in one's own study. Before going into specific theories, it may be a good idea to know what is a theory and how it is different from a model.

What Is a Theory?

Before identifying and analysing the theories of health behaviour, it may be a relevant step to explain the very concept of 'theory'. In the simplest term, a theory is a construction of an 'idea' that explains a phenomenon through all the known variables and experiences related to the phenomenon. Kerlinger (1986) defined a theory as "a set of interrelated constructs (concepts), definitions and positions that present a systematic view of phenomenon, by specifying relationships among variables, with the purpose of explaining and predicting the phenomena" (p. 9). Concepts are the major components of a theory. Concepts need to be understood in the context of the theory. The meaning outside the context of the theory may vary. For example, Freud's concept of 'ego' has a different connotation outside his theory of personality. When concepts are specifically developed in the context of a theory or adopted for a theory, they are called constructs (Kerlinger, 1986). For example, 'conservation' is a construct in Piaget's theory of cognitive development. Every construct in the theory must have a precise definition. The construct of 'conservation' is defined in the context of Piaget's theory of cognitive development. It refers to a logical thinking ability that enables a person to determine that changing the form of a substance or object does not change its amount, volume or mass. However, the meaning of the term is totally different outside the context of the theory. The constructs need to be operationalized in terms of variables that can be empirically measured. Thus, the variables open up the scope for evaluating a theory through research.

There is a difference between a theory and a 'model'. A model is built by drawing inputs from a number of theories and empirical findings. Some complex phenomena such as health behaviour cannot be explained by a single theory. In such instances, the phenomena are explained through models. The Health Belief Model, Ecological Model, Precede-Proceed Model and Social Marketing Model are examples in the context of health promotion.

Theories and Their Usefulness

There is a close interlink between the theory, research and practice. They can be viewed as a continuum. "The best theory is informed by practice; the best practice should be grounded in theory", write Glanz, Rimer and Viswanath (2008). While theories are developed based on basic research, they need to be empirically tested through research. Thus, theories, research and practice mutually aid and strengthen each other. Hence, it may be right to state that theories are useful ingredients to research and practice, while they also function as feeders to continuously develop or improve a theory.

Interventions are usually based on theories, particularly in the context of behavioural science. Theories contribute significantly to planning, designing and implementing interventions. They are useful guides in evaluating the interventions. Theories provide answers to 'why, what and how' in the context of planning, implementing and evaluating interventions. For example, in the event a national health care scheme did not succeed in attracting the beneficiaries, the theories provide an answer for 'why' people behaved in a particular way (declining the scheme), 'what' is it that the policy should consider before designing a scheme and 'how' or in what 'form' and 'context' should it be offered in order to optimize its acceptability.

With the above essential knowledge, we now explain various theories/models of health behaviour.

Health Belief Model (HBM)

The Genesis

The Health Belief Model is perhaps the oldest and the most tested model of health behaviour. The origin of the Health Belief Model can be traced back to the failure of a public health programme in the US during the 1950s. It was noticed that people were not inclined to accept and adopt the screening tests for early detection of some asymptomatic diseases like tuberculosis, cervical cancer, dental diseases, rheumatic fever, polio and influenza. This happened despite the fact that these screening services were offered at low or no cost. What later gave a shape to the model was an attempt by a group of social psychologists working in the field of public health to explain why people failed to avail of the services.

The Health Belief Model was first conceived by Rosenstock (1966) and later developed, modified and refined by Becker (1974). In view of the backdrop, the major focus of the model at initial phases remained illness preventive behaviour, which was later extended and applied to a broader context.

The Health Belief Model (HBM) is identified as a cognitive model. The model can be conceptualized better with a clear understanding of the constructs explained below.

Perceived Susceptibility: Susceptibility refers to vulnerability. Perceived susceptibility refers to the beliefs about one's likelihood of contracting the disease or the condition. For example, a woman whose mother and sister were diagnosed with breast cancer will believe that she is more vulnerable to get breast cancer than a woman who has no family history.

Perceived Severity: This refers to the seriousness of the health problem. The seriousness of the person attributes to the physical consequences (e.g. pain, deformity or death) and social consequences (e.g. impact on one's job, family and social relatives) if the individual contracts the disease or if the person already contracted the disease that left untreated. For example, if an individual is communicated about the diagnosis of throat cancer in stage 3, the seriousness of it is assessed in terms of the expected pain, deformity, complications, financial implications, disruption to family commitments, emotional turmoil to the family etc. Perception of susceptibility and severity together pose a perceived threat.

Perceived Benefits: This refers to the individual's assessed beliefs about the relative benefits one reaps by engaging in preventive behaviour or health-seeking behaviour. The benefit assessment includes direct health benefits such as 'early detection enhances the probability of cure' and 'pleasing the spouse by consenting for screening test'. For example, when a patient with hypertension is advised by the doctor to adopt regular physical exercise to avoid possible cardiovascular complications, one may assess the benefits such as keeping oneself physically fit and regaining the body shape while evaluating the positive impact of averting serious health adversities. One may also consider the benefit of possible socialization while joining the tennis club in the community.

Perceived Barriers: This refers to the potential hurdles in taking up the recommended health behaviour. For example, a patient advised to bring changes in lifestyle by stopping smoking behaviour may think 'I can stop smoking, but how do I handle my stressful situation?' Similarly, a patient advised to walk for at least one hour every day may think 'Well, I love walking but it means that I need to start my day early, which is difficult'.

Self-efficacy: This factor was not present in the original model but was later added by Rosenstock, Strecher and Becker (1988). The concept has been borrowed from Bandura's (1977) Social Cognitive Theory of learning. Self-efficacy refers to belief in one's ability to execute a given behaviour.

Perceived Control: This construct is rarely mentioned except a few like Ogden (2007). It refers to the belief that based on past experience in health issues and having external or internal control over them could affect health.

The perceived benefit and perceived barriers normally lead to a cost-benefit analysis that either contributes to or prevents action. Thus, the perceived benefits, barriers, self-efficacy and perceived control culminate in health motivation.

Cues to actions. The cues are reminders or prompts to initiate action in congruence with intentions. The cues can be internal or external. Internal cues can be manifestation of a symptom (e.g. a reeling sensation in the head) or external (e.g. a reminder call from the doctor's clinic) to take a blood pressure reading, which was being put off for quite some time.

The Health Belief Model can be summarized in the following way. People will change their existing behaviour (health risk behaviour or the absence of health risk behaviour) to a more desirable health promotive and health protective behaviour depending on their perceptions and beliefs. In order to change the behaviour, they should perceive a potential threat in their existing behaviour. In addition, they need to believe that the benefits from changed behaviour overweigh the loss or inconveniences or pain. Further, they also should believe that they are capable of successfully implementing the change in health behaviour and that they can have control over their health. This disposition for a positive change can be augmented by a suggestion from a friend or exposure to a media campaign in initiating the behavioural change. The model was initially used to explain illness preventive behaviour, but later extended to other aspects of health behaviour (Figure 5.1).

The Model

The diagram explains the model in three categories, viz. modifying factors, individual beliefs and actions. The components of perceived susceptibility, seriousness, benefits, barriers, self-efficacy

122 *Theories of Health Behaviour*

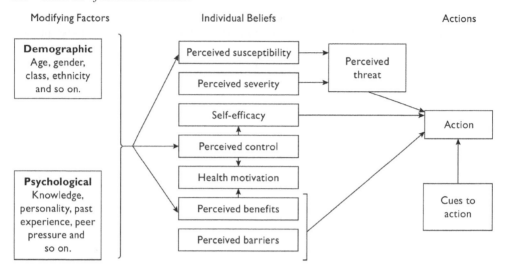

Figure 5.1 Health Belief Model.

and control are the individual beliefs. These beliefs are influenced by the demographic factors such as age, gender, cultural background on the one hand and psychosocial factors such as personality, knowledge, past experience, on the other. For instance perceptions vary based on the knowledge level. A patient with adequate knowledge about the risk factors for uncontrolled hypertension perceives the condition as very serious compared to the one who is ignorant about it. A woman who holds control over the menu of family meals may not perceive too many barriers in following a high-fibre/low-carbohydrate diet, while a man may perceive relatively stronger barriers. A cardiac patient from a poor family may perceive treatment cost as a major barrier for the advised Coronary Artery Bypass Grafting (CABG) compared to the one who comes from a sound financial background. An introvert may not perceive scope for socialization in joining a yoga group to comply with physical exercise as medical advice, while an extrovert will. Thus, all the beliefs related to health behaviour are shaped by demographic and psychosocial factors through the socialization process.

An individual who believes that he/she is vulnerable to a disease is more likely to respond positively to the call for a screening test.

Though one perceives susceptibility to a disease, only when it is combined with a belief that the consequences of the disease or condition would be severe in terms of one or a combination of consequences like severe pain expensive treatment, social stigma and family burden, one is likely to perceive a threat. The perception of threat, which is a combined outcome of susceptibility and severity perception, refers to personal health stake and negative consequences of it that are detrimental enough to cause a disruption. The negative balance between susceptibility and severity has to be high enough to create the threat. The cognitive imbalance generated by the threat perception pushes the person towards action and also contributes to the motivation for initiating appropriate health behaviour.

While the individual with threat perception is inclined for action, he/she also engages in a cost-benefit analysis. The sort of logical reasoning is a cognitive action. Only when the balance sheet of benefits and barriers weighs towards the benefits, does the person feel motivated to initiate action.

Apart from the perceived benefits and perceived barriers, there are other factors that contribute to motivation for action. They are self-efficacy and perception of control. An individual even after weighing the benefits and barriers will be successful in initiating a behaviour (change) only if he/she has the conviction in his/her personal ability to do so, and only when he/she believes that the issues related to personal health are under his/her control. This contributes to the motivation to initiate the behaviour.

The individual disposed to act is likely to start the action quicker when there is a propeller in the form of what is termed as 'cue to action'. A person after the cognitive exercise in assessment of the situation comes to a conclusion that the outcome of action is beneficial and the benefit has a personal value almost decides on the action. Translating this intent into concrete action happens with a trigger in the form of chance reading of an article about the impact of lifestyle on NCDs, or an experience of breathlessness while climbing stairs.

In short, the Health Belief Model explains that health behaviour depends upon the beliefs related to health, which in turn are influenced by a number of demographic and psychosocial factors. In order to bring a change in health behaviour, one needs to operate on the belief system related to health. Thus, intervention aimed at public health measures is likely to get optimal outcome if public perception is targeted.

Application

Research in general proved that people who go for regular health check-ups, follow discipline in their dietary habits and exercise regularly are likely to believe that they are susceptible to health problems, which have serious consequences, and the benefits of preventing the same are better than the inconveniences involved in following a healthy lifestyle compared to those who do not. Research also proved that people who have high adherence to medicines and medical advice related to their health problems believe that their health condition is susceptible to progression for the disease and complications, which will have bad repercussions compared to those who have low or no adherence.

Now let us examine the application of the Health Belief Model in specific contexts. The model has been used in the context of a broad range of health behaviour related to various health conditions and a broad range of subjects. The context of its application can be classified under three broad categories, viz. preventive health behaviour, comprising of health promotion (e.g. diet, exercise, screening), health risk behaviour (e.g. smoking, binge drinking), sick role behaviour (e.g. adherence to medication and medical advice during a phase of illness) and use of clinic (e.g. visit to clinics/hospitals for different reasons).

The earliest empirical study closely related to the Health Belief Model was by Hochbaum (1958). He studied the individual's beliefs about their susceptibility to tuberculosis and the benefits they believed to reap by subjecting themselves to screening for early detection. The findings revealed that 82% of people who believed that they were vulnerable to the disease and endorsed the benefits of early detection volunteered for chest X-ray. On the contrary, among those who did not perceive personal susceptibility and benefit out of early detection, only 21% volunteered for chest X-ray as a process of screening.

Starting with Hochbaum in 1958, until now, the Health Belief Model is applied in the context of preventive behaviour and found helpful in predicting the behaviour. Kim, Ahn and No (2012) applied the model to study the nutrition behaviour of college students. The results revealed that objective knowledge about nutrition, perceived benefits and perceived barriers of eating healthy food predicted the behavioural intention of eating nutrition food.

Studies found that knowledge intervention enhanced the motivation and thereby participation in screening tests as a preventive measure. This is possible only when the perception of susceptibility and seriousness are increased and perception of barriers is decreased. The knowledge intervention needs to be designed to target these cognitive components. Jeihooni et al. (2016) studied the nutritional behaviour related to the prevention of osteoporosis in 120 Indian women in a quasi-experimental design applying the Health Belief Model. The participants were randomly distributed into experimental and control groups. All the participants were administered a questionnaire measuring the constructs of the Health Belief Model and underwent a Bone Mineral Density Test (BMD) in the pre-intervention and post-intervention phase. The experimental group was exposed to knowledge intervention. It was found that the knowledge intervention impacted in increasing the perception of severity, benefit, motivation and self-efficacy and reduced the perception of barriers and susceptibility. A six-month follow-up showed a marginal non-significant increase in BMD in the experimental group and a decrease in the same in the control group.

In a quasi-experimental study on screening test for colorectal cancer, Moattar et al. (2014) equally divided 156 adults into experimental and control groups. The experimental group received knowledge intervention in line with the HBM. In the post-intervention, screening for colorectal cancer by Fecal Occult Blood Test (FOBT) and Colonoscopy was offered. Though there was a general reluctance in volunteering for screening, the participation of the experimental group in screening was significantly high compared to the control group.

Application of the Health Belief Model in the context of sexual behaviour was not very encouraging. Wiggers, De Wit, Gras, Coutinho and Hock (2003) investigated the psychosocial factors influencing the use of condoms in a sample of 537 men and women. The subjects were interviewed. It was found that the condom use was reported as consistent to 23% in primary partnership and 77% in casual partnership. Components in the HBM such as perceived susceptibility and severity of HIV, perceived benefit of condom use and cues to action did not influence the use of condom. Thus, the application of the HBM did not predict the protective sexual behaviour.

Limitations

Though the HBM is one of the most applied models in health behaviour, the limitations of it have also been pointed out. The model has been criticized on the following grounds:

1 **Fails to explain health-promoting habits:** It was pointed out that not all health behaviour can be viewed as an outcome of conscious cognitive processing. Certain health behaviour such as brushing the teeth in morning and night, having bath every morning, washing hands before eating are habits inculcated in the child-rearing process. One imbibes these health behaviours (preventive in nature) without weighing the benefits and barriers and without assessing susceptibility and seriousness. The model does not explain such behaviour that gets converted into 'habits'.

2 **Role of social influence ignored:** The entire emphasis of the HBM is on the individual. The behaviour is predicted based solely on the individual's assessment of the disease or condition and the pros and cons of initiating the behaviour advocated. However, many a time the health-promoting and health risk behaviours are the outcome of mere social influence rather than any conscious cognitive process. For example, children's high

adherence to medication is influenced by the adults, while adherence among adolescents is poor because of a shift in the social influence from the adults to the peer group. Similarly, sustenance of health risk behaviour such as smoking and rash driving is often the result of peer pressure than the cognitive process among the adolescents and young adults. The model is silent on whether health beliefs have a role in breaking habits that pose a health risk.

3 **Failure to operationalize the constructs and confusion over measurements:** Rosenstock (1966) did not specify the manner of interaction of variables with each other. He stated that the components operate independently and could be added to each other in a useful manner. This created a scope for confusion. The measurement of constructs in a model depends upon the clarity gained through operationalization of the same. There was a problem doing it because of the suggestion that susceptibility and severity are combined under the construct of threat and similarly benefits and barriers, weighed against each other. Having said that there was no specific direction in measuring the constructs, it creates a confusion as to whether the severity and susceptibility be added or multiplied to arrive at the threat index, or whether the two need to be measured separately. For example, HIV/AIDS is considered a serious illness by a 20-year-old person. However, his volunteering for a screening test will happen only if he perceives himself vulnerable to the disease. Some researchers suggested that severity figures in health decision only when it has certain magnitude even after reaching a decision on health behaviour based on perception of susceptibility. Similarly, whether to measure benefits and barriers separately or to combine them in a single index raised a confusion. The questions that arise are, is it right to combine the constructs that are qualitatively different? For example, how correct is it to combine the scores of perceived barriers relating to concrete realities such as financial constraints with perceived benefits such as avoidance of hypertension, which is hypothetical.

   The critiques (Ogden, 2007) posed a question as to whether the model is linear or multifactorial.

4 **Failure to take into account role of emotions:** Susceptibility relates to the perception of vulnerability to a disease. A number of studies validated its predictive value of health behaviour. Interventions targeting perceived susceptibility should design a health message wherein the personal vulnerability of the target population is emphasized. If health promotion messages overused to target susceptibility factor run the risk of provoking fear, the emotion of fear in the context of vulnerability to a disease may lead to denial, which is counterproductive to desirable change in health behaviour.

5 **Beliefs assumed to be static:** The HBM describes that beliefs occur simultaneously. There is no scope for the change in the dynamic process of belief. In reality, beliefs are dynamic and susceptible to change.

6 **No standardized measurements:** The model is tested by different studies in the context of different diseases predicting different health behaviours. The researchers used their tailor-made tools to measure the variables in the model. This is the consequence of not having a standard tool of measurement.

The limitations discussed above should not be viewed as the reasons for rejecting the model. The model is not wrong, but has a few shortcomings. Normally, the shortcomings of a theory/model are taken care of by a subsequent one, which is developed with an aim to address the loopholes in the model.

Box 5.1 Researcher's Box

The Health Belief Model is well tested in various contexts of health. Despite this, there is still wide scope of research related to this model.

- The whole model can be tested by fitting all variables as predictors of health behaviour or 'action'.
- Specific age groups like adolescents, young adults, can be compared on the influence of demographic factors on health beliefs.
- Sample from specific target groups like patients going for specific surgery or suffering from common NCDs can be chosen. All the variables under modifying factors, health beliefs and action can be studied by applying independent assessment tools. The entire model can be tested by identifying mediating and moderating variables and track the pathway from modifying factors to action.
- Cues to action are identified as a significant variable in the model. A study can be designed to assess the contribution of cues to action on the health behaviour. The sample of people who have been smokers at least for the past 24 months can be drawn. The sample should be tested on all the modifying and health belief variables. The entire sample should be divided into two equal groups following the randomization technique. One group has to be exposed to intervention that provides cues to action, while the other has to be treated as the control group. The sample should then be tested on 'action'. A comparison of the groups and appropriate statistical analysis gives an insight into the relative contribution of cues to action and the perceived threat to the health behaviour.
- Intervention studies can be designed by manipulating knowledge (to influence threat perception and the perception of benefits and barriers) and self-efficacy in control group studies to examine the impact in isolation and their interactions.
- Longitudinal studies with intervention package on children in high school stage in fact will be very valuable in influencing children in adopting a healthy lifestyle. These studies can identify either one or a combination of health risk behaviour. An intervention package exposing the children to the severity and consequences of these behaviours at preset intervals will constitute the independent variable. Follow-up on the sample until their late adulthood and examining the presence or absence of these behaviours at different stages help in standardizing the health intervention for various cultures, regions and age groups. Comparisons can also be planned taking counterparts of different cultures, regions or age groups.

Box 5.2 Practitioner's Box

Patients with non-communicable diseases need to change their lifestyle. Bringing a change in lifestyle is not possible with a pill or a surgery. It calls for changing the behaviour of the patients. Following are some aspects to be applied in health care:

- Health risk behaviour needs to be replaced with health-promoting behaviour. At the outset, take record of the modifying factors. Assess the patient's health belief and identify the strengths and weaknesses. In case of low scores on perceived severity

and susceptibility or benefits, the knowledge base needs to be assessed. In case of low scores, knowledge intervention has to be provided in an appropriate measure and method. Functional knowledge needs to be emphasized. If the score on self-efficacy is found to be below, counselling sessions aimed at enhancing self-efficacy need to be planned. If the perceived barriers are found to be high, the rationality of the same may be assessed. If necessary, family counselling may be offered.
- Group interventions for the patients with the same health problem will be very effective for knowledge enhancement, as well as strengthening self-efficacy. This is because of the efficiency of peer learning.
- Exposure to success stories through face-to-face interaction with those who changed lifestyle or video clippings for the group followed by a group discussion may not only change the health belief but also help in strengthening self-efficacy.

Protection Motivation Theory (PMT)

Background

Rogers (1975) is the founder of the Protection Motivation Theory (PMT): The original intention of Rogers was to explain the way people cope with fear appeals. Later in 1983, he extended it to persuasive communication. Thus, it was more a communication theory in its roots. The ideas of the theory are based on the work of Lazarus (1966) and Leventhal (1970), which concentrated on people's coping with stress. Thus, the major thrust of the theory is on cognitive appraisal and coping appraisal. PMT can also be viewed as an extension of the HBM in using the same constructs as perceived susceptibility and perceived severity as major components in explaining and predicting health behaviour.

Description of PMT

The Protection Motivation Theory assumes that the individual's intention is to protect health and embrace health protective behaviour. However, 'protection motivation' depends upon two appraisal processes, viz. appraisal of threat and appraisal of coping behaviour. The response in terms of health behaviour can be adaptive response (intent to protect oneself) or maladaptation response (behaviour that is contrary to health protection).

Protection Motivation Theory identified four basic components that are crucial for the intention to protect oneself:

1 Perceived severity of a threatened event (e.g. a cardiac arrest)
2 Perceived susceptibility of oneself to that event (e.g. the chances of facing cardiac arrest)
3 Perceived response efficacy (e.g. the efficacy of the recommended behaviour of stopping smoking in protecting from the occurrence of cardiac arrest)
4 Perceived self-efficacy (e.g. level of confidence in one's own ability to give up smoking)

Similar to the Health Belief Model, the constructs of PMT also are individual's perception. These perceptions are related to a number of factors comprising of information from various sources. The theory assumes that the sources of information can be broadly classified into two:

1 Environmental
2 Intrapersonal

Environmental sources are the verbal persuasions and observational learning of the individual about the specific health behaviours in question. Intrapersonal sources relate to the individual's personality variables and the past experience.

Taking inputs from these sources, the individual estimates the severity and susceptibility of the specific disease or health condition. A combination of these two estimates is called 'threat appraisal'. The individual also makes another appraisal, viz. 'coping appraisal'. This is a combination of assessment of 'response efficacy' (i.e. the expectancy of the individual that the recommended behaviour has the potential to insulate or protect him/her from the said disease or health condition) and assessment of self-efficacy (the confidence in one's ability to execute the recommended behaviour). The threat appraisal and coping appraisal together determine the 'behavioural intention' and thereby the 'behaviour'. This is explained in Figure 5.2.

The complexity of the model lies in the cognitive mediating process, which explains the entire process of cognitive assessment. In explaining the cognitive process, the following components need to be understood.

1. Fear: This refers to the emotional response triggered by the two sources of information. The information is not an input to trigger only the cognition. The contents also may trigger the affect, particularly when it is internalized. Thus, there is a role of emotion in the process.
2. Rewards: Rewards are intrinsic or extrinsic. They refer to the incentives the individual receives in continuing a (health risk) behaviour or not initiating a (health-promoting) behaviour. Thus, they refer to the factors that reinforce the sustenance of a wrong behaviour or maintaining the status quo.
3. Response costs: This refers to the evaluation of the gain or loss one sees in initiating or ceasing a behaviour compared to maintaining the status quo.

The Protection Motivation Theory with the cognitive mediation process is presented in Figure 5.3.

The figure shows two pathways between the information and the behavioural outcome, viz. the threat appraisal pathway and the coping appraisal pathway. Both the pathways lead to 'protection motivation', i.e. the intention to initiate a (health-promoting) behaviour or inhibit a (health risk) behaviour. The intention triggers the action. The threat appraisal pathway starts with the individual comparing the intrinsic and extrinsic rewards of the maladapted behaviour with the threats associated with the behaviour, i.e. severity and susceptibility perceived against

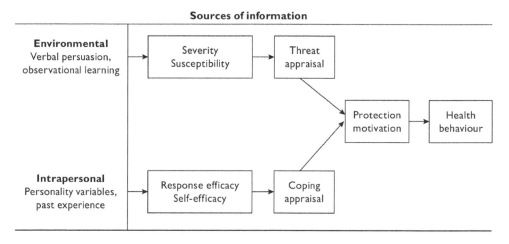

Figure 5.2 Fundamentals of Protection Motivation Theory.

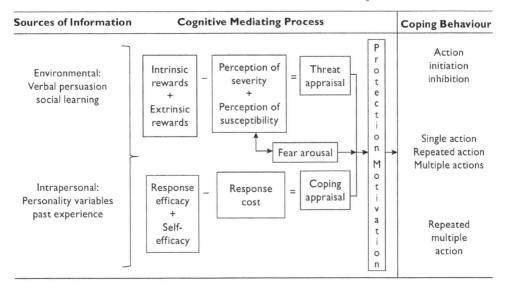

Figure 5.3 Protection Motivation Theory with Cognitive Mediation Process and Behavioural Outcome.

the knowledge background one has. In case the said maladaptive behaviour is associated with strong intrinsic and extrinsic rewards than the perceived threat, the intention of continuing the maladaptive behaviour will be high. The model also mentions the arousal of fear based on the information, which affects and also is affected by the threat appraisal.

The coping appraisal pathway starts with the individual's perception of the potential of the recommended behaviour in preventing the disease or health condition (response efficacy) and his/her own ability to successfully implement the recommended behaviour (self-efficacy). These efficacies are now compared with the cost of the recommended behaviour.

The threat appraisal and coping appraisal independently contribute to protection motivation, i.e. the intention of the behaviour. If the rewards are perceived as high and severity and susceptibility are perceived low, the threat appraisal is low. In such case, intention of continuing the maladaptive behaviour is high. On the contrary, if the efficacy is perceived high and response cost is perceived low, the probability of having intention of initiating adaptive behaviour is high. Thus, evolved protection motivation helps in triggering the health-promoting behaviour or stopping the health risk behaviour.

The coping thus evolved has the possibility of initiating the health behaviour first as a one-time action. Depending upon the cognitive mediating process and the outcome strength of it, the health behaviour may repeat itself, and evolve as multiple acts, which may subsequently strengthen and sustain as repeated multiple acts.

Though the Protection Motivation Theory refers to the component of fear, it does not explain much about this component. Further, Rippetoe and Rogers (1987) stated that fear aroused by communication has no direct impact on attitudes and behaviour. Hence, thus created fear is treated as "insignificant byproduct of threat appraisal" (Tanner, Hunt, & Eppright, 1991, p. 2).

Earlier research findings on communication had indicated the significance of fear. Studies by Ray and Wilkie (1970) found that communication that aroused an moderate level of fear enhanced the drive. Studies that followed also investigated the impact of optimal fear, role of personality variables in determining the impact of fear, social impact of fear etc., which failed to provide any conclusive evidence of the role of fear in behaviour. However, one cannot refute

130 *Theories of Health Behaviour*

that fear appeals sometimes influence the health behaviour. Tanner, Hunt, and Eppright (1991) presented what is termed as 'Ordered Protection Motivation Schema' (OPM). In OPM, the state of fear is assumed to bring the advantage of enhanced attention and the believability. This in turn enhances the probability of involving in coping appraisal because experience of emotion (fear) triggers the secondary appraisal, i.e. coping behaviour.

The OPM includes a component called Behaviour Repertory Appraisal as a factor contributing to threat appraisal. The current behaviour may have both adaptive and maladaptive coping, out of which any one may be employed in a situation. Hence, in addition to the four components used in cognitive appraisal, the Behavioural Repertory is also added.

The second component that is added is the 'social context'. It is argued that the arousal of fear may increase the drive for adopting effective and practicable coping. However, this effective coping behaviour is found to be guided by the social implications.

The OPM model also explains the intermediate states of emotion and motivation during cognitive process and between cognitive process and the health behaviour as an outcome.

The OPM model (Figure 5.4) depicts that the threat appraisal is influenced by the present behaviour of the individual, which has the contribution to social norms and values. The threat appraisal leads to fear, which in turn influences the perception of response efficacy and self-efficacy. The threat appraisal simultaneously contributes to coping appraisal, and the outcome is health behaviour. Similarly, the social norms and values have their influence in the coping appraisal and the final health behaviour in addition to the Behaviour Repertory. While the model calls the threat and coping appraisals as cognitive processes, the period between the two is identified as 'intermediate emotional state'. Similarly, the phase between the coping appraisal and the outcome behaviour called coping behaviour is called the intermediate state. This state assumes significance for 'protection motivation' or the intention for adaptive or maladaptive behaviour.

Application

The theory has been applied in a number of fields such as reducing the use of tobacco and alcohol, enhancing the lifestyle, and preventing sexually transmitted diseases, coronary heart disease and cancer.

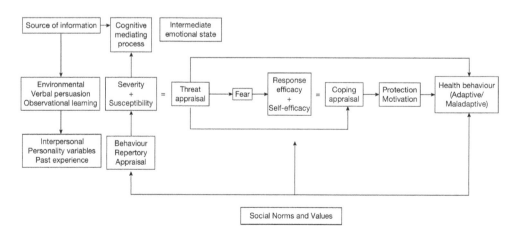

Figure 5.4 Ordered Protection Motivation Schema.

Yan et al. (2014) applied PMT in the context of smoking behaviour. The participants were 553 students from a vocational high school in China. They were administered a 21-item PMT scale measuring the constructs on a 7-point scale. They measured the four perceptions, viz. perceived threat, perceived rewards, perceived efficacy and perceived costs. In addition, they also measured the threat appraisal pathway and coping appraisal pathway. Further, they recorded the past smoking behaviour and intention of smoking behaviour. The results supported the theory, by finding that smoking behaviour was predicted by PMT. The results found that high perceived severity and susceptibility, and high self-efficacy and response efficacy explained avoidance of smoking behaviour intentions. On the contrary, high perception of rewards from smoking behaviour and high costs estimated from avoidance of smoking predicted maladaptive intentions of continuing smoking behaviour. However, the PMT measures differed in their strength of predicating the behaviour.

Grindley, Zizzi and Nasypany (2008) applied the theory on the patients advised physiotherapy for four to eight weeks. The sample comprised of 229 adults. The participants were assessed on the positive and negative affect, response efficacy and costs at the base level apart from the adherence to the physiotherapy session. The results revealed that affect was related to adherence to physiotherapy session. Dropout from the physiotherapy was predicted by affect, severity, self-efficacy and age.

Limitations

The PMT has been less criticized compared to HBM. However, many of the criticisms of the HBM also apply to PMT. Similar to the HBM, PMT considered the individuals as cognitive processors and did not quite explain the habitual behaviour. The social influence on behaviour is not taken into account. The impact of fear is not conclusive.

Box 5.3   Researcher's Box

- Testing the model: The model can be tested taking all the variables into consideration and evaluating the mediation role of the cognitive process.
- Quasi experimental designs can introduce the interventions through verbal persuasion and observational learning as environmental sources of information. Keeping the content and the exposure time constant, the relative impact of them on threat appraisal, fear arousal and coping appraisal and the subsequent influence on behaviour can be assessed.
- The impact of social learning with differential thrust on negative affect and self-efficacy can be studied.
- Intervention packages differing in their emphasis may be designed. One intervention package should have a thrust on the self-efficacy, overcoming hurdles and successfully bringing in a behavioural change. The second intervention package should have thrust on the 'severity' factor and the serious repercussions of non-adherence. The two packages may be so designed in the form of video films on two real-life models. Two groups of sample should be exposed to one of the two packages. The groups should be evaluated on threat appraisal, coping appraisal and health behaviour. The design can also be increased in complexity by adding one control group and a fourth group with exposure to both the intervention packages. The pre-post, multiple group comparison on adherence behaviour will throw light on the relative efficacy of the intervention packages. A follow-up on the sample also would throw light on the fear arousing 'severity' thrust intervention in sustenance of adherence.

132 *Theories of Health Behaviour*

Box 5.4 Practitioner's Box

Patients prescribed to disengage health risk behaviours such as smoking, drinking, binge eating, taking junk food or those advised to practise health-promoting behaviours including yoga in daily routine, following sleep hygiene, adhering to specific health-related diet require assessment at baseline and intervention in the said area followed by post-intervention assessment.

- The initial assessment that includes intrapersonal factors such as personality and post-experience may be helpful in planning interventions.
- Patients may be advised to draw a balance sheet on the positive and negative reinforcements of the existing health risk behaviour. Once completed, similar exercise may be given on the prescribed behaviour.
- The practitioner can manipulate the information through social models with adequate content and data based on severity and susceptibility.
- The patient may be assessed on perceived threat.
- Intervention aimed at enhancing self-efficacy can be provided. This should be followed by a short-term goal (varying from one to four weeks based on the patient's choice) of abstinence of health risk behaviour or practice of health-promoting behaviour. The length of the period can be marginally increased in every review meeting.
- After experimentation with the prescribed behaviour, the patient may be asked to draw the balance sheet of positive and negative outcomes of practising the behaviour during the experimental phase. The practitioner may have discussion or counselling sessions based on the differences between the balance sheet at the baseline and post-experimentation.

Theory of Reasoned Action (TRA)

The Theory of Reasoned Action was developed by Fishbein and Ajzen (1975). As indicated by the nomenclature, the theory speaks about the 'action' or behaviour that is an outcome of 'reasoning', hence 'Reasoned Action'. This core theme of the theory can be understood through the way it is explained. According to this theory, reasoning as antecedent of behaviour involves attitudes, believes, social norms and the value the subject associates with them. It explores the cognitive processes involved between the attitude and the behaviour, and identifies the social influence playing a significant role in determining the behaviour.

The components that construct the Theory of Reasoned Action are behavioural intention, subjective norm, attitude towards behaviour, normative belief, motivation to comply, outcome expectancy and outcome value. Figure 5.5 explains the way these components are linked in predicting the behaviour.

Behavioural intention refers to the readiness or the conscious predisposition of the individual to initiate a behaviour. The theory assumes that behavioural intentions proximally precede a behaviour.

The behavioural intentions are influenced by the individual's attitude towards the behaviour on the one hand and subjective norms on the other. The individual's attitudes towards a behaviour are formed taking the contributions from outcome expectancy of the behaviour and the evaluation of the outcome by the individual. Outcome expectancy refers to the individual's beliefs about the outcome of the proposed behaviour. These beliefs can be positive or negative.

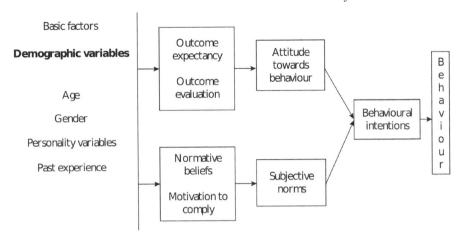

Figure 5.5 Theory of Reasoned Action.

Normative beliefs refer to the individual's belief about the attitude of important people towards the behaviour, i.e. the individual's perception of social pressure related to the behaviour. For example, in the context of alcohol consumption the normative beliefs could be, my family members want me to stop drinking and my close friends want me to continue drinking. Now, which of the two social pressures weighs heavy for one determines the behaviour one chooses to comply with, which refers to the motivation to comply. The perception of social norm and the pressure one feels to comply with lead to the subjective norm. The subjective norm is the outcome of the individual's evaluation of the importance of people whose approval or disapproval matters. The model states that the intention of behaviour is decided by a person weighing his/her personal attitudes towards a behaviour against the subjective norms. It may so happen that the individual who thinks that withdrawal syndrome is too painful and I don't like it (negative attitude) may still have intentions to give up alcohol if his subjective norm (my family will be happy if I stop smoking and my family's approval and happiness is important for me) is strongest.

The subjective norm assumes high significance in affiliation-oriented cultures like India, where decisions are normally taken with due consideration on the impact of it on the significant others. This does not negate the role of one's own independent assessment of the recommended behaviour. Thus, the behaviour is the outcome of two parallel reasoned processes. The behaviour need not necessarily be the 'right' one. The reasoning process involves two kinds of individual beliefs related to the recommended behaviour, viz. behavioural beliefs and normative beliefs. The behavioural beliefs are the individual's independent assessments of the likely outcomes of the behaviour. The normative beliefs are the individual's assessment about whether the significant others in one's life think that one should or should not perform the behaviour. Evaluation of these beliefs assumes significance, because they are crucial in deciding how ready or willing the person is in performing the behaviour. The evaluation of behavioural beliefs involves how good or bad are the likely consequences of the behaviour. The evaluation of normative beliefs is how important are the people who wish or do not wish that the person initiates the behaviour.

The Theory of Reasoned Action was subsequently developed by adding other constructs and called the Theory of Planned Behaviour. Hence, most of the applications reported in literature refer to both the theories in combination.

134 *Theories of Health Behaviour*

Application

TRA has been applied in preventive sexual behaviour, exercise and vaccination apart from smoking, alcohol consumption etc. Albarracin et al. (2001) applied the theory to predict the use of condoms. Results revealed a significant correlation between behaviour and intentions of behaviour. Intentions were predicted by attitudes towards condom use and the subjective norms. Doswell, Braxter, Cha and Kim (2011) used the framework of TRA to explain the sexual behaviour of African American adolescent girls. The behavioural intentions contributed to the sexual behaviour. Further, the results revealed that the behavioural intentions for early social behaviour were related to their pre-existing attitudes and the subjective norms of the peers.

Limitations

The TRA has been challenged on several grounds:

1. The model is developed initially to be applied on volitional behaviour (behaviour performed out of one's own will and choice) without examining the self-efficacy factor that is highly relevant as a prerequisite of volitional behaviour.
2. Most of the health behaviours are not volitional. Addictive behaviours such as smoking, alcoholism, and sexual behaviours such as use of condoms need not be volitional.
3. The TRA has not specified the transaction between attitude, subjective norm, intention and behaviour. It is possible that the attitudes are sometimes shaped by the behaviour. Thus, the cause-effect relationship between attitudes and behaviour is challenged.
4. Behavioural intentions are shaped by a number of factors other than attitudes and subjective norms. Operation of one's conscience, i.e. one's sense of right and wrong and the moral obligations, may influence the intentions.
5. Despite behavioural intentions, one may not execute a behaviour because of the habituation of past behaviour.
6. The relationship between intentions and behaviour appears to be short term.

Box 5.5   Researchers' Box

- Correlational designs can study the contribution of the basic factors on outcome expectancy, outcome evaluation, normative beliefs and motivation to comply.
- The outcome expectancy, outcome evaluation and normative beliefs and motivation to comply can be taken as predictor variables, and their independent and combined contributions to behavioural intention and behaviour can be studied.
- Comparisons of groups can be carried out after exposing them to different interventions influencing one aspect such as outcome expectancy or normative beliefs or a combination of the two.
- The model of Reasoned Action and Planned Behaviour can be assessed on improved efficacy of adding control beliefs and perceived behavioural control. This is possible by application of the Hierarchical Regression Model on the data from the same sample.

Box 5.6 Practitioner's Box

- The practitioner can effectively make use of the normative beliefs and subjective norms. Patients measuring high on these two aspects are likely to feel the pressure for change. These measures may coincide with high perceived social support. These patients need to be strengthened on the outcome expectancy and outcome evaluation. For this, a sound knowledge intervention can be planned.
- Patients measuring high on outcome expectancy and outcome evaluation but subnormal on normative beliefs need to be strengthened on this aspect. Planned sessions with family and significant others identified by the patients may be of good help.
- Patients not showing strength on control beliefs and perceived behavioural control may be encouraged to make short-term contracts on the behavioural change in order to gain confidence and consolidate their perception on behavioural control. This systematic progressive measure is essential for specific behavioural change in a phased manner.

Theory of Planned Behaviour (TPB)

The Theory of Planned Behaviour (TPB) is an extension of the Theory of Reasoned Action. The improvement on the Theory of Reasoned Action came in response to the criticism that the theory could explain only the behaviour that is volitional, while there may be a number of situations where despite the intentions to initiate a behaviour, one may fail because of several factors such as want of skills, abilities, opportunities, time or other material resources. Hence, unless the behavioural intentions are built upon the pragmatic considerations, they may fail to predict the behaviour. The modifications incorporated are with an intention to allow enhanced accuracy and reliability in predicting the behaviours, which is well deliberated and planned at a cognitive level.

Description

The core assumptions of the Theory of Planned Behaviour are same as that of the Theory of Reasoned Action. The assumptions are recapitulated briefly under the following points:

1. Intentions of behaviour are influenced by two pathways, viz. behavioural beliefs and normative beliefs.
2. Behavioural beliefs of the individual contribute to the individual's attitude towards the behaviour in question.
3. Normative beliefs influence the subjective norm.
4. The attitude towards the behaviour and the subjective norm contribute to the behavioural intentions, which in turn predict the actual behaviour.
    While the above points are common between the TRA and TPB, the following salient point is added in TPB.
5. Apart from the attitudes and subjective norms, there is a third factor that influences the behavioural intentions. This factor is called perceived behavioural control.

The understanding of TPB rests on the comprehension of this additional factor, viz. perceived behavioural control. Hence, there is a need to explain this concept at length.

Perceived Behavioural Control

The core factor of the TPB is the intention for behaviour. 'Intention' has a motivational connotation. Hence, it is inferred that the higher the intention, the higher the likelihood for the performance of the behaviour. Contrarily, very often the actual behaviour is found to depend on a number of non-motivational factors such as resource availability, support of social agents connected with the behaviour, the presence or absence of personal skills in performing the behaviour. These factors collectively represent the actual control over the behaviour in question. The presence or absence of these factors boosts or inhibits the behaviour. The individual's perception of behavioural control has an impact on both the intention and the behaviour in question.

In order to bring clarity to the concept of behavioural control, there is a need to explain it with a reference to the other related concepts.

Behavioural Control & Locus of Control

The concept of behavioural control is different from Rotters (1966) locus of control. Perceived behavioural control refers to the ease or difficulty one perceives in performing a particular behaviour in question. Perceived locus of control is a generalized perception that relates to whether the control over events in one's life lies within self (internal) or outside the self (external).

Behavioural Control & Achievement Motivation

Achievement motivation (Atkinson, 1964) is defined as the probability of succeeding in a given task. Behavioural control is one's perception of control over the specific behaviour based on objective consideration of the internal and external resources.

Behavioural Control & Self-Efficacy

Self-efficacy (Bandura, 1977, 1982) refers to the confidence one has in his/her ability in executing a particular behaviour. Such belief in one's ability influences a number of factors associated with the behaviour itself. Self-efficacy has an influence on the choice of activity, preparation for it, thoughts and emotions related to the activity, as well as the efforts one would invest in executing the activity. The concept of behavioural control is closely associated with this concept. The perception of 'internal' control factors refers to one's abilities and skills. Further, the individual's perception of control over behaviour influences other factors such as the individual's attitudes, subjective norms, intention and the behaviour itself.

The operation of the model is described with the help of Figure 5.6. According to the Theory of Planned Behaviour, the actual behaviour can be predicted by behavioural intentions and perceived behavioural control. Perceived behavioural control can predict the behavioural intentions and the behaviour itself. Perceived behavioural control is influenced by one's control beliefs. The control beliefs have two dimensions:

1. Beliefs about Internal Controls: This refers to the individual's perception of their own self being in control in performing the behaviour. It relates to one's assessment of himself/herself in knowledge, skill, ability and discipline required to perform the behaviour (Kraft, Rise, Sutton, & Røysamb, 2005). This concept is close to self-efficacy.
2. Beliefs about External Controls: This refers to a number of factors other than oneself. It includes cooperation of other people, availability of material resources such as money, time, opportunity.

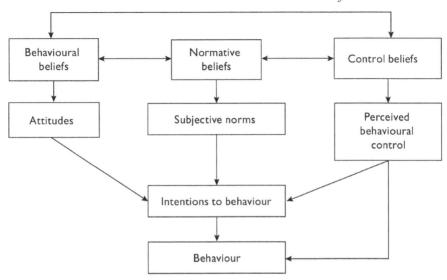

Figure 5.6 Theory of Planned Behaviour.

As shown in the figure, beliefs about internal and external control over behaviour influence and also are influenced by the behavioural beliefs, i.e. the expectancy of the outcome of the behaviour and the value of the same are assessed by the persons. Simultaneously, they also influence and are influenced in the normative beliefs, i.e. the perception of the person about the approval or disapproval of the behaviour by the significant others in the person's life.

The behavioural intentions are influenced by the subjective norms, attitudes and perceived behavioural control.

The difference between the Theory of Reasoned Action and Planned Behaviour is that in the Theory of Planned Behaviour, apart from the attitudes and subjective norms the behavioural intentions are also influenced by the perceived behavioural control. Secondly, while in the Theory of Reasoned Action the behaviour is predicted by the Intentions for Behaviour, in the Theory of Planned Action, the behaviour is predicted both by behavioural intentions and by perceived behavioural control. Further, the Theory of Planned Behaviour assumes the existence of mutual influence between the control beliefs, normative beliefs and behavioural beliefs.

Application

The empirical studies that validated the Theory of Reasoned Action hold good in testing the Theory of Planned Behaviour with regard to the variables common in both theories. The real application value of the Theory of Planned Behaviour lies in testing the predictive value of the added construct, viz. perceived behavioural control, and the way it correlates with other variables in the model.

Mok and Lee (2013) applied the theory of Planned Behaviour to predict the physical activity of adolescents in Hong Kong. Their sample constituted 486 adolescent students in the age group of 11–18 years. They measured the past physical activities and the attitude, subjective norm and behavioural control related to physical activity in the participants. The results revealed that about 75% of the sample failed to meet the norms of physical activities prescribed by the government. Subjective norms and perceived behavioural control predicted 53.1% of behavioural intention for physical activities.

Huchting, Lac and Labrie (2008) conducted a study to predict behavioural intentions and the behaviour of alcohol consumption among sorority women of Greek college students using the Theory of Planned Behaviour. They included a sample of 247 women in the sample. The participants responded to a questionnaire that measured four variables of TPB, viz. attitudes, subjective norms, perceived behavioural control and intentions to drink. The drinking behaviour was measured one month later. The statistical analysis of the structural equation model tracked the pathways to drinking behaviour. Results revealed that behavioural intentions (to drink) mediated between the attitude and norms on drinking behaviour. Subjective norms, more than the attitudes or behavioural control, predicted the intention to drink. Behavioural control was found to be a better predictor of behaviour than behavioural intentions.

Limitations

The Theory of Planned Behaviour was criticized on the following grounds:

1 **Weak prediction of behaviour:** There is sufficient evidence from the meta-analysis that prediction of actual behaviour by the variables in the model is far weaker compared to prediction of intention for behaviour. This indicates that there may be other (unidentified) variables contributing to the actual behaviour.
2 **Connect between variables has no universality:** It has been pointed out by researchers that the performance of a behaviour is not linked to attitudes, particularly in instances where the cognitive effort is the least. Similarly, the behaviour is not always linked to the behavioural intentions.
3 **Norms other than subjective norms as motivators:** Few studies (Evans & Norman, 2003; Manstead, 2000; Conner & Armitage, 1998) indicated the role of moral norms in predicting the behaviour and intentions. Some of the health behaviour such as sexual behaviour involving a partner in performing are motivated by moral norms than the subjective norms.
4 Behaviour guided by self-identity or label: Some health behaviours (e.g. eating behaviour) are found to be guided by the way an individual has 'labelled' oneself. For example, a person who has labelled oneself as a 'green activist' increases the intentions to consume organic food.
5 Self-efficacy rather than behavioural control was found to be a stronger predictor.

Transtheoretical Model (TTM)

This is otherwise known as the 'stages-of-change' model. This model was developed by Prochaska and DiClemente (1982, 1983, 1984). It is a synthesis of 18 therapies with the description of process of change in behaviour and its maintenance (Ogden, 2007). It integrates key constructs from other theories to explain the process of intentional behavioural change. It is called a model than a theory because it draws inputs from various theories to explain volitional behavioural change. The model evolved through studies on the smoking behaviour—people who quit smoking on their own. The model was developed on the basic assumption that change in behaviour does not occur quickly or decisively (especially when the behaviour in question is a habit), but the change is continuous through the cyclic process. The theory has its roots in studying smoking behaviour and can be applied to a variety of behaviour and various settings and can be applied on a wide variety of population. That is the reason it is called Transtheoretical Model (TTM). The model assumes that change in behaviour happens across stages, hence the nomenclature 'the Theory of Stages-of-Change'.

Stages of Change

The stages of change constitute the nucleus of the model. The stages refer to a temporal dimension, which is unique to the model, ignored by other theories. When the other theories explained behavioural change as an 'all-or-none' phenomenon where either the behaviour changed or the status quo continued, the TTM explained the change as dynamic; this is considered the great strength of the theory.

The unfolding of the change in behaviour over time is explained as an incremental progressive process that happens across five sages. Though the stages are explained as hierarchically organized, the model clearly states that the change in behaviour need not necessarily follow linear progression. Very often, individuals are found to regress to an earlier stage. The model provides sufficient scope for it, calling itself a spiral model.

The stages of change proposed by TTM can be viewed as 'motivational readiness' (Morrision & Bennett, 2006) as described below:

1 Pre-contemplation (not ready for change)
2 Contemplation (getting ready for change)
3 Preparation (ready for change)
4 Action (changing)
5 Maintenance (changed)

The description of TTM is shown in Figure 5.7 and the time period associated with each stage is presented in Table 5.1. Application of the model in a real-life situation is depicted in Figure 5.8.

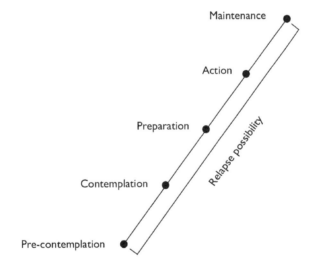

Figure 5.7 Transtheoretical Model.

Table 5.1 Temporal details of the stages of the TTM

Stage	Pre-contemplation	Contemplation	Preparation	Action	Maintenance	Relapse
Time	> 6 months	Next six months	Next one month	Now	≥ 6 months	Anytime

140 *Theories of Health Behaviour*

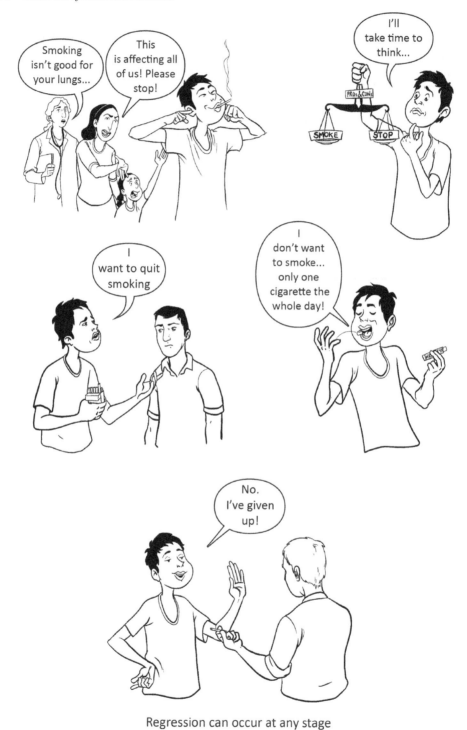

Figure 5.8 Stages of Transtheoretical Model in Real Life.

Temporal Details of the Stages of TTM

While the original model had the five stages, the following two were added later. They cannot be called stages in a strict sense (Figure 5.8).

6 Termination (change established)
7 Relapse (regression in change)

Let us examine each of these stages.

1 **Pre-contemplation:** This is a stage where people are 'not ready' for a change in behaviour. According to Prochaska and DiClemente (1983), the person in the stage has no intention to change the behaviour in the foreseeable future. They even measure the 'foreseeable future' as the 'next six months'. The reason for the lack of readiness could be their ignorance or inadequate knowledge about the adverse consequences of the behaviour they have been performing. Alternatively, they may be the individuals who, in the past, attempted change and faced failures, which in turn could have demoralized them. Persons belonging to either of the two categories will have resistance to any inflow of information with regard to their health risk behaviour. People in this stage are more likely to underweight the advantages of changing the behaviour and overestimate the costs or barriers of changing behaviour. This unmotivated and demoralized group of people was not included in the design of traditional theories.
2 **Contemplation:** This stage is characterized by people's readiness to change. People's intentions to change are given a time frame of 'next six months'. Unlike the first stage, people in this stage are aware of the advantages of changing the behaviour. They engage in weighing the pros and cons of changing the behaviour. However, in their calculations the pros and cons are likely to weigh equal, thus creating an ambivalence in them. From the point of view of advantages, the change in behaviour may appear attractive, while the comfort zone of continuing the present behaviour and not opting for change also may appear comfortable. They are in the process of deciding which of the two choices outweighs the other in their pros (Scholl, 2002). A person in the process of decision-making may get stuck in this process for a prolonged period. This phenomenon is called 'chronic contemplation' or 'behavioural procrastination'. The person in this stage still continues the health risk behaviour albeit the knowledge about the adverse consequences. However, the individual continues the contemplation as an effort to resolve the dilemma. The person, who finally perceives the pros of changing behaviour outweighing the continuation of the present behaviour, will move to the next stage, i.e. preparation.
3 **Preparation:** In this stage, the person is ready for change. The person is ready to take action in the next one month. Typically, a person in the stage is often found to have taken some initiative to change in the past year, though unsuccessfully. This person may feel nervous and may not know how to go about in initiating the change and may not be sure of one's own ability to make the right beginning. Sometimes, one may take small steps that they consider right in making a healthy beginning. For example, one may tell the people close to him/her that he/she wants to change. People in this stage need to be handled with encouragement. Intervention in the form of a plan of action to eliminate or significantly reduce the health risk behaviour may help the individuals in this stage to move to the next stage.
4 **Action:** This is a stage where the behavioural change is in present continuous tense. This is a stage where the individual is seen to have put in efforts to bring in overt changes in the behaviour in the past six months. The efforts to change are observable in terms of modification in their behaviour, environment and experiences. A word of caution about this stage is that the observable action needs to be construed only as 'trying to change' but not the change

itself. The actual change in behaviour has to qualify certain scientific criteria. For example, a heavy smoker in this stage reducing the number of cigarettes considerably was formerly considered as in this stage of 'action'. However, following the scientific criteria as 'sufficient to reduce the risk of problem behaviour', the consensus of scientists and professionals is only total abstinence but not reduction. This is because reduction in the number of cigarettes has the higher risk of regressing to old problem behaviour.

Persons in this stage need to learn techniques to strengthen their commitment to change and fight the temptations to regress. Interventions in the form of substituting the risk behaviour with positive and harmless behaviour (e.g. chewing herbs with strong tastes in place of smoking) will be of help. Further, training in the methods of avoiding people and situation that may induce temptations to relapse to old behaviour also will be of help. Counselling related to how a one time lapse should prevent a relapse also will constitute good intervention. The individual who perceives evidence of the advantages of the changed behaviour in terms of improved performance, experience of positive psychological state and positive social feedback is more likely to move to the next stage of sustaining the change.

5 **Maintenance:** This is a stage where one can say that the behavioural change has occurred. Overt modification in the behaviour/lifestyle is evident. The individuals work for prevention of relapse. This stage sees the person more confident to sustain the change and less likely to give in to temptations of relapse. A person is considered to be in the maintenance stage if he/she is able to be out of the problem behaviour for more than six months during which he/she is able to participate in new behaviour that is incompatible with the problem behaviour. Maintenance is not characterized by the mere cessation of the risk behaviour but has to be qualified by continuation of the change.

6 **Termination:** This is a stage where the behavioural change has been maintained for an adequate time so that the individual feels no desire to return to the health risk behaviour. The individual in this stage has a strong belief in one's self-efficacy in maintaining the changed behaviour. This stage is one that is not reached very often. Hence, the intervention programmes do not take it into cognizance.

7 **Relapse:** This is a stage where the person returns to the original health risk behaviour. This is not a stage by itself but can happen at any stage. This is highly applicable for people who say "Quitting smoking is not at all difficult; I have done it many times". Persons who have high addiction to health risk behaviours like smoking, drinking or taking other intoxicants are more vulnerable to relapse. They need to receive additional intervention at every stage in the form of continuous support from family, psychologist, employers and peer group to prevent relapse. Many a time, a single instance of lapse (performing the health risk behaviour) at the stage of action or maintenance may drive a person to regress. Hence, it is very important to prevent lapse converting to relapse.

The progress from one stage to the other is not smooth. It is like a snake and ladder game. For example, individual in the stage of preparation may slide back to the contemplation stage. He/she may remain for a prolonged period, before moving back to preparation stage again. Similarly, a person in the action stage may suffer a setback of temptation and regress to the contemplation stage with repeated incidents of lapses. The model recognizes such recycling, for which it is also known as the 'spiral model'.

The stages are characterized with cognition, affect, motivation and behaviour. The first two stages, i.e. pre-contemplation and contemplation, are generally defined by cognition, motivation and emotion. This stage of the preparation stage is marked by motivation and intentional behaviour or volitional behaviour. The stage of maintenance is process of behavioural change.

The model explains the psychological process that is in operation to help the individual progress along the stages. Some of these psychological processes are action in more than one stage. Prochaska and DiClemente (1983) explained the process of change. According to them, the process involves activation of cognitive, affective and behavioural domains. Understanding these processes is important because this helps to match the intervention to the appropriate stage based on the process involved in the stage. The stage-matched interventions are more effective as they are process-appropriate and boost the shift to the next stage. The theory identified ten processes that received support from empirical studies. Out of these, the first five processes are related to the early stages. They are called 'experiential'. The last five processes relate to the later stages and are called 'behavioural'. Table 5.2 shows the process of change across stages.

1 **Consciousness Raising:** This is a process in which the individual needs to attempt to enhance the knowledge and awareness related to the causes, negative consequences and the remedies of the problem behaviour. Interventions at the individual level through counselling, psychoeducation, cognitive therapy or at the mass level through media campaigns help in enhancing the knowledge. This process, in simple terms, is 'getting the facts'.
2 **Dramatic Relief:** Affect is the highlight of this process. The individual needs to experience and express the feelings and emotions in association with the problem behaviour. It includes the persons' fears, anxieties and worries related to the health risk behaviour. It may also include positive affect like feelings of inspiration on hearing success stories of people who changed their risk behaviour to healthy behaviour. Negative life events such as death of a family member due to the problem behaviour may induce the negative emotions. Positive life events where a family member or a close friend successfully changed to a healthy behaviour from the problem behaviour may elicit positive affect. Such emotions play a significant role in contributing to the outcome of behavioural change.
3 **Environmental Reevaluation:** This can be called a social cognition process. This involves the individual's perception and covert endorsement of the way the problem behaviour impacts others around. It also includes how the person through positive behaviour could be a role model for others. For example, an individual who smokes heavily understands how this smoking behaviour places his family members into high risk for cancer for being the passive smokers. It may also include the realization that his/her adolescent child may imbibe the risk behaviour taking the parent as a role model. Instead by changing the behaviour, one could be a passive role model for the child. Interventions such as documentaries, empathy training will be of help in moving the person to the subsequent stage.

Table 5.2 Process of change across stages of behavioural change

	Pre-contemplation	Contemplation	Preparation	Action	Maintenance
Process of change	Consciousness rating Dramatic relief Environmental reevaluation Social liberation Self-reevaluation	Self-liberation	Contingency management Helping relationships Counterconditioning Stimulus control		

Source: Adapted from https://en.wikipedia.org/wiki/Transtheoretical_model

4. **Social Liberation:** This is a process where the individual notices the public support. The individual realizes that society is supportive of healthy behaviour. For example, the individual with smoking behaviour realizes that the opportunities and alternatives for the non-problem behaviour have better support from society. For example, advocacy empowerment and policies to protect the health of minorities such as transgenders, socially marginalized population send a clear message about the support of society for health protective behaviour of the socially oppressed. In the same light, provision may be created for healthy behaviour. For example, public places identified as smoke-free zone, installation of free condom vending machines in red light areas etc. also send a clear social communication about the support for positive health behaviour.

5. **Self-Reevaluation:** This involves creating new self-image. There is a realization that the positive behaviour forms a significant aspect related to who they are and who they want to be. The self-reevaluation is a cognitive and affective process of realizing and assessing one's own self with and without the risk behaviour. For example, an alcoholic may assess oneself as an intelligent, sociable and affectionate person. But under the influence of alcohol, one may perceive oneself indulging in verbal and physical violence directed at the family members. Thus, one perceives one's own self with and without the risk behaviour in question. The contrast of this is likely to make them aware of the guilt associated with the negative behaviour. The self-reevaluation assumes significance in the movement of the person from the stage of contemplation to preparation. Interventions include corrective emotional experience and healthy role models.

6. **Self-Liberation:** The individual operates on the belief that he/she has the ability to change. This triggers their commitment to take action. New year or birthday resolutions, public testimony etc. are found to enhance the motivation and will power. Research evidence suggests that the commitment is stronger when the individual chooses from multiple alternations in giving up the risk behaviour.

7. **Contingency Management:** The health risk behaviour has been continuing with the individual because the behaviour provided some reward. For example, the 'relaxed feeling' that follows consumption of alcohol is what is the reward for the behaviour of consumption. The behaviour continues because of the rewarding outcome associated with it. Contingency management refers to managing things in a way where the individual perceives the change in behaviour more rewarding than the problem behaviour. For that, the rewards associated with health risk behaviour must reduce, while the rewards for the positive health behaviour must increase. Contingency management though considered punishment as an option of weakening the negative behaviour chose not to include it because self-changers depend more on rewards than punishments. The stage model operates on the philosophy of working in harmony with natural change than inducing the change forcibly. Interventions such as self-contract (e.g. If I do not smoke for the whole week, I will go on a weekend trip with my friend), overt and covert reinforcement recognition in the group etc. are recommended. The fit-bit worn on the sleeve to give feedback on health behaviours such as physical activities, calories burnt functions as a good automated reward to strengthen health behaviours like physical exercise, eating behaviour. These rewards help in repetition of positive behaviour.

8. **Helping Relationships:** This refers to getting help from supportive sources. The individual needs to identify those who are in support of their behavioural change and be open with them. Those who are actively involved in the process of changing the risk behaviour constitute the major source of support for the change. Confiding in them helps in weakening of any temptation to relapse to the old negative behaviour. Further, they constitute a strong source of reward through appreciation and recognition of positive behaviour.

Theories of Health Behaviour 145

9 **Counterconditioning:** This is related to the process of substitution. The individual learns to replace the unhealthy or health risk behaviour with healthy behaviour. The process has an assumption that the unhealthy behaviour continues because it is conditioned. In order to quit the unhealthy behaviour, the healthy behaviour needs to be conditioned to elicit the same outcome. For example, the 'strong oral sensation' one experiences with consumption of '*ghutka*' (a form of tobacco chewed) is the reason for which the health risk behaviour continues. In place of '*ghutka*', if the person is given healthy herbs to chew that provides similar oral sensation, the person gets counterconditioned. Similarly, counterconditioning can happen in other situation with therapeutic interventions such as relaxation, desensitization, assertion, thought substitution.

10 **Stimulus Control:** Managing one's own environment involves reorganizing one's own physical and social environment with a specific goal of enhancing the positive behaviour and reducing the negative behaviour. This can be done by arranging the cues appropriately so that there is support and encouragement for the positive, healthy behaviour. At the same time, there has to be efforts to remove any objects or situations from the environment that may encourage going back to the negative behaviour. Restructuring one's social support network so as to increase the frequency and duration of contact with those who support the behavioural change is one of the measures of stimulus control. Organizing and planning the activities in a way that compels the positive behaviour is yet another measure. For example, a person who has resolved to increase physical exercise may decide to park the car 2 km away from the workplace so that it becomes imminent for one to walk the distance every day. A person abstaining alcohol deciding to shift the residence to a state where prohibition is in force in fact is applying stimulus control.

The model assumes active participation and involvement of the individual throughout the progression of behavioural change. The involvement of the individual is seen in convert and overt action, assessing the relative advantages and disadvantages of the behavioural change. The progress in behavioural change is influenced by two major factors:

1 Decisional balance
2 Self-efficacy

1 **Decisional balance:** Decision-making involves constant comparison of the pros and cons of a decision. This involves drawing a mental balance sheet. In the context of the Transtheoretical Model, the individual has to constantly compare the pros and cons of adopting the proposed positive, healthy behaviour against that of the pros and cons of giving up the health risk behaviour.

   The individual's balance sheet of pros and cons is found to change across stages.

   a During the pre-contemplation stage, the pros of the health risk behaviour outweigh the cons.
   b During the contemplation stage, the pros and cons of the health risk behaviour and those of the proposed positive behaviour appear same, thus rendering the decision-making difficult.
   c During the action and maintenance stages, the cons of the health risk behaviour appear greater than the pros.

2 **Self-efficacy:** The concept of self-efficacy is borrowed from Bandura's theory. It refers to the confidence of the individual in his ability to perform an action in question. In the context of the TTM, the construct of self-efficacy is defined as the situation-specific confidence that an individual can cope with high-risk situations and not relapse back to the problem behaviour (Fallon & Hausenblas, 2004). It is considered an important factor that facilitates progressing movements

to the higher stages of behavioural change. In the pre-contemplation stage, where there are no intentions to change behaviour, the people are likely to report low self-efficacy. In the stage of contemplation, what the person perceives the pros and cons of problem behaviours and positive behaviours is almost equal. Self-efficacy plays a significant role in tilting the decision, motivating the person to the stage of preparation. Similarly, in the stage of preparation when the person starts to make up the small moves towards the positive behaviour, there is a possibility of feelings of uncertainty in plunging into action. Self-efficacy plays a crucial role because it instils confidence in the person that he could successfully initiate the change in behaviour.

During the earlier stages, there in a high probability of the individual to yield to the temptation and either not initiate behavioural change or relapse to the old behaviour. Self-efficacy and temptation are inversely related. An individual with high self-efficacy is very difficult to succumb to temptations compared to the one with low self-efficacy. Thus, self-efficacy helps in propelling the person to transit from one stage to the next.

Applications

The TTM has a number of variables to test the stages and process. It is difficult to accommodate all these aspects of the model in single studies. That could be the reason why studies applying the TTM limited themselves to select variables. The Transtheoretical Model was applied in the context of physical activity, risk behaviour and clinical adherence for specific illnesses.

Holmen et al. (2016) tested the TTM on patients diagnosed with type 2 diabetes. They included a sample of 151 adults above the age of 18 years with their HbA1c level 7.1% or more. Stages of change was categorized as 'pre-action' and 'action'. Self-management and quality of life were measured in the sample. Results revealed that 58% were in the pre-action stage for physical activity change and 79% were in the pre-action stage for change in diet. Higher scores of self-management were related scores in the 'action' stage. Higher body mass index was associated with reduced chances of being in the action stage.

Liu, Kueh, Arifin, Kim and Kuan (2018) studied the physical activity of university students applying the TTM. A total of 562 students were included in the sample. The decisional balance, self-efficacy, process of change, stages of change were the constructs measured. Apart from these, the participants' engagement in physical activities was also measured. The results revealed that among all the variables, only process of change had a direct significant effect on physical activity. Pros and cons of stages of change explained the process of change and self-efficacy.

The model was applied and found effective across different population in various health contexts like smoking cessation, weight control, high-fat diet, condom use, sun-screen use, mammography screening to have a few.

Limitations

1 Prochaska and DiClemente (1983) in their theory proposed a time frame for every stage. However, there is no evidence on this aspect.
2 Bandura (1997) criticized the model on the ground that human behaviour is rather too multidimensional and versatile to be placed into specific stages.
3 Bandura remarked that the stages of pre-contemplation and contemplation are only different in degree of intention for behaviour, while preparation, action and maintenance differ only in regularity or duration of behaviour but not in kind of behaviour. Kraft, Sutton, and Reynolds (1999) felt that the whole thing can be explained in two stages—pre-contemplation and the rest combined into one.

Despite the criticisms, the TTM is a widely used model in predicting behavioural change. It is very useful in planning appropriate interventions to match the process involved in different stages.

Box 5.7 Researcher's Box

- One aspect on which this theory was criticized was the time frame suggested for each stage. Research can be designed to verify the time frame for the stages. Sample with a specific health risk behaviour like smoking can be followed up for two years after exposing them to a well-designed intervention targeting the hazards of the behaviour. Following them up either through self-maintained diary or a questionnaire administered at frequent intervals helps trace the point or phase of transition from one stage to the other. However, it would be a highly challenging research because of the probability of subject dropout and possibility of relapse at any stage. In view of this, the sample size should be planned with provision for heavy subject loss.
- Various types of intervention packages varying in content, tone and form can be tested at various stages for establishing relative efficacy.
- Studies can be planned to identify factors influencing relapse, and preventive measures can be designed and tested.

Box 5.8 Practitioner's Box

- Proper assessment of the client to ascertain the stage in which he/she is very important
- Stage-appropriate intervention packages play a significant role in helping hem move forward
- Counselling, psychoeducation and cognitive therapy for patients at the pre-contemplation stage will be of help in triggering the thought process. The programme must include not only the repercussions of behaviour on self but also on immediate physical and social environment
- Contemplation stage may put the individual through flood of thoughts associated with specific and vague apprehensions. Encouraging one to express, ventilate and clarify the fears and anxieties would aid in leading one forward to a higher stage
- The interventions through psychoeducation and counselling would be effective if the micro-level positive behaviour is linked to the macro-level support system in society. For example, the public support one receives for wearing a helmet while riding a two wheeler and the public opposition when not wearing it enable one to perceive the contrast of support for positive and negative health behaviours
- A practitioner can adopt motivational interviewing for helping transition from one stage to the other
- The individual at the preparation stage needs to be encouraged and the perception of self-efficacy strengthened. Encouraging the person to openly discuss the plans, contingency plans and of hurdles and strategies to cope with external hurdles and internal temptations would be of help in shaping the action at the next stage by revising the plans that may not be realistic

- Training the patient on stimulus control helps in preventing possible lapses and relapse
- The person at the action stage requires reinforcement from the practitioner. Effective supervision and mid-term evaluation and correction by the practitioner constitute strong support to guide one to maintain the behaviour
- The practitioners need to apply the skills of counsellor in the action and maintenance stage. Condoning sporadic lapses and helping the client overcome the temptation of turning occasional entropy to a total retract are essential in these stages

Precaution Adoption Process Model (PAPM)

This is a stage theory developed by Weinstein, Rothman and Sutton (1998). The theory is based on the following assumptions:

1. Stages need to be defined in terms of category or system. Though the stages are basically theoretical constructs where the boundaries are not as clear as suggested in theories, they are useful to researchers.
2. It is assumed that people pass through all steps before they perform the behaviour. However, progressing to the stage above is not essential. Similarly, there is also possibility of regressing to the previous stage. An individual's time at each stage is not standardized. It may so happen that the movement from one stage to another is so fast that it is not even taken to cognizance.
3. Issues at each stage are by and large uniform. Hence, interventions can be designed to suit the stage.
4. Different stages pose the challenges of different barriers.

Description of Stages

The theory explains individual's adoption of new precaution that involves decision-making through conscious awareness and translating the decision into action. The theory explains the process of adopting such precaution. The behaviour involved here is a new precaution or giving up an old health risk behaviour.

The model is explained in terms of seven stages. The initial stages preceding action are defined in terms of mental states, and later stages in terms of behaviour. Though the stages are labelled by numbers, the numbers have no arithmetic value.

Stage 1: 'Unawareness' is a predominant characteristic of this stage. This is a stage where the person is 'unaware' of the risk associated with a behaviour. This is a stage marked by the individual's ignorance about the threat posed to health by a behaviour.

Stage 2: This stage is marked by 'un engagement'. When people learn for the first time about the risks involved in a behaviour, they are no longer ignorant or unaware. Yet, they are not yet engaged by it. For example, one may say 'I know smoking is bad for lungs, but I do not smoke so much to be vulnerable to it'. This is unrealistic optimism or 'optimistic bias'.

Stage 3: In this stage, people are aware of the issue and also are engaged in it. They are in the process of considering a response. This stage closely resembles the stage of contemplation. The outcome of this stage has three possibilities. They may be undecided about change and continue to remain in stage 3 for some time, suspending their decision. Secondly, they may decide not to change and move to a different direction of stage 4. Thirdly, the engagement in the issue may help them to take a decision for change in which case they move forward to stage 5. In stage 3, the person considers a number of factors associated with the decision. All these factors compete among themselves for the limited time and attention that though one is fairly aware of the risks, it is only the beginning of considering whether an action of change is called for or not.

Stage 4: This stage brings uniqueness to this model. This stage sets a possibility of a decision for no change despite the awareness about severity and susceptibility. Some people may consciously take a decision not to take any precaution even against the backdrop of knowledge about the risk. This is different from 'behavioural intention not leading to actual behaviour'. Here, the person takes an 'informed decision' for no behavioural change. They step aside without moving to stage 5. Others who lean towards 'action' after a considered thought in stage 3 will move to stage 5. Thus, strictly speaking stage 4 is not a 'stage' in real sense because it is not a step indicating decision for progression towards the behavioural change.

Stage 5: This is a stage characterized by the 'decision to act'. People in stage 3 behaviourally differ from people in stage 5. In stage 3, when people are still undecided about whether to change or not, they are likely to be more open to information and knowledge about the issue. On the contrary, people in stage 5 who decide to act may not require or seek any further inputs on the issue because the decision to act has already emerged.

Stage 6: This is the stage of action. Here, the individual initiates the behavioural change.

Stage 7: This final stage is marked by maintaining the changed behaviour. This stage while relevant to behaviours like cessation of smoking may not apply to decision like going for a screening test or taking a vaccination (Figure 5.9).

Application

PAPM has been applied in the context of variety of health behaviour such as prevention of osteoporosis, screening for cancer, taking vaccine for hepatitis B, smoking cessation and red meat consumption.

Elliot, Seals, and Jacobson (2007) conducted a unique study on a sample of epileptics to predict their osteoprotective behaviour. The background of the study is the well-established fact about the epilepsy patients' vulnerability to fracture. The objective of the study was to investigate how knowledge related to the significance of calcium intake and exercise, health beliefs, self-efficacy impacts the osteoprotective behaviour among the epilepsy patients. The sample constituted 94 epilepsy patients between the age ranges of 19 and 78 years. The participants were administered a questionnaire based on Precaution Adoption Process Model (PAPM),

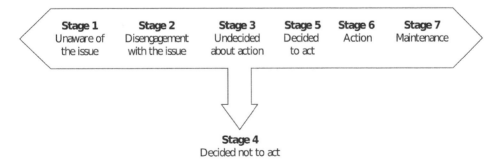

Figure 5.9 Stages of Precaution Adoption Process Model.

150 *Theories of Health Behaviour*

Osteoporosis Knowledge Test, Osteoporosis Behaviour Scale, Osteoporosis Self-efficacy Scale and Epilepsy Self-efficacy Scale. The results revealed that the knowledge for exercise was predictor for higher stages of dietary calcium and exercise behaviour, indicating that promoting knowledge and exercise motivated them to commit to make changes in lifestyle. Perceived susceptibility and age predicted higher stages of calcium supplement and screening behaviour. Self-efficacy was also found to be the predictor of higher stage of dietary calcium adoption.

Weinstein, Sandman and Blalock (2008) applied the model in a situation of home testing of radon, an invisible odourless radioactive gas produced by the decay of natural uranium in soil. This gas was found to enter homes through cracks in the foundation. It is supposed to be highly hazardous in causing cancer. They studied the behaviour of testing the homes for radon. The findings indicated that perceived susceptibility predicted the transition from stage 3 (undecided) to stage 5 (deciding to act). However, the intervention matched to the stage failed to move people from stage 5 (decided to act) to stage 6 (action) of buying a home radon testing kit.

The literature search indicated that this is not a model that has been utilized widely.

Box 5.9 Researcher's Box

- Stages 3, 4 and 5 in this theory evoke special attention. It may be of research interest to identify various psychosocial correlates that predict the maintenance of the status quo in stage 3 for a prolonged period, slip away to stage 4 characterized with a decisive inaction and move forward to stage 5 of action towards positive change. Identification of factors contributing to these changes helps contemplate appropriate intervention.

Box 5.10 Practitioner's Box

- Knowledge interventions to suit the education level for those in stage 1 where they are ignorant about the health risk behaviour or health-promoting behaviour would set the beginning of the treatment process.
- Once the awareness is created, the practitioners need to make the awareness personally relevant for the person. Until this is achieved, the disengagement continues.
- Practitioners must be cautious in handling those in stage 3. It is important not to push them hard for behavioural change, lest they turn defensive and slip to stage 4.
- Any thoughts related to positive change need to be openly reinforced in persons in stage 3 so that they decide to act.
- Expression of intent to act should be taken as the cue, and the practitioner may help the person to turn them into aim and then formulate goals and subgoals.
- The practitioner may help the individual transit from decision to act to real action by helping him/her to translate the goals into specific strategies. This can be attained by having brainstorming sessions with the person in framing specific strategies of action.
- Helping the person to identify the forces in the social environment that facilitate the maintenance of changed behaviour through reinforcements would go a long way in instilling confidence and setting the environment to his or her advantage. All these can be done through counselling sessions.

Health Action Process Approach (HAPA)

This model was developed by Schwarzer (1992). The model has convergence of ideas from different theories and models preceding this. In addition, it also attempts to fill in the gaps that the preceding models suffered. As the name suggests, HAPA suggests that adoption, initiation and maintenance of health behavioural change have to be viewed as a 'process', but not an event.

As assumed by a number of theories, HAPA reiterates that a number of illnesses are caused because of health risk behaviours (smoking, alcoholism, binge eating, driving without seat belt/helmet, unsafe sexual practices etc.). Such health-compromising behaviour needs to be eliminated and replaced with health-enhancing behaviour. This involves a process. The process consists of phases involving getting motivated to change the behaviour, take initiative for the change through appropriate planning and then implement the behavioural change. HAPA identifies the difference between the 'intention to change' (behavioural intention) and the 'change' (behaviour) itself. Hence, it explains the model in the 'pre-intentional'/'motivational' phase and the post-intentional/volition phase.

Description

The model refers to the following psychological constructs. It will be easy to explain the model once the constructs are understood.

Risk Perception: The trigger to replace health-compromising behaviour with health-promoting behaviour originates from a cognition or awareness of the risks involved in the prevailing health behaviour. Perception of a threat to health comes from two sources, viz. the severity of consequences of such behaviour and the individual's susceptibility or vulnerability to the consequent repercussion. These two factors together lead to the risk perception of the prevailing health-compromising behaviour. More often than not, people indulging in health-compromising behaviour are aware (at least superficially) of the threats posed to themselves by such indulgence. However, while rating their vulnerability to the threat, more often than not people are found to underestimate the probability of them being the victim to the threat. Accurate communication with appropriate database by an authentic health professional may be helpful in creating risk perception in the individual.

Outcome Expectancies: This refers to the awareness of the positive outcome of substituting the health hazard behaviour with health-promoting behaviour. When the individual finds the outcome expectancies of discontinuing a prevailing health-compromising behaviour to be positive, the motivation for the desirable change in behaviour is triggered contributing to the intention to change.

Intentions: It refers to felt motivation by the individual to change his/her own behaviour. Behavioural intention is considered an indispensable variable in explaining and predicting behaviours. In explaining motivation, 'intention' is considered as a watershed between goal-setting and goal-pursuit phases.

Self-Efficacy: The construct of self-efficacy refers to the individual's beliefs in their capabilities to exercise the control on the challenging demands over their functioning. The HAPA advocates that the construct of self-efficacy differs at various points. In other words, the meaning of self-efficacy depends on a particular situation in which the individual operates (Figure 5.10).

HAPA identifies three types of self-efficacy:

1 Action self-efficacy
2 Maintenance self-efficacy and
3 Recovery self-efficacy

152 *Theories of Health Behaviour*

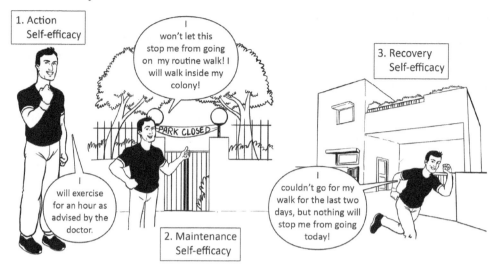

Figure 5.10 Three Types of Self-Efficacy.

Action self-efficacy is otherwise known as task self-efficacy. This refers to the individual's belief in his/her ability to change the prevalent negative health behaviour in the first phase of the process when the individual has not yet initiated any action. It is just the initial stage of motivation to act with a foundation with a belief in one's own ability to act. Persons with high action self-efficacy imagine success. They expect positive outcomes and have higher probability to initiate action towards the behavioural change. Those with low self-efficacy apprehend failures, nurture self-doubt and have a tendency to defer action towards behavioural change.

Maintenance self-efficacy is also known as coping elf-efficacy. It refers to the individual's belief about one's own ability to handle and overcome the hurdles and obstacles in sustaining the changed behaviour. Initiating a change in behaviour is easier than sustaining it. Very often, the resolve for the change breaks because of a number of external hurdles like unsupportive or disruptive social environment, one's own impulse to retract to the old behaviour that was rewarding in some way or failure to cope with the internal and external consequences of the changed behaviour (e.g. withdrawal symptoms, expenditure on joining a new yoga centre). An individual who has high maintenance self-efficacy responds to such consequences with a higher level of confidence, investing more effort and applying varying strategies, and would show prolonged persistence.

Recovery self-efficacy refers to the individual's belief in one's own ability to spring back to the desirable behaviour after a lapse. This refers to the belief in one's own ability to save a lapse from becoming a relapse.

Action self-efficacy is said to predict the intention, while maintenance self-efficacy and recovery self-efficacy predict the behaviour.

Planning: Planning refers to preparatory strategies for executing a task. HAPA identifies two types of planning:

1 Action planning
2 Coping planning

Action plan is the details of executing the task that answers 'when? where? and how?' It is distinguished from the expression of 'Aim' or behavioural intention by including situational cues. For example, 'I will quit drinking alcohol' is an intention and 'I will talk to my wife on the Saturday to communicate my consent to accompany her for a consultation in the de-addiction centre' is an action plan.

Action plans are likely to encounter a number of obstacles and challenges, which sometimes may prevent a successful execution. A sound resolve, hence, should have a backup of contingency plans or ways of overcoming the possible obstacles. Coping plans are contingency plans put in reserve for operation after the first choice of action plan renders unrealistic or meets with a failure due to the obstacles.

Coping plan and action plan go hand in hand. Once the action plan is made, people while imagining success also imagine or remember the possible hurdles in executing the task. Hence, it is difficult to separate the effects of these two plans.

Self-Monitoring/Action Control

According to HAPA, behavioural change is a process. During the process, there is a need to monitor oneself so that the direction of change is sustained making the goal attainment possible. Self-monitoring or action control refers to the self-regulatory strategy to constantly evaluate the ongoing behaviour on the parameter of a standard. It comprises of three components, viz. awareness of standard, self-regulatory effort and self-monitoring.

HAPA Mechanism Explained

The mechanism of HAPA can be explained in two phases, viz. the motivation phase and the volition phase. The motivation phase is related to setting the goal, while the volition phase relates to engagement in pursuit of goal. The various psychological factors in operation during these phases are explained in Table 5.3.

The process of action for behavioural change starts with the awareness related to behaviour. The individual, when gains awareness about the severity of a health condition that results out of the prevailing negative health behaviour and the chances of oneself being a victim (susceptibility) to the condition, perceives the risk involved in the behaviour. Alongside this, when the person gains the knowledge related to the positive outcome of discontinuing the behaviour, he/she will feel motivated for the change in behaviour. The motivation for behavioural change is a combination of risk perception and outcome expectancy. The outcome expectancy

Table 5.3 Two phases in HAPA

	Motivation	*Action*
Goal setting	• Risk perception • Outcome expectancy • Action self-efficacy • Intention	
Goal pursuit		• Coping self-efficacy • Recovery self-efficacy • Action planning • Coping planning • Self-monitoring/action control

also has a positive input from action self-efficacy, i.e. the belief of the person in his/her ability to initiate the behavioural change. Thus, a combination of perception of risk, outcome expectancy and action self-efficacy contributes to the intention of changing behaviour. This intention is very crucial because the individuals who have an informed intention to change are more likely to change than those who initiate change as a knee-jerk reaction. Thus, the person through the pre-intentional motivation process reaches the point of behavioural intention. The process that sees the risk perception, outcome expectancies and action self-efficacy culminating in behavioural intention operates in what is called the 'motivation phase'. All these are covert actions.

One of the unique features of HAPA is the explanation of process between the behavioural intention and the actual behaviour through concrete covert action, which marks the transition from the motivation phase to the volition phase. The volition phase can be explained in terms of two subdivisions, viz. planning process and action process. The planning process consists of two types of planning, viz. action planning and coping planning. The individual who reaches the stage of behavioural intention engages in planning the execution of the behavioural change, with minute action points of 'what to do, when to do, where to do, how to do'. Apart from this, the person also reserves coping planning or the contingency plans in the event of difficulty in operating the original plan in the event of obstacles or failure midway. The intention contributes to this planning. Individuals with stronger motivation and intentions have better plans. In addition, action self-efficacy contributes to planning. A person with high action self-efficacy is likely to have good planning. Apart from action self-efficacy, coping self-efficacy contributes to planning. Thus, intention, action self-efficacy and coping self-efficacy help in the process of planning, which is the first part of the volition phase.

It is a sound planning that leads to concrete overt 'action'. The action substage of the volition phase comprises of 'initiation, maintenance and self-monitoring' of action. Adopting a health behaviour is not achieved and sustained merely by having a strong 'will', but involves skills of self-regulation to ensure the goal attainment. Initiating the action demands strategies to fight procrastination. Health behaviour is not a one-time 'performance' but has to get integrated into lifestyle. Hence, the behavioural change has to be successfully transformed into an integral part of living. In this process, one may encounter intrapersonal problems such as lowered motivation, health setback or external problems such as social obligations, professional commitment, climate change, major life event, which may temporarily pose a problem in implementing the action. This demands a number of skills like drafting attainable goals, setting subgoals, creating incentives and structuring appropriate social support to sustain motivation. Besides, one also requires proper strategies of coping, compensating for a loss, enlisting and implementing alternative action in case of failure so that a one-time lapse does not lead to complacence. Thus, action includes not only initiating action but also maintenance of the health behaviour by protecting it from a number of possible deviations, distractions and disruptions.

The obstacles in implementing action pose a major challenge in sustaining the health behaviour. Many people tend to give in to the situation, thereby retracting to old negative health behaviour. Techniques to prevent this one-time deviation from sliding to old behaviour call for different sets of competence from bringing oneself to initiate action. Restoration of health behaviour, harm minimization, renewal of motivation are essential skills in relapse management.

Self-monitoring or action control plays a crucial role in maintaining the behaviour. Continuous self-assessment of the quantity and quality of the changed behaviour contributes to initiate mid-term changes to keep up the standard set for goal attainment is an important aspect of

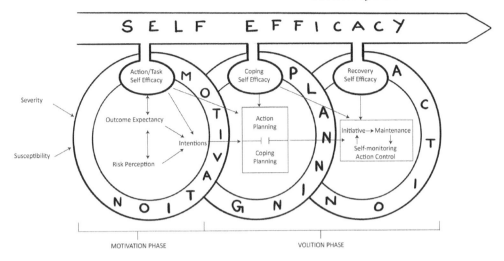

Figure 5.11 Health Action Process Approach (HAPA).

action. Initiation, maintenance and recovery are enabled by planning, coping self-efficacy and recovery self-efficacy. Planning, considered as a meta-cognitive activity, helps in completing the action and suppressing the tendencies of distractions that have the potential either to cease the behaviour prematurely or to cause interruption by competing intentions that are contrary to the set goal. Coping self-efficacy again is a cognition that highlights the individual's belief in one's own ability to encounter challenges of intrusion of factors with potential to abort the behaviour or cause disruption that contributes to maintenance of behaviour. Recovery self-efficacy, the belief in one's ability to recover from a setback, helps in quick restoration of the healthy behaviour in the event of a deviation of disruption (Figure 5.11).

Principles of HAPA

The HAPA model operates on five principles.

Principle 1: Behavioural change can be divided into two phases: (1) motivation phase and (2) volition phase.

Principle 2: The volition phase is subdivided into two to accommodate two types of individuals. There are individuals who have translated their intentions to actions (Actors). There are also individuals who have not yet translated their intentions to actions (Intenders). Based on where the individual is positioned in the continuum of behavioural change process, individuals can be categorized into three types—Pre-intenders, Intenders and Actors.

Principle 3: In volitional, pre-action stage, planning operates as a mediator. Intenders positioned in volitional or pre-action stage have the adequate motivation to change, but have not yet initiated any action towards the change because of the lack of appropriate skill to translate the intention into action. Planning assumes a crucial role. As a meta-cognition, planning providing the strategy for action assumes a mediating role between intention and behaviour.

Principle 4: Planning can be divided into two: action planning and coping planning. While action planning is crucial in initiating a change behaviour, coping planning assumes significance both in initiating and in maintaining the behavioural change.

Principle 5: Perceived self-efficacy runs across the entire process. However, the characteristics of self-efficacy differ at every phase. The individual faces different challenges as he/she progresses in health behavioural change. The type of self-efficacy at different points relates to the challenge encountered at a particular point. The process of behavioural change involves several actions such as goal setting, planning, initiation, action maintenance and relapse management. Each of them poses challenges unique for the action. Hence, there is a need to distinguish between action self-efficacy (also called task self-efficacy), coping self-efficacy and recovery self-efficacy. Coping self-efficacy and recovery self-efficacy are combinedly called as 'maintenance self-efficacy'.

Application

Schwarzer (2016) stated that HAPA is not an easily testable theory. According to him, "it is an open architecture framework that serves to guide research and practice". In view of this, studies vary in their choice of constructs tested. Very few studies employed all the constructs.

In a pre-post group comparison study, related to vaccination for flu on Thai sample, Payaprom, Bennett, Alabaster and Tantipong (2011) found knowledge intervention based on the HAPA model to be effective. The sample comprised of 201 participants from Thailand. Out of this, 99 were given a leaflet on the flu vaccination based on HAPA. They were asked to form action plan on when, where and how they would seek vaccination. The second group consisting of 102 participants received the leaflet that provided the standard information by the government. Results revealed that HAPA intervention brought significant changes in risk perception, outcome expectancies, self-efficacy and intentions when compared to the standard government information. Stronger intentions to seek vaccination were predicted by changes in outcome expectancies, self-efficacy and planning. However, when it came to the actual behaviour of seeking vaccination the HAPA group did not significantly differ from the comparison group that was exposed to standard government information.

Zhou et al. (2016) conducted an interesting study on the use of filtering face mask respirators to reduce exposure to pollution among Chinese participants. The sample consisted of 164 young Chinese adults. He tested the HAPA model by studying the sample at three time points (baseline, at two weeks and four weeks) referred to as time 1, time 2 and time 3. At the baseline, i.e. time 1, self-efficacy, risk perception, outcome expectancies and intention were studied. Planning and action control were studied at time 2. Face mask use was studied at time 3. Results revealed that at time 1, self-efficacy and risk perception combinedly predicted intentions. Planning and action control at time 2 combinedly predicted the behaviour of face mask use at time 3. Planning and action control were found to play a mediating role between the intentions at time 1 and behaviour of face mask use at time 3. Thus, the results were found to have a perfect sync with the theoretical model of HAPA.

Criticisms

The major criticism of HAPA is that human beings are not conscious processors of information. The social environment has a significant role in behavioural change, which is not explained in the model.

The second criticism is that the theory cannot be falsified.

Despite the criticisms, the HAPA model is unique in filling the gap between the intention and behaviour. Further, the model highlighted the importance of self-efficacy through its consistent presence throughout the process. Thus, it qualifies to be rated as more elaborate and complete in explaining behavioural change.

Box 5.11 Researcher's Box

There is wide scope for research on HAPA.

- Tools can be constructed, and psychometric properties can be established for the tools related to each construct. A universal tool to measure health-compromising behaviour and health-promoting behaviour can be constructed and validated.
- Non-communicable diseases (NCDs) to a large extent demand changes in lifestyles. The HAPA model can be adopted in creating health awareness interventions (in print, audiovisual or direct interaction mode), and the efficacy of it can be tested by measuring and comparing the changes in psychological constructs (HAPA) with a control group.
- Pre-post quasi-experiments can be designed to evaluate the influence of interventions using the HAPA model to measure the impact of knowledge intervention in bringing behavioural change in any specific behaviour like changing the diet pattern, monitoring the blood glucose level, adopting proper household waste management as a step towards environmental hygiene.
- Studies tracking the process of behavioural change across motivation and volition stage to establish the strength of sequentially ordered variables in predicting the succeeding variables go a long way in validating the model. For example, after exposing the sample to the knowledge about diabetes, the consequences of uncontrolled diabetes, the risk perception, outcome expectancy, intention, planning and the behaviour of adopting the diabetic diet and exercise regimen can be tracked. The predictability of intention to change and the behaviour by the variables shown as contributing factors to them can be studied.
- Control group studies can be designed to examine the impact of the motivation phase on the volition phase in relation to alcohol consumption. For example, divide the sample into the study group and the control group by randomly distributing sample into the two groups. Administer tools to study their perception of severity, vulnerability of alcohol consumption, outcome expectancy, self-efficacy and intention of quitting alcohol. Expose the study group to the information on the chosen health risk behaviour (consumption of alcohol). The second group has no exposure. Compare the two groups on pre-test-post-test using the same tools to measure the perceived severity vulnerability outcome expectancy and self-efficacy and intention related to alcohol consumption. Apply multiple regression analysis to predict the 'intentions' taking all the other variables as predictors of behaviour of alcohol abstinence.
- A unique research can be designed to determine the ideal time gap between the intention and behaviour. This requires a follow-up of the participants until they make a final decision either to change or not to change. Such design helps in identifying a time range within which the intention has the possibility of translating into action.
- Follow-up after the action is initiated also provides new insight into the time required for a health behaviour to get integrated into a lifestyle. This may vary for different groups depending upon various factors such as age, gender, length of health risk behaviour, personality, social support. Each of this can be considered as an independent variable.
- Designing and standardizing the knowledge intervention package for each NCD will be a huge research task. Further, designing separate packages to suit the educational level will have a great utility value.

Box 5.12 Practitioner's Box

- Assessment of the individual on the knowledge component related to the (a) behaviour and (b) disease condition as a consequence of continuing the behaviour is an essential prerequisite. The knowledge component needs to include the essential functional knowledge related to what is normal physiological functioning, what disruptions are caused due to the risk behaviour or disease condition, the time required for return to normalcy, consequences of continuing risk behaviour or unattended disease condition.
- Based on the knowledge level, the intervention has to be chosen. It will be beneficial to have a choice of knowledge intervention packages. The packages can vary in content, language and form. For example, there should be packages varying in their emphasis on various aspects of knowledge. This enables to suit the package for the client. Further, if packages designed in print, audio and audiovisual forms are made available in different languages, there will be possibility of optimizing the impact.
- Face-to-face psychoeducation can supplement the packages.
- Post-intervention assessment on psychological parameters at the motivation level gives an insight about the impact of intervention.
- In case the impact is not satisfactory, there is a need to reinforce the intervention by changing the package. A re-assessment is always better after the repeat of intervention.
- If the assessment shows an impact of intervention, it reflects in perception of risk and outcome expectancy. In case the risk perception and outcome expectancy are high but the individual measures low on self-efficacy, counselling sessions to boost the self-efficacy will do good.
- If the individual is unable to translate the intention to action, counselling that involves drafting the agenda for lifestyle change, brain storming sessions for action plan and coping plan may be of help.
- People in the 'maintenance of action' phase need to be apprised that occasional deviations are not abnormal. However, caution needs to be taken so that such appraisals are not construed as 'permissions' for lapse.
- Accountability of recovery from minor lapse needs to be fixed on the individuals.
- Broad skill training in self-monitoring and blaming oneself from the setback of limited downward slide in behaviour work as a prophylactic.

Self-Determination Theory (SDT)

Self-Determination Theory is primarily a general theory of motivation that explained human behaviour in a number of contexts, such as education, organization, industry, sports, politics, religion, family and health care. The application of Self-Determination Theory in the context of health, and specifically in explaining, predicting and facilitating health behaviour, is of relevance in this chapter. For clarity in understanding, we will first discuss the theory in general, and then explain its application in predicting health-related behaviour.

The innate human tendency is to tread the path of development. Investment of energy, commitment, skill and talent towards this goal is thus normative than exceptional. Yet, it is often observed that contrary to this natural phenomenon, the apathy, dampened spirit, complacence, lethargy or procrastination pulls the individual back from adopting behaviour that leads to growth and development. Accordingly, human nature can be categorized as active or passive, constructive or indolent. It is of significance to identify the intrapersonal factors, and social factors that contribute to motivating the individuals to initiate and sustain behaviour relevant to growth and development.

Initiation and sustenance of a behaviour are explained by underlying motivation. Individuals differ in their motivational orientation. Further, there may be the influence of contexts on motivation. Based on the motivational orientation and the contextual influence, the trigger for the behaviour could be internal (the satisfaction derived from the very behaviour) or external (the reward one receives for the behaviour or the punishment imposed for not adopting the behaviour). The Self-Determination Theory examines the two types of motivation, their causal loci, factors regulating them and the process involved. Its application on health behaviour examines the strength of the behaviour based on the types of motivation and in terms of initiation and sustenance. Thus, the explanation involves the impact of the quality of motivation on health behaviour.

Subtheories of Self-Determination Theory (SDT)

Self-Determination Theory is in fact a meta-theory comprising of five subtheories:

1. Cognitive Evaluation Theory (CET)
2. Organismic Integration Theory (OIT)
3. Basic Psychological Needs Theory (BPNT)
4. Causality Orientation Theory (COT)
5. Goal Contents Theory (GCT)
6. Relationship Motivation Theory (RMT)

These theories were developed to explain the phenomena having its base on motivation. They evolved out of research in laboratories or the field. Each of these mini-theories refers to one aspect of motivation or related personality factor.

Cognitive Evaluation Theory (CET)

This mini-theory is related to intrinsic motivation. It explains the factors impacting intrinsic motivation, such as rewards, interpersonal control factors and ego-involvement. CET also explains the positive impact of support from social context to competence and autonomy to foster intrinsic motivation.

TYPES OF MOTIVATION

People are driven to a particular action (behaviour) because of various reasons, each of which constitutes a motivation. For example, let us discuss the action (behaviour) of your reading in this part of the text. You may be reading this chapter because you enjoy learning the theories of health behaviour. It is also possible that you are reading the text because you value gaining knowledge. You may also be reading this text because your teacher promised a reward for the best presentation of the theory in the whole class. It is not farfetched that you may be reading this part for fear of failing the forthcoming exam on theories of health behaviour. Whether you are reading this text out of your own interest and enjoyment or because of your value or your reading the text is because of external factors such as gaining a reward, high marks or fear of failure in the examinations holds high significance. The reason is, if you read the text because of internal factors related to reading such as interest, enjoyment, the focus on the behaviour,

160 *Theories of Health Behaviour*

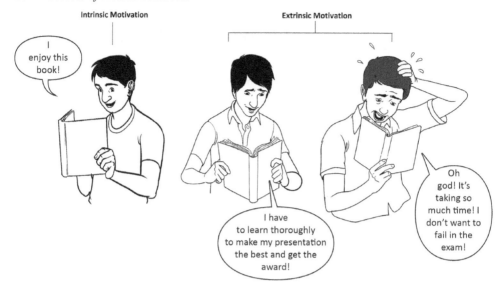

Figure 5.12 Types of Motivation.

excitement generated by the behaviour, and the confidence with which you read is likely to reflect not only in your high perseverance, in vitality (Nix, Ryan, Manly, & Deci, 1999), in reading but also in the quality of your performance, the self-esteem (Deci & Ryan, 1991; Sheldon, Ryan, Rawsthrone, & Illardi, 1997) and general wellbeing (Ryan, Deci, & Grolnick, 1995). Thus, the type of motivation at the base of behaviour plays a crucial role in the strength of behaviour in terms of performance and sustenance on the one hand and the outcome of wellbeing on the other. When external factors such as rewards and punishment trigger a behaviour, the behaviour is said to be guided by 'extrinsic motivation'. When the person performs a behaviour because of the satisfaction derived from the very act, the guiding force is said to be 'intrinsic motivation' (Figure 5.12).

INTRINSIC MOTIVATION

The construct of intrinsic motivation is related to the natural human tendency to extend, explore and learn by using one's capacities. This natural and inherent tendency propels an individual to act, move, do and accomplish not for any specific concrete reward but for the very joy and satisfaction derived from the action. This phenomenon vital for growth and development can be observed in infants constantly striving to attain developmental milestones one after the other because of the propelling force from within. However, the natural phenomenon is not something that is universally present across human beings and also not all along life in the same person. Intrinsic motivation is active and sustained or subdued and diminished by a number of factors. Cognitive Evaluation Theory examines the conditions that impact intrinsic motivation.

Deci and Ryan (1985) propounded the Cognitive Evaluation Theory. They enumerated three essential elements of the theory:

1 Human beings have inherent potential to be proactive
2 By virtue of being human, they seek growth, development and integration.
3 The inherent potential to optimize the growth and development does not happen automatically.

A conducive social environment functions as nutrients to realize the inherent potential of humans for optimal growth and development. The environment can be construed as conducive if it satisfies the three basic needs that function as a fuel to intrinsic motivation. These basic needs are competence, autonomy and relatedness. All the three are significant.

Competence refers to the feeling of being effective in bringing desired outcomes and exercising one's own capacities. The social environment that encouraged the feelings of competence through communication and feedback and restrains demeaning negative feedback contributes to intrinsic motivation. Competence and competence-promoting social environment alone are not sufficient to enhance intrinsic motivation. It needs to be accompanied by autonomy.

Autonomy refers to 'perceived internal causality'. It means the individual must perceive oneself as the cause of an action. There is a need to perceive their behaviour as 'self-determined'. The very perception that one is the cause of one's own behaviour contributes to intrinsic motivation. In such case, the probability of the individual repeating the behaviour is high simply because the person enjoys being the initiator of the behaviour. The need for autonomy will be satisfied by appropriate environmental factors that prohibit, intruding into one's autonomy. Threats, deadlines, evaluations, directives and goals imposed on task also are detrimental to intrinsic motivation because they have the potential to create a feeling of 'control from outside', which is the opposite pole of 'internal causality' of the behaviour.

The third need 'relatedness' is the universal need to be connected to others and experience the caring for others. It also includes the 'will to interact' feeling of being respected, understood and cared for by others. The need for relatedness and secure relational base contribute to high intrinsic motivation.

The Cognitive Evaluation Theory suggests that intrinsic motivation–based behaviour shows stronger initiative, greater perseverance, higher performance and is accompanied by greater self-confidence, self-esteem and feelings of wellbeing.

It is very important to understand that intrinsic motivation can be invoked only when the task (behaviour) is perceived as interesting and appealing because of either the associated challenge, novelty or the value it holds for the individual.

Organismic Integration Theory (OIT)

The focus of this theory is extrinsic motivation. Human experience and observation reveal the fact that not every action of individuals originates from intrinsic motivation. As the infant develops into a child and adult, the social norms and pressures come into operation, demanding compliance. As a result, there is likely to be a progressive increase in the number of activities executed not because of any personal interest or pleasure, but to abide by the social norms, discharge responsibilities, receive incentives for the action itself or because the action leads to a valued incentive. For example, as the infant grows up to join school, there is an obligation to groom one's behaviour in compliance with the school rules, similarly as an adult when one joins a job in an organization, and one has to abide by the organizational code of conduct. When an individual (child or adult) falls sick, there is a need to follow medical advice. Thus, when an individual encounters such situations where one has to foster a behaviour, the motivation for adopting the behaviour may vary from 'amotivation' (state of unwillingness) to active commitment, none of which has the characteristic of autonomy explained in the Cognitive Evaluation Theory.

The Organismic Integration Theory explains the process by which the value and the regulation of the prescribed behaviour get internalized and integrated. 'Internalization' in this context refers to the way the value of the behaviour is 'taken in'. Integration refers to further transformation of that value and regulation whereby it is considered as 'one's own', which subsequently brings in the feeling of autonomy. Thus, the Organismic Integration Theory explains the process related to extrinsic motivation changing in autonomy, i.e. the way a non-intrinsically (extrinsically) motivated behaviour can change into 'self-determined' or intrinsically motivated.

An extrinsically motivated behaviour may vary in its causality. For example, a student who is reading this text because the teacher has given it as a handout and wanted all students to go through the chapter during the class is extrinsically motivated. Another student who is reading the text because he/she understands the value of this knowledge in performance in the exams and thereby the career ahead also is extrinsically motivated. In both cases, the reading behaviour is guided by an instrumentality that is different from reading the text because of the enjoyment or the pleasure it provides.

However, in the first case, the 'compliance behaviour of reading' is controlled by 'external regulation', while in the second instance, the reading behaviour is guided by personal choice and endorsement of value. In both cases, the reading behaviour is intentional, but they differ in the feelings of autonomy.

According to the Organismic Integration Theory, the motivation for an adopted behaviour can be amotivation, extrinsic motivation or intrinsic motivation. Amotivation is characterized with not valuing the behaviour, the absence of feelings of competence and the absence of desired outcome expectations. This amounts to unwillingness to act. Extrinsic motivation refers to adopting a behaviour for an external reward (or avoidance of punishment) rather than the pleasure derived from the behaviour.

Extrinsic motivation explained in terms of varying causality of adopting the behaviour covers the continuum from 'amotivation' to 'intrinsic motivation'. They vary in their degree of autonomy.

External Regulation: The behaviour that originates from externally regulated extrinsic motivation is performed to comply with some external force or imposition. They have the least autonomy. For example, having to take the antibiotics as intramuscular injection three times a day has no autonomy for a patient diagnosed with gastrointestinal infection.

Introjected Regulation: The individual adopts the behaviour voluntarily but without accepting it as one's own. The adoption of behaviour is guided by avoidance of guilt, anxiety or to establish a sense of pride. Thus, the causality is closely related to one's own self-esteem. For example, a person put under weight reduction programme goes to gym at 5 am every day fighting his temptation to sleep till 8 am in the morning. This is because exercise in the gym constitutes an important aspect of the treatment regimen about which the physician expressed doubts of compliance since it is the early morning slot. The person adopts this behaviour lest he may feel guilty for wasting the money or because he wants to prove his resolve to the physician who had expressed doubts. The feeling of autonomy here is higher than in externally regulated motivation. The behaviour here is more control-regulated and less autonomously regulated.

REGULATION THROUGH IDENTIFICATION

The individual adopts a behaviour because he/she attaches a value for it. The behaviour is considered personally important. The individual believes that the outcome of the behaviour matches with one's own behavioural goal.

INTEGRATED REGULATION

When the basis of a behaviour is integrated regulation, the person adopts a behaviour because the behaviour has been thoroughly evaluated and is convincingly found to be in congruence with one's value system and needs. The behaviour is owned up. Behaviour guided by integrated regulation has qualities close to intrinsic motivation. However, they cannot be classified as intrinsic motivation because the causality is the outcome of the behaviour that is separate but not the enjoyment of the behaviour itself. With increasing internalization of regulation, the individual experiences greater autonomy in behaviour. People may progress to internalization in stages, but it is not mandatory.

Though the extrinsic motivation is explained in terms of a continuum connecting amotivation on the one end and intrinsic motivation on the other, the attainment of motivation with higher autonomy is not hierarchical. There is a possibility of a behaviour being guided by any of the extrinsic motivation without passing through the previous ones.

Research has proved the association between higher autonomous extrinsic motivation and better performance, higher quality of behaviour and more engagement. Greater internalization was found to be associated with higher level of adherence, maintenance, participation in treatment and prognosis.

Basic Psychological Needs Theory (BPNT)

The mini-theory of Basic Psychological Needs (Deci & Ryan, 2000) is connected to Organismic Integration Theory. The theory advocates that self-determined motivation originates from the individual's propensity to satisfy the three basic psychological needs, viz. autonomy, competence and relatedness.

The Basic Psychological Needs Theory suggests that the behaviour that has higher autonomy at the base is more likely to be repeated and maintained. The environment that promotes autonomy by providing choice and volition satisfies the need for autonomy. However, as already indicated there are a number of actions that are performed due to external force or the reward associated. These behaviours are typically not interesting or enjoyable. What sustains such behaviour? The major reason for initiating such behaviour is because such behaviours are proposed, demanded, prompted or modelled by people with whom one has attachment, which is valued. This is what is called 'relatedness'. The need for belongingness or affiliation constitutes an important factor in promoting internalization.

Apart from relatedness, internalization of behaviour is also influenced by satisfaction of competence needs. Individuals are more likely to adopt the behaviour valued by significant others with whom they share an attachment or affection only when they feel confident about performing the behaviour.

Satisfying relatedness and competence needs does not ensure internalization. The social environment also should be congenial to autonomy. The autonomy needs are satisfied when the environment facilitates the exercise of choice, volition, and protection from excessive pressure and coercion to adopt a behaviour. This helps the person to own up the behaviour, internalize and integrate the same into the self.

Internalization is a function of satisfaction of all the three psychological needs. Satisfaction of these needs across life span is likely to result in integrity and wellbeing in the individual.

Causality Orientation Theory (COT)

The Causality Orientation Theory explains individual differences in terms of tendencies to relate to environment and regulate the behaviour. This helps in predicting the extent to which they are self-determined in their motivation in general across various situations. The theory identifies three types of orientations.

i Autonomous Orientation: This is the outcome of satisfaction of the three basic needs, viz. autonomy, competence and relatedness. People with autonomous orientation adopt a behaviour out of interest or the value they attach to it.

ii Controlled Orientation: This is related to satisfaction of competence and relatedness needs, but not autonomy needs. People with controlled orientation adopt a behaviour guided by external control and direction. Such persons are likely to have rigid functioning and low wellbeing.
iii Impersonal Orientation: When the basic psychological needs are not satisfied, the individual has impersonal orientation. A person with impersonal orientation finds it beyond his control to attain the desired outcome. This is characterized by poor functioning and a state of ill-being.

Goal Contents Theory (GCT)

Goal Contents Theory is a subtheory that explains individual differences on the basis of their life goals. People are classified into two on the basis of their emphasis on the type of goals and their potential for satisfying psychological needs.

i Intrinsic Goals: The emphasis of intrinsic goal is on personal growth, affiliation and community that satisfy the basic needs of autonomy, competence and relatedness. This is positively related to a number of wellbeing factors such as self-esteem, self-actualization.
ii Extrinsic Goals: The emphasis is on wealth, fame, position, power, image, which at best satisfy the needs indirectly. Focus on extrinsic goals was found to be negatively associated with wellbeing factors.

Relationship Motivation Theory (RMT)

'Relatedness' is one of the basic psychological needs. This refers to the development and maintenance of close personal relationships with family and friends. Relationship Motivation Theory advocates that some interaction with significant others in one lives is not only desirable but is also essential for wellbeing as it satisfies the relatedness need. It not only satisfies the relatedness need but also satisfies the other two needs for autonomy and competence. Close relationships in which there is mutual support for autonomy and competence flourish and contribute towards internalization and integration of behaviour that promotes wellbeing.

THE MODEL THAT INTEGRATES ALL THE MINI-THEORIES

Integrating the mini-theories, the Self-Determination Theory postulates that an individual has three basic psychological needs, viz. the need for autonomy, the need for competence and the need for relatedness. Adoption and maintenance of any behaviour depends upon the satisfaction of these needs. The social environment that supports and satisfies these needs, the personality orientation of the individual and the life goal of the individual contribute to satisfying or depriving the persons' three psychological needs.

The behaviour is triggered either by intrinsic motivation or by extrinsic motivation. The extrinsic motivation is of four types based on the causality and regulatory process. Causality refers to the individual's perception of the causal agent of the behaviour as oneself or external agents. The behaviour that is triggered by motivation with an internal locus is more likely to be strong and sustains compared to the ones where the locus of cause is perceived to be external. The four types of extrinsic motivation, viz. external regulation, and Introjected regulation, Identified regulation and Integrated regulation, are spaced on a continuum that connects to intrinsic regulation (associated with intrinsic motivation). On the extreme left of the continuum lying next to external regulation is 'Non-Regulation' associated with amotivation where the individual has no intention for action, i.e. has no motivation. The movement on the continuum, from amotivation to intrinsic motivation, is in positive direction indicating higher probability for the strength of the behaviour and its sustenance. The degree of autonomy progressively increases in its locus from external regulation to intrinsic regulation. Similarly, the regulatory process of behaviour moves from sheer compliance to external force to inherent satisfaction and enjoyment of the task involved in behaviour. The theory argues that the more the social environment is organized in a way to satisfy the three needs, the more will be the perception of the internal causality and higher will be the probability of the behaviour getting closer to be triggered by intrinsic motivation.

MODEL OF SELF-DETERMINATION THEORY EXPLAINED IN THE CONTEXT OF HEALTH BEHAVIOUR

The self-Determination Theory is explained in Figure 5.13 with reference to health behaviour. Central to the theory are the three basic psychological needs—autonomy, competence and relatedness. The factors influencing the satisfaction of these needs are explained in three layers, viz. the health care climate, causality orientation and life goals, all of which have both facilitating and debilitating influence in satisfaction of these needs. The facilitating influences are shown to the left part of the needs, while the debilitating influences are shown to the right of the needs. The health behaviour is predicted based on the three influencing factors.

Health Care Climate: Satisfaction of the psychological needs depends on the climate of health care, which consists of the physical infrastructure and social medical environment constituted by health care professionals, and the system that refers to the health policy adopted by the organization. Based on all these factors, the health care climate is either autonomy supportive or

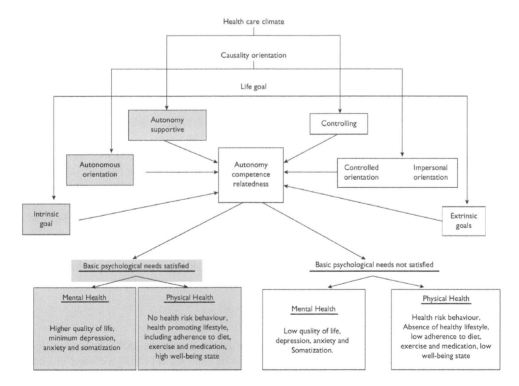

Figure 5.13 Self-Determination Theory in Health Behaviour Context.

controlling. According to Markland and Tobin (2010) and Williams (2002), respecting the perspectives of patients and providing them with a choice contribute to patient autonomy. Keeping the information channel open, and accepting and respecting even when the choice of the patient is against pursuing the advised treatment create a climate that supports autonomy. On the contrary according to Ryan and Deci (2000), the use of tangible rewards and exercising pressure on the patients to pursue a particular action for specific outcome create a controlling health care climate. While an autonomy supporting climate helps in satisfying the needs, the controlling climate thwarts the need satisfaction.

Causality Orientation: Apart from the health care climate, the need satisfaction is also influenced by the personality aspects related to the causality orientation. Deci and Ryan (1985) theorized that people who are autonomy-oriented regulate their behaviour based on their personal interest, values and enjoyment of the particular behaviour. Such persons are expected to have motivation to adopt positive health behaviour and wellbeing to change to health-promoting behaviour. The reason is autonomy orientation helps in satisfying the autonomy needs supported by competence and relatedness needs.

People with controlled orientation regulate their behaviour based on directions or pressure from outside. Such people are likely to look for specific direction and instruction from their health care professionals. They comply with the behaviour because of the pressure. They are not likely to behave out of any conviction and hence are not likely to own the behaviour. As a result, the involvement and commitment may be to the extent of obliging the pressurizing agent. The motivation here is to satisfy the controlling authority.

People with interpersonal orientation are those who are not motivated to initiate a behaviour. They are the ones whose behaviour is beyond intentional control. Persons belonging to the categories of controlled orientation and interpersonal orientation are less likely to avail opportunities or adopt behaviour to satisfy the basic psychological needs.

Life Goals: The third layer of influence on the basic psychological needs is the life goals set by the individual. Life goals can be intrinsic or extrinsic. People with intrinsic goals seek personal growth and development, community involvement and physical fitness. Individuals with such goals are likely to operate on intrinsic motivation and satisfy the three needs. On the contrary, people with extrinsic life goals seek achievement of wealth, fame, image, power and position. The pursuit of such goals is relatively less likely to satisfy all the needs. Autonomy needs, in particular, are less likely to be satisfied when the behaviour is adopted for such external rewards. The guiding motivation is extrinsic.

The outcome of the influence of the three factors in satisfying the needs is seen on the mental health and physical health. Ryan, Huta and Deci (2008) proposed that the positive influence of these factors satisfies the needs and results in positive mental health. Positive mental health is characterized by high quality of life, lower anxiety and depression levels. The negative influence is characterized by low quality of life, the presence of anxiety and depression. Similarly, the positive influence of the factors that satisfy the needs also leads to a higher state of wellbeing. This is attained because the intrinsic motivation for health-promoting behaviour is more likely to be adopted and sustained resulting in no health risk behaviour, positive lifestyle and physical fitness.

APPLICATION

There is a progressive increase in the prevalence of NCDs across the globe demanding long-term management. Almost all the NCDs demand lifestyle changes indicating a change in a number of health behaviour dimensions. The Self-Determination Theory advocates that adoption and maintenance of the behavioural change depends upon the extent to which the health care climate supports the satisfaction of need for autonomy, competence and relatedness, because internalization of the behaviour and autonomy perceptions leading closer to intrinsic motivation is possible with such climate. Health behavioural changes such as adherence to medication or complying to a restricted diet or cessation of smoking or alcohol are not strictly the 'enjoyable' behaviour for a patient, and hence, it may not be pragmatic to expect these behaviour to be guided by intrinsic motivation. However, it is possible to induce value for such behaviour, which is internalized by the patients. The more they are internalized or integrated, higher is the probability of the adoption and maintenance of such behaviour.

Edmunds, Ntoumanis and Duda (2006) investigated adherence and wellbeing of overweight and obese patients on a prescribed exercise regimen by applying the Self-Determination Theory. The sample consisted of 49 overweight or obese persons. They were prescribed to join a physical exercise scheme where the instructor developed tailor-made exercise schemes to suit the condition of the patients. The participants responded to questionnaires at the point of induction (baseline), one month later and at the end of three months, i.e. the time of termination of the exercise scheme. At the baseline, the participants were assessed on body weight, perceived autonomy support, psychological need satisfaction, and motivational regulation in the context of exercise, self-reported exercise, self-efficacy and wellbeing. In the following two assessments at the end of one and three months, in addition to the same assessment, they were assessed on commitment to scheme, behavioural intention of continuing the regimen and the weight. The participants' attendance was rated by the instructor. Results revealed that higher adherence to exercise was related to greater satisfaction of relatedness need. Satisfaction of needs contributed to self-determined regulation and together the need satisfaction, and self-determined regulation contributed to general wellbeing. Thus, the study strengthened the SDT's postulate that the desirable health behaviour is strengthened by need-satisfying services.

In an attempt to apply SDT to bring change in smoking behaviour, Niemiec, Ryan Deci and Williams (2009) conducted an intervention study on 1006 smokers who participated in the study as volunteers. The participants were assigned to intervention (70%) and comparison (30%) groups randomly. The study continued for 30 months. The intervention group interacted with a counsellor who took their inputs on their smoking history, and attitude towards smoking, life aspiration and the way they perceived the smoking behaviour contributing to life aspiration. The counsellors explained to the participants the benefits of stopping smoking. The counsellors were non-judgemental and encouraged the participants to interact with them. Thus, the interaction created autonomy supportive climate. The participants were asked if they wished to quit smoking. If the response was affirmative, they were provided competence support. If the response was negative, they were asked to return in two months to continue the discussion. The participants in the comparison group were provided community care. They were asked to meet the physician and provided information on various smoking cessation resources. The participants were tested on their tobacco cessation behaviour. Based on the criteria of cessation behaviour, they were placed in the category of primary tobacco outcome, secondary tobacco outcome or tertiary tobacco outcome. Results showed that the intervention group maintained the aspiration for physical health over 18 months compared to the community care group. This maintained importance of life aspiration was found to relate positively to health behavioural change, i.e. cessation of smoking. The relation between autonomy support climate, maintenance of life aspiration and tobacco abstinence was limited to the tertiary tobacco outcome that referred to the longest number of days without tobacco use. Thus, the results indicated the relationship between life aspiration and tobacco cessation. The findings have relevance for practitioners.

Box 5.13 Researcher's Box

The theory opens scope for research using survey design, correlational design and quasi-experimental design.

- The relationship between types of motivational and demographic variables can be investigated. This provides an insight into the gender and age group manifesting certain typical motivation orientation if any.
- Different intervention modules varying in content/form can be compared on their impact in need satisfaction and type of health care climate it creates.
- Measuring the sample on all the constructs, in the theory the mediation and moderation variables can be found specific to certain health behaviour.
- The model can be specifically tested in the context of adherence among chronic illness patients such as diabetes, hypertension, pulmonary diseases or in HIV/AIDS patients.
- The theory can be applied in regulating behaviour related to social media gadgets. In fact, the theory would best fit in the context of internet and mobile phone addiction where the behaviour is best expected to be regulated with autonomous regulation.

Box 5.14 Practitioner's Box

Self-Determination Theory helps the practitioners in the right way by suggesting that they consciously create a psychosocial environment that supports desirable health behaviour.

- Quality of Communication: The quality of communication between the patients and health care providers needs to create a climate that supports autonomy, competence and relatedness. This is possible with the following guidelines
  - Explain the disease, the function of medication, diet and other behaviour in simple language avoiding jargon
  - Handle expression of diffidence carefully by delineating the strengths in the patient
  - Respect patient participation in the decision for treatment allowing to choose from options

- It would highly benefit to have an assessment of the patient (particularly those with NCDs) on their psychological needs, causal orientation, type of motivation and life aspiration at the baseline. This helps in identifying their position, which in turn facilitates patient education and counselling

Social Cognitive Theory (SCT)

Social Cognitive Theory of behaviour, as the name suggests, explains the behaviour in the context of social influences and cognitive processes. The social learning theory of Bandura (1962) developed into social cognition theory in 1986. We will first look at the theory in general and then explain it in the context of health behaviour.

This theory suggests that human behaviour can be explained by a triangular interaction between the person, the environment and the behaviour, each influencing the other. Bandura

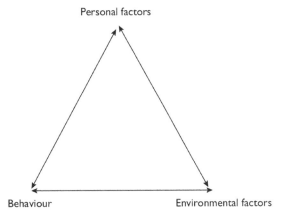

Figure 5.14 Social Cognition Theory.

called it 'reciprocal determinism'. The 'Person' includes all personal variables such as biological makeup, cognition and emotions. The 'environment' includes socio-structural factors related to social norms. The 'behaviour' refers to the actions of the individual. The environment plays a major role in contributing to the personal factors such as cognition and emotional reactions. At the same time, the environment also influences the behaviour of the person. Simultaneously, the environment is influenced by the individual's personal factors and behaviour.

The personal factors have a major role in determining the behaviour. At the same time, the individual's perception of his/her behaviour also impacts the cognitive, emotional factors of the individual. The reciprocal relationship between the three factors is presented in Figure 5.14.

Social cognition theory argues that behavioural change needs to take into cognizance not only merely the initiation of behaviour, but also the more significant aspect of maintaining the behaviour. Maintenance of the behaviour is contingent on the reinforcement. A reinforcement helps in maintaining the behaviour, while a punishment weakens the behaviour as a consequence of which maintenance of the behaviour is less likely.

The theory can be explained through the following constructs:

- Self-efficacy: This refers to the belief one has in his/her ability to successfully perform a behaviour.
- Outcome Expectations: This refers to the persons' anticipation of the outcomes of the behaviour. The domain of the outcome includes the impact on self, on the significant social agents and on the value one attaches to the outcome.
- Reinforcements: This refers to the response to the behaviour (that may be internal or external), which, with its positive or negative characteristics, has the power to decide whether the behaviour is strengthened (continued) or weakened (discontinued).
- Observational Learning/Modelling: This explains the reproduction of behaviour in a person based on observation of such behaviour in another person. People adopt new behaviour by observing someone who performs a behaviour successfully and be rewarded by the society or deriving pleasure from the behaviour.

Explanation of the Theory in General Context

The Social Cognitive Theory argues that any behaviour to be adopted and maintained is influenced by two factors, viz. the cognition of the individual and the social environmental structure. In turn, the individual's behaviour also contributes to these two factors.

Personal Factors: The self-efficacy and outcome expectation may be considered as personal factors, involving perception and cognitive evolution of the self, social environment and the behaviour in terms of outcomes. These personal factors are influenced by a number of cognitive, affective and social factors such as the past experience of success in performing such behaviour, the vicarious feelings of a model's success, failure, ease or difficulty in performing the behaviour, the social expectations of performance, and the evaluation of stress one is likely to experience in adopting the behaviour, encountering the obstacles and handling the possible failure or underperformance in case of worst consequences.

Social Environmental Factors: The behavioural goals are set based on whether the social environment is conducive to the behaviour or not. The social environment is perceived in terms of facilitation and impediments set in its structure for the proposed behaviour. The higher the facilitating factors, the greater is the probability of setting the behavioural goals. The structure of social environment contributes to placing a positive or a negative reinforcement for the behaviour. The behaviour positively rewarded by the social environment is strengthened and is likely to continue and maintain.

The reinforcement comes from the environment and from within. The behaviour is predicted by the strength of the goal. Besides the goal, the outcome expectation and self-efficacy directly contribute to the adoption and maintenance of behaviour.

The Theory Explained in the Context of Health Behaviour

Change in health behaviour assumes that individuals have adequate knowledge about health risk behaviour and health-promoting behaviour in terms of their advantages and disadvantages respectively. Thus, knowledge constitutes the prerequisite for behavioural change. However, knowledge alone cannot bring the desirable change in health behaviour. In addition, a number of internal and external factors play a crucial role in bringing in and sustaining the health behavioural change.

Self-efficacy occupies a significant place in Social Cognitive Theory. The belief in one's own ability to bring a desired change in behaviour itself operates as an incentive to initiate and persevere in the face of obstacles. This demands acquisition and the use of skills adequately and appropriately. Self-efficacy includes the belief in oneself to learn and apply the skills in overcoming the hurdles in bringing about a behavioural change. For example, a patient diagnosed with hypertension and diabetes is medically advised to bring about a positive change in lifestyle. The sedentary life has to be replaced with a prescribed level of physical activities with practice of certain '*yogasanas*' and regular walks. The patient's indulgence in food has to be regulated with low fat, low salt, high fibre and sugarless diet in prescribed quantity. He is advised to abstain from smoking. Adopting these behavioural changes requires to learn specific physical skills (learning *yogasanas*), behavioural skills (stimulus control in diet), assertiveness training in saying 'No' to attractive offers for food, activity substitutes to avoid company of peer group who meet chat and smoke during weekends. Unless the individual believes that he has the ability to learn these new skills, the probability of initiating the behavioural change is almost nil.

The four factors that positively contribute to the self-efficacy are success, model, social persuasion and stress. The past experience of success in accomplishing abstinence (e.g. alcohol), quitting a favourite diet (e.g. meat) and learning a physical activity (e.g. swimming) helps in enhancing self-efficacy. The vicarious experience of a valued model (e.g. an elder sibling) changing the lifestyle helps in having high self-efficacy. Social persuasion in the form of a valued friend endorsing that one has the 'fire' required to bring in the change in behaviour helps in adding to self-efficacy. The fourth influence of stress or affect needs to be handled effectively. Some persons tend to overestimate the physical strain, craving, withdrawal symptoms or consequent negative affect of changing behaviour. This in turn gives rise to stress. Thought substitutions with rationality, reinterpretation of the outcome expectation, and actions for affect change and mood enhancement help in bringing higher self-efficacy.

High self-efficacy and realistic outcome expectations contribute to perseverance of behaviour. Bandura (1997) observed that people's expectation of stress and their perception of self-efficacy in coping with the anticipated stress directly contributed to the health status. Experiments (Bandura, 1992, O'Leary & Brown, 1995) proved that when people were directly exposed to stress without perceived self-efficacy, the physiological arousal was evident in terms of catecholamine and opioids. But when the self-efficacy of coping was strengthened, they coped with the stress without physiological arousal. Low self-efficacy to cope with stress resulting in cortisol secretion has a detrimental impact on the immune system, thereby the health status. Coping self-efficacy helps in physiologically strengthening the individual and managing stressful situations arising in the process of changing the health behaviour.

Beliefs of self-efficacy relate to controlling and regulating health-related habits. It is not just related to initiating a health-related behaviour, but also related to the belief in sustaining it, and successfully handling the occasional relapse by exercising appropriate behavioural control that constitutes self-efficacy related to health behaviour. The stronger the self-efficacy, the higher is the probability of goal setting for behavioural change by abstinence from health risk behaviour and adoption of health-promoting behaviour.

While impacting the goal setting for behavioural change, self-efficacy also influences the outcome expectations. The outcome expectations of changed health behaviour can be at three levels, viz. physical, social and self-evaluation. For example, an individual who is advised to have vitamin D supplementation that provides relief from the symptoms may expect to have reduced feelings of fatigue and exhaustion, at the physical level. The outcome expectation also includes lessening the worry of one's parents who were constantly concerned about their easily fatigued young offspring. Finally, the person also takes into consideration the self-evaluation of the behavioural change. If the general fatigue lowers and energy levels are increased, the accomplishment may be high. Thus, it qualifies self-worth.

The outcome expectations related to a health risk behaviour follow the same line. For example, a person advised to quit smoking in view of the cardiac condition has outcome expectations related both to his smoking behaviour and to the proposed abstinence behaviour. The physical outcome expectation associated with smoking behaviour may include experience like oral stimulus, feeling of relief, and remaining active, contrasted with worsening of cardiac condition, susceptibility to cardiac arrest and feeling of increasing breathlessness. Contrarily, abstinence of smoking may have outcome expectation at the physical level that includes withdrawal syndrome, possibility of increased appetite and overeating leading to undesirable weight gain. But on the positive side, the improvement in cardiac condition, breathing problem and fitness in general also emerge as outcome expectations. On the social level, making the family members happy and gaining their approval add to the probability of behavioural change goals. Finally, the evaluation of self on the changed behaviour and the value of the proposed change in health behaviour through abstinence contribute to outcome expectations. These outcome expectations contribute to the individual's setting of a goal to quit smoking if he/she finds more overall positive outcomes than the negative ones. Simultaneously, the outcome expectations also directly contribute to initiation of behavioural change and its sustenance.

The stronger the self-efficacy and more positive the outcome expectations, the sooner is the initiation of behavioural change and better will be the perseverance of the same. Self-efficacy functions as an internal reinforcement for the positive behavioural change in the person. Besides internal reinforcement, goals and behaviours are also reinforced by external factors.

172 *Theories of Health Behaviour*

The social norms and sanctions have an influence on the behavioural goals and the behaviours. The behavioural goals and behaviours in congruence with the social norms get rewarded, while those that violate social norms elicit social disapproval, sanctions or censure, which function as negative reinforcement weakening the behaviour. For example, drug abuse by the young student in the university elicits social disapproval and punishments from university authorities. Now, when the medical advice is to deaddict oneself, the outcome expectations and the social support system works in favour of choosing deaddiction programme. Here, if the student beliefs in self-efficacy in going through the de-addiction programme and the peer group and family volunteer their support if the student chooses to consent for deaddiction programme, they function as positive reinforcement for setting the goal and cessation of the habit. The external rewards and punishments rest on the socio-environmental structure. The socio-environmental structure may have factors that facilitate the health behaviour and also those that debilitate the behaviour. For example, a hypertensive, diabetic patient advised to follow a fat-free, sugar-free diet has a family that has to prepare food for six members and finds it difficult to accommodate a menu that suits the patient who has an impediment in social environment that stands in the way to adhere even if he/she intends to. If the patient has the self-efficacy to cope with such situation by making any alternative arrangement by cooking for himself/herself or appointing a cook, the adherence behaviour gets regulated by handling the external barriers. Sometimes, the barriers can be auto-generated. For example, the same patient, who is served the special diet in every meal, feels that it is difficult to consume because it is not appetizing; the impediment is said to be from within. The self-efficacy needs to include coping with such personal impediments too in regulating the desirable health behaviour. The adopted health behaviour is sustained through such continuous regulation.

The explanation fits well into the person-environment-behaviour triangle. Self-efficacy and outcome expectations are the 'Person' factors. Socio-environmental structure is the 'Environment' factor, while the goal and behaviour are the 'Behaviour' factor. The reciprocal process of their operation is explained in Figure 5.15.

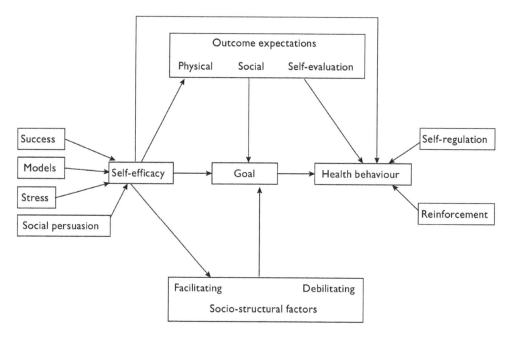

Figure 5.15 Social Cognitive Theory & Health Behaviour.

Application

The major constructs of the theory that were applied in research are self-efficacy, outcome expectations, behavioural goals and actual behaviour.

Wallace, Buckworth, Kirby and Sherman (2000) applied Social Cognitive Theory to predict exercise behaviour among college students. They recruited 937 undergraduate students in the study. The participants responded to a mailed questionnaire that measured personal, environmental and behavioural variables. The association between stage of exercise behavioural change and three sets of variables was examined. The results revealed an association between exercise self-efficacy and stage of exercise. Gender differences were identified in predictors of exercise. The stage of exercise behaviour in girls was predicted by exercise self-efficacy and family support for physical activity. In case of boys, exercise self-efficacy, friend's social support for physical activities and physical activity history contributed to stage of exercise behavioural change.

Limitations

- The theory explaining the dynamic interplay between person, environment and behaviour is unclear about the extent of their influence on behaviour.
- The two important factors of emotion and motivation playing their role in behaviour need better treatment.

Despite the limitations, it has to be kept in mind that it is the contribution of the construct of self-efficacy in Social Cognitive Theory that facilitated the emergence of a number of other theories that used the construct as a central focus.

Box 5.15 Researcher's Box

- The role of self-efficacy in enhancing health behaviour has been reiterated by a number of research findings. There have been a number of correlational studies establishing the predictive value of self-efficacy on behavioural goals and behaviours. Similar designs can be replicated in the context of various non-communicable diseases that predict relevant health behaviour related to diet, exercise and medication adherence. There are fewer studies related to self-monitoring and consultation visits.
- Intervention studies related to self-efficacy and behaviour performance will be of great relevance with application values on the patients diagnosed with NCDs. This calls for two stage studies—first, developing and validating intervention packages aimed at enhancing self-efficacy, and second, application for establishing the efficacy of these intervention packages by adopting control group quasi-experimental studies.
- The intervention packages can make use of one or combinations of the factors impacting self-efficacy, such as past success (highlighting the past success in changing behaviour), use of models, social persuasion (through video clippings or direct interaction) or stress management techniques.
- The methods of the intervention package can use interview, simulations (in quasi-experiments), exposure to knowledge, sharing of experience by models through video programmes or direct interactions, exposure to role play, street plays or sharing of real-life success stories through print medium.

- Research can be planned in examining the relative efficacy of the methods, modes and techniques in enhancing self-efficacy and its influence on the health behavioural change.
- Follow-up studies can be planned to measure the sustainability of the impact, and further plan to block or arrest the factors negatively impacting the behaviour maintenance.

Box 5.16 Practitioner's Box

The Social Cognitive Theory emphasizes on three factors—Person (self-efficacy and outcome expectation), Environment (socio-environmental factors) and Behaviour. It explains the process of regulating health behaviour based on reinforcement contingencies from within and from outside. Based on the above, the practitioner intending to bring about a healthy lifestyle through behavioural change in the patient should focus on the following factors to bring in desirable results.

- Enhancing the self-efficacy: This can be done through a series of counselling sessions and training programmes.
- Restructuring social environment: Social support significantly contributes to bring in the desirable health behaviour. Identifying and handling the probable impediments in social environment that may constitute barriers for initiating and sustaining health promotive behaviours in the patient can be made possible through family counselling sessions. Similarly, identification of factors facilitating and strengthening the behavioural change is possible through family counselling. This in a way helps in setting the external reinforcements for the positive health behaviour.
- Training the patient in stress management skills helps in enhancing self-efficacy.
- Short experiments on ceasing the health risk behaviour under the supervision of the practitioner set the path for instilling confidence, and also inculcating simple skills in handing temptation for retreating to old behaviour may help the patient.
- It is of great importance for the practitioner to keep in mind that proper assessment to ascertain various factors is an essential prerequisite to introduction of any intervention.

Self-Regulation Model (SRM)

This model is one that of illness cognition and behaviour. This is also known as the Common-Sense Model. Self-Regulation/Common Sense Model is conceptualized by Leventhal et al. (1984, 1997). Self-Regulation is defined as 'any efforts, undertaken to alter one's behaviour' (Sniehotta, Scholz, & Schwarzer, 2005). The model explains the health behaviour in terms of cognitive affective process, with the knowledge or information related to the illness at the foundational base. The model is explained more with reference to illness than health. The model explains the process related to perception and interpretation of an illness through regulating the cognitive and emotional aspects and the coping behaviour with it until the equilibrium is restored. The entire process involving cognition, affect and behaviour is regulated by oneself, hence the nomenclature of 'Self-Regulation Model'.

Basic Constructs

Let us understand the following constructs associated with the model.

Illness Representation: This refers to the mental models of illness. They may be called schemas. In simple terms, 'illness representation' refers to the way an illness is conceptualized by the person. This conceptualization or construction of schema happens with the following material or content.

a **Identity:** This refers to the way an illness is recognized, by the symptoms or the label. More often than not an illness has the identity with its symptoms.
b **Cause:** This constitutes the beliefs of the individual with regard to the origin of the illness. The causal attribution may be external, internal or one's own behaviour.
   The casual attribution assumes significance because it contributes to the individual's participation in type of treatment process. The attribution may or may not be factually valid.
c **Time line:** This refers to the beliefs of the individual about the duration of the illness. Illnesses are classified as acute (transient), chronic (long lasting) or cyclic (follow a pattern in their appearance and disappearance) based on the duration for which they last.
d **Control/Cure:** This refers to the individual's beliefs related to the extent that the illness can be arrested or completely cured.
e **Consequence:** This refers to the individual's beliefs related to the impact of illness in his/her physical psychological and social life. This is related to the perception of severity of the illness.

Description:

The five aspects of illness representation play a crucial role in determining health behaviour. Wide interpersonal variation is observed in illness representation. The reason could be a number of factors influencing the perception, such as personal experience, vicarious experience, exposure to knowledge that may vary in content, form, correctness, quality and quantity, the individual's ability to perceive, assimilate and apply it to the context to name a few. Depending on these factors, the cognitive base, the affective and behavioural responses change.

Figure 5.16 explains the Self-Regulation Model. The entire process starts with the stimulus of knowledge input. The source of this knowledge could be personal experience, experience of others, exposure to information in written or electronic media or a direct communications from another individual (the physician or a health professional or any other individual having the knowledge). Once the individual has the knowledge base related to an illness, it simultaneously triggers the cognitive and the affective process in the person. Let us explain these two processes.

The knowledge base helps trigger the cognitive process that includes the illness representation, problem-focused coping to address the issues related to the illness (involving the health-seeking behaviour with the objective of controlling curing or arresting the progression of illness) and the appraisal of outcome of the coping behaviour. The mental representation once formed is integrated into long-term memory and helps in predicting coping behaviour. To elaborate the same, the cognitive process involves forming a schema about the illness and its symptoms. Further, there is also a knowledge base that helps in understanding the cause of the illness. The individual may attribute to self (e.g. his/her past/prolonged indulgence in health risk behaviour) or external factors such as job stress or environmental pollution. When the causal attribution is internal, at least partially so, the cognition on controllability through active participation is likely to be high. For example, an individual who attributes his diagnosis of primary hypertension to the sedentary job and obesity would think of compensating it with deliberate physical

176 *Theories of Health Behaviour*

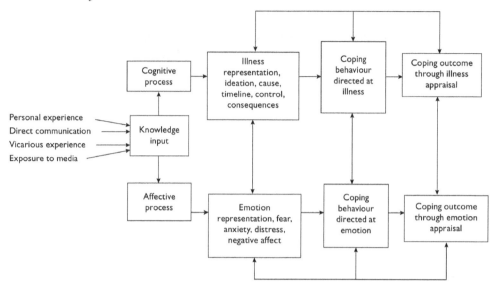

Figure 5.16 Self-Regulation Model.

activity by allocating specific time for it in a day. The motivation for such change in lifestyle also is influenced by the perceptions of the consequences of illness in terms of its seriousness. For example, the individual's cognition that left unattended and the hypertensive condition may affect vital organs like kidney, liver, which could be fatal contributes to strengthening the intentions of allocating dedicated time for physical exercises in daily routine. Thus, the illness representation concerning the ideation, cause, control and consequences influences the individual in changing the lifestyle. The other illness representation refers to 'time line'. Based on the knowledge input, the individual develops conceptualization on the duration of an illness. An individual whose knowledge base is factual would cognizize that the condition of his/her primary hypertension stays lifelong and hence has to be managed for the whole life. This, in combination with the illness representation related to serious consequences, helps in leading to high adherence to medication, diet and exercise, which again can be labelled as a coping behaviour with a focus on the problem. The outcome of such coping behaviour is assessed in terms of the disease condition following the behavioural change. Illness representation, coping behaviour and coping outcome have a mutual relationship among themselves. Change in any point has the potential to bring on commitment change in others. For example, if the illness representation has any flaw in any component (e.g. if the perception of control on hypertension is negative), it impacts the coping behaviour (e.g. there would be no initiative to change the lifestyle). Similarly, if the coping outcome is found to be suboptimal, there is a possibility of the individual reviewing the coping behaviour and mental representation and revising one or both of them.

The knowledge input parallelly triggers the affective process. The inputs about an illness with its representation on the dimensions of ideation, cause, control, timeline and consequences give rise to the emotional reactions like fear, anxiety, distress or negative mood. In adequate proportion, this may function as a motivator for the coping behaviour in the right direction. The illness representation has an interlink with the emotional representation as already explained. There is also an interlink between the coping behaviour related to the problem of illness per se and coping with the emotions. Similarly, the outcome appraisal of coping with the disease and coping with emotions is mutually related. For example, when the illness representation is constructed of facts related to ideation, cause, timeline, control and consequences, the coping behaviour in terms of health-seeking behaviour is likely to include active participation in treatment and adherence to the same. The probability of the outcome appraisal is positive in such case. However, alongside the factual illness representation, if there is elicitation of emotions such as fear and distress, the same is likely to get back to normalcy when the coping with illness through compliance brings in positive outcome. This brings in restoration of balance. In case the balance is not restored, the cycle of the process resumes incorporating necessary revisions at the points of representation or coping behaviour.

Thus, the model suggests that the behavioural change happens through self-regulation.

Application

Assessing illness cognition not only allows research into how patients understand and respond to illness but also offers a theory-based intervention target to improve outcomes. Petrie et al.'s trail of an individually tailored psychological intervention in patients with a myocardial infarction is exemplary in this respect (Petrie et al., 2002). A brief hospital-based intervention designed to alert negative cognitions resulted in quicker return to work and improved functional outcomes following myocardial infarction. In other words, negative consequence beliefs in patients with dizziness have been shown to predict sustained activity restriction and these beliefs have been shown to be modifiable by therapy (Yardley & Redfern, 2001).

Leventhal et al. (1997) found that combining two patients awaiting surgery in a room facilitates sharing their fears related to the images of surgery involving the chest being cut open, the heart assaulted etc. On the contrary, combining a patient awaiting surgery with another who successfully survived the surgery in the same room helped in reassuring the patient. Thus, the emotion-focused coping can be facilitated through simple manipulating of hospital situations.

Box 5.17 Researcher's Box

- A number of ideas can be generated by taking the five components as independent variables and coping behaviour as dependent variable following the correlational design. This is possible with every chronic or acute disease, as well as victims of accidents.
- Surveys can be conducted on population to measure the five components of the illness representation of highly prevalent NCDs or any sudden onset of viral/infectious disease (e.g. dengue, swine flu, chikungunya etc.), as well as their coping behaviour in facing the illness. Alongside this, the affect of fear, anxiety and distress can be measured.
- Intervention studies can be planned designing the intervention package varying the emphasis on the five components of illness representation, either in isolation or in combinations. The coping behaviour may be measured as a dependent variable.
- Follow-up studies can be designed on patients with NCDs, after exposing them to knowledge interventions. The cognitive interventions may aim to enhance illness representations. The health behaviour such as adherence to medication, cessation of health risk behaviour (like smoking) and coping with hurdles in sustaining the behaviour can be measured.

Box 5.18 Practitioner's Box

- The model clearly indicates that self-regulation starts with illness representation. The practitioners need to necessarily integrate suitable form and content targeting to enhance illness representation of the patients.
- Affect state of the patient is normally left unattended. It is essential to address the fears and anxieties of patients. More often than not the fear and affect are the results of either incorrect, inadequate or over-information. It is not uncommon for patients to experience severe anxiety as a consequence of browsing the net on their symptoms or diagnosis. It is essential for the practitioner to verify this and address related issues so as to help the patient formulate a cognitive base on facts.
- Patients awaiting major surgery normally experience anxiety during the waiting period and on recovery from anaesthesia effect. It goes a long way in helping the patient to cope well with post-surgical trauma by apprising them on the probable physical and psychological experience post-surgery even before they undergo surgery.
- The practitioner, by helping the patient have correct illness representation, creates a mental readiness. If this is combined by stimulating the thoughts on coping behaviour, the patient is helped to think in a right direction.
- Encouraging the patient to ventilate all apprehensions helps both the patient and the practitioner because once the fears are addressed, there is likely to be better focus on the cognitive aspects leading to problem-focused coping that involves behavioural change to handle the illness effectively.
- When the diagnosis of a NCD is communicated to the patient for the first time, there is a need to educate the person about the five components of the illness (constituting illness representation). This can be done by exposing the patient to a video clipping (designed to suit the age, education and language of patients) of not more than 30 minutes. It would be better to share this video with the patient for repeated viewing even after leaving the clinic. The video exposure should be necessarily followed by the interaction session to address specific concerns, fears and anxieties of the patient. Following this, one or two more review meetings in a gap one week or more to continue the interaction would help in strengthening the cognitive based about the disease and weakening the unfound fears and anxieties. This therapeutic intervention sets a good foundation for long-term management of the disease that involves behavioural change.
- If the treatment process involves assessment of illness representation before treatment, it helps the practitioners to plan the number of review sessions.
- For the patients low in self-efficacy and internal locus of control, training session to enhance self-efficacy helps in strengthening patient's active participation in treatment regimen.

Theories of Health Behaviour 179

Table 5.4 Theories of health behavioural change at a glance

S. No.	Theory	Proponent(s)	Salient features	Unique features	Criticism/limitations
1	Health Belief Model (HBM)	Rosenstock (1974), and Becker (1974)	• Perceived severity • Perceived susceptibility • Self-efficacy • Perceived control • Perceived benefits • Perceived barriers • Cues to action • Behaviour/action	• Perceptions of the seriousness, personal stakes, cost-benefit analysis and internal or external cues together bring change in behaviour	• Model fails to explain habits acquired from childhood • Role of social influence and emotions ignored • Confusion over measurement of constructs
2	Protection Motivation Theory (PMT)	Rogers (1975)	• Perceived severity and susceptibility constitute threat appraisal • Response efficacy and self-efficacy constitute coping appraisal • Motivation to protect from health risk (Protection motivating) is influenced by threat appraisal and coping appraisal • Protection motivation influences the health behaviour	• Cognitive evaluation of the threat, and the outcome of the possible behavioural change and one's own capability initiating the change trigger the motivation and thereby bring in the behaviour (change)	• Individuals are not systematic, mechanical cognitive processors • No explanation of health behaviour inculcated as habit
3	Theory of Reasoned Action (TRA)	Fishbein and Ajzen (1975)	• Behaviour is triggered by behavioural intentions • Behavioural intentions are influenced by attitudes towards behaviour and subjective norms • Attitudes towards a behaviour are formed by the expected outcome of the proposed behaviour and the value of it • Subjective norms are formed by perceptions of significant other's approval/disapproval of proposed behaviour and the value attached to the significant others	• Intents for behaviour are formed not merely by cognitive assessment of the present behaviour or situation, but by assessment of the probable outcome of the proposed change and the social response to the proposed change • Addition of social cognition relevant to affiliation-oriented societies like Indian society	• Not all health behaviours are voluntary • Transaction between variables not explained • Behavioural intentions are influenced by a number of other factors • Behavioural intentions need not lead to behaviour

(*Continued*)

Table 5.4 (Continued)

S. No.	Theory	Proponent(s)	Salient features	Unique features	Criticism/limitations
4	Theory of Planned Behaviour (TPB)	Fishbein and Ajzen (1975)	• Behaviour is predicted by perceived behaviour control and behavioural intentions • Attitudes, subjective norms, perceived behavioural control predict behavioural intentions • Perceived behavioural control is influenced by control beliefs • Behavioural beliefs, normative beliefs and control beliefs are mutually connected	• An extension of Theory of Reasoned Action • The additional features to Theory of Reasoned Action are behavioural control and control beliefs	• Behaviour predictions are weak • Interconnection between the variables lacks universality • Self-efficacy a better predictor than behavioural control
5	Transtheoretical Model (TTM)	Prochaska and DiClemente (1982–1984)	• A Cognitive Behavioural Model • Behavioural change occurs across five stages • Stages are pre-contemplation, contemplation, preparation, action and maintenance. Each stage is connoted by a time frame • The process of change across stages is explained in terms of ten factors • Two aspects operating in the process are decisional balance and self-efficacy. They help in decision-making and progress along stages • The progress along stages need not be linear. There is scope for relapse to earlier stage	• Behavioural change related to health is a conscious decision calling for consideration of various factors • A number of factors internal and external influence the cognitive process • The decision to change behaviour and implement the change is a gradual process, which is featured in this theory	• Time frame for the stages is not supported by evidence
6	Precaution Adoption Process Model (PAPM)	Weinstein, Rothman, and Sutton (1998)	• Behavioural change has 7 stages, viz. unawareness, unengagement, undecided, decided not to act, decided to act, action and maintenance • After stage 3, i.e. undecided one-way side step to stage 4 'decided not to act' or move forward to ecide to act'	• The stages featured are progressive in nature with a provision for side stepping and informed decision of inaction • The person progresses from indecision to decision based on awareness	• Not applied widely

(Continued)

Theories of Health Behaviour 181

Table 5.4 (Continued)

S. No.	Theory	Proponent (s)	Salient features	Unique features	Criticism/limitations
7	Health Action Process Approach (HAPA)	Schwarzer (1992)	• Risk perception, outcome expectancies, action self-efficacy predict intention. • Intention, action self-efficacy and coping self-efficacy and predict planning. • Planning coping self-efficacy and recovery self-efficacy predict behavioural change initiative to leading maintenance. • Behavioural change is sustained by self-monitoring. All these happen in two phases, called Motivation phase and volition phase	• Self-efficacy with different characteristics at different points is present throughout the process • The model fills the gap between the intention and behaviour	• Human being is not a conscious processor of information • The model cannot be falsified
8	Self-Determination Theory (SDT)	Deci and Ryan (1985)	• Adoption and maintenance of health behaviour depends on the motivation type that triggers behaviour, satisfaction of basic psychological needs, health care climate and life goals. • Higher the satisfaction of needs, more the behaviour is likely to have internal regulation and higher the likelihood of adopting health-promoting behaviour leading to good physical and mental health	• The emphasis is on maintaining the health behaviour	

(*Continued*)

Table 5.4 (Continued)

S. No.	Theory	Proponent(s)	Salient features	Unique features	Criticism/limitations
9	Social Cognitive Theory (SCT)	Bandura (1986)	• The personal factors environmental factors and behaviour have a triangular relationship • Self-efficacy plays a major role in setting the goal and health behaviour on the one hand, and in handling the socio-structural factors and in outcome expectations on the other • The health behaviour is influenced not just by behavioural intentions (goal) but by self-efficacy, outcome expectations, reinforcement, socio-structural factors and goals • Thus, the model includes all possible factors in influencing health behaviour	• The triangularity of relationship between person, environment and behaviour • The powerful role of self-efficacy	• The emotional reactions are not included in the model
10	Self-Regulation Model (SRM)	Leventhal et al. (1984, 1997)	• Knowledge input triggers the cognitive and affective processes simultaneously • Illness representation comprising of ideation, cause, time line, control and consequences influences the problem-focused coping in relation to the illness • The emotions of fear, anxiety, distress trigger emotion-focused coping that handles emotion • The outcomes of both problem- and emotion-focused coping are evaluated	• The main reference of the model is illness than health behaviour • By explaining the health behaviour with reference to cognition and emotion, the model is more complete compared to many other cognitive models	

References

Albarracin, D., Johnson, B. T., Fishbein, M., & Muellerleile, P. A. (2001). Theories of reasoned action and planned behaviour as models of condom use: A meta-analysis. *Psychological Bulletin, 127*(1), 142.

Atkinson, J. W. (1964). *An introduction to motivation*. New York: Van Nostrand.

Bandura, A. (1962). Social learning through imitation. In: M. R. Jones (Ed.), *Nebraska Symposium on Motivation*. Lincoln: University of Nebraska Press.

Bandura, A. (1977). Self-efficacy: Towards a unifying theory of behavioural change. *Psychological Review, 84*(2), 191–215.

Bandura, A. (1982). Self-efficacy mechanism in human agency. *American Psychologist, 37*(2), 122.

Bandura, A. (1986). *Social foundations of thought and action: A social cognitive theory*. Englewood Cliffs, NJ: Prentice-Hall.

Bandura, A. (1992). Self-efficacy mechanism in psychobiologic functioning. In: R. Schwarzer (Ed.), *Self-efficacy: Thought control of action* (pp. 355–394). Washington, DC: Hemisphere.

Bandura, A. (1997). *Self-efficacy: The exercise of control*. New York: Freeman.

Becker, M. H. (Ed.) (1974). The health belief model and personal health behaviour. *Health Education Monographs, 2*, 324–508.

Conner, M., & Armitage, C. J. (1998). Extending the theory of planned behaviour: A review and avenues for further research. *Journal of Applied Social Psychology, 28*(15), 1429–1464.

Deci, E. L., & Ryan, R. M. (1985). *Intrinsic motivation and self-determination in human behaviour*. New York: Plenum.

Deci, E. L., & Ryan, R. M. (1991). A motivational approach to self: Integration in personality. In: R. Dienstbier (Ed.), *Nebraska symposium on motivation. Perspectives on motivation* (Vol. 38, pp. 237–288). Lincoln: University of Nebraska Press.

Deci, E. L., & Ryan, R. M. (2000). The "what" and "why" of goal pursuits: Human needs and the self-determination of behavior. *Psychological Inquiry, 11*(4), 227–268.

Doswell, W. M., Braxter, B. J., Cha, E., & Kim, K. H. (2011). Testing the theory of reasoned action in explaining sexual behaviour among African American young teen girls. *Journal of Pediatric Nursing, 26*(6), e45–e54.

Edmunds, J., Ntoumanis, N., & Duda, J. L. (2006). A test of self-determination theory in the exercise domain. *Journal of Applied Social Psychology, 36*(9), 2240–2265.

Elliott, J. O., Seals, B. F., & Jacobson, M. P. (2007). Use of the precaution adoption process model to examine predictors of osteoprotective behaviour in epilepsy. *Seizure, 16*(5), 424–437.

Evans, D., & Norman, P. (2003). Predicting adolescent pedestrians' road-crossing intentions: An application and extension of the theory of planned behaviour. *Health Education Research, 18*(3), 267–277.

Fallon, E. A., & Hausenblas, H. A. (2004). Transtheoretical model of behaviour change: Does it take five years to reach termination. *American Journal of Health Studies, 19*, 35–44.

Fishbein, M., & Ajzen, I. (1975). *Belief, attitude, intention, and behaviour: An introduction to theory and research*. Reading, MA: Addison-Wesley.

Glanz, K., Rimer, B. K., & Viswanath, K. (Eds.). (2008). *Health behaviour and health education: Theory, research, and practice*. San Francisco: John Wiley & Sons.

Grindley, E. J., Zizzi, S. J., & Nasypany, A. M. (2008). Use of protection motivation theory, affect, and barriers to understand and predict adherence to outpatient rehabilitation. *Physical Therapy, 88*(12), 1529–1540.

Hochbaum, G. M. (1958). *Public Participation in Medical Screening Programs: A Socio-Psychological Study* (No. 572). US Department of Health, Education, and Welfare, Public Health Service, Bureau of State Services, Division of Special Health Services, Tuberculosis Program.

Holmen, H., Wahl, A., Torbjørnsen, A., Jenum, A. K., Småstuen, M. C., & Ribu, L. (2016). Stages of change for physical activity and dietary habits in persons with type 2 diabetes included in a mobile health intervention: The Norwegian study in renewing health. *BMJ Open Diabetes Research and Care, 4*(1), e000193.

Huchting, K., Lac, A., & LaBrie, J. W. (2008). An application of the theory of planned behaviour to sorority alcohol consumption. *Addictive Behaviours, 33*(4), 538–551.

Jeihooni, A. K., Hidarnia, A., Kaveh, M. H., Hajizadeh, E., & Askari, A. (2016). Application of the health belief model and social cognitive theory for osteoporosis preventive nutritional behaviours in a sample of Iranian women. *Iranian Journal of Nursing and Midwifery Research, 21*(2), 131.

Kerlinger, R. (1986). *Foundations of behavioral research*. New York, NY: Holt, Rinehart, & Winston.

Kim, H. S., Ahn, J., & No, J. K. (2012). Applying the health belief model to college students' health behaviour. *Nutrition Research and Practice, 6*(6), 551–558.

Kraft, P., Rise, J., Sutton, S., & Røysamb, E. (2005). Perceived difficulty in the theory of planned behaviour: Perceived behavioural control or affective attitude? *British Journal of Social Psychology, 44*(3), 479–496.

Kraft, P., Sutton, S. R., & Reynolds, H. M. (1999). The transtheoretical model of behaviour change: Are the stages qualitatively different? *Psychology & Health, 14*(3), 433–450.

Lazarus, R. S. (1966). *Psychological stress and the coping process.*

Leventhal, H. (1970). Findings and theory in the study of fear communications. *Advances in experimental social psychology, 5,* 119–186. Academic Press.

Leventhal, H., Benyamini, Y., Brownlee, S., Diefenbach, M., Leventhal, E. A., Parker-Miller, L., & Robitail le, C. (1997). Illness representations: Theoretical foundations. In: K. J. Petrie and J. Weinman (Eds.), *Perceptions of health and illness: Current research and applications* (pp. 19–45). Amsterdam: Harwood Academic.

Leventhal, H., Nerenz, D. R., & Steele, D. J. (1984). Illness representation and coping with health threats. In: A. Baum, S. E. Taylor and J. E. Singer (Eds.), *Handbook of psychology and health* (pp. 219–252). Hillsdale, NJ: Lawrence Erlbaum.

Liu, K. T., Kueh, Y. C., Arifin, W. N., Kim, Y., & Kuan, G. (2018). Application of transtheoretical model on behavioural changes, and amount of physical activity among university's students. *Frontiers in Psychology, 9.* https://doi.org/10.3389/fpsyg.2018.02402

Manstead, A. S. (2000). The role of moral norms in the attitude-behaviour relation. In: Terry, D. J., Hogg, M. A. (Eds.), *Attitudes, Behaviour and Social Context.* Mahwah, NJ: Lawrence Erlbaum Associates.

Markland, D., & Tobin, V. J. (2010). Need support and behavioural regulations for exercise among exercise referral scheme clients: The mediating role of psychological need satisfaction. *Psychology of Sport and Exercise, 11*(2), 91–99.

Moattar, M., Roozitalab, M., Gholamzadeh, S., Firoozi, M. S., & Zare, N. (2014). Practical application of health belief model to enhance the uptake of colorectal cancer screening. *Journal of Community Medicine & Health Education, 4*(297), 4.

Mok, W. K., & Lee, A. Y. (2013). A case study on application of the theory of planned behaviour: Predicting physical activity of adolescents in Hong Kong. *Journal of Community Medicine & Health Education, 3*(5), 100231.

Morrison, V., & Bennett, P. (2006). An introduction to health psychology. Pearson/Prentice Hall. Niemiec, C. P., Ryan, R. M., Deci, E. L., & Williams, G. C. (2009). Aspiring to physical health: The role of aspirations for physical health in facilitating long-term tobacco abstinence. *Patient Education and Counseling, 74*(2), 250–257.

Niemiec, C. P., Ryan, R. M., Deci, E. L., & Williams, G. C. (2009). Aspiring to physical health: The role of aspirations for physical health in facilitating long-term tobacco abstinence. *Patient Education and Counseling, 74*(2), 250–257.

Nix, G. A., Ryan, R. M., Manly, J. B., & Deci, E. L. (1999). Revitalization through self-regulation: The effects of autonomous and controlled motivation on happiness and vitality. *Journal of Experimental Social Psychology, 35*(3), 266–284.

O'Leary, A., & Brown, S. (1995). Self-efficacy and the physiological stress response. In: James E. Maddux (Ed.), *Self-efficacy, adaptation, and adjustment* (pp. 227–246). Boston, MA: Springer.

Ogden, J. (2007). *Health psychology: A textbook.* Maidenhead: Open University Press.

Payaprom, Y., Bennett, P., Alabaster, E., & Tantipong, H. (2011). Using the Health Action Process Approach and implementation intentions to increase flu vaccine uptake in high risk Thai individuals: A controlled before-after trial. *Health Psychology, 30*(4), 492.

Petrie, K. J., Cameron, L. D., Ellis, C. J., Buick, D., & Weinman, J. (2002). Changing illness perceptions after myocardial infarction: An early intervention randomized controlled trial. *Psychosomatic Medicine, 64*(4), 580–586.

Prochaska, J. O., & DiClemente, C. C. (1982). Transtheoretical therapy: Toward a more integrative model of change. *Psychotherapy: Theory, Research & Practice, 19*(3), 276.

Prochaska, J. O., & DiClemente, C. C. (1983). Stages and processes of self-change of smoking: Toward an integrative model of change. *Journal of Consulting and Clinical Psychology, 51*(3), 390.

Ray, M. L., & Wilkie, W. L. (1970). Fear: The potential of an appeal neglected by marketing. *Journal of Marketing, 34*(1), 54–62.

Rippetoe, P. A., & Rogers, R. W. (1987). Effects of components of protection-motivation theory on adaptive and maladaptive coping with a health threat. *Journal of Personality and Social Psychology, 52*(3), 596.

Rogers, R. W. (1975). A protection motivation theory of fear appeals and attitude change. *The Journal of Psychology, 91*(1), 93–114.

Rosenstock, I. M. (1966). Why people use health services. *The Milbank Memorial Fund Quarterly, 44*, 94–127.

Rosenstock, I. M. (1974). The health belief model and preventive health behavior. *Health Education Monographs, 2*(4), 354–386.

Rosenstock, I. M., Strecher, V. J., & Becker, M. H. (1988). Social learning theory and the health belief model. *Health Education Quarterly, 15*, 175–183.

Rotter, J. B. (1966). Generalized expectancies for internal versus external control of reinforcement. *Psychological Monographs: General and Applied, 80*(1), 1.

Ryan, R. M., & Deci, E. L. (2000). The darker and brighter sides of human existence: Basic psychological needs as a unifying concept. *Psychological Inquiry, 11*, 319–338.

Ryan, R. M., Deci, E. L., & Grolnick, W. S. (1995). Autonomy, relatedness, and the self: Their relation to development and psychopathology. *Ariel, 128*(151.189), 155.

Ryan, R. M., Huta, V., & Deci, E. L. (2008). Living well: A self-determination theory perspective on eudaimonia. *Journal of Happiness Studies, 9*, 139–170. doi: 10.1007/s10902-006-9023-4.

Scholl, R. (2002). *The transtheoretical model of behaviour change*. University of Rhode Island.

Schwarzer, R. (1992). Self-efficacy in the adoption and maintenance of health behaviours: Theoretical approaches and a new model. In: R. Schwarzer (Ed.), *Self-efficacy: Thought control of action* (pp. 217–242). Washington, DC: Hemisphere.

Schwarzer, R. (2016). Health Action Process Approach (HAPA) as a theoretical framework to understand behaviour change. *Actualidadesen Psicología, 30*(121), 119–130.

Sheldon, K. M., Ryan, R. M., Rawsthorne, L. J., & Ilardi, B. (1997). Trait self and true self: Cross-role variation in the Big-Five personality traits and its relations with psychological authenticity and subjective well-being. *Journal of Personality and Social Psychology, 73*(6), 1380.

Sniehotta, F. F., Scholz, U., & Schwarzer, R. (2005). Bridging the intention_behaviour gap: Planning, self-efficacy, and action control in the adoption and maintenance of physical exercise. *Psychology and Health, 20*, 143–160.

Tanner Jr, J. F., Hunt, J. B., & Eppright, D. R. (1991). The protection motivation model: A normative model of fear appeals. *Journal of Marketing, 55*(3), 36–45.

Wallace, L. S., Buckworth, J., Kirby, T. E., & Sherman, W. M. (2000). Characteristics of exercise behaviour among college students: Application of social cognitive theory to predicting stage of change. *Preventive Medicine, 31*(5), 494–505.

Weinstein, N. D., Rothman, A. J., & Sutton, S. R. (1998). Stage theories of health behaviour: Conceptual and methodological issues. *Health Psychology, 17*(3), 290.

Weinstein, N. D., Sandman, P. M., & Blalock, S. J. (2008). The precaution adoption process model. In: K. Glanz, B. K. Rimer and K. Viswanath (Eds.), *Health behaviour and health education: Theory, research and practice* (4th ed., Ch 3, pp. 123–147). San Francisco: Jossey-Bass.

Wiggers, L. C., de Wit, J. B., Gras, M. J., Coutinho, R. A., & Hoek, A. V. D. (2003). Risk behaviour and social-cognitive determinants of condom use among ethnic minority communities in Amsterdam. *AIDS Education and Prevention, 15*(5), 430–447.

Williams, G. C. (2002). Improving patients' health through supporting the autonomy of patients and providers. In: E. L. Deci and R. M. Ryan (Eds.), *Handbook of self-determination research* (pp. 233–254). Rochester, NY: University of Rochester Press.

Yan, Y., Jacques-Tiura, A. J., Chen, X., Xie, N., Chen, J., Yang, N., ... & MacDonell, K. K. (2014). Application of the protection motivation theory in predicting cigarette smoking among adolescents in China. *Addictive Behaviours, 39*(1), 181–188.

Yardley, L., & Redfern, M. S. (2001). Psychological factors influencing recovery from balance disorders. *Journal of Anxiety Disorders, 15*(1–2), 107–119.

Zhou, G., Gan, Y., Ke, Q., Knoll, N., Lonsdale, C., & Schwarzer, R. (2016). Avoiding exposure to air pollution by using filtering facemask respirators: An application of the health action process approach. *Health Psychology, 35*(2), 141.

6 Human Physiology

Nervous System

Imagine a typical day in your life. It was a Friday morning. You have a morning class at 9.00 am. Since you had a late-night party on Thursday, you found it difficult to wake up to your alarm. On opening your eyes, you realized that you have very little time to get ready for the class. You skipped your breakfast and barely managed to reach the class on time. You made notes while listening to lecture. As the class progressed, you started feeling hungry and gradually felt drowsy. As a result, you could not be attentive for the rest of the time. Soon after the class you rushed to the canteen and had your breakfast. On your way back while crossing the road, a huge truck emerged from a bye line and was almost close to you. Without any thinking, you took a few quick steps backwards; otherwise, it could have hit you. You felt palpitation and were sweating. The very thought was fearful and increased your heartbeat. You went to the library and spent about two hours reading article relevant for the review paper that you have to submit. You decided to leave the library because you were disturbed by the annoying noise from the floor above where construction activity was going on. You recognized the sound as the wood cutting machine. As the evening approached, you started looking forward to meeting your girlfriend and the visit to the riverside with her. The very imagination gave you a lot of pleasure. Before leaving the library, you headed towards the washroom. There was a ring on your phone. You stopped and answered the phone. Your friend informed that your professor has announced that she would take the class on Saturday on the request of two of your friends. 'Why did you do it without consulting others? How can this be planned so suddenly'? You shouted at him. 'This is not the right way to make decision', you fumed. You argued quite a bit without giving a chance to your friend to explain. You hung the phone in a huff and walked out of the library. As you started walking towards your hostel, you suddenly realized that in the anger towards your friend, you left the library without using the washroom. You started walking faster towards hostel to reach the washroom.

What do you think facilitated all these activities/responses of yours during the day? A single answer to this is your 'nervous system'.

Your feeling 'sleepy' or attentive is associated with the activity of a part of the brain called 'thalamus'. Your hunger and eating behaviour are controlled by a centre called 'hypothalamus'. Your emotion of anger and fear is associated with the 'limbic system'—an area in the brain. You could concentrate in reading in the library because of the 'frontal lobe' in the brain. You could identify the noise in the library as 'wood cutting machine' because you were assisted by your 'temporal lobe'. You could escape the serious accident on the road because of your 'spinal cord'.

Thus, from the most 'taken-for-granted' action like breathing essential for our survival to the complex activity of 'problem solving' is possible because of our nervous system. The simple reflex action like closing the eyelid when an insect is close to the face, motor action like moving our limbs to enjoying a taste or an aroma to complex cognitive activity like solving a mathematics problem or real-life problem, or an emotion or the experience of hunger or other biological needs and outburst can be traced back to various bidirectional communication centres in the nervous system. Thus, it will not be an exaggeration to say that the central nervous system is the 'head office of our existence'. The knowledge about the nervous system is an ocean. Exploration in the area of neuroscience continues. What we know about Central Nervous System (CNS) may appear 'huge', but what we are yet to know constitutes a larger area.

What we discuss in this part is just the fundamentals of the nervous system.

It is called the 'nervous system' because it is a complex collection of 'nerves' connecting every nook and corner of the body to brain and spinal cord, functioning as a communication channel. It can be compared to electrical wiring in the body. The communication in the body is carried out through this 'wiring system'. What initiates and transmits the communication in the body is 'neuron'. Hence, it may be a good beginning to initiate the study on the nervous system with an understanding of the structure and function of a neuron.

Neurons

Neurons are individual cells. Thus, they can be construed as a basic unit of the nervous system. They process and transmit information. Depending upon their functions, neurons are in different shapes and sizes. However, the structural components of the neurons are by and large the same.

Structure of a Neuron

The structure of a basic neuron is represented in Figure 6.1

A neuron has four regions, viz. (1) cell body or soma; (2) dendrites; (3) axon; and (4) terminal buttons.

Cell body/Soma: This is like a generic cell. It contains nucleus and other elements necessary for the process of a cell.

Dendrites: The term dendrites originated from 'Dendron', the Greek word for free. The dendrites are the extensive branches from the cell body that resemble a tree. The dendrites receive information from other neurons. This message is passed on in the direction of the cell body. This message is called 'action potential'. The action potential is like a fraction of a pulse.

Axon: The axon is a slender tube–like structure extending from the tapered portion of the cell body (called axon hillock) to the opposite end of the cell body. The axons are covered by 'myelin sheath', which functions as protective insulation from one another. The myelin is 80% fat and 20% protein. Not all axons are protected by myelin sheath. Further, the axon does not have the cover of myelin sheath continuously. The bare portion of axon uncoated by myelin sheath is called 'node of Ranvier'. The myelinated axon looks like a string of elongated beads. The information received from the dendrites called action potential travels through the axon.

Terminal Buttons: They are also called end bulb. They are tiny knobs at the end of the axon. They release neurochemicals called neurotransmitters. The neurotransmitters either excite or inhibit the receiving cell. This in turn decides whether an action potential occurs in the axon or not.

A single neuron is connected to the terminal buttons of axons of several other neurons. The junction between the terminal buttons of an axon and the membrane of a dendrite or soma of another neuron is called a 'synapse'.

188   *Human Physiology*

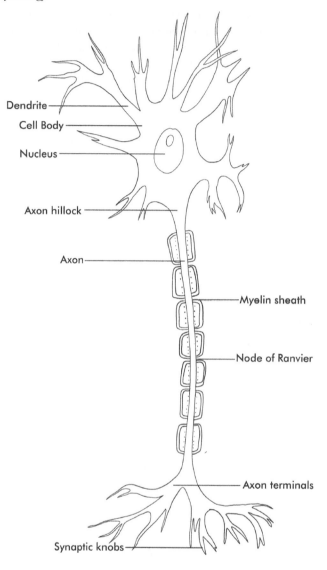

Figure 6.1 Structure of the Neuron.

Types of Neurons

Neurons can be classified into different types based on their structure or functions. Structurally, neurons are classified as multipolar, bipolar and unipolar neurons.

The **multipolar neuron** has the somatic membrane, and gives only one axon but many dendrites. Most of the neurons in brain and spinal cord are multipolar. **Bipolar neurons** are different in structure. Here, there is one axon and one dendrite starting from soma but going in two opposite directions from soma. They are found in retina, inner ear and the pathway of smell. In **unipolar neurons,** there is only one stalk. It starts from soma, and after a little distance, it divides into two branches. Unipolar neurons are found transmitting information from sense organs to the brain and spinal cord.

Based on their functions, neurons are classified into (1) **afferent neurons** (sensory neurons), (2) **efferent neurons** (motor neurons) and (3) **interneurons** (association neurons). Afferent refers to 'moving towards', and efferent refers to 'moving away'. Thus, these two names are with reference to brain and spinal cord. Afferent neurons respond to sensory stimulus from environment such as light, sound, odour, touch, temperature and carry the information from the sense organs to the spinal cord and brain. Efferent or motor neurons carry messages from the brain and spinal cord to muscles and glands causing motor response or activate the gland. Interneurons are found within the brain and spinal cord. As the name suggests, they connect neurons to other neurons.

Reflex Arc: Now that we know about the three types of neurons discharging their assigned functions, it is of relevance to understand the reflex arc. A reflex arc is the route to and from the brain and spinal cord conducting impulses. The well-known reflex arc is of three neurons consisting of an afferent neuron, an interneuron and an efferent neuron. The afferent neuron conducts impulses from sense organs to the spinal cord and brain, while the efferent neurons conduct impulses from the brain and spinal cord to the muscles and glands activating them. In between, the interneurons conduct impulses from afferent neurons to efferent neurons or towards efferent neurons. The three of them an arc constitutes a pathway to conduct information.

Support for Neurons: Neurons receive immense support from glial cells. They hold the neurons in place by surrounding them. In addition, they provide nutrients to the neurons. Further, they supply the chemicals used by the neurons for transmitting information. If a neuron is destroyed because of any injury or disease, the glial cells clean up the dead cells. Glial cells also help in insulating the neurons in brain and spinal cord from getting glued to other (thus creating a mess in information processing) by creating myelin sheath around axons. The same function is done by Schwann cells for the neurons in the rest of the body.

Neural Communication as Function of Neuron

We will try to understand the functions of the neuron from the behavioural perspective. From this angle, it is important to understand the communication process of the neural network, which determines minor and major behaviour. We will try to understand the neural communication and the consequent behavioural response with the help of two hypothetical contextual examples.

Example 1: You are in the kitchen on the job of making rotis for yourself. While doing so, you are also speaking on the phone. While putting the roti on the pan, your palm contacts the pan, but in no time you withdraw your hand. All these happens in what appears 'a fraction of a second'.

The neural networking and the communication that happened in this 'fraction of a second' are explained in Figure 6.2.

When your hand contacted the hot pan, the sensory neurons on your palm detected the painful stimulus. The dendrites receiving the painful stimulus sent the information down the axon to the terminal buttons. These terminal buttons located in the spinal cord release neurotransmitters, which excite the interneuron. The interneuron in turn transmits this message down its axon to terminal buttons. The terminal buttons of the interneuron release neurotransmitters. The interneuron connected to the motor excites it. The axon of the motor neuron joins a nerve that travels to the muscle in the hand. When the terminal buttons of the motor neuron release the neurotransmitter, it stimulates the muscle cells to contract, leading to the withdrawal of the hand from the pan. Yes, all these activities are completed within that 'fraction of a second'.

190 *Human Physiology*

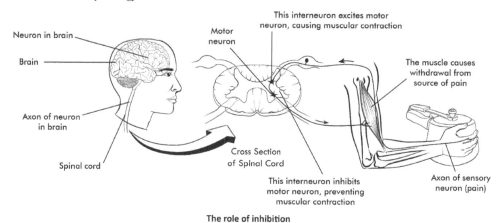

Figure 6.2 Neural Networking and Communication.

Example 2: You have invited your friends home and wanted them to have an experience of your culinary expertise. You have prepared 'Alu Mutter Paneer'. You shifted the dish to a serving container and are carrying it from the kitchen to the dining room holding the container with a thin cloth. As you start walking, the heat of the container starts to pass through the thin cloth and your hand starts feeling the heat. However, you do not drop the container, but walk fast to the dining table continuing to hold the container until you placed it on the table. In this case though the fingers felt the pain of the heat of the pot, and you felt like dropping the pot, you hold the pot bearing the heat until you reach the destination. How is this behavioural response different? What neural networking prevented you from dropping the pot?

As in case of your reflex actions of withdrawing your hand from the pan in previous example, the sensory neuron receives the painful stimulus of heat and transmits this message through its axon to the spinal cord. The interneuron in turn carries this message to motor neuron, which subsequently sends the message to the muscles. However, before the withdrawal of the hands from the pot, an axon from the neuron in the brain reaches the spinal cord. Here, its terminal buttons join interneurons, which are inhibitory. The neuron from the brain excites the inhibitory interneuron. This interneuron releases inhibitory neurotransmitter. This in turn reduces the activity of the motor neuron that otherwise would have excited the muscle to withdraw the hand and drop the pot. Because of the inhibitory neurotransmitter, the reflex response of withdrawing hands from the pot is blocked.

For the sake of understanding, the explanation is given in terms of a single neuron, though in reality hundreds of neurons are activated to provide a sensory input or a motor response. The neural networking is responsible for all our involuntary and voluntary responses.

Masses of these neural tissues constitute the nervous systems. Now that we have understood the neuron—the basic element in the nervous system—we are ready to explore into the vast area called the nervous system, which is made of hundreds of thousands of neurons. It can be described as a complex interdependent organization of sensory and motor nerve fibres, receiving inputs from the environment and from within and responding to these stimuli in a simple and complex way. The complex nervous system is depicted in a simple way in Figure 6.3.

The whole nervous system is divided into two—central nervous system (CNS) and peripheral nervous system (PNS). The central nervous system consists of the brain and spinal cord. The peripheral nervous system is divided into the somatic nervous system and the autonomic

Human Physiology 191

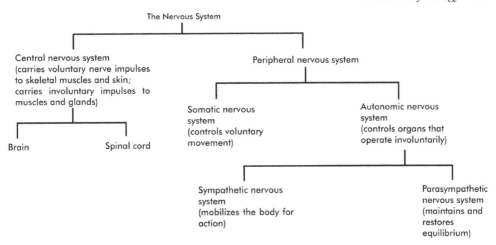

Figure 6.3 Components of the Nervous System.

nervous system (ANS). Some scholars have identified the enteric nervous system as a separate classification. The autonomic nervous system is further divided into the sympathetic nervous system and the parasympathetic nervous system. Each of these systems explains the coordinated functioning of a specific segment. The structure and function of the nervous system leave one in awe because of the complex coordinated functioning and about creation. Let us try to understand the systems.

The stepping stone to understanding the nervous system is to conceptualize the basic terms used in describing or explaining the locations and functioning of various parts. Figure 6.4 explains the meaning of terms such as 'dorsal' (top of head and back), 'caudal' (tail), 'ventral' (front), 'anterior' (in front), 'posterior' (in back), 'lateral' (away from middle) and 'medial' (towards middle).

The Central Nervous System (CNS)

The central nervous system (CNS) consists of the brain and the spinal cord. It acquires the tag of 'Central' because it is 'Central' to the regulatory processes. It integrates the inputs from sensory nerves and the outputs of motor action. It regulates the human responses by evaluating the changes in the environment so as to maintain the homeostatic balance.

Natural Protection to Brain

Brain is one of the most delicate organs in the human body. It is very soft and slimy. It is so delicate and jelly-like that it is extremely difficult to remove it from a deceased body without causing any damage to it. The approximate weight of the brain is 1.4 kg. The weight and the delicate structure of the brain are a combination that suggests its vulnerability to damage and injury. In order to protect this structure in every way, this organ is given natural protection that is sound and robust. In fact, both brain and spinal cord, the two parts of the CNS, have this natural protective covering. The multiple factors protecting the CNS are described below.

The outermost protective covering for the brain and the spinal cord is the skull and the vertebral column, the bony protection.

192 *Human Physiology*

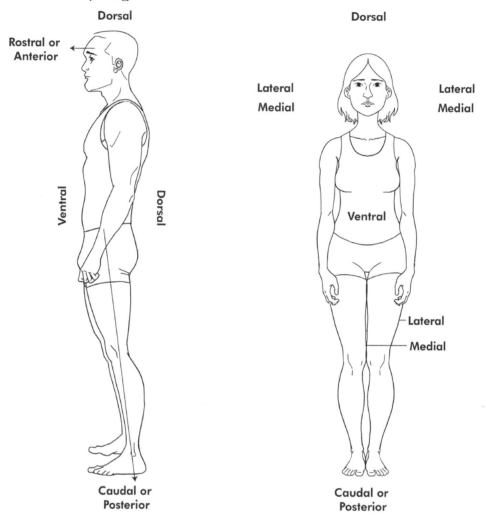

Figure 6.4 Basic Concepts of Locations/Positions.

Meninges

The brain and spinal cord are protected by outer sheaths called 'meninges'. This has three layers of covering called (1) dura mater, (2) arachnoid and (3) pia mater. Dura mater is the outer cover that is hard and tough. It is a layer made of a hard fibrous tissue white in colour. The term 'dura mater' connotes 'hard mother'. The second layer arachnoid membrane has a web-like appearance. This is spongy and soft. The innermost of the three layers is pia mater meaning 'Pons mother'. This layer is transparent. It contains the blood vessels of the brain and spinal cord. It sticks to the outer surface of the brain and spinal cord. The pia mater does not stick to the arachnoid membrane. There is a space between the arachnoid membrane and pia mater. This gap is called subarachnoid space. This space is filled with a liquid substance called cerebrospinal fluid (CSF).

Cerebrospinal Fluid (CSF)

The 1.4-kg brain does not rest on a hard or soft surface. It floats in the cerebrospinal fluid that fills the subarachnoid space. Because of this, the weight of the brain in its position is reduced to 800 g. The floating condition of the brain thus decreases its pressure on the base. This itself constitutes a good protection for the brain from any shock caused due to swift head movements or impact on the head.

Cerebrospinal fluid is (extracted) from the blood. It is produced in the four ventricles of the brain by a special tissue that is rich in supply of blood. This tissue, called choroid plexus, protrudes into the four ventricles of the brain. The ventricles of the brain refer to the series of hallow, interconnected chambers in the brain. These ventricles are presented in Figure 6.5.

Lateral ventricles on the either side of the brain are the largest chambers. Though they are also known as first and second ventricles, they are normally referred to as lateral ventricles. The lateral ventricles are connected to the third ventricles located at the midline of the brain. The third ventricle in turn is connected to the fourth ventricle through a long tube known as cerebral aqueduct. The cerebrospinal fluid is continuously produced. The total volume of the fluid is about 125–140 mL (Carlson, 2005; Khosla, 2017). It takes about three hours to replace about half of the cerebrospinal fluid with freshly produced fluid. The cerebrospinal fluid produced in lateral ventricles flows to third and fourth ventricles where more of this is produced. From the fourth ventricle, the CSF flows out through a small opening to the subarachnoid space. Then flowing through the subarachnoid space, it gets reabsorbed into the blood stream.

Within this protective structure lies the brain. Now let us broadly discuss the structure and functions of the brain.

Major Anatomical Map of the Brain

From the point of anatomy, the brain can be subdivided into three major parts, viz. forebrain, midbrain and hindbrain. They acquired the names based on their position. The forebrain is further subdivided into telencephalon and diencephalon. Cerebral cortex, limbic system and basal ganglia are the parts that come under telencephalon. Diencephalon that covers the third

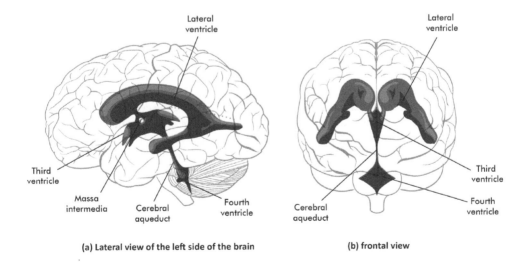

Figure 6.5 Ventricular System of the Brain.

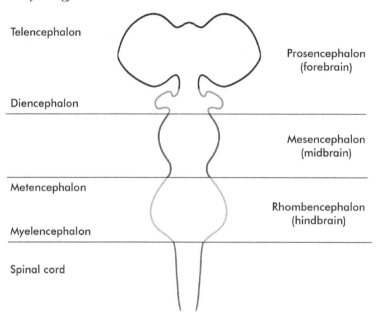

Figure 6.6 Brain: Its Anatomical Divisions and Subdivisions.

ventricle covers the thalamus and hypothalamus. The midbrain is also known as mesencephalon. It surrounds the cerebral aqueduct. It has two major parts called tectum and tegmentum. The hindbrain surrounds the fourth ventricle and consists of two major parts, viz. metencephalon and myelencephalon. Metencephalon consists of cerebellum and pons, while myelencephalon consists of medulla oblongata. The division and subdivision are depicted in Figure 6.6 for a clear conceptualization.

The Forebrain: Under the forebrain—telencephalon—we will discuss the location, structure and function of cerebral cortex, limbic system and basal ganglia.

Cerebrum: This is the largest part located at the uppermost part of the brain. It is systematically divided into two halves each of which is called a 'hemisphere'. Thus, it has a left and right hemisphere. These left and right hemispheres control the opposite side of the body. Though they control the opposite side of the body, they function in perfect coordination. The two halves are connected by a large bundle of axon called 'corpus callosum'. The surface of the cerebrum is called cerebral cortex. Cortex means 'bark'. It is called so because the cerebral cortex surrounds the two hemispheres like a bark of the tree. It has few millions of neurons where the axon terminals synapse with dendrites and cell bodies of other neurons. These cells present in millions in the cerebral cortex give it a colour of grey-brown. The appearance of the cortex is several bulges and grooves. The small grooves are called sulci, while the large grooves are known as fissures. The bulges are called 'gyri'. It is said that about 2/3rd of the cortex area is hidden in the grooves (Carlson, 2005). The total surface area of the cortex measures 2.5 ft^2, while the thickness is 2–4 mm (Carlson, 2005; Khosla, 2017).

Depending upon their specific sensory or motor control, the cerebral cortex is divided into four areas. Each area is called a 'lobe'. Each lobe is named after the bone in the skull that covers the area. The lobes are formed by the fissures in the cerebral cortex. These lobes are frontal lobe, temporal lobe, parietal lobe and occipital lobe. The fifth lobe 'insula' is not visible on the surface (Khosla, 2017).

Frontal lobe: The entire area in front of the central sulcus anterior of the cerebral cortex is called frontal lobe. The frontal lobe controls the voluntary movements, fine motor movements such as movement of a finger or toe.

The most anterior part of the frontal lobe is known as the prefrontal cortex. Integration of huge information happens in this part. Frontal lobe is involved in a number of behaviours that involve concentration, problem solving and speech production.

Temporal lobe: They are located on either side of the cortex, besides the temple area of the head. The lateral fissure demarcates the temporal lobe separating it from other lobes. Temporal lobe has the primary auditory area. It controls complex visual functions such as perception of movements and recognizing faces. Important for the students of psychology is to know that temporal lobes are also associated with emotional and motivational behaviour. Temporal lobes help in interpretation of sensation, and visual and auditory memory.

Parietal lobe: Parietal lobes are located just behind the central sulcus posterior to the frontal lobe that they are known for interpretation of body sensations like heat, cold, touch, pressure and pain. It has a general interpretation area. It facilitates understanding speech and use of words (Norris & Siegfried, 2011).

Occipital lobe: Occipital lobe is situated at the back of the cerebral cortex posterior to temporal and parietal lobes. This lobe is associated with vision and visual recognition of objects.

The picture of the brain with different lobes and fissures is depicted in Figure 6.7b. Though the cortex is described in terms of the four types of lobes, it is important to remember that they are not functional water-tight components. They function in perfect coordination.

The primary sensory areas of the cerebral cortex send information to 'sensory association cortex'. Here, the neural circuits analyse the information received from the primary sensory cortex. This makes perception possible. These perceptions are stored as memories. For example, the area closest to the primary visual cortex in occipital lobe receives the visual input that is stored as visual memory. Sensory association areas located far from the visual cortex in occipital

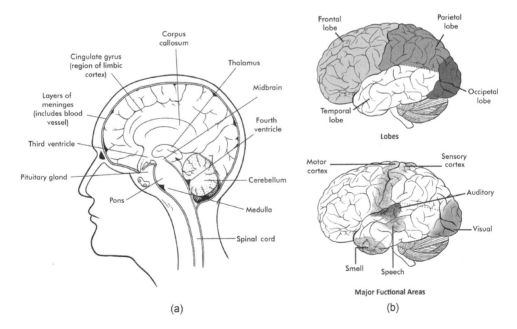

Figure 6.7 (a) Major Parts in the Brain. (b) Lobes in the Brain.

lobe receive inputs from other sensory systems such as auditory system. They are involved in perceptions and memory associated with multiple sensory systems, making it possible to integrate them and associate them with the single stimulus. For example, when we get the aroma of jasmine from somewhere we can associate it with the sight and touch of the flower.

As has been already mentioned, the left and right hemisphere of the brain and the lobe on the sides are connected to the opposite sides of the body. Hence, any damage through injury to the area on the left affects the right part of the body and vice versa. Patients of hypertension who suffer haemorrhage to the right side of the brain suffer paralysis on the left and vice versa. If the haemorrhage damages the left side of the brain that includes the temporal lobe, the patient suffers from problems in speech.

The second part of telencephalon is the limbic system.

Limbic System: Limbic in Latin means 'border'. This refers to an area that forms a curve like borders around corpus callosum. The most important parts of the limbic system are 'amygdala' and 'hippocampus'. They are located besides the lateral ventricle in the temporal lobe. A bundle of axons called 'fornix' connects hippocampus with other regions in the brain such as 'mammillary bodies' and hypothalamus. The limbic system is found to be associated basically with emotion and motivation. Feelings and expression of emotions, recognition of emotional signs in others, and emotional memories are associated with the limbic system. Apart from these, especially, the hippocampal area is found to be associated with hearing and memory.

Basal Ganglia: This refers to a collection of nuclei located deep inside the white matter of each hemisphere. It is a thin layer of grey matter. The limited knowledge gained on the functions of basal ganglia reveals its regulatory role in muscular contraction required for activities like maintaining posture and walking.

Diencephalon: This is the second major division of forebrain. It is located around the third ventricle. Its two constituent parts of brain are thalamus and hypothalamus. Let us discuss the structure and functions of these two parts of diencephalon of the forebrain.

Thalamus: The meaning of the word 'thalamus' in Greek is 'inner chamber'. Thus, the name of this part indicates the location of it. Thalamus constitutes the paired gray matter structure of the diencephalon located near the centre of the brain. Its location is in the middle of the cerebral hemisphere. The shape can be compared by and large with a dumbbell. It is made of a number of nuclei giving it the look of a mass of grey matter.

Thalamus is known as the 'Relay centre' of the brain. It receives impulses from axons from other different parts of the nervous system such as the spinal cord, cerebellum, basal ganglia, brain stem and various thalamic nuclei and synapse with dendrites whose axons carry impulses from thalamus to almost all parts of the cerebral cortex.

Recognition of various sensations happens in thalamus. Except olfactory sensation, the neurons from other sensory areas have their dendrites and cell bodies in the nuclei of thalamus. They form synapse with dendrites of other neurons, which pass on the information to the relevant sensory areas in the cerebrum. Any lesion or injury to thalamus leads to coma and death.

Hypothalamus: Hypothalamus is located below the thalamus forming the floor of the third ventricle. It is a tiny structure weighing about 7 g (Khosla, 2017). The location of thalamus and hypothalamus is shown in Figure 6.8.

Though small in structure, hypothalamus plays a significant role in survival. It exercises control over the autonomic nervous system and the endocrine system. Behaviours essential for basic survival such as Feeding, Fighting, Feeling and Mating (known as the four 'F's) are controlled by hypothalamus. It plays a significant role in maintaining homeostasis of the body. It ensures the balance of the body, and temperature and water levels in the body. Hypothalamus is also responsible for maintaining the waking state arousal and alertness in the body. This can

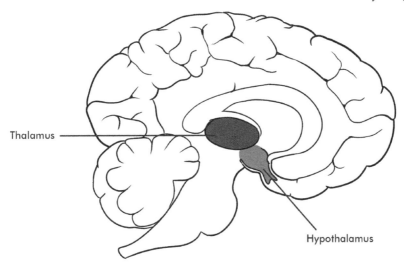

Figure 6.8 Location of Thalamus and Hypothalamus.

be stated that the behaviours that satisfy basic physiological needs (for survival) and escape or encountering danger (for survival) are controlled by hypothalamus. Any lesion in the hypothalamus impacts these basic survival behaviours like eating, sleeping and sexual behaviour. Animal experiments have proved that lesion in hypothalamus results in essential eating or starving behaviour in the animals.

The Midbrain: The part surrounding the aqueduct is called midbrain. It is also called 'mesencephalon'. It has two major parts, viz. tectum and tegmentum.

Tectum: Tectum is located in the dorsal part of the midbrain. Each side of the tectum has a bump. They are called 'superior colliculus' and 'inferior colliculus', referring to the visual and auditory systems respectively.

Tegmentum: Tegmentum is located beneath the tectum. It covers several structures in the midbrain like reticular formation, red nucleus, substantia nigra and periaqueductal grey matter.

Reticular Formation: This is a net-like structure. 'Reticulum' means 'little net'. This is a network consisting of many interconnected neurons with their dendritic and axonal processes. This network occupies core of the brain system starting from the lower border of medulla to the upper border of midbrain. Sensory information reaches reticular formation from various pathways. From here, the axons are projected to cerebral cortex, thalamus and spinal cord. It has a major role to play in a number of responses like sleep, arousal attention, muscle tone, movement and vital reflexes.

Red Nucleus: A bundle of axons originating from red nucleus is one of the two major fibre systems that carry message from the cerebrum and cerebellum to the spinal cord. It constitutes an important component in the motor system.

Substantia Nigra: It contains neurons whose axons project to basal ganglia. It is the major source of dopamine in the brain. Dopamine plays a significant role in extrapyramidal motor behaviour (Khosla, 2017).

Periaqueductal Grey Matter: The name is acquired for two reasons: 'grey matter' because it consists of the cell bodies of the neurons giving a grey colour to it; and 'periaqueductal' because it surrounds the aqueduct while it travels from third to fourth ventricles. The 'grey matter' consists of neural circuits that control the sequence and movements of behaviour typical to species in their fighting and mating behaviours.

Hindbrain: The hindbrain is the posterior part of the brain with two major divisions called 'metencephalon' and 'myelencephalon'.

Metencephalon: This consists of cerebellum and pons.

Cerebellum: This is known as 'little brain' located in the posterior part of cerebrum. Transverse fissures separate cerebellum from cerebrum.

Just as cerebrum, the outer surface of cerebrum is covered with grey matter, while the interior is covered with white matter. Cerebellum also has several sulci and fissures. Thus, it is an abridged version of cerebrum.

Cerebellum is important for three functions:

1 It maintains body balance and coordinates movements.
2 It coordinates with cerebrum and produces skilled movements.
3 It helps in controlling postures.

Cerebellum smoothens your movements by comparing and converging the intent with performance in direction rate and force. Injury to cerebellum results in jerky movements. This condition is called 'ataxia', where simple movements like walking become jerky.

Pons: Pons is located above medulla. It consists of white matter and reticular formation. The fibres on pons give it a bulge. It functions as a regulator of respiration and is associated with eye movements, chewing and facial expressions (Sarafino, 1994).

Myelencephalon Medulla Oblongata: This connects brain to the spinal cord. It contains part of the reticular formation. Its known function includes control of vital functions such as regulation of cardiovascular, respiratory and skeletal muscle functions. Hence, injury to medulla is considered fatal.

Spinal Cord: The second part of the CNS is the spinal cord. It stretches from foramen magnum at the bottom of the brain stem to the lower border of lumbar vertebrae. The length of the spinal cord in an average human body is about 45 cm (Khosla, 2017), and thickness is close to the little finger of an adult (Carlson, 2005). Spinal cord is located within the protective vertebral column, which is made of 33 vertebrae located in cervical (neck) thoracic (chest) and lumbar sacral coccygeal (lower back) regions. These vertebrae are so organized to create a continuous column through which the spinal cord runs. It is important to note that the length of the spinal cord is only 2/3rd of the vertebral column. The other 1/3rd consists of spinal roots that compose what is known as 'cauda equina' (horse's tail). There are two bulges in the spinal cord, one in the cervical region and the second in the lumber region. The afferent and efferent neurons pass through the spinal cord.

Figure 6.9 shows the cross-section of the spinal cord.

As can be seen from the figure, from either side of the spinal cord (from dorsolateral and ventrolateral surface) small bundles of fibres emerge out. Groups of these bundles converge giving rise to 31 paired sets of dorsal roots and ventral roots. They all join together while entering the intervertebral foramens and become spinal nerves.

The spinal cord is similar to brain in having the grey matter and white matter. However, it differs in location. Unlike brain, the outer side of the spinal cord has white matter, while the inner side has grey matter. This is because the outer part has the ascending and descending bundles of axons, which have myelin sheaths white in colour, while the inner side consists of neural cell bodies and unmyelinated axons. The cross-section of the spinal cord shows 'H'-shaped grey matter.

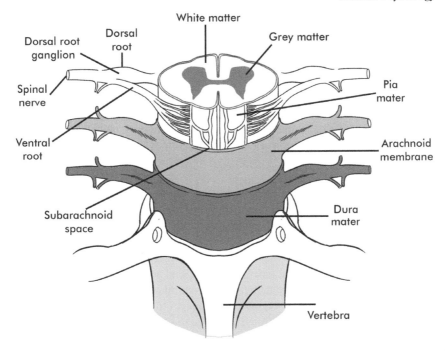

Figure 6.9 Spinal Cord: Cross-section.

The spinal cord assumes two important functions:

1 It provides a two-way route for the neurons to and from the brain.
2 It functions as a reflex centre.

There are ascending and descending tracts for the neurons. The impulses to the brain carry impulses to the brain up the spinal cord, while the descending tracts carry impulses from the brain down the tract. The ones that carry impulses to the brain conduct sensory impulses, while the descending tracts carry motor impulses.

The reflex actions are also the result of the function of the spinal cord. The synaptic junction between the sensory and motor neuron in the spinal cord constitutes the 'reflex arc'. As a result of this, the sensory impulses that reach the spinal cord become the outgoing motor impulses, resulting in snap action (e.g. sneezing, withdrawing hand from a piercing pin, closing eyelids when an insect approaches). Reflex arcs also exist when the sensory and motor neurons are connected through an interneuron.

Peripheral Nervous System (PNS)

The peripheral nervous system relates to the nervous system that reaches all over the body. They carry information from CNS and to CNS. The sensory inputs from different parts of the body and the environment are carried to the brain, and the commands from the brain for motor actions are carried to various muscular regions and glands to activate them. The majority of peripheral nerves pass through the spinal cord.

They add up to 31 pairs of spinal nerves and 12 pairs of cranial nerves. They are on either sides of the body. They help in maintaining homeostasis by sensing changes in the body and the environment.

The 12 pairs of cranial nerves emerge from brain, leave the cranial cavity and reach their destinations to carry out the functions. They are named after their destination. They are classified into three—viz. mixed cranial nerves, sensory cranial nerves and motor cranial nerves. As the names suggest, the mixed cranial nerves contain the axons of both sensory and motor neurons, while the other two cranial nerves have the axons of their respective types of neurons. The 12 cranial nerves are listed below with their respective numbers as labels.

- Olfactory Nerve (I): These nerves carry the sensory input of smell.
- Optic Nerve (II): They carry visual inputs from the eyes. Two optic nerves (one from each eye) join together after entering the cranial cavity and form into what is called 'optic chiasma'. The optic chiasma is where fibres of each nerve reach the opposite side and continue in the optic tract of that side. The majority of optic tract fibres end in thalamus. From thalamus, two fibres reach the occipital lobe where the visual area is located.
- Oculomotor Nerve (III): They originate from the ventral part of midbrain and reach various external eye muscles. They help in regulating the penetration of light into the eye. They cause all cycled movements of the eye.
- Trochlear Nerve (IV): This is responsible for eye movements. It innervates only a single muscle.
- Trigeminal Nerve (V): The name 'trigeminal' because it braches out to three. The sensory neurons of the branches carry message from the skin and mucosa of head and teeth to trigeminal ganglion and from there to pons. They are associated with the sensation of head, face and chewing. They control the jaw muscles.
- Abducens Nerve (VI): This is a motor nerve and is associated with eye.
- Facial Nerve (VII): Starting from the lower part of pons, this nerve reaches superficial muscles of the face and scalp through several branches. Facial expressions, tears, salvation and sensation of taste are associated with the nerve.
- Vestibulocochlear Nerve (VIII): It is a combination of two, viz. vestibular and cochlear nerves. It is an auditory nerve. The cochlear nerve is responsible for hearing, balancing of body and equilibrium.

The cranial nerves are given a pictorial representation in Figure 6.10.

- Glossopharyngeal Nerves (IX): This nerve supplies fibres to tongue, pharynx and carotid sinus. It is associated with sensations in tongue, salivary secretion, swallowing and reflex control of blood pressure.
- Vagus Nerve (X): It is a mixed nerve consisting of sensory and motor neurons. Most of the motor neurons in this nerve are autonomic. This nerve is associated with functions related to a wide spectrum of organs such as pharynx, larynx, trachea, heart, lungs, bronchi, oesophagus, stomach, small intestine and gallbladder.
- Accessory Nerve (XI): This acquires the name because it is considered an accessory to the vagus nerve. This is associated with movements in the shoulder, turning of head, visceral movements and voice generation.
- Hypoglossal Nerve (XII): This is involved in the movement of tongue.

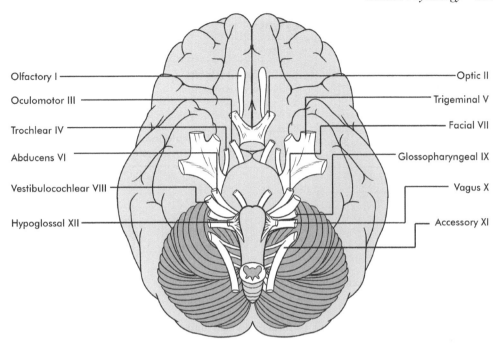

Figure 6.10 12 Pairs of Cranial Nerves.

It should be remembered that the cranial nerves emerge from the brain stem, while the spinal nerves emerge from the spinal cord. The PNS comprises of all pathways outside the brain and spinal cord. Both afferent and efferent nerves constitute the PNS. The efferent or motor nervous system is further divided into somatic and autonomic nervous system. The autonomic nervous system (ANS) is divided into sympathetic and parasympathetic nervous system. The division of the peripheral nervous system is presented in Figure 6.11.

We have already discussed that the afferent nervous system comprises of sensory neurons, while the efferent nervous system refers to motor nerves. The efferent nervous system consists of the somatic nervous system and autonomic nervous system.

Somatic Nervous System

These are voluntary motor pathways outside the central nervous system. This implies that these pathways operate voluntarily. The somatic nervous system receives sensory information sent from the sense organs. Depending upon the information, they trigger the movements of skeletal muscles.

Autonomic Nervous System: The autonomic nervous system is an important constituent of the peripheral nervous system. The term 'autonomic' connotes 'self-governance'. Thus, the autonomic nervous system is unique in the sense that on its own, it regulates smooth muscles, cardiac function and glandular secretion in such a way to maintain homeostasis.

To give examples of contraction of smooth muscles, the autonomic nervous system contracts and regulates the internal organs without a conscious effort. For example, it regulates the sphincters of gallbladder, urinary bladder etc. Thus, it controls the vegetative process in the body through controlling these muscles.

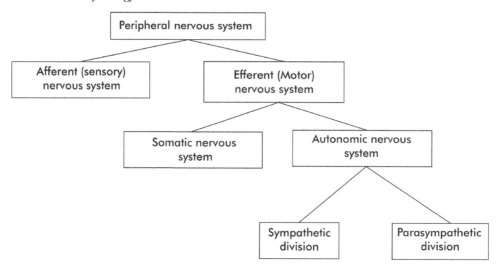

Figure 6.11 Structural Representation of the Peripheral Nervous System.

The autonomic nervous system is further divided into sympathetic nervous system and parasympathetic nervous system. We shall discuss these two systems from their functional perspectives.

Sympathetic Nervous System

Sympathetic nervous system is involved in expenditure of energy. When the person is excited, the sympathetic nervous system gets activated increasing the outgoing signals rapidly. The body's defence mechanism takes over by enhancing the sympathetic activities. Sympathetic activities include a group of responses that are triggered simultaneously, reading the body to encounter the threat and cope with the stress that requires energy. There are increased blood flow to the skeletal muscles, faster conversion of glycogen into glucose that flows into the blood, enhanced heartbeat, dilated bronchi and dilated blood vessels facilitating easy and faster flow of blood. The sympathetic impulses also stimulate the adrenal glands located above the kidneys, which in turn release adrenaline, noradrenaline and cortisol into the blood. All these changes lead to what is popularly known as 'fight-or-flight' response that demands the person either to confront the situation or to escape from the spot, both of which demand additional energy. The fight-or-flight response includes two types of reactions. The first is enhanced activity of heart through cardiac muscle contraction, faster blood flow through dilation of blood vessels and skeletal muscles, respiratory system, enhanced function of sweat glands. The second is controlled activity. This is done by constriction of blood vessels to all digestive organs. By this way, it slows down the regular activities of the digestive system. That is the reason one does not feel hungry when one has to run away to escape an engulfing fire.

During the normal condition, the sympathetic nervous system helps in normal functions of the body. It confronts the parasympathetic system that tends to slow down the heart function and sustain the normalcy.

The parasympathetic nervous system concentrates on functions that create and conserve body's energy. For example, it helps in secretion of saliva and gastric juices for digestion and assimilation. The body organs associated with sympathetic and parasympathetic systems are depicted in Figure 6.12.

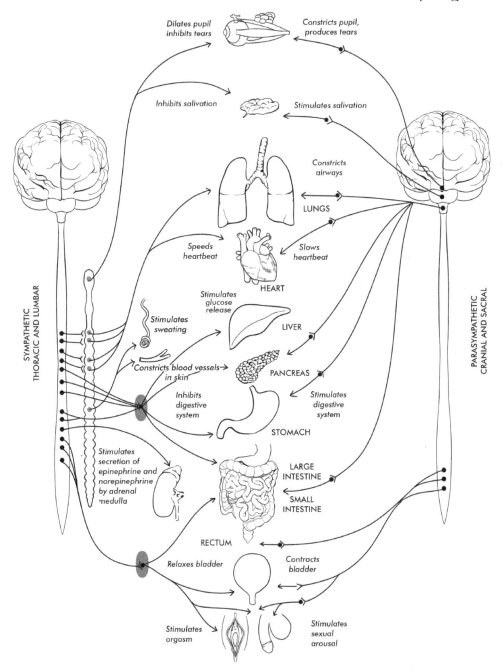

Figure 6.12 Functions of the Autonomic Nervous System.

Endocrine System

The endocrine system refers to a number of ductless glands located in different parts of the body-releasing hormones into the blood that are essential for the human survival. The endocrine system plays a role in regulating the growth and development, tissue functions, body metabolism, mood, sexual functions and reproductive process.

204 *Human Physiology*

The endocrine system works in close association with the nervous system. The difference between the two is that the nervous system sends both electrical and chemical messages, while the endocrine system sends only chemical messages. Further, the nervous system controls the faster processes such as breathing and body movements, while the endocrine system is in control of slow body processes such as growth and development.

We shall explain the various glands and the hormones they secrete and their major functions.

Before discussing various glands and their hormones, it is necessary to understand basic aspects related to hormones. A hormone is an endogenous substance. It means it is produced within the body. They are produced by one gland and released to the blood stream. They travel through the blood and reach their target cell. The receptors in the target cell bind to the hormone and induce a response. The coordination of the endocrine system with the nervous system can be explained in simple terms—while the glands in the endocrine system produce the hormones, the instructions for the production and its pace come from the nervous system.

There are three types of hormones based on their source, viz. lipid hormones, peptide hormones and amine hormones.

Lipid Hormones: They are derived from fatty acids, e.g. steroids such as oestrogen, progesterone, testosterone and cortisol, which originate from cholesterol.

Peptide Hormones: They are short chains of amino acids, e.g. antidiuretic hormone (ADH), thyrotrophic-releasing hormone (TRH) and oxytocin.

Amine Hormones: They originate from amino acids, e.g. thyroxin, adrenaline and noradrenaline.

The Control Centre of Endocrine System:

As already mentioned, the instructions to the endocrine system come from the nervous system. The connection of these two systems is facilitated by the connectivity between the hypothalamus and the pituitary gland. The hypothalamus sends chemical message to the pituitary gland. This stimulates the pituitary gland to release pituitary hormones, which in turn selectivity trigger other glands in the system to secrete hormones.

The various glands in the endocrine system and their location are depicted in Figure 6.13.

Pituitary Gland: Pituitary gland is located at the base of the brain, below the hypothalamus and close to the optic nerve. It controls the release of hormones in the entire endocrine system following the stimulation from hypothalamus. Because of this, it is popularly known as the 'master gland'.

The pituitary gland has two lobes—the anterior pituitary lobe and the posterior pituitary lobe. Let us explain the hormones secreted by these two lobes. Receiving the message from the hypothalamus, the anterior pituitary lobe secretes four types of hormones:

1. On encountering stress, the hypothalamus stimulates the anterior lobe, which releases a hormone called 'adrenocorticotrophic hormone' (ACTH). This gets released into the blood and travels to the adrenal glands located on top of the kidneys and stimulates them to release adrenaline, noradrenaline and cortisol. We shall discuss the functions of these hormones when we explain the functions of adrenal glands.
2. The anterior lobe of pituitary gland also releases the growth hormone (GH) also known as somatotrophic hormone (STH). This growth hormone is responsible for the growth of tissues in the body, including muscles and bones. Gonadotrophic hormones released by the anterior pituitary gland are responsible for growth and development of glands (testes and ovaries) (Taylor, 2006).

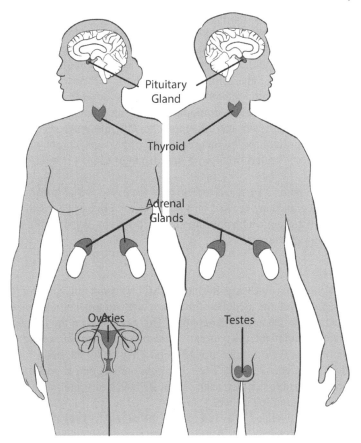

Figure 6.13 Endocrine System.

3 The third hormone produced by the anterior pituitary lobe is 'prolactin'. This is helpful in production of milk by targeting the mammary glands.
4 The fourth hormone produced by the anterior pituitary lobe is 'thyroid-stimulating hormone' (TSH). This hormone triggers the thyroid gland that in turn releases two hormones called 'calcitonin' and 'thyroxin'.

The posterior lobe of the pituitary gland produces two hormones, viz. 'oxytocin' and 'vasopressin', which is known as 'antidiuretic hormone' (ADH).

1 Oxytocin released by the posterior pituitary lobe is a hormone that is very helpful for females during labour and lactation. It helps uterine contraction during child birth. It also stimulates the mammary glands that release milk. In males, it is found to help in contraction of sperm ducts during ejaculation.
2 The second hormone that is released from the posterior pituitary lobe is 'vasopressin' or antidiuretic hormone (ADH); when the water level in the body is low, thus disturbing the equilibrium, it stimulates the kidneys to reabsorb the water content. This prevents dehydration in the body.

Thyroid Gland: The thyroid gland is located in the anterior part of the neck. It is described as having the shape of a butterfly shading the trachea with the wings of the butterfly on the two sides of trachea. Two hormones called 'thyroxin' and 'triiodothyronine' are produced in thyroid. When the posterior pituitary gland releases 'thyroid-stimulating hormones' (TSH), which in turn trigger the thyroid gland, the two thyroid hormones absorb the protein molecules in the cells and release them into the blood. Thus, thyroxin helps in the growth and development of the tissues. This is particularly important among children and adolescents, which are known as critical stages of growth and development. The hormones secreted by the thyroid gland are considered important for the metabolic rate of proteins, carbohydrates, fat minerals and vitamins. Hormones secreted by thyroid are also significant for development of mental processes.

Adrenal Gland: The name 'Ad-renal' refers to its location. 'Renal' means kidney, and 'ad' means 'near'. Adrenal glands are located on the top of each kidney. Adrenal glands have two parts, viz. medulla and cortex, which are functionally different. We will discuss the hormones secreted by each of these parts.

1 Adrenal Medulla

   The adrenocorticotrophin-releasing hormone (ACTH) from the anterior pituitary gland reaches the adrenal gland, the medulla of the adrenal gland gets stimulated and releases two hormones called adrenaline and noradrenaline. This occurs when the individual encounters a stressful condition and perceives a threat. These two hormones are called catecholamines. They are hormones, as well as neurotransmitters. They ready the body for 'fight-or-flight' response in the face of emergencies. These hormones are by and large similar in their functions. They are responsible for increasing the heart rate, heart 'contractility' (how hard the heart), contracts and blood sugar level.

2 The Cortex of Adrenal Gland: The cortex of the adrenal gland secretes three types of hormones.

   a Glucocorticoids: The glucocorticoids released from the adrenal cortex include 'hydrocortisol' commonly known as 'cortisol'. This is a steroid hormone. Its main function is to convert proteins, fats and carbohydrates into glucose.
   b Gonadocorticoids: Basically, these are sex hormones secreted by the adrenal cortex. However, what is secreted by the adrenal cortex is only a fraction of gonadal source. Its levels in body rise years prior to the onset of puberty. It stimulates sexual instincts.
   c Mineralocorticoids: This hormone secreted by the adrenal cortex regulates the electrolyte balance in the body. It facilitates the excretion or reabsorption of sodium and potassium by kidneys, and salivary and sweat glands, depending on the need of the body.

Gonads: Gonads are reproductive glands. These glands in females are called ovaries and in males testes. They produce sex hormones in males and females, which are essential to stimulate sexual behaviour. These hormones are called 'oestrogen', 'progesterone' and 'testosterone'. Oestrogen and progesterone are female hormones, while testosterone is a male hormone. However, traces of oestrogen are found in male, while traces of testosterone also are found in female urine samples. By and large, these hormones are gender-specific facilitating the gender-specific structure and functions in males and females. Let us try to have a broad understanding of their role in sexual behaviour and reproduction.

Oestrogen: Oestrogen is produced by the ovaries in females. During adolescent age, the growth and development of the girls manifest in secondary sexual characteristics. Oestrogen facilitates the process of puberty and the concomitant developments such as breast enlargement, growth in height, bones, muscles and skin. It is oestrogen that helps in widening of the pelvic bones in girls so that the body is prepared for the child birth. Oestrogen is also responsible for fat around the female body. Oestrogen levels are high during pubertal age. Hence, we see a growth spurt in girls who gain in height and weight during this period.

Progesterone: This is also released by ovaries. Progesterone plays a vital role in strengthening the uterus. It helps in storing nutrients in uterus lining. It prepares the uterus to allow implantation of embryo. This is done by creating changes in the uterine wall.

Testosterone: This is basically a male sex hormone secreted by testes. The levels of testosterone are high during pubertal stage of boys. This hormone causes secondary sexual characteristics in boys. One can see the growth in muscle tissues, hair on the face, chest and underarm. This stimulates sexual behaviour in male.

Pancreas: Located in the abdomen, it occupies space near kidneys, stomach and small intestine. Pancreas plays duel function, viz. a digestive function and an endocrinal function. We shall now focus only on its endocrine function.

Pancreas produces two hormones—insulin and glucagon.

Insulin and glucagon work in good coordination to balance the glucose level in the blood. Let us elaborate on this. Glucose travels in the blood to be available to all the cells as energy. But there has to be a balance in the glucose level in the blood. Otherwise, excess supply of glucose can be harmful for the small blood vessels, particularly in kidneys, eyes and extremities of the body. The insulin and glucagon produced by the pancreas function in coordination to check the glucose level in blood within acceptable levels. The job of the insulin is to lower the level of glucose in the blood, while the role of glucagon is to rise it. When the blood glucose level rises, pancreas releases insulin to stimulate the cells to increase the burning of it so that the level of glucose in the blood is reduced. Insulin also helps glucose storage in liver, muscles and fatty tissues. Once the level is reduced, the secretion of insulin is also reduced. When the glucose level in the blood drops, the pancreas secretes glucagon. Glucagon pulls into the blood stream the glucose stored in the cells.

Thus, the two pancreatic hormones—insulin and glucagon—are responsible for maintaining homeostatic of blood glucose, and also responsible for all actions calling for energy investment.

Dysfunction of pancreas or disturbance in the coordinated function of these two hormones results in excess or reduced glucose level in the blood causing diabetes or hypoglycaemia.

Pineal Gland: This is located between the two hemispheres of the brain. The area of its location is called 'epithalamus'. It is one of the last glands discovered. It used to be known as the 'third eye'. The pineal gland secretes a hormone called 'melatonin'. This hormone is responsible for the circadian rhythm of the body. Secretion of melatonin depends upon the exposure to light. Perception of light inhibits the secretion of melatonin, which is produced in large amounts when there is no light and one is placed in dark environment. That is the reason why we need to switch off the lights to fall asleep. Again, exposure to electronic screens like mobile phones or television or computer before bedtime hampers our sleep because they interfere in melatonin secretion.

Secretion of melatonin is said to be healthy for blood pressure and healthy cardiac function.

Melatonin plays an inhibitory role in production of reproductive hormones from the anterior pituitary gland that helps in development and functioning of reproductive organs.

Parathyroid Glands: These glands, as small as rice granules, 6 mm/3–4 mm, are located in the neck of the thyroid gland. They secrete two hormones, viz. 'parathormone' and 'calcitonin'. The main function of parathyroid hormones is to regulate calcium levels in the blood, by acting

208 Human Physiology

on bones, intestines and kidneys. When the calcium levels in the blood reduce, the parathyroid hormones bring up its level by the following means:

1. They stimulate the bones to release stored calcium into the blood.
2. They increase the calcium absorption in the intestine.
3. They minimize the loss of calcium in urine.

Thus, every gland in the endocrine system contributes to one or more vital function of the body.

Table 6.1 provides a summary of the various glands in then endocrine system, the hormone secreted by them and the role of the hormone.

Table 6.1 Important glands in the endocrine system, their location, the hormones, and functions

S. No.	Gland	Location	Hormone	Functions
1	Pituitary gland	Base of brain below hypothalamus, close to the optic nerve		
1 a	Anterior of the pituitary gland	Front of the pituitary gland	Adrenocorticotrophic hormone (ACTH)	Stimulates secretion of corticosteroids by adrenal cortex
1 a(I)	Anterior of the pituitary gland	Front of the pituitary gland	Growth hormone (GH)/somatotrophic hormone (STH)	Stimulates growth of bones and tissues
1 a(II)	Anterior of the pituitary gland	Front of the pituitary gland	Prolactin	Targets mammary glands to stimulate production of milk
1 a(III)	Anterior of the pituitary gland	Front of the pituitary gland	Thyroid stimulating hormone (TSH)	Stimulates the thyroid gland to produce and release calcitonin and thyroxin
1 b(I)	Posterior of the pituitary gland	Back part of the pituitary gland	Antidiuretic hormone	Stimulates kidneys to reabsorb water to prevent dehydration
1 b(II)	Posterior of the pituitary gland	Back part of the pituitary gland	Oxytocin	Uterine contraction during child birth and release of milk through mammary glands in females and contraction of sperm duct during ejaculation
2	Thyroid gland	Anterior part of neck	(a) Calcitonin	Regulates the calcium level in blood by targeting the bones, kidneys and the intestines
			(b) Thyroxin	Increases metabolic rate in tissues. Regulates growth and development
3	Adrenal glands	Top of the kidneys		
3 a	Medulla of the adrenal gland	Top of the kidneys	Adrenaline and noradrenaline	Stimulates the heart and other muscles during stressful emergencies, increases glucose in blood
3 b(I)	Cortex of adrenal glands	Top of the kidneys	Glucocorticoids	Helps in the formation of glucose from fats and proteins

(*Continued*)

Table 6.1 (Continued)

S. No.	Gland	Location	Hormone	Functions
3 b(II)	Cortex of adrenal glands	Top of the kidneys	Glucocorticoids	Stimulates sexual instincts
3 b(III)	Cortex of adrenal glands	Top of the kidneys	Mineralocorticoids	Targets kidney cells to reabsorb sodium and excrete potassium to keep electrolyte balance
4	Ovaries	Held by a membrane besides uterus on each side of lower abdomen	(a) Oestrogen	Stimulates the maturation and release of ova Works on muscles, bones and skin to develop secondary sex characteristics
			(b) Progesterone	Prepares uterus for implantation of embryo and maintains pregnancy
5	Testes	Within the scrotum that hangs outside the body	Testosterone	Stimulates sperm production in testes. Helps in male sex characteristics by targeting skin, muscle and bone
6	Pancreas Pancreas	Behind the stomach in the upper left abdomen Behind the stomach in the upper left abdomen	(a) Insulin (b) Glucagon	Prompts liver, muscles and fat tissues to store glucose so as to lower the blood glucose level Prompts liver, muscles and fat tissues to release glucose into the blood stream
7	Pineal gland	Back of the third ventricle in the brain	Melatonin	Maintains body's biorhythm by targeting a variety of tissues
8	Parathyroid glands	Behind thyroid gland	Parathyroid hormone (parathormone and calcitonin)	Helps increase the blood calcium level by stimulating cells in bones, kidneys and intestines

Cardiovascular System

Cardiovascular system is also known as the circulatory system. The circulatory system explains the circulation of blood in the body. The purpose of the blood circulating in the body is to keep the organism alive by taking care of every cell in the body. The blood carries the necessary nutrients, oxygen and other gases to the cells that are essential for their survival. It also carries the carbon dioxide and the other unnecessary elements discarded by the cells back to the heart and then the lungs for purification and recirculation. The circulatory system is also known as the 'cardiovascular system' where 'cardio' refers to the heart and 'vascular' refers to the blood vessels. Thus, the three main parts of the system are the heart and the blood vessels and the blood itself. Let us first understand the structure and function of heart.

The Heart: The heart is a soft muscle. The size of the heart is about a fist. It weighs about 280–340 g in men and 230–280 g in women. The dimensions of heart are roughly 12 cm long, 9 cm wide (across its broadest point) and 6 cm thick. It is located between the two lungs behind the sternum and above the diaphragm (a dome-shaped muscular membrane separating thoracic and abdomen regions). Heart being a very delicate and vital organ, its location protects it very well. A fibrous covering celled 'pericardium' gives a protective covering around the heart. It also provides a good anchoring so that the heart sits well in the thoracic area allowing it a safe expansion when it is full. The pericardium has two layers, viz. 'visceral layer', which directly covers the outside of heart and 'parietal layer', a sac that is the exterior layer. This sac contains serous fluid produced by pericardium called pericardial fluid', which protects the heart from any friction with the surrounding areas, and also serves as a good lubricant.

Heart Walls: The heart is made up of three layers. These layers are nothing but connective tissues.

Epicardium: This is the outermost layer of the heart, which constitutes the inner wall of pericardium. This is thin membrane that lubricates the outer part of the heart and protects it.

Myocardium: This is the middle layer. It is a thick membrane. It helps in pumping activity of the heart.

Endocardium: This constitutes the innermost layer of the heart chambers. It covers the valves of the heart. This is the layer that is in contact with the blood in the heart. It presents the blood from sticking and forming clots.

Chambers of the Heart: The heart has four chambers. We can describe them in two ways—the right and left heart or the top and bottom chambers. The right and left parts are divided by a membrane called 'septum'. The top chambers are called 'atria' (right and left atrium). The bottom two chambers are called 'ventricles' (right and left ventricles). The atria are the receivers of the blood to the heart. The ventricles are 'senders' of blood from the heart. The left atrium receives purified blood from the lungs and sends to the left ventricle. The left ventricle pumps this purified blood to all over the body. The right atrium receives the impure blood from the body and sends it to the right ventricle. The right ventricle in turn pumps out this impure blood to the lungs for the purpose of infusing oxygen. The left side of the heart is slightly larger compared to the right. The ventricles have much thicker walls, which facilitates the work of pumping the blood.

Heart Valves: The heart valves are fibrous tissue flaps. They are located between the chambers of the heart to ensure the flow of blood in one direction preventing any retraction into the opposite direction.

Atrioventricular Valves: These valves are located between the atrium and the ventricle on either the left and right side of the heart. The atrioventricular valve in the right side is called 'tricuspid valve', and the one on the left side is called 'mitral valve'.

Semilunar Valves: The name 'semilunar' connotes the 'half-moon' shape of these valves. The left semilunar valve is located between the 'aorta' and left ventricle. The right semilunar valve is located between the 'pulmonary artery' and right ventricle.

Blood Vessels: The second important component of the circulatory system is blood vessels. We find major blood vessels entering and leaving the heart and all over the body. The blood vessels are transporters of blood between the heart and other body parts. There are three types of blood vessels, viz. arteries, veins and capillaries. Veins carry deoxygenated blood from different parts of the body and enter the right atrium of the heart through 'superior vena cava' and inferior vena cava. They also carry oxygenated blood from lungs to the heart. 'Arteries' carry oxygenated blood from heart to different parts of the body. They also carry deoxygenated blood from heart to lungs. 'Capillaries' are the minuscular network of arteries. They are present in the lungs and muscles as the smallest blood vessels. Most capillaries are thinner than the hair. They are so thin that only one blood cell can move at a time.

The major blood vessels connecting to the heart are shown in Figure 6.14.

As can be seen in the diagram, the main blood vessels entering and exiting the heart are 'aorta', 'the superior vena cava', 'the inferior vena cava', 'the pulmonary artery', the 'pulmonary veins' and 'coronary arteries'.

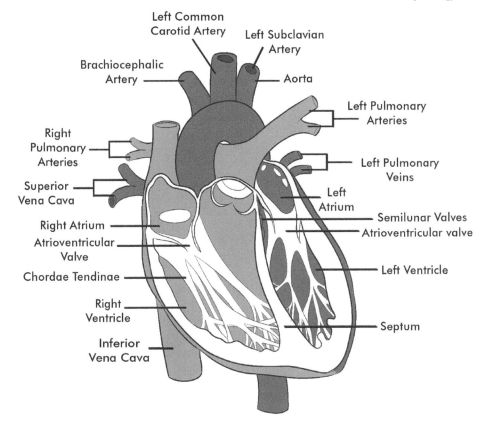

Figure 6.14 Structure of Human Heart.

The aorta begins in left ventricles. It is an artery. Like most of the arteries, it supplies the oxygenated blood to the body parts.

Superior vena cava is the large vein that receives deoxygenated blood from the upper parts of the body such as head, neck, thorax and upper extremities and empties it into the right atrium.

Inferior vena cava is the large vein carrying deoxygenated blood from lower parts of the body and empties it into the right atrium. This runs posterior in the abdominal cavity.

Pulmonary artery originates at the base of the right ventricle. At this point, it looks short and wide and is known as 'pulmonary trunk'. As it leaves the heart, it branches into two. Based on their position, they are called right pulmonary artery and left pulmonary artery. The right pulmonary artery enters the right lung, and the left pulmonary artery enters the left lung. Unlike the other arteries that carry oxygenated blood, the pulmonary arteries carry blood from heart to lungs, which are low in oxygen levels.

Pulmonary Veins: The pulmonary veins originate in lungs and enter the left atrium of the heart. Two pulmonary veins emerge from each lung. Thus, there are four pulmonary veins. Unlike the other veins that carry deoxygenated blood, the pulmonary veins carry the oxygenated blood from the lungs and empty it into the left atrium.

Coronary Arteries: These arteries are found wrapped around the outside of heart and diving into the heart muscles. They are the arteries that supply nutrients and oxygen to heart muscles. The Left Main Coronary Artery (LMCA) supplies blood to the left side of the heart muscle, while the Right Coronary Artery (RCA) supplies blood to the right side of the heart muscle.

There is a small muscle like tissue that looks like a knot located on the back wall of the right atrium close to the place where the superior vena cava enters the heart. This is called the 'sinoatrial node'. This is the pace maker of the heart that initiates the electric impulses, which generates the 'heartbeat'.

Following are the main arteries that carry oxygenated blood to different parts of the body. The names of these arteries are related to the body organs. They carry nutrients.

- Coronary arteries—heart muscle
- Carotid arteries—neck and head
- Hepatic artery—liver and stomach
- Mesenteric artery—intestines
- Renal arteries—kidneys
- Femoral arteries—legs

A total of 20 major arteries branch out into smaller vessels called 'arterioles'. Arterioles branch into thin capillaries. It is the capillaries that deliver nutrients and oxygen to the cells. After delivering the nutrients and oxygen, they pick up carbon dioxide and other waste and move the blood back through what is called 'venules'. These venules join the veins, which carry the deoxygenated blood to the heart.

The Blood: The blood is the third important factor in the cardiovascular system. The average adult has about 5.7 litres of blood in the body. Human blood has 92% water. The remaining 8% consists of 'plasma proteins', salt ions, oxygen and carbon dioxide, glucose, amino acids and fats (major nutrients), hormones, enzymes and waste products such as 'urea'. The various cells that blood consists are 'red blood cells', 'white blood cells' and 'platelets'.

Cardiac Functioning

The functioning of the heart is continuous. It pumps around 5.7 litres of blood in a day. As part of this process, on an average the heartbeats about one lakh times a day and three billion times during life time.

The right and left sides of the heart that are the atria and ventricles of the heart work in good coordination. The right heart receives deoxygenated blood from different parts of the body and sends this to the lungs. The left side of the heart receives oxygenated blood from the lungs and sends the same to different parts of the body.

The contraction and relaxation of the atria and ventricles, and closing and opening of the atrioventricular valves and semilunar valves with absolute precision enable the pumping of the blood by the heart. Let us now explain it in a sequential order.

The right atrium receives the deoxygenated blood into it through superior and inferior vena cava. Once it is filled with blood, the right atrium contracts, the right atrioventricular valve opens, and the blood passes into the right ventricle soon after which the valve closes. Now the right ventricle filled with blood contracts and pumps in the blood into the pulmonary trunk and later branches into right and left pulmonary. These pulmonary arteries carry blood into the lungs. In the lungs, the arteries branch into capillaries. These capillaries come in contact with small air sacs called 'alveoli'. Through this contact, there is exchange of oxygen and carbon dioxide. The capillaries take in oxygen and release carbon dioxide. This process facilitates oxygenation of blood.

Thus, oxygenated blood enters the pulmonary vein originating from the lungs. The pulmonary veins carry the oxygenated blood to the left atrium and empty blood into it. Once the atrium is filled, it contracts opening the mitral valve and blood enters the left ventricle. Soon after this, the left ventricle contracts and the mitral valve closes. Contraction of left ventricle allows the flow of oxygenated blood to flow into aorta through the aortic valve. The aorta branches and sends the blood to all parts of the body through arteries that branch into capillaries to reach every cell.

The blood circulation in the cardiovascular system is of two types, viz. 'the systemic circulation' and 'the pulmonary circulation'. The systemic circulation refers to the circulation of oxygenated blood from the heart to different parts of the body through arteries and transportation of deoxygenated blood from the body to the heart through veins. The pulmonary circulation refers to the flow of deoxygenated blood from the heart to the lungs where the carbon dioxide and impurities are expelled and oxygenated blood from the lungs is carried back to the heart.

Cardiac Cycle

The process of the contraction and relaxation of heart muscle is the 'heartbeat'. The sound is usually described as 'lubb—dubb'. The sequence of events that happen in one complete beat of the heart is called 'cardiac cycle'.

The process of heart function as described has two states of the cardiac muscle, viz. the state when it is pumping and active and the other when it is relaxed. The pumping phase is called 'systole', while the relaxing phase is called 'diastole'. Let us examine the cardiac cycle.

At the beginning of the cardiac cycle, both the atria and ventricles are in non-pumping relaxed stage, i.e. diastole state. This is the phase all chambers of the heart receive blood and are in relaxed state. Now, the left and right atria contract and push blood into the ventricles. This is 'atrial systole'. Now that the two ventricles are filled with blood, the left and right ventricles contract pumping blood out of them into aorta and pulmonary trunk respectively. This is 'ventricular systole'. During ventricular systole, the atria are relaxed and receive blood. During the ventricular systole, the atrioventricular valves close to prevent retraction of blood into atria.

At the same time, the semilunar valves are open to allow blood into aorta and pulmonary trunk. Once the blood is pushed out of the ventricles, the ventricles are relaxed causing 'ventricular diastole'. The semilunar valves close. Once again, the atria and ventricles are in the diastole stage. This is one cardiac cycle. The sound of 'lubb—dubb' is the consequence of closure of the valves. The first sound of 'lubb' is to be associated with the closure of atrioventricular valves, and the second sound of 'dubb' is because of closure of semilunar valves. These are the sounds of normal heartbeats. When the sound is not this but a 'murmur', it indicates possibility of problems in heart valves.

We are aware about the measurement of blood pressure in the body. The blood pressure (BP) is measured in terms of systolic pressure and diastolic pressure. Diastolic pressure (expressed as denominator) is the pressure of blood when the heart is on the relaxed phase, while the systolic pressure (expressed as numerator) is the pressure of blood when the heart contracts and pumps in the blood, e.g. 120/80.

The Electrical System of the Heart

In order to facilitate normal blood circulation between the heart and different parts of the body or between the heart and lungs, the functioning of the cardiac muscle has to be in perfect coordination at different levels such as contraction of chambers, opening and closure of the valves, flow of the blood in right volume at the right direction with the right pressure. This calls for some method of signalling and monitoring system.

214 *Human Physiology*

To coordinate the complex functioning of the heart, there is an electrical system. The sinoatrial node situated on the posterior wall of right atrium discharges the function of initiating the electrical signal for the heart to contract. The sinoatrial node, which is known as the pace maker, generates electrical impulse, which triggers the atria to contract. Subsequently, when the blood flows into the ventricles, the electrical impulse is passed on to the ventricles causing them to contract. These electrical impulses spreading over the heart can be measured through an instrument called 'Electrocardiogram' (ECG).

Box 6.1   Summary of the Circulatory System or Cardiovascular System

- The circulatory system or cardiovascular system refers to the heart, blood vessels and the blood itself that circulates from the heart to the whole body through blood vessels.
- Heart, the vital organ is a cardiac muscle.
- It has four chambers, out of which the upper chambers are atria and the lower ventricle.
- Heart is divided into right and left by a membrane called septum.
- The heart is well protected by three layers of tissues and pericardial fluid.
- The heart pumps nutrients and oxygen to all parts of body.
- The oxygenated blood is pumped into left atrium to the left ventricle, aorta and then arteries to various parts of body. The capillaries supply oxygen and nutrients to the cells in the body and carry back waste and carbon dioxide from the cells and flow through the veins back to the right atrium, right ventricle and from there to pulmonary arteries, which carry deoxygenated blood to the lungs. The blood gets oxygenated and expels carbon dioxide in lungs. This oxygenated blood is transported back to through pulmonary veins to the left atrium.
- The atrioventricular valves between atria and ventricles open and shut in coordination with contraction and relaxation of atria. The semilunar valves open and shut in coordination with contraction and relaxation of the ventricles. The contraction of the atria and ventricles is triggered by the electrical impulse from the sinoatrial node.
- By default, the arteries carry the oxygenated blood, while the veins carry deoxygenated blood with an exception of pulmonary arteries and vein where it is the reverse.
- Aorta is the largest artery. The arteries break into minute vessels called capillaries.
- The blood contains 92% of water, oxygen, carbon dioxide, proteins and other nutrients. It also has red blood cells, white blood cells, plasma.

Respiratory System

Every cell in the body requires oxygen for its survival and reaction. It is the respiratory system that is responsible for drawing in the oxygen into the body. Breathing is the activity that happens 12–20 times in a minute and about 17,000 times a day on a rough average. This activity of breathing that is involuntary is not taken into cognizance every time it happens.

Respiratory system serves the following functions:

1 Ventilation (breathing in and out)
2 Exchange of oxygen for carbon dioxide in blood
3 Maintenance of blood pH levels (acid/alkalinity of blood) by coordinating with other systems
4 Facilitation of speech

Following are the organs that constitute the respiratory system (Figure 6.15):

Nose
Pharynx
Larynx
Trachea
Bronchi
Lungs

Nose: Nose, which a prominent part of the face and considered to be one of the organs whose shape and size contributes to the 'beauty' of the face, is the outermost organ involved in respiration. The air passes through the two nostrils. The nostrils have tiny hair. Just beyond the nostrils is the 'nasal septum' (referred to as nose bridge) that separates the nasal cavities.

The in-built protective system in the nose prevents minor dust particles entering into the system. At the first level, the tiny hairs inside the nostril function as a filter and obstruct dirt or bacteria from gaining an entry. Inside the nasal cavity, the respiratory mucosa has miniscule hair-like structures called 'cilia'. This helps in removing the dirt-laden mucus towards the nostrils. Apart from acting as the first line of defence, the hairs in the nostrils and cilia in the nasal cavity provide humidity to the air that is inhaled.

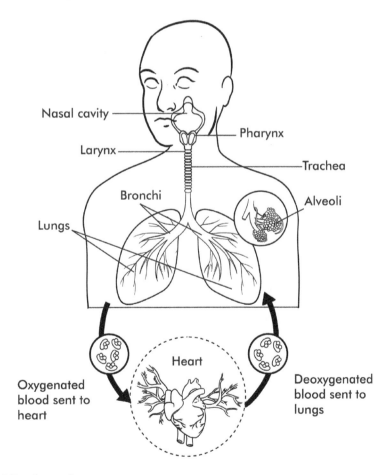

Figure 6.15 Respiratory System.

Pharynx: The wide hollow space into which the nasal chambers open is called the 'pharynx'. It is located behind the mouth and nasal cavities. It is considered to be a part of digestive system, as well as the conducting zone of the respiratory system. It is called so because it helps the passage of air that is breathed in, and it filters, warms and moistens it before conducting it to the lungs. The pharynx is made of pharyngeal muscles, which lie in circles in the outer layer and longitudinally in the inner layer. These muscles facilitate swallowing of food. Pharynx has three major functions, viz. conduction of air, facilitation of swallowing and vocalization.

Larynx: Larynx is located in the anterior part of neck. It is in a place below the pharynx towards its front and above the 'trachea'. It is made of three cartilages, viz. 'cricoid', 'thyroid' and 'epiglottis'. Larynx is also called the 'voice box' or 'Adam's apple'. Its main function is to protect the trachea by closing it abruptly to prevent entry of food into it while swallowing. The other function is production of sound.

Trachea: This is also known as 'wind pipe'. This is a tube that originates below the larynx and runs down the neck. It extends till the breast bone and splits into two bronchi directing towards each lung. The walls of trachea are made of semi-circular rings made of cartilage. This helps in the expansion of trachea and also provides it the required hardness.

Bronchi: When the trachea splits into two each going into one lung, it is called 'bronchi' (singular is bronchus). Each bronchus on entering the lung is divided into secondary and tertiary bronchi. The primary bronchi are in the upper portion of lungs, the secondary in the centre and the tertiary near the bottom of lungs. As they get closer to the lung tissue, the tertiary bronchi become smaller, and these smaller parts are called 'bronchioles'. The bronchioles are further divided into minute air sacs called 'alveoli'. It is these alveoli that facilitate exchange of oxygen for carbon dioxide in the lungs.

Lungs: Lungs are the prime centres of the respiratory system. Being the vital organ, this pair of large spongy organs is located in a well-protected manner. It is placed in the thoracic cavity, on the either side of the heart. They are based on the strong muscular membrane called the 'diaphragm', which is connected to lower ribs, sternum and lumbar vertebrae.

Protection for Lungs

Each lung is well protected in the close wrap of 'pleural sac'. This pleural sac consists of two layers of membranes. The outer membrane is 'parietal pleura'. This is attached to the thoracic wall. The inner membrane called 'visceral pleura' is attached to the inner surface of the lung. In between these two layers is the pleural cavity, which contains 'interpleural fluid'. This fluid with its adhesive characteristic keeps the lungs attached to the thoracic wall. This fluid also serves the purpose of keeping the two membranes moist.

The right lung is relatively larger in size. It has three lobes—the right inferior, the right middle and the right superior lobes. The left lung has two lobes, viz. the left inferior and the left superior lobes.

The inner surface of the lungs has the bronchi divided into bronchioles and 'alveoli'. The terminals of smallest bronchioles have small bulb-like structures. These are called 'alveolar sacs'. Each of these sacs contains a number of alveoli. The human body consists of more than 300 million alveoli. The walls of alveoli consist of epithelium and elastic tissue that constricts and expands as we breathe. Each of this is covered with capillaries carrying deoxygenated blood from the heart. The walls of the capillaries also contain epithelium. Now, there is an interface between the epithelium of the alveoli and pulmonary capillaries called 'respiratory membrane'. It is through this respiratory membrane that the capillaries take in the oxygen from the alveoli and expel carbon dioxide into the alveoli. The carbon dioxide travels to the bronchi and pharynx and is exiled through the nose.

Respiratory Cycle: 'Breathing' comprises of inhalation and exhalation, when oxygen is breathed in and carbon dioxide breathed out. During the process of respiration, a host of activities happen in the respiratory system.

a **Muscular Function:** The major muscle responsible for the expansion and contraction of lungs is the diaphragm. Diaphragm is a dome-shaped muscle on which the lungs are based. Diaphragm separates the right lung from the liver and on the left side separates the lung from stomach and spleen. When air is inhaled, the diaphragm contracts, causing the expansion of lungs. Thus, the air rushes into the lungs through bronchi, finally resulting in the inflation of the alveoli. The exchange of gases happens between alveoli and capillaries. Now, the diaphragm relaxes causing the lungs to deflate. When air is exhaled, the alveoli deflate releasing carbon dioxide into the bronchi, which travels back to be expelled through nostrils.
b **Intercostal Muscles:** The intercostal muscles are located between the ribs. When air is breathed in, the intercostal muscles make the ribs move up and outwards. This expands the thoracic cavity creating more space to accommodate the expansion of lungs when it is filled with air. During exhalation, the intercostal muscles cause the ribs to move down and inwards as the diaphragm moves up. The lungs deflate pushing out the air.
c **Accessory Muscles:** There are several muscles that do not directly contribute in the process of respiration but play a supportive role. Abdominal muscles and muscles near the collar bone are included in this group.

Breathing and the Control Centre

The activity of the diaphragm (contraction and release), which triggers the expansion and depletion of lungs, is controlled by the brain stem (medulla) of the autonomic nervous system. The diaphragm receives impulses from a pair of spinal nerves called 'phrenic nerves'. They regulate breathing in systematic rhythm is such a way to maintain 12–20 breaths a minute in an average healthy person.

There are times when this normal rate of breathing is violated. Following are the conditions that deviate from the normal rate of breathing:

1 During physical exercise when the tissues demand more oxygen
2 In situation where the level of carbon dioxide in the blood rises
3 The individual is under stress
4 Respiratory infections

In such instances, the medulla sends more impulses to the diaphragm, which contracts and releases at faster pace so that we breathe in more air and expel more frequently.

Breathing Mechanism—Pressure Relationship

Breathing activity was explained in terms of muscular activity and autonomic nervous system's impulses. It is now explained in terms of air pressure.

Inspiration and expiration are associated with the difference in air pressure in the atmosphere and lungs. When molecules in the air move freely and collude with each other, it generates a

218   *Human Physiology*

pressure. Air moves from an area of high pressure to the area of low pressure. This movement is called 'bulk flow'. Let us explain the activity of breathing in terms of 'bulk flow'.

When the air is inhaled, the diaphragm contracts and presses down on the abdomen and lifts the thorax. This creates an additional space in the rib cavity. Simultaneous with this, due to the contraction of intercostal muscle, the rib cage expands horizontally creating additional space all around.

We know that the (outer) parietal layer of pleura is attached to the diaphragm and the thoracic wall. When the diaphragm contracts, the parietal layer also moves with it. As a result, the pressure in the interpleural space falls. As a result, the (inner) visceral layer of the lungs also follows the movement. Since the visceral layer is attached to the lungs, with its movement the lungs expand increasing their volume. Now that the air in lungs has less space to full the pressure of air falls. This produces a vacuum. As a result of this, more air is sucked in by 'bulk flow'. The flow of air continues to fill the lungs until the pressure in the lungs is same as atmospheric pressure.

During expiration, the diaphragm and intercostal muscles get back to their position. As a result, the volume of the chest cavity is decreased. Subsequently, the volume of the lungs also decreases. This results in squashing air in the lungs, and the air is expelled out by 'bulk flow' until the pressure in the atmosphere equals the pressure in lungs.

Breath Control: Breathing is an involuntary function controlled by an autonomic nervous system. However, the normal rhythm of breathing is regulated to facilitate certain behaviour unique to humans. The two functions, speaking and singing, require some control over breath. The rate of expiration has to be far lower for these activities. During these processes, the breath control is regulated as per the requirement (voluntary).

Voluntary Control over Breath

Very often, we encounter situations that force us to hold our breath. For example, when we sense bad odour in the air or while swimming under water, we have to hold our breath. In such situations, the cerebral cortex sends signals to the diaphragm and intercostal muscle to ignore signals from the medulla for the time-being. Even during this period, the metabolism and exchange of oxygen and carbon dioxide continue to take place. However, the carbon dioxide concentrate in the body increases, when the concentrate crosses a certain threshold level posing a threat to damage to the brain due to the lack of oxygen, the chemoreceptor of the respiratory centre gets stimulated and overrides the message from the cerebral cortex. In extreme cases, one may become unconscious when the voluntary control of holding the breath is lost and then the respiration resumes.

Voluntary control over breathing is also recommended in yoga to enhance the physical and psychological wellbeing.

Summary

- Respiratory system works in good coordination with the circulatory system, muscular system and autonomic nervous system.
- Respiratory system has a built-in protection against external dirt and bacteria, which are filtered by the hairs and cilia in the nostrils and nasal cavity.
- The air is breathed in through the nostril, pharynx, trachea and bronchia into the two lungs.
- The bronchi split into bronchioles and alveoli.
- The alveoli are in contact with the capillaries that come from heart carrying oxygenated blood, and pass on the oxygen to capillaries, and the carbon dioxide is carried back and exhaled.

- The lungs expand and deflate in sync with the contraction of diaphragm, which acts as per the impulses from the medulla controlled by the autonomic nervous system.
- An average healthy human being breathes 12–20 times in a minute.

Digestive System

Digestive system can be conceptualized as a long 20-ft tract into which the ingested food travels, halting at places along way for physical and chemical processing. This digestive tract is also known as 'alimentary canal' or 'gastrointestinal tract'.

What precedes the digestion process is ingestion or eating behaviour. Ingestion of food starts as a reflex behaviour at the time of birth and later is guided by a number of factors such as age, region, sociocultural affiliation, personal experiences, emotional state and biological factors such as allergic reactions.

Keeping aside the sociocultural factors, we shall explain the purely biological process of digestion here. This biological process starts from the time the food enters the mouth till the waste product is excreted. In between, the food travels from mouth through the food pipe, and then to stomach. The process of digestion starts in the mouth itself, then continues in the stomach and small intestines. The process of digestion includes assimilation of nutrients into the body.

The following are the organs involved in the process of digestion:

1 Mouth
2 Pharynx
3 Oesophagus
4 Stomach
5 Small intestines
6 Large intestines
7 Pancreas
8 Liver

Of the above, pancreas and liver are called accessory organs. They are located outside the gastrointestinal (GI) tract and aid the process of digestion.

Right from the mouth till the end point of large intestine, the entire system has a lining of mucous membrane. This membrane assumes significance in many ways. First, it protects the digestive organs from any corrosion due to the food particles and the acidic digestive juices. Secondly, the secretion from the mucosa maintains the GI tract moist, soft and slippery facilitating the movement of food. Thirdly, the tissues and cells on mucous membrane secrete gastric acid, hormones, enzymes and neurotransmitters. Finally, it is through the mucous membrane that the nutrients are transferred to blood to be transported to various parts of the body. The digestive mucosa is referred with different labels in different locations of the GI tract. We will refer to these names in the context of discussing the organ.

The Mouth: As soon as (the sight, odour or the thought of food) the food is placed in the mouth, saliva is secreted. From where does this saliva come? As mentioned earlier, the mouth region is covered with mucous membrane, which in this location is called 'buccal mucosa'. The salivary glands having their ducts secrete and release saliva, mucous and a digestive enzyme called 'amylase' through this membrane to the oral cavity. Saliva helps in softening the food that is chewed by teeth facilitated by the tongue movements. The process of digestion begins in the mouth itself. The amylase converts the starch into sugar as you continue to chew. That is why you feel the sweet taste of starchy food such as rice while you chew. The preliminary process of digestion makes the food into soft rounded lumps called 'bolus'.

Oesophagus: Located posterior to mouth, pharynx connects to oesophagus. When the bolus travels down the pharynx, it bounces off 'epiglottis', a piece of cartilage, so that the trachea is closed and the bolus enters oesophagus. The food travels down the oesophagus because of a wave-like muscular contraction called 'peristalsis'. The digestive process is proactive. By the time the food centres the oesophagus, the stomach readies itself to receive it by secreting small amounts of gastric juice.

Stomach: Propelled by the peristalsis, the bolus drops into the stomach.

Stomach is a 'J'-shaped organ starts at the end of oesophagus and ends where the small intestine begins. The stomach when empty is only the size of a fist. However, when it stretches it can hold about 4 litres of food. Like rest of the GT tract, the stomach has four layers in it. The outermost layer is 'adventitia', also known as 'serosa'. Next to this layer is 'muscularis propria'. This layer is followed by 'submucosa', and the innermost layer is 'mucosa'.

Adventitia or serosa contains blood vessels, lymphatics and nerves. Muscularis propria is a smooth muscle layer. This is useful for peristalsis. The submucosa has larger blood vessels, lymphatics and nerves, and has glands that secrete mucous. Mucosa, the innermost layer of stomach, has a lining of epithelium. It consists of mucous cells, which secrete mucus that is alkaline. This has a number of 'gastric pits', which are the entry points to gastric glands, which secrete gastric juice.

The muscularis has three layers of muscle fibres. The shape of these fibres is oblique, circular and longitudinal. This enables the stomach to churn when it is filled with food. The stomach has four major parts, viz. 'cardia', 'fundus', 'body' and 'pylorus'. Figure 6.16 indicates these parts.

The point where the oesophagus connects to stomach is called 'cardia'. Above the cardia and to its left is 'fundus'. The 'body' is below the fundus. The narrow end of the stomach is called 'pyloric canal'. Pyloric canal connects the stomach to the duodenum. When the stomach has no food, it deflates. With this, the mucosa and submucosa create a fold, which is known as 'rugae'.

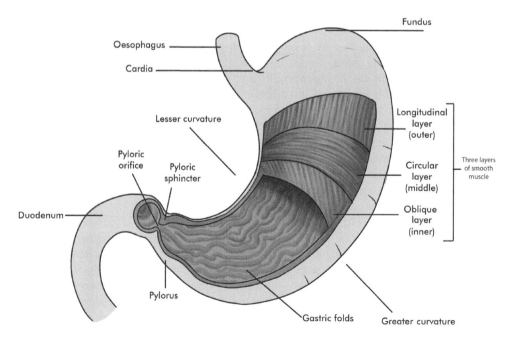

Figure 6.16 Anatomy of Stomach.

Functions of stomach: Stomach has three main functions—

1. It stores food and releases it to small intestine at a pace that is congenial for digestion and absorption.
2. It secretes hydrochloric acid and pepsin. Hydrochloric acid helps in killing the microorganisms that enter along with food. Pepsin initiates the digestion of protein.
3. By churning the food that enters, it mixes it with gastric secretion and produces a thick mixture called 'chyme'.

As soon as the food enters the stomach, it gets mixed with hydrochloric acid and the stomach starts mixing the food. The process of mixing continues for three to four hours. This semi-liquid chyme is passed into the duodenum, the top part of the small intestine (through the pyloric canal). Thus, contrary to the common notion, the prime job of the stomach is not digestion of food but storing of food.

The Small Intestine

The intestines are divided into small and large intestines based on their width. The width of the small intestine is about 1 inch and that of large intestine 2.5 inches. The average length of the small intestine in an adult is about 5 m (Standring, 2015). The length varies between 3 and 6.7 m depending on the height of the person.

Structurally, the small intestine is divided into three parts—the 'duodenum', 'jejunum' and 'ileum'.

Duodenum is the short 'C'-shaped structure that is at the beginning of the small intestine. It surrounds the pancreas head. The duodenum has the 'Brunner's glands'. These are submucosal glands. They secrete mucus-rich alkaline consisting of bicarbonate.

The intestines lie in the abdominal cavity. The fibrous layers of peritoneum hold it in place. There are two layers of muscle tissues that are longitudinal and circular. This helps peristalsis.

The intestinal mucosa has some areas that produce hormones, enzymes and neurotransmitters in the lumen (the inner space). The intestinal lumen has finger-like projections called villi. This increases the surface area used for exchange. The villi have capillaries. Each villus (singular of villi) has capillary assigned to it. The capillaries absorb the nutrients.

The small intestine is both an endocrine gland and a digestive organ. Its walls have cells that secrete the hormones called 'secretin' and 'cholecystokinin' (CCK). These hormones stimulate the pancreas and liver to release pancreatic juice and bile respectively.

The duodenum receives chyme from the stomach. Stimulated by the hormones, the digestive enzymes from pancreas and bile from the liver are released into the duodenum. The digestive enzymes break down the protein in the food, while the bile breaks down the fat into molecules. Here, the carbohydrates, proteins and fats are broken into molecules of glucose, amino acids, fatty acids and glycerol. The shortest chain fatty acids are directly transported to capillaries through villi. The villi transport the long-chain fatty acids to the lymphatic system. The long-chain fatty acids join to create a compound called 'triglycerides'. Glycerol is absorbed by liver, which converts it into glucose. From here, the chyme, almost digested, moves to jejunum and ileum. The amount of flow of chyme into the duodenum is regulated by pyloric sphincter.

By the time process in the small intestine is completed, the nutrients from the chyme are absorbed into the blood by the capillaries. Finally, in the last part of small intestine, i.e. ileum, the remaining matter is passed into the large intestine.

The intestines (small and large) are depicted in Figure 6.17.

The Large Intestine: The large intestine is also called as 'colon'. It is about 2 m long. It surrounds the small intestine like a frame. The part that joins it with the small intestine is called

222 *Human Physiology*

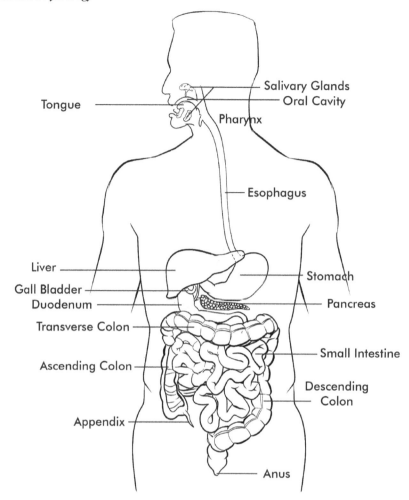

Figure 6.17 Digestive System.

'caecum'. From the caecum, the large intestine move upwards. This part is called 'the ascending colon'. It continues across the abdomen horizontally. This part is known as 'transverse colon'. The continuation of large intestine from here is downwards. This part is called 'descending colon'. This finally ends in what is called 'sigmoid colon' and rectum.

From the small intestine, the chyme is pushed into the caecum of large intestine. Now the label of the matter changes to 'faeces'. The walls of the large intestine absorb the water content from the faeces into the capillaries. Once the water component is removed, the faeces sets into the colon compactly. The yellow brown colour of the faeces is because of the bile pigments, bacteria and the broken-down haemoglobin.

The intestines harbour million of bacteria. Some of these bacteria are of help. They produce vitamin K that helps in clotting of blood.

The faeces moves to the rectum due to the peristalsis. When the rectum consists of about 5–8 ounces of faeces, the 'stretch receptors' send a signal to the brain that there is a need for defecation.

It may be stated that while the stomach does the little bit of mechanical digestion, the intestines carry out the real chemical digestion.

Pancreas

Pancreas is located behind the stomach next to the duodenum. It is placed in upper left abdomen. It is flat, fish-shaped spongy structure that is 6–10 inches long. The head of the pancreas is close to the duodenum. About 95% of pancreas has 'exocrine tissue', which produces the pancreatic enzymes. The remaining tissues have endocrine cells.

Pancreas executes two major functions, viz. exocrine function (that helps in digestion) and endocrine function (that regulates blood sugar). In this context, we will focus on exocrine function.

The pancreatic enzymes consist of 'trypsin and 'chymotrypsin'. They are useful in digestion of proteins. The pancreatic enzymes also have 'amylase' and 'lipase'. Amylase helps in digestion of carbohydrates, while lipase breaks down the fats. These enzymes released by pancreas are carried by the pancreatic duct. The pancreatic duct joins the common bile duct and opens to the duodenum. The enzymes help in digestion of carbohydrates, proteins and fat in the food.

The Liver

The liver is the largest organ. It is also a gland. The liver of an average adult weighs about 1.4–1.6 kg. This pinkish-brown triangular organ is located under the diaphragm, above the stomach on the right side of the abdomen. Liver receives its blood from hepatic artery, as well as hepatic portal vein. Hepatic artery supplies oxygenated blood to the liver from aorta, while hepatic portal vein from small intestine supplies blood rich in nutrients.

The tricone-shaped liver consists of four lobes, viz. right lob, left lobe, quadrate lobe and caudate lobe. The lobes of the liver consist of thousands of 'lobules'. Every lobule is made of million of hepatic cells. The lobules are connected to small ducts. These small ducts connect to a hepatic duct. The hepatic cells secrete bile. The common hepatic duct carries the bile generated in liver to the duodenum and gallbladder. The bile in the duodenum is used for digestion of food, while the gallbladder stores the bile.

Functions of Liver

1. Bile production: One of the functions of liver as explained above is production of bile, which is directly sent to duodenum for immediate use in digestion and also to gallbladder where it is stored and supplied to duodenum on demand. Apart from bile production, the liver carries out many other functions.
2. Processing and elimination of toxins: The toxic contents of medicines and even of alcohol reach the liver through the portal vein. They are processed and sent to intestine for elimination.
3. Processing and elimination of metabolic waste: A number of red blood cells die regularly. The liver removes these dead blood cells and converts the haemoglobin into bilirubin. This is transported to intestines and expelled with faeces.
4. Storage of Glucose: The liver converts glucose into glycogen and stores it. It reconverts this into glucose to be released in times of need when the blood glucose levels fall. Insulin and glucagon from pancreas aid in this function.
5. Other functions: It produces a number of proteins, protein hormones and those proteins that help in clotting of blood.

As has already been mentioned, the pancreas and liver do not constitute the main gastrointestinal tract but are known as accessory organs that play a significant role in the process of digestion.

Box 6.2 Summary of the Digestive System

- The process of digestion starts in the mouth where the amylase converts starch into sugar.
- The chewed food called bolus moves from mouth to pharynx and oesophagus through peristalsis and reaches the stomach.
- The stomach produces hydrochloric acid and pepsin, which give an acidic character and partly digest protein. The stomach churns the food and converts it into 'chyme', which is passed into the duodenum, the beginning of small intestine.
- Pancreatic enzyme and bile are supplied into the small intestine at the point of duodenum. They break down the proteins and fat into molecules. Part of the fat is absorbed into blood in the small intestine. In the small intestine, the food nutrients are absorbed into the blood capillaries. Most of the food is digested and absorbed in the small intestine. The remaining 'chyme' is transported to large intestine.
- The large intestine helps in absorbing water from the faeces and excretes the waste matter.

Renal System

The renal system is crucial for the body as it carries out several functions that are important for survival. The metabolic wastes produced by the body are toxic and hence need to be excreted. The urinary system is one of the systems that carries out this function. Apart from that, the system also carries out a number of other functions. We will examine the role of this system in sustaining the health of the individual.

Structure of Renal System

The renal system is compactly structured with a definite start point and an end point—all connected by tubes. The urinary system includes the following parts:

1 Kidneys
2 Ureters
3 Urinary bladder
4 Urethra

All the four constitutes what is called 'urinary tract', which functions as a good plumbing system to drain out the toxins and wastes in the urine. Let us explain their structure.

Kidneys: The pair kidneys are the size of a fist (4–5″), shaped like a bean and situated on the posterior walls of abdominal cavity, touching the muscles of the back. They are protected by a tough connective tissue layer (renal fascia) and perirenal fat capsule. It helps to hold the kidneys in place. The colour of the kidneys can be described as reddish-brown. They are elongated oval shape with a depression or a curve that brings a concavity to it giving it a shape of a bean. The large concave part is called 'hilum'. We can see a number of vessels entering and existing the kidneys through this part. They include ureter, renal artery, renal vein, lymphatic vessels and nerves. The kidneys are said to be protected by the peritoneum adipose, the back muscles and lower part of ribs. Yet, they are located at a very vulnerable place.

In the kidney, the various tissues are so arranged to give concentric layers. The outermost layer is 'cortex'. Below the cortex is 'medulla'. This is a series of a fan-shaped structure with a membrane that has several folds. These folds give it a structure of pyramid, conical in shape. They are called 'renal pyramids'. The innermost layer in kidney is 'renal pelvis'. The various parts of kidneys are shown in Figure 6.18.

Microscopic Parts in Kidney

Each kidney consists of around one million 'nephrons'. Nephrons are microscopic units of kidney. Each nephron consists of a renal 'corpuscle' and a renal 'tubule'. Every corpuscle has a tuft of capillaries, is called 'glomerulus' and is surrounded by 'Bowman's capsule'. This capsule is a tiny sack in the shape of a cup. The glomerulus is positioned inside the 'capsule'. The renal tubule extends out of the capsule. The tubule and capsule are made of epithelial cells. Tubules are surrounded by capillaries and flittering cells.

Ureters: The ureters originate from the renal pelvis and go down to terminate in urinary bladder. They are 10–12 inches long and run on right and left sides of the vertebral column. The function of ureters is to carry urine from the kidneys to the bladder. The walls of ureters have muscular layers that move in wave-like motion called peristalsis. When they terminate in urinary bladder, their ends are sealed at the entry of the bladder with a valve called 'ureterovesical valves'. This prevents reflux of urine.

Urinary Bladder: It is located in the pelvic cavity posterior to the pubic bones and anterior to rectum. It is a funnel-shaped hollow organ. The outer protective membrane has a number of layers of muscles in opposite direction. The inner layer is mucus membrane. The mucosa

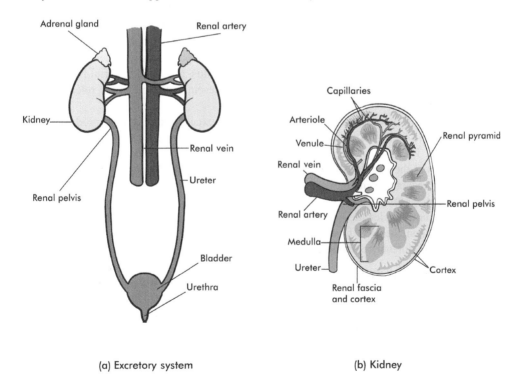

Figure 6.18 Renal System and Kidney (a and b).

consists of special epithelial tissues called 'transitional epithelium'. This facilitates the cells to change shape to accommodate larger volume of urine.

When the bladder gets full, the stretch receptors in the muscle layer communicate to brain through impulses.

Urethra: This is a tube that originates in urinary bladder terminates as the opening out of the body or elimination of urine. In females, it is 2 inches long originating from the bladder and ends between the clitoris and the vagina. In males, it is 8–10 inches long originating from bladder and terminating at the tip of penis. In males, it also functions as a reproductive organ, which carries sperm through the penis.

The sphincter muscles control the flow of urine. The sphincter muscle in the inner layer is made of smooth muscles. When the bladder reaches certain threshold of volume, it opens involuntarily. This creates a sensation of need to urinate. However, the skeletal muscles of the external sphincter have a voluntary control. Thus, it can help in holding the urine and withstands a delay in urinating.

The Process of Filtration: The urine is produced by a process of filtration. This process occurs in the kidney. It involves filtering from blood the water, toxins, ions and other wastes that are harmful for the body. Let us now explain the process.

The renal artery enters each kidney anteriorly (pelvis of kidney). They deliver blood to capillaries. The nephrons help in filtration in a two-step process. The nephrons consist of tufts of capillaries called glomerulus located inside the Bowman's capsule. When blood flows through the glomerulus, the capsule collects much of the plasma into it from the capillaries. This is the first step of filtration. The remaining small amount of plasma and blood cells continue to travel through the capillaries. Now the liquid filtrate collected in the capsule flows into the series of tubules. The tubules are lined with filtering cells. A blood vessel runs alongside tubules. The major job of the tubule is facilitating reabsorption. A beautiful exchange mechanism takes place here. The cells around the tubules absorb water and other nutrient substance from the filtrate in the tubule. This absorption is highly selective with the aim of maintaining the electrolyte balance in the body. Thus, absorbed material is returned to the capillaries. At the same time, the waste products present in the blood are released to the filtrate in the tubules.

By the end of this process, the tubules have just water, excess ions and waste products, called 'urine'. The blood that exits the kidneys has all nutrients, ions and water to the needed level absorbed into it. The filtered blood flows back into the heart through renal veins.

The urine from the nephrons reaches ureter and travels to the bladder. When the bladder is full, the stretch receptors send message to the brain indicating the need for urination.

Maintenance of Homeostasis:

Kidneys function under the hormonal control of the endocrine system. This empowers the kidneys to maintain chemical homeostasis in blood and other fluids in the body. The major aspects related to maintenance of homeostasis are discussed below.

1 **Blood Pressure:** The kidneys consist of a special cell called 'juxtaglomerular cells' that monitor the blood pressure as blood flows through the kidneys for filtration. When the blood pressure is high, the kidneys can reduce the blood pressure by reducing the blood volume. How does this happen? It is simple. When the blood pressure is high, the kidneys reduce the reabsorption of water into blood, the second step of filtration. This leaves higher volume of water in the form of urine. The reverse is done when the blood pressure is very low. The kidneys reabsorb more water into the kidneys, thus increasing the volume of blood. In such cases, the water content in the urine is reduced.

The second way the kidneys help in maintaining blood pressure is by releasing a hormone called 'renin' when the blood pressure is very low. This triggers a chain of reactions in the body. Renin acts on a circulating layer called 'angiotensinogen' and produces 'angiotensin'. The blood converts it into angiotensin I and then angiotensin II. The latter sends signals to blood vessels to constrict. This in turn signals the heart to work harder and pump blood. Angiotensin II simultaneously signals to release a hormone called 'aldosterone'. This in turns initiates absorption of more fluids and sodium into the blood. Once this happens, there is more volume of blood demanding the heart to work harder.

2 **Chemical Balance:** The body needs to maintain the balance of chemicals in the body. Kidneys, during the filtration, excrete a number of chemicals (electrolytes) like sodium, potassium, calcium, magnesium, phosphate and chloride ions. When the blood composition has these chemical in levels higher than what is required, they may harm the body. In such cases, kidneys filter out more of these chemical ions into the urine. The reverse is done when their concentration is low in the blood.

3 **Acid-Alkaline Balance (pH):** The body metabolism produces acids and alkalis as products or byproducts. Acids are produced out of digesting fat, capillary exchanges and muscular activities, and also are consumed with food. This disturbs the pH levels in blood. The kidneys respond to changes in blood pH levels. When the acid content is high, kidneys excrete more acidic ions into the urine.

4 **Osmolarity:** The kidneys maintain the osmotic balance in the body. This is done by regulating the amount of water filtered out of blood into urine. When the body is dehydrated due to any reason such as exposure to heat, the kidneys absorb less water from the blood and there is less volume of water in urination. On the contrary, when a person drinks lot of water, more water is absorbed from blood into urine, thus increasing the volume of water in the urine.

Box 6.3 Summary of the Renal System

- The urinary system consists of kidneys, ureters, bladder and urethra.
- Kidneys are bean-shaped, fist-sized reddish-brown pair of organs in the posterior of abdominal cavity.
- Renal veins, renal arteries, ureter, lymphatic vessels are seen entering/existing the hilum of kidneys.
- Kidneys have layers called cortex, medulla and pelvis.
- The kidneys filter the blood and remove water, toxins, minerals and other waste materials from the blood.
- The filtration happens at two levels. In the first level, the capsule takes in much of plasma into it. The remaining blood travels through capillaries. The liquid filtrate travels through tubules where reabsorption of nutrients and water from the tubules to capillaries and release of further waste matter from capillaries to tubules happen.
- The water and waste from tubules travel to ureters, then to bladder. From bladder, they travel through urethra and excreted.
- Kidneys also discharge other functions such as maintaining the blood pressure, electrolyte balance, osmotic balance, pH balance, essential for body's homeostasis.

Reproductive System

When we discussed the nervous system, endocrine system, circulatory, respiratory and gastrointestinal systems, the structure and functions were discussed for the human being where it is uniform with no gender difference. The reproductive system has to be discussed with reference to the male and female separately in terms of their unique features and functions.

The special characteristics of the reproductive system are the 'sexual maturity', which occurs at the time of puberty. The system functions under endocrinal control. While the control centre and process of sexual development are the same for both genders, the outcomes of this are different in boys and girls.

Let us start the explanation of the system from puberty and sexual development.

Puberty is the time of sexual maturity for boys and girls. The girls have it between 10 and 14 years, while the boys have it between 12 and 16 years. Puberty is the consequence of coordinated function of hypothalamus and pituitary glands. Around the age of eight years, the hypothalamus begins to increase its secretion of 'gonadotrophin-releasing hormone'. This triggers the anterior pituitary to release a hormone known as 'luteinizing hormone' (LH) and 'follicle stimulating hormone' (FSH). This causes gradual enlargement of gonads that produce high levels of sex hormones, 'testosterone' and 'oestrogen'. These two hormones are responsible for development of secondary sex characteristics in boys and girls. Boys and girls have different secondary sex characteristics. Table 6.2 presents the secondary sex characteristics of boys and girls.

The growth spurt in girls starts around 9–11 years during which the girl grows about 3 inches in height every year. In boys, the growth spurt occurs between 11 and 13 years. The growth in height in boys is about 4 inches per year during this phase.

The ages mentioned above are only suggestive. Besides the age, a number of factors contribute to sexual maturity. Genetic and environmental factors, nutritional factors and stress levels are some of the determinants. There are studies that indicate an association between fat and set of menarche (Khadgawat et al., 2016, Kelly et al., 2017; Surana et al., 2017). The average age of onset of menarche in girls is found to be dropping gradually. The age of Indian girls attaining menarche used to be 13.83 years, while 80% of urban girls are now found to attain menarche at 11 years. A drop in the age of onset of puberty and menarche age was also reported among population of a number of countries in Europe, North America, and developing countries from Asia, Africa and Latin America (Pathak, Tripathi, & Subramanian, 2014).

The onset of puberty is accompanied by a number of new behavioural initiatives such as increasing attention to bodily changes, new interest in the heterosexual peers due to the hormonal changes. A number of cultural factors foster and regulate such behaviour so as to be acceptable in the social norms.

Table 6.2 Secondary sex characteristics

Boys	Girls
• Enlarging and strengthening of skeletal structure • Increase in musculature • Larynx elongation and drop in voice pitch • Growth of facial hair • Growth of pubic hair and hair in other parts of body (chest, armpit, legs) • Growth of penis and scrotum	• Enlarging and strengthening of skeletal structure • Broadening of hips • Change in skin texture • Growth of public hair, axillary hair • Development of breast

Male Reproductive System

The organs of other systems like cardiovascular, respiratory and gastrointestinal systems are located within protective layers of skin muscular tissues and other fluids. So, is the case with the organs of female reproductive organs. However, the male reproductive organs are exceptions in this respect. These organs have an exposed location. The main parts of male reproductive system include prostate glands, testes, scrotum and penis.

Testes and Scrotum: Testes are a pair of oval bodies with a length of one and a half to 2 inches. They are primary sex organs of males. Sperm is produced in testes.

Inside the testes, there are compartments formed by the fibrous tissues. These compartments have what is called 'seminiferous tubules', which are long and coiled. These are the sites for development of sperm. The immature sperm called 'spermatogonia' occupy the walls of seminiferous tubules in thousands. The seminiferous tubules also consist of 'Sertoli cells' that provide nourishment to these immature sperm so that they develop.

The top of each testis has a long cord-like structure called 'epididymis'. This epididymis becomes 'vas deferens', a site for maturation of sperm. It is vas deferens that is the continuation of epididymis that connects to the penis.

Scrotum is the sac that holds the testes below and outside the abdomen. The muscles in the scrotum contract on sensing cold temperature and pull up the testicles close to the body for the warmth. This helps to provide the right temperature for the sperm.

Prostate Gland: It is located between the bladder and the penis. The size of prostate gland is that of a walnut. It secretes fluid for protection and nourishment of sperm.

The urethra passes through the centre of the prostate from urinary ladder and terminates in penis carrying the urine that flows out of the body. At the time of ejaculation, the prostate squeezes the fluid it secretes for sperm to enter the urethra. The sperm is expelled along with this fluid.

Penis: It is a sponge tissue consisting of a duct and a tip called 'glans penis'. The urethra passes through the penis and opens to the tip or 'Glans penis'. During ejaculation, the semen passes through the urethra and comes out through the opening in the tip of penis. The urethra and its opening also carry urine from the bladder. However, during ejaculation, a sphincter closes the bladder so that urine does not flow into urethra and mix with semen.

The Female Reproductive System

The female reproductive system comprises of ovaries, uterus, fallopian tubes, vagina, vulva and breasts.

Ovaries: They are a pair of almond-shaped structures that are 2–3 inches in length and 2 inches in width. They are located either side of the pelvic cavity. They are supported by the extension of peritoneum called 'mesovarium' that connects ovaries to broad ligament. The ovarian ligament connects ovaries to uterus.

Ovaries are the primary sex organs in the female reproductive system. The outer covering of ovaries has dense tissue covering called 'tunica albuginea'. Below this is the cortex. The cortex is made of a framework of tissues, which is called 'ovarian stroma'. The ovarian stroma facilitates the production of 'oocytes', which are the 'gametes' (gametes are mature reproductive eggs in ovaries that unite with other gametes of sperm). Each oocyte is surrounded by a number of cells called 'follicle'. Below the cortex is the medulla of the ovary. This is the place where there are blood vessels, lymph vessels and nerves of the ovary. The ovulation process starts at puberty. The mature oocytes are released one per month from menarche to menopause.

The ovaries play a major role in sending signals to endocrine system for production and regulation of hormones associated with sexual activity and reproduction.

Uterus: It is a muscular organ that is about 3 inches long and 2 inches wide. It is in the shape of an inverted pear. It has three sections. The part above the opening of the uterine tube is called 'fundus'. The middle part is called 'body of uterus'. The narrow lower portion that projects to vagina is called 'cervix'. The cervix produces mucus, which facilitates the movement of sperm along the reproductive tract. The cervix opens wide during child birth to enable the foetus to move downwards from the uterus.

Uterus has three layers. The exterior layer is called 'perimetrium'. It consists of epithelial cells. The middle layer is called 'myometrium'. It has thick smooth muscles and helps in contraction of uterus, which happens during mensuration and labour and also ovulation. The innermost layer is called 'endometrium'. There are two structural layers in endometrium, viz. 'stratum basalis' and 'stratum functionalis'. Stratum basalis is adjacent to myometrium. Stratum functionalist provides site for implantation of a fertilized egg. In case of no fertilization, the layer is shed during mensuration.

Fallopian Tube: This pair of tubes is also known as uterine tube. They run from the ovaries to the uterus. They are not joined to the ovaries but hang over them. They are used as conduits that carry oocytes to the uterus during the monthly cycle. In case of conception, they carry the 'pre-embryo' to the uterus.

Vagina: It is a muscular canal of 3–4 inches long. Like the other organs, the outer layer is fibrous, the middle layer has smooth muscles, and the inner layer has mucus membrane having transverse folds. These layers facilitate the expansion of vagina for sexual intercourse and child birth. A thin layer called 'hymen' is located around the vaginal opening. This can be ruptured in sexual intercourse or rigorous physical exercise.

Vulva: Vulva is the name given to the combination of three external genitalia, viz. 'labia majora', 'labia minora' and 'clitoris'. 'Labia' connotes 'lips'. Labia majora extends towards anus from the pubic mound. Post-puberty, it is covered by pubic hair. Labia minora is beneath labia majora. It is the skin fold that covers the opening of vagina. It continues upwards and covers the clitoris constituting its foreskin. Clitoris is that sensitive part of vulva located above vaginal opening and urethra. It has erectile tissues, which fill with blood during sexual stimulation.

Breasts: Breasts are accessory organs of the reproductive system. The main function of breasts is production of milk by the mammary glands for nourishment of the infant. Externally, the breasts include nipples surrounded by 'areola', an area that is pigmented and dark. This region has small areolar glands. They secrete lubricating fluid during lactation.

There are about two dozen lobules filled with milk-secreting cells in clusters called 'alveoli'. The alveoli contribute to the ducts, which merge at nipples. These lobules and ducts are formed during puberty but are protected by the adipose deposit under the skin. This also serves the purpose of giving a shape to breasts.

Function of Female Reproductive System:

A woman is in her reproductive stage, from menarche till menopause. During this phase, the primary reproductive organs, ovaries, are active. The readiness of the ovaries for reproduction follows a cycle of approximately 28 days. This cycle consists of two interrelated processes, viz. 'oogenesis' (production of female gametes) and folliculogenesis (growth and development of ovarian follicles).

At puberty, a girl has about 4,00,000 oocytes present in her. The initiation of release of oocyte from ovary is called ovulation. This marks the transition in the life of a female by being ready for reproduction. From the time of menarche, the female passes through cycles of 28 days (approximately) that prepares the ovum and uterus for reproduction. These cycles are triggered by activation of hormonal release as a result of endocrinal regulation.

The 28-day ovarian cycle plays a crucial role by producing the relevant hormones, which control the uterine cycle.

The functions of the female reproductive system can thus be explained in terms of two interrelated cycles—viz. ovarian cycle and uterine cycle.

Ovarian Cycle: Ovarian cycle is of 28 days approximately. The onset of menstrual bleeding is counted as day 1. This begins when the levels of oestrogen and progesterone are the lowest. The low levels of oestrogen communicate the message to hypothalamus, which then releases gonadotrophin-releasing hormone (GnRH). This travels and stimulates the pituitary gland to produce gonadotrophins, which are called follicle stimulating hormone (FSH) and luteinizing hormone (LH).

From day 1 and day 13, FSH helps in development of follicles. Follicles are the basic units of the female reproductive system. Each follicle contains an immature ovum called 'oocyte'. The LH stimulates the oocyte to mature in one of the ovaries. The secretion of FSH and LH is at the peak when the follicle is fully developed and the oocyte is ready to be released. The oocyte is released on day 14. The process of this release of oocyte is called ovulation. Post-ovulation, an oocyte lives for 12–24 hours only.

During ovulation, the pituitary gland secretes luteinizing hormone (LH). Because of this, the follicle after releasing oocyte becomes 'corpus luteum'. The corpus luteum secretes 'progesterone'. When adequate progesterone is secreted, the message to hypothalamus is sent. Hypothalamus in turn sends message to pituitary to stop further secretion of LH. Once the secretion is stopped, the corpus luteum starts shrinking and disappears around day 26. Once the corpus luteum is gone, the oestrogen and progesterone are in the lowest level. The menstruation starts at this time. This completes one full cycle, and the cycle starts all over again. When the hypothalamus receives the message of low oestrogen, it stimulates the pituitary gland by releasing gonadotrophin-releasing hormone (GnRH). In turn, the pituitary gland secretes FSH and LH.

Uterine Cycle: The uterine cycle coincides with the ovarian cycle. Just recall the three layers of uterus. The innermost layer called endometrium readies itself for implantation of fertilized egg, in the absence of which its tissues are torn apart rupturing the blood vessels, which passes out of vagina during the menstrual cycle. This process occurs between days 1 and 5 of the cycle.

After the menstrual cycle, the secretion of oestrogen starts and gradually increases. During the time when follicle start developing in ovaries, due to the secretion of oestrogen, the tissues in the inner lining of uterus starts regenerating, once again building endometrium. This process is on from days 6 to 14, when there is ovulation. By the time the ova are released, the endometrium is regenerated ready for the implantation and nourishment of the fertilized egg—the embryo.

While discussing the ovulation cycle, we referred to the ovulation time when the LH produces a lot of progesterone. The progesterone contributes to thickening of endometrium. During this time, the glands in uterus also secrete thick mucus. The thick endometrium and the mucus function as the 'trap' for the fertilized egg. In case there is a fertilized egg, it gets implanted in the uterus. This is the beginning of the process of pregnancy. Once it happens, the corpus luteum secretes oestrogen and progesterone until placenta is formed. Once the placenta is developed, it takes once the secretion of oestrogen and progesterone. If fertilization fails to occur, the corpus luteum shrinks and the production of oestrogen and progesterone decreases and the endometrium is shed.

Thus, for the pregnancy to occur, the opportunity for fertilization should coincide with ovulation.

Menopause: A woman's reproductive system ovulates roughly about 400 times during the life time. When a woman enters menopause, the stage when the ovulation stops, her ability to conceive ends. There is a general slowdown in other processes. Cellular metabolism slows down. As a result, replacement of structural protein in the skin is slowed down creating wrinkles in the skin. Bones lose their strength. The most commonly referred 'hot flashes' are experienced by women due to faulty signals from parasympathetic nervous systems disrupting the body's ability to monitor the body temperature accurately.

The Reproduction and Preparation for the Body

The process of reproduction passes through several stages. The initial phase calls for certain coincidence of timing to suit the woman's ovulation. Let is briefly explain the process of reproduction.

It may be recalled that the process of ovulation releases the oocyte from the ovary. The oocyte now travels along a fallopian tube. If the intercourse occurs, the semen from the male body ejaculates into vaginal of the female. A few million sperm find way through cervix and fallopian tube. The oocyte is already in the fallopian tube.

When at least one sperm penetrates into the oocyte, the cell division called 'Meiosis II' is initiated. When the nucleus of the sperm fuses with ovum, there is fertilization and it is called a 'zygote'. The fertilization depends upon the timing of the intercourse because the developed oocyte stays in the body for a very short period of 12–24 hours.

Soon after fertilization, the zygote divides itself moving down the fallopian tube. When the embryo reaches the uterus and implants itself successfully on the endometrium, it is called 'pregnancy'.

The embryo successfully embedded in the endometrium is called 'blastocyte'. It produces a hormone called 'human chronic gonadotrophin' (HCG). This helps in maintenance of 'corpus luteum', which shrinks in the event of no fertilization. Corpus luteum produces oestrogen and progesterone. Because the levels of oestrogen and progesterone are high, menstruation does not happen. The presence of HCG in the urine is tested to confirm pregnancy.

The uterus expands about five times its size during the entire period of pregnancy and reaches its optimum in 38 weeks. The expanded uterus accommodates the foetus, placenta, umbilical cord and amniotic fluid. The placenta produces large amount of oestrogen and progesterone. This causes a number of changes in maternal body.

Towards the end of pregnancy, the cervix becomes soft. The mucus glands in the cervix produce what is called a mucus plug. This helps in protecting the foetus from infections.

The ovulation process is suspended during pregnancy.

During the pregnancy, the breasts enlarge in size. The areolas of the nipples enlarge and become dark. The breasts begin to produce 'colostrum'.

The labour process begins with the contraction of smooth muscles in the uterus. This results in the cervix becoming thinner and wider. There is rupture of amniotic membrane. The continuation of contraction pushes the foetus down. Gradually, the baby comes out of the birth canal with the head emerging out first. The umbilical cord is cut to separate the baby from the placenta. The contraction continues until the placenta comes out and the uterus gets back almost to its original size.

The reproductive system is one that is closely associated with changes in the body state and behaviour. These changes are concomitant with the changes in hormonal levels. Further, the sexual behaviour has significant influence of sociocultural factors and is guided by social norms, values, morals and ethics. Thus, one may say that the reproductive system is closely associated with biopsychosocial aspects such as antecedents and consequences.

Box 6.4   Researcher's Box

- A population survey to identify the age of puberty for boys and girls differing in socio-economic status and region.
- An interdisciplinary study can be designed to find out the relationship between pubertal age and diet and stress levels. For this, a survey design can help. A survey of population of age group between 6 and 16 years can be planned. A questionnaire, for diet survey, physical anthropometry measures and a scale for measuring stress levels among children constitute the tools. Appropriate statistical analyses help identify the onset of puberty and factors contributing to early/late pubertal age.
- Values associated with reproductive behaviour can be compared among the adolescents from various countries, cultures within the nation, socioeconomic classes.
- Changes in states among girls coinciding with ovarian cycles can be studied. This can be done by following up a sample of girls who have attained menarche, for a period of full cycle. The affect state of the day can be assessed. The measurement tool can be a scale and also a dairy or a combination of both.

Box 6.5   Summary of the Reproductive System

- The reproductive system is closely associated with the endocrine system.
- The reproductive system of males has organs like testes, scrotum, prostate glands and penis, while the organs for females are ovaries, uterus, fallopian tubes, vagina, vulva and breast.
- The organs show spurt of growth and development during puberty, which is 9–11 years in girls and 11–13 years in boys. Secondary sexual characteristics develop during this period.
- The male reproductive system produces sperm, while the female system produces ovum. Fusion of these two causes fertilization.
- Reproduction occurs because of a beautiful coincidence between the female reproduction system readiness and the sexual intercourse when the ovum is released on the 14th day of ovarian cycle and meets the sperm and the zygote gets formed.
- The female reproductive system functions as ovarian cycle and uterine cycle, which are interrelated. Ovarian cycle develops and releases the ovum, while the hormones released by the ovarian cycle help build the uterine environment for implantation of the fertilized egg.
- The fertilized egg develops into a foetus and is delivered. Again, the hormonal secretion prepares the uterus for labour, delivery and lactation.

The Immune System

The immune system is different from other systems in the human body. While the other systems are made of a number of organs, the immune system is made of a combination of special organs, cells and chemicals. While the other systems have a dedicated function such as digestion, excretion, respiration, the dedicated function of the immune system is to protect these systems and others from the attack of antigens such as bacteria, fungi, protozoa and viruses, with the help of the special organs, cells and chemicals.

The immune system is one of the systems that is still being explored. It is as recently as 1970s that knowledge about immune system was found in a significant way (Sarafino and Smith, 2005): However, whatever knowledge gathered until now has certainly made a significant contribution to medical science.

Human Vulnerability to Microbes

The human body is vulnerable to microorganisms that invade through many ways. They may be transmitted to people in the following four ways (Taylor, 2006):

- Direct transmission through bodily contact, e.g. hand shake, kissing, sexual intercourse
- Indirect transmission through air, water, soil or food., e.g. drinking contaminated water or food
- Biological transmission through mosquitos, e.g. mosquitos pick up microbes and release them to the human body after changing its form causing illness like chikungunya, malaria
- Mechanical transmission. Here, the transmission happens through an agent that carries and transmits the disease but not directly affected by the disease, e.g. flies carrying microbes infecting your food, rats and mice that carry the microbes

Antigens: They are substances that initiate response from the immune system. If you conceptualize the immune system as 'You', any substance that is not 'you' but trying to make way into you is bound to create a response from you by way of resistance. Thus, antigens can be described as substances that are 'not self', trying to invade. An antigen can be a foreign body from the environment that includes bacteria, fungi, virus or protozoa, or it can even be produced by one's own body.

Bacteria are microorganisms that exist in huge numbers in the environment. They cause diseases such as tuberculosis, food poisoning, leprosy—to name a few.

Fungi are organisms that attach themselves to some organic host and absorb nutrients from there. Some skin diseases like ring worm are the result of fungal infections.

Protozoa are like amoeba—single-celled animals. They thrive in water and insects. Drinking water contaminated with protozoa can cause amoebic dysentery.

Viruses are very tiny antigens, smaller than cells. A virus attaches to a cell by getting in. Once it slips in, it takes over the work by issuing its own genetic instructions. This forces the cell to abandon its own metabolic activities and converts itself into a 'factory' of producing viruses. The viruses thus produced tear away the cell and spread themselves to infect other cells. Viruses have the characteristic of being dormant in the human body for some time and then emerge as infections.

Immune System and Its Parts: The immune system is constituted with a combination of body organs, cells and chemicals. Following are the main parts of the immune system:

1 Lymphatic system
2 Spleen
3 Bone marrow
4 Thymus
5 While blood cells
6 Antibodies

Let us now try to understand each of them.

Lymphatic System: The lymphatic system comprises of lymph, lymph vessels, lymphatic ducts and lymph nodes.

In the circulatory system, when the blood is circulated all over the body, the capillaries supply the oxygen and other nutrients to the cells, and carry away the waste products. The exchange of oxygen, ions, glucose, proteins, hormones and other nutrients is pushed out of the capillary cells in watery solution. This water solution is called 'interstitial fluid'. This is also called 'extracellular fluid' as it flows between cells. Most of this is reabsorbed into the blood. Rest of it goes into the lymphatic system. What goes into the lymphatic system is called 'lymph'.

The lymph is carried in 'lymphatic vessels'. The lymphatic vessels start as lymph capillaries, and become vessels and then lymphatic ducts. They run all over the body alongside the blood vessels. The lymphatic ducts drain into large veins.

Lymph nodes are bean-shaped structures situated along lymph vessels. This is not true because these nodes do not secrete any hormone, hence cannot be identified as glands. Their location is quite prominent in pharynx, armpit and groin. They are also located in the digestive system and other places. Every lymph node is within a 'capsule' made of a fibrous cover. Filtration of lymph happens in the node. The afferent lymphatic vessels bring lymph into the node, while the efferent vessels carry the filtered lymph out of the node.

The Spleen: The spleen is located to the left of the stomach. It is an oval-shaped organ. It can be construed as a large-sized lymph node because it performs the function of a lymph node by filtering blood and segregating the pathogens and other foreign matters, as well as exhausted RBC. The 'leucocytes' present inside the spleen help in this filtration. It also initiates production of 'antibody'.

Bone Marrow: The soft tissue inside the bone is bone marrow. It produces red blood cells and white blood cells and platelets. White blood cells are also referred to as 'leucocytes'. There are five types of leucocytes. Out of this, 'lymphocytes' are produced in bone marrow. From her, the lymphocytes migrate to one or two other organs where they mature. Thymus is one such organ where they mature.

Thymus: This is a gland below the neck and between the lungs. Thymus is relatively large in childhood, and with age, the size decreases. It produces a hormone called 'thymosin'. This stimulates the differentiation and maturation of one kind of lymphocyte called 'T' cells. The major part of processing of lymphocytes happens at the prenatal stage itself.

White Blood Cells (WBC) or Leucocytes (May Be Spelt Two Ways)

White blood cells are the main component of the immune system. It is called leucocytes because it means 'white cells'. The name is because these cells appear white under the microscope. Both red and white cells develop from haematopoietic stem cells in the red marrow. White the red cells contain haemoglobin and iron (that are absent in leucocytes), the leucocytes unlike RBC continue to have their nuclei, organ cells and cytoplasm throughout their life cycle.

The leucocytes are broadly divided into two groups based on the presence or absence of granules in their cytoplasm—granulated and agranulated. Granulated leucocytes are three types, viz. 'basophil', 'neutrophil' and 'eosinophil'. Agranulated leucocytes are of two types, viz. 'lymphocytes' and 'monocytes'. Based on their functions, leucocytes are of two types—phagocytes and lymphocytes.

1 **Phagocytes:** These are the cells that carry out patrolling of the body. When there is an antigen, they surround, absorb, break them down and eat them. The job of phagocytes is to clean the blood of any 'invading' substance. Hence, they are also called 'the scavengers'.

Phagocytes do not discriminate or choose the 'foreign elements' invading the body. Anything that does not belong to the blood stream, tissues or lymphatic system is destroyed by phagocytes. The active phagocytes in the lungs go on consuming the duct particles and the black smoke stains. Thus, by responding to any kind of antigen, the phagocytes are labelled as 'non-specific' cells. Phagocytes are of different types.

  a Neutrophils: They are the most common type of phagocytes accounting to about 40%–70% of leucocytes. They are found in active operation in circulatory and lymphatic system. They squeeze into the capillaries and infected tissues and consume the bacteria.
  b Monocytes: They play a very unique role similar to stem cells. They divide to produce two types of immune cells called 'macrophages' and 'dendritic cells'. Production of these cells is based on the demand for homeostasis. When the body has any inflammation, monocytes travel to the site to produce its cells.
  c Macrophages: The meaning of 'macrophage' is 'big eater'. They are large phagocyte cells that attach and consume the antigens and the dead cells.
  d Mast Cells: They help in healing the wounds in addition to fighting the antigens.

2 **Lymphocytes:** The lymphocytes are identified as T cells, B cells and NK cells. The origin of all lymphocytes is red marrow. The B lymphocytes and NK lymphocytes complete the process of differentiation in the marrow and join the circulatory and lymphatic systems. However, the T cells are carried to the thymus gland. Their differentiation takes place in the presence of the hormone, thymosin. Once differentiated, the T cells travel to medulla of the lymph node where they get further differentiated as helper T cells (T_H), cytotoxic T cells and suppressor T cells depending on their specific immune function.

Lymphocytes engage in specific immune processes. They are tailored to attack specific antigens. Specific immune process is of two types, viz. cell-mediated immunity and antibody-mediated 'humoral immunity' (Sarafino, 1994).

Cell-mediated Immunity: Lymphocytes called 'T cells' are the fighters. They operate at the level of cells. They acquired the name T cells because they are matured in the 'thymus gland' (R for thymus). The T cells are of different types. Each type has their assigned functions. The types of lymphocytes are depicted in Figure 6.19.

Killer T Cells: The job of the killer T cells is to destroy the harmful elements. They attack and kill those tissues that do not belong to the body and considered 'foreign'. Thus, the tissues that are transplanted into the body are the targets. The second target is the cancerous cells growing in the body, and the third target is the cells that are invaded by antigens such as viruses.

Memory T Cells: Memory T cells remain in the body for a long period in human life that may be even for decades. This long life of memory T cells is with a purpose. When the individual is first infected or affected by a particular infection or illness caused by a specific antigen (like a bacterium causing typhoid or infection like mumps caused by a virus), the memory T cells remember the features of this antigen, which is imprinted in them. With this 'memory', the T cells and their offspring stand as a defence against such antigens in future and protect the body against them.

Delayed Hypersensitivity T Cells: These cells are assigned two specific functions. The reaction of these cells takes several days (Warrington et al., 2011). The response is one where there is an interaction between T cells, monocytes and macrophages. "They are involved in delayed immune reaction, particularly in allergies such as of poison ivy, in which tissue becomes inflamed" (Sarafino, 1994, 99.61).

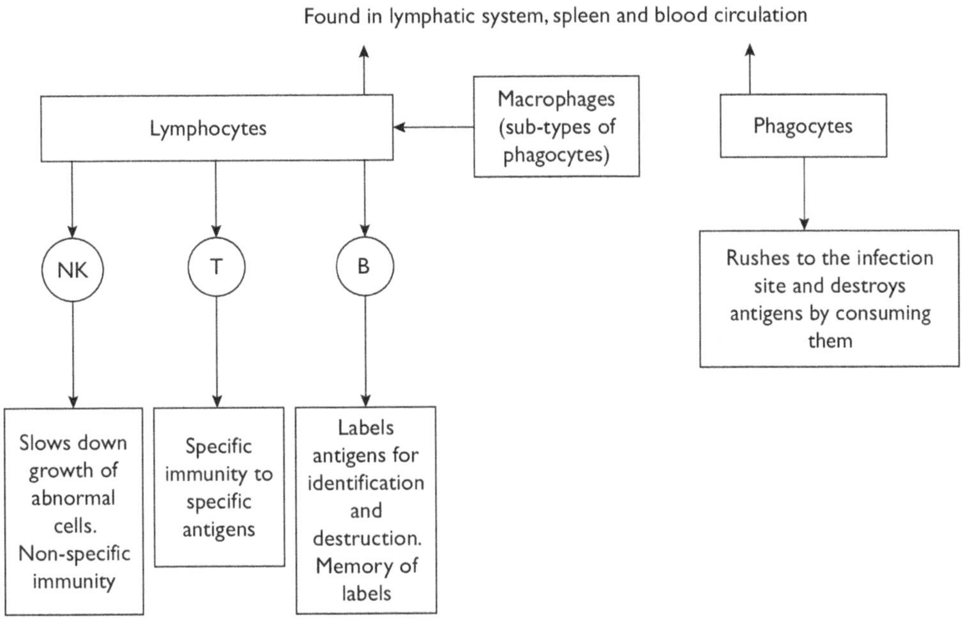

```
                    Found in lymphatic system, spleen and blood circulation
                              ↑                                    ↑
  ┌─────────────────────────────┐   ┌──────────────┐   ┌──────────────┐
  │                             │   │ Macrophages  │   │              │
  │       Lymphocytes           │◄──│(sub-types of │   │  Phagocytes  │
  │                             │   │  phagocytes) │   │              │
  └─────────────────────────────┘   └──────────────┘   └──────────────┘
         │        │       │                                    │
         ▼        ▼       ▼                                    ▼
       (NK)     (T)      (B)                        ┌────────────────┐
                                                    │Rushes to the   │
                                                    │infection site  │
                                                    │and destroys    │
                                                    │antigens by     │
                                                    │consuming them  │
                                                    └────────────────┘
  ┌──────────┐ ┌──────────┐ ┌──────────┐
  │Slows down│ │ Specific │ │  Labels  │
  │growth of │ │immunity  │ │antigens  │
  │abnormal  │ │to specific│ │for ident-│
  │cells.    │ │ antigens │ │ification │
  │Non-spec- │ │          │ │and       │
  │ific      │ │          │ │destruction│
  │immunity  │ │          │ │Memory of │
  │          │ │          │ │labels    │
  └──────────┘ └──────────┘ └──────────┘
```

Figure 6.19 Immune System: Functions.

Helper T Cells: On receiving the entry of the antigens in the body, the helper T cells travel fast to the spleen and lymph nodes and stimulate the production of lymphocytes for attack.

Suppressor T Cells: When the leucocytes initiate attack on antigens and successfully destroy them, they should know to stop further attack. The suppressor T cells carry out this function. When the infection is gone and the antigens are attacked, the suppressor T cells slow down or stop the process.

The second type of lymphocytes as mentioned is the antibody-mediated 'humoral immunity'. These lymphocytes attack the antigens much before they invade the cells in the body. They target the antigens when they are in body fluids. The attackers are the B cells. These B cells produce 'antibodies'. "An 'antibody' is a protein molecule with immune function" (Norris & Siegfried, 2011). They are called 'immunoglobulin' (IG). When the B cells sense the invasion of antigens, they produce antibodies or immunoglobulin. The B cells produce thousands of antibodies. Each antibody is produced in response to one antigen.

The lymphocytes are covered with receptors of various antigens. Some of them could be totally new. When a B cell comes in contact with an antigen, the receptor on the cell binds the antigen. Now the B cell multiples very fast. All the cells thus produced get engaged in producing antibody specific to that antigen. The antibodies bind and disable the target antigen. Once the antibody binds an antigen, the antigen ceases to be active. This inactive or destroyed antigen is removed out by other immune system in the body. When the antibodies find new antigens, they form memory B cells. They are used in future for labelling these antigens and fighting them. Thus, antibodies are useful in neutralizing the antigens. They are compared to 'arms' in the war.

Researchers have identified five types of antibodies. They are immunoglobulin (Ig)A, IgD, IgE, IgM and IgG. They are found in blood and other body fluids. Their presence in the blood helps in diagnosis of bacteria- and viral-infected diseases. Antibodies of the IgM group present in the body fluid indicate that the infection is recent, while IgG suggests that the infection has been in the past.

> **Box 6.6   Summary of the Immune System**
>
> - The important constituents in the immune system include lymphatic system, spleen, bone marrow, thymus, white blood cells and antibodies.
> - Bone marrow and spleen are the production sites of immune cells called leucocytes.
> - The lymph nodes are filtering agents.
> - The leucocytes include phagocytes and lymphocytes.
> - Phagocytes are non-specific defence functionaries.
> - There are T cells and B cells, which carry out specific defence functions.
> - The T cells are of five types, each with specific functions.
> - B cells are producers of antibodies.
> - When an antigen enters the body, the body's defence gets activated and puts up a fight with it by directly destroying it or destroying the cells it invaded.
> - The memory cells remain in the body for decades so that they label any invaders using their earlier memory.

Operation of the Body's Defence System

The body's immune system functions as a defence against the invasion of any antigen (foreign body) that may cause damage to the body. However, the first line of our defence is our own skin. The mucus membrane and the hair follicles (in the nostrils, for example) present any foreign body entry into the system. The mucus, antibodies and antimicrobial substances in the mucus membrane stand as barriers against any invaders. However, despite these primary defences, the antigens sometimes manage an entry. When they manage the entry, they have to encounter the second line of defence. As already discussed, they may fall victim to the phagocytes, which destroy and eat up the invaders indiscriminately. This non-specific immune response of phagocytes is very useful when there is a new antigen and the memory cells have not yet got their imprint. The phagocytes also present the antigens to T cells and B cells. Responding to this and the helper T cells, the B cells produce the required antibodies. The antibodies do their job of binding the antigen to make the antigen a target to phagocytes.

In case the antigen wedges through even this second line of defence, they will face the third line of defence. Phagocytes present them to T cells. Here, they are destroyed by the killer T cells. Once the invasion of antigens is stopped, the suppressor T cells slow down the process and stop it. The memory T cells and B cells are now flowing in the body and other fluids, and ready to identify the antigens when they try entry and invasion next time.

Stress levels play a significant role in determining the level of efficiency with which the immune system functions. This will be discussed in detail in the section on stress and coping.

References

Carlson, N. R. (2005). *Foundations of physiological psychology* (6th ed.). Boston, MA: Pearson Education New Zealand.

Kelly, Y., Zilanawala, A., Sacker, A., Hiatt, R., & Viner, R. (2017). Early puberty in 11-year-old girls: Millennium Cohort Study findings. *Archives of Disease in Childhood, 102*(3), 232–237.

Khadgawat, R., Marwaha, R. K., Mehan, N., Surana, V., Dabas, A., Sreenivas, V., … & Gupta, N. (2016). Age of onset of puberty in apparently healthy school girls from Northern India. *Indian Pediatrics, 53*(5), 383–387.

Khosla, M. (2017). *Physiological psychology: An introduction*. New Delhi: SAGE Publications.
Norris, M., & Siegfried, D. R. (2011). *Anatomy and physiology for dummies*. Hoboken, NJ: John Wiley & Sons.
Pathak, P. K., Tripathi, N., & Subramanian, S. V. (2014). Secular trends in menarcheal age in India-evidence from the Indian human development survey. *PLoS One*, *9*(11), e111027.
Sarafino, E. P. (1994). *Health psychology: Biopsychosocial interactions*. Canada: John Wiley & Sons.
Sarafino, E. P., & Smith, T. W. (2005). *Health psychology: Biopsychosocial interactions*. Canada: John Wiley & Sons.
Standring, S. (Ed.). (2015). *Gray's anatomy e-book: The anatomical basis of clinical practice*. Elsevier Health Sciences.
Surana, V., Dabas, A., Khadgawat, R., Marwaha, R. K., Sreenivas, V., Ganie, M. A., & Mehan, N. (2017). Pubertal onset in apparently healthy Indian boys and impact of obesity. *Indian Journal of Endocrinology and Metabolism*, *21*(3), 434–438.
Taylor, S. E. (2006). *Health psychology*. New Delhi: Tata McGraw-Hill Education.
Warrington, R., Watson, W., Kim, H. L., & Antonetti, F. R. (2011). An introduction to immunology and immunopathology. *Allergy, Asthma & Clinical Immunology*, *7*(1), S1.

7 Stress and Illness

What Is Stress?

When I asked this question to various groups of students, and trainees from different professional groups, the few common responses were as follows: stress is more work, difficult work, harassment by boss, conflict with others, failure in achievement, having to take humiliation, not getting recognition for merit, breakup in relationship, inability to balance work and home, being evaluated on core competence or having a strained relationship. Few other responses also named factors such as fast heartbeat, shivering of body, headache, ill health. Organizing these responses, it was found that some referred to an event (examination) or a person (hostile boss/teacher), some others referred to one's own internal responses (fast heartbeat, inability), and yet others referred to a continuing process (going through a strained relationship).

Thus, it can be summarized that for some who viewed stress as an event, situation or another person, it is a stimulus. For those who viewed stress as physiological changes in self or a behaviour itself, it is a response. Yet for others who viewed it as a combination of a specific situation and an internal response, it is a transaction.

From the perspective of Health Psychology, the definition of Baum (1990) sounds very appropriate. He defined stress as a "Negative emotional experience accompanied by predictable biochemical, physiological, cognitive and behavioral changes that are directed either towards altering the stressful event or accommodating to its effects".

This definition appears to have its emphasis on the 'response' and 'transaction' perspective of stress. The stimulus perspective of stress is equally significant and calls for a space in a definition to be qualified as inclusive. Taking all the perspectives, stress may be defined in the following terms.

Stress refers to a negative emotional condition, accompanied by biomedical and physiological changes in the body, preceded by a cognitive appraisal where the individual perceives the demands on self, exceeding the resources, and followed by a behavioural initiative to change the situation or adapt to it.

The above definition lays emphasis on five components. Let us elaborate on these six factors—

1. Demands on Self: Stressful situation is one where the individual perceives high demands on oneself. These demands may originate from external sources (e.g. competition in the academic field) or from within (e.g. aspirations to top the university examination).
2. Limited Resources: Resources refer to external and internal resources. External resources are one's financial state, power, position or social support network. Internal resources refer to one's personal abilities, personality disposition, personal competency, self-efficacy, cognitive base, emotional intelligence, cognitive, motivational and social competence and so on.

The individual experiences stress when he/she perceives that the available resources are not adequate in meeting the demands. This perception could be real based on objective judgement or unrealistic due to judgement errors.

3 Cognitive appraisal: When the individual encounters a demand either from the external environment (e.g. completion of a task against a time line) or from within (e.g. to crack the Junior Research Fellow Test and acquire a seat in Ph.D.), he/she would match the demand with the resources (internal or external) available. When one perceives a balance between the two, it does not generate any stress. However, when the cognitive appraisal indicates a mismatch between the demand and resources, there is a perception of imbalance. In instances where achievement of goal by encountering the demands involves significant stakes, and the goal is highly attractive and essential in fulfilling important needs, the individual feels the pressure of attaining it. Secondly, when the individual perceives an obstacle between the goal and oneself and there is a strong demand from within to attain the goal, yet, the resources are found to be inadequate in reaching the goal as per the cognitive appraisal, and the individual experiences stress.

4 Biochemical and physiological changes in the body: When a block to the goal is perceived either in the form of another individual, stringent rules in the system, limited abilities or any other situation, it triggers a negative emotion and a concomitant change in the neuroendocrinal functioning. The endocrinal system gets stimulated, and results are secreting some hormones that flow into the blood stream. This brings in biochemical changes in the body.

The message of perception of a block to the goal or mismatch between the demand and the resources is transmitted to the brain. The hypothalamus activates the sympathetic nervous system, which in turn brings about a number of physiological changes in the body that include fast heartbeat, breathing, stimulation of sweat glands, flushing of more glucose to the muscles, dilation of pupils. These biochemical and physiological changes coexist with negative emotional state of the individual.

5 Negative emotional state: The individual's cognitive appraisal of the situation suggests either a harm (a loss that already occurred) or a threat (a potential for loss) to the individual. This harm or threat may relate to one's security, affiliation or self-esteem causing stress. Stress is always characterized by a negative emotional state. This could be fear, anxiety, anger or depression. These emotions are unpleasant.

It is evident that stress induces a state of disequilibrium on all dimensions of the individual such as physiological, biochemical, emotional and cognitive functions. Whenever there is disequilibrium, the natural tendency is to restore the equilibrium and attain homeostasis. Hence, the individual would now be motivated to initiate action to restore the balance in all dimensions either by changing the situation (e.g. attempting to remove the block to the goal), by mobilizing additional resources or by reconciling to adapt to the situation either by altering expectation levels and the goal or by changing attribution to the goal itself. In this process, the individual invests some efforts. Depending upon whether the efforts invested are commensurate with the value of the outcome in terms of the goal, the individual opts whether to change the situation or to adapt to the situation. In either case, the homeostasis is restored and the stress is minimized.

Models of Stress

The phenomenon of stress is studied through different approaches. The study of stress can broadly fit into three different models—viz. medicophysiological model or response model, the engineering or stimulus model and the interactional or transactional model. These models are elaborated under their respective heads.

Stress as a 'Response'—The Medicophysiological Models

This relates to two early theories of stress popularized by two physiologists, named Walter Canon and Hans Selye. Before going into the models propounded by the two physiologists, it is relevant to understand the physiological and endocrine response system to stress. This helps in understanding the models better.

The Sympathetic Adrenomedullary Response System (SAM)

This involves the response of the sympathetic division of the autonomic nervous system. When the individual encounters a stressful situation and perceives a threat and is frightened, the hypothalamus immediately sends the message to the adrenal gland located in the kidneys. The adrenal gland medulla gets stimulated and secretes catecholamines called adrenaline and noradrenaline into the blood. The adrenaline and noradrenaline reach the internal organs along the blood stream and activate several functioning. They have the same effects on target organs as direct stimulation by sympathetic nerves. Apart from these, the mental activity also is heightened. Figure 7.1 depicts the Sympathetic Adrenomedullary System.

As a consequence, the following changes occur:

- The reaction of adrenaline with beta receptors increases the heart rate and the force in contraction of heart muscles. The outcome of enhanced force in contraction is an increased blood flow to the muscular regions of the body.
- Noradrenaline in particular creates widespread vasoconstriction. When the blood vessels are constricted, there are a resistance to the blood flow and an increased pressure of blood in the arteries. Overall, there is an increased blood pressure.
- Dilation of bronchioles results in added pulmonary ventilation. This causes increased breathing.
- The fat cells in the body get stimulated for lipolysis. Lipolysis is the process where the adipose or fat is split into fatty acids and glycerol. This provides energy in many tissues and helps in conserving the reserves of glucose in the blood.
- In response to the hormone, adrenaline secreted into the blood stream reaches every part of the body. There is an increase in consumption of oxygen and heat production in the body. Further, the catecholamines also result in breaking down the glycogen in skeletal muscles, which results in more glucose for enhanced energy to the skeletal and muscular system. This indicates an increased metabolic rate.
- While the catecholamines result in enhanced activity of certain organs, it also functions as an inhibitor of certain processes that are not essential in a stressful situation. For example, gastrointestinal function is inhibited during stress.

Apart from reaction to stress, catecholamine secretion is found when the individual experiences hypoglycaemia and haemorrhage and while involved in exercise.

The Hypothalamic-Pituitary-Adrenal (HPA) Axis Response System

The second physiological response to stress is hypothalamic-pituitary-adrenal (HPA) axis activation. On encountering the stressful situation, the stress message reaches the brain, and the hypothalamus is stimulated. The hypothalamus releases a hormone called corticotrophin-releasing hormone (CRH) or corticotrophin-releasing factor (CRF). This released into the blood system stimulates the pituitary gland. The pituitary gland on being stimulated releases adrenocorticotrophic hormone (ACTH). The adrenocorticotrophic hormone through blood circulation reaches

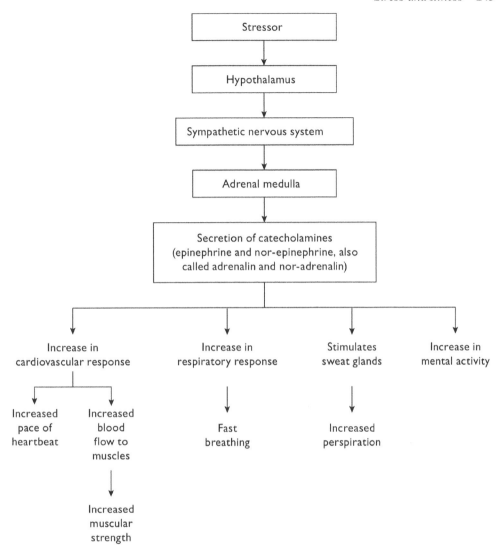

Figure 7.1 Sympathetic Adrenomedullary System (SAM).

the adrenal cortex of the adrenal gland located in the kidneys. The adrenal cortex releases glucocorticoids. The term 'glucocorticoids' can be better understood and remembered if we break it into two, where 'gluco' refers to glucose, which is the main carbohydrate. The second part 'corticoid' refers to the 'cortex' of adrenal gland that secretes it. On release of glucocorticoids into the blood stream, the body's glucose levels increase. The increased glucose is used by body cells for additional energy to combat a stressful situation.

The most important glucocorticoid in the body is cortisol, also called 'stress hormone'. Cortisol regulates the metabolism of carbohydrate and has an anti-inflammatory effect on the body. Thus, the immediate effect of cortisol in the body is to enhance access to energy store, and decrease inflammation. For example in a combat situation when a soldier is fighting with the enemy, and got injured in the foot, the cortisol helps in preventing an inflammation and also enhancing the energy levels so that the soldier continues to fight. This is possible because the

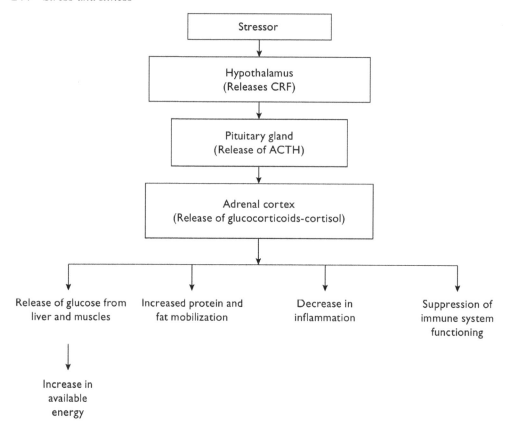

Figure 7.2 Hypothalamic-Pituitary-Adrenal (HPA) Axis Response to Stress.

cortisol triggers excess energy stored in liver and muscles, and breaks them into glucose to be used by brain and muscles.

The process is depicted in Figure 7.2.

In addition to enhancing energy reserve, the cortisol also destroys the B and T lymphocytes, thus lowering the functioning of the immune system.

Fight-or-Flight Response

Cannon (1932) is the proponent of this model. He explained stress as a fight-or-flight response on encountering an emergency threatful situation. His explanation was in the context of perception of danger. When animals or humans perceive any dangerous situation, the message reaches the brain and the sympathetic adrenomedullary system is activated. As a consequence, the adrenal gland secretes adrenaline and noradrenaline setting the sympathetic nervous system to action. This in turn induces the body to an arousal state and mobilizes the additional energy. Both are essential prerequisite, either to fight the situation or to flee the situation.

This response can be classified as adaptive because it mobilizes the individual to react immediately. However, the state of high arousal, if prolonged, can be harmful to health. The major criticism of the fight-or-flight model came from Taylor. It was argued that animals and humans do not limit themselves to fight-or-flight. The other important reaction during stressful situation is affiliation. Animals are seen to herd together on perceiving danger. Human beings encountering major natural disaster also try to be with each other and find supportive behaviour. This is often seen in females. Thus, Taylor and colleagues (2000) argued that in addition to fight-or-flight, individuals also respond with 'tend-and-befriend' response to stress. They also traced the physiological basis for this natural reaction to stress among females, pointing out that a hormone called oxytocin is responsible for eliciting this response in female gender.

General Adaptation Syndrome (GAS)

Hans Selye (1956, 1976, 1985) built upon the research of Cannon. While Cannon's research initiated by secretion of catecholamine, Selye explored the stress response based on adrenocortical secretion.

Selye believed that resistance and adaptation are the life's basic prerequisites. All vital organs actively participate in these processes. Further, Selye assumed that the physiological response to stress is universal and it never varies with the type of stressors. He stated that the explanation of his theory involved the disciplines of physiology, biochemistry and medicine.

The initial work of Selye was on rats. He was studying the impact of stress hormones on their physiological functioning. Subsequently, he got interested in the stress that his intervention seems to have created in rats. He exposed the experimental animals in the laboratory to various stressors such as high or low temperatures, insulin injections, exercise and X-rays for long period of times. His experimental rats exposed to stressors like extreme cold or fatigue showed similar physiological responses. The result of exposure to stress, irrespective of stressors, was enlarged adrenal cortex, shrinking of the thymus gland and lymph gland, ulceration of stomach and duodenum (Taylor, 2006).

Since the stress response was universal, he perceived a general way in which the body adapts to stress. Since the adaptation was observed in several dimensions, he called it a 'syndrome'. Hence, his model is named as 'General Adaptation Syndrome'. The basic assumptions of General Adaptation Syndrome are as follows: on encountering a stress, the organisms mobilize itself for action. The physiological response to stressor is non-specific; i.e., the response pattern is the same for all stressors. Repeated exposure to stress results in the wear and tear of the system.

General Adaptation Syndrome (GAS) consists of three stages, viz. alarm, resistance and exhaustion. The GAS model is presented in Figure 7.3.

Alarm Reaction

This is the first stage after encountering the stress. It is very similar to fight-or-flight response. As an immediate reaction to stress, the body secretes the relevant hormones (explained under SAM syndrome and HPA axis) into the blood stream, and gets ready for action. The body is in intense state of arousal. It is very difficult for the body to maintain this intense arousal/alarm state. Animals and human beings who continued in such alarm state for prolonged periods died within hours or days.

There was a case of kidnap of a child in the state of United Andhra Pradesh. The father was a business man. The police were searching for the child. There was continuous live telecast of the reactions of family for a couple of days. There were observable shock and high level of stress in the parents. On the second day, there was a breaking news telecast that the child was brutally murdered. The father collapsed and died on hearing the news, which was also telecast live by the television crew present in their house.

It was observed by the measure of blood pressure that at the very beginning of alarm stage, there is a momentary below normal drop in the arousal, after which it peaks above normal. Towards the end of this stage with the fast pace of endocrine secretion and biochemical, physiological changes, the body is fully mobilized to resist the stress.

246 *Stress and Illness*

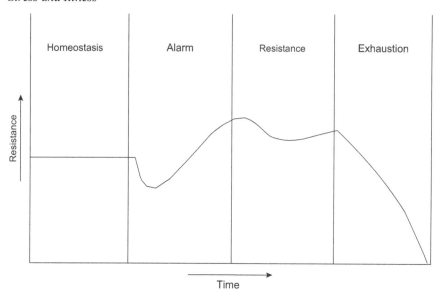

Figure 7.3 General Adaptation Syndrome (GAS).

Stage of Resistance

This stage is characterized by the body's attempts to adapt to the stress. Before entering this stage, the physiological arousal and body's mobilisation of energy are at the peak. In the resistance stage, the physiological arousal shows a decline, from its peak though it continues to be above normal. At the biochemical plane, the body replenishes the hormones released by adrenal glands. At the behavioural level, despite the high level of arousal, few outward stress signs are shown. The organism makes efforts to cope with the threat. While there is an attempt to adapt to stress, it appears superficial, and the person for a long period loses the ability to resist any new stressor. This impairment makes the individual susceptible to a number of illness, such as ulcers, viral, bacterial infection, high blood pressure, asthma. According to Selye, this increased vulnerability to diseases is called 'diseases of adaptation' (Sarafino, 1994a,b).

Stage of Exhaustion

If the stress continues, the physiological arousal state prolongs. It uses up the body's energy reserves. As a result, the immune system is weakened, the vital organs are overfunctioned, and the resistance drops. At this point, the stage of exhaustion begins. The body's defence being very low, the likelihood of physiological damage and diseases is very high, sometimes leading to death.

Criticism

Selye's General Adaptive Syndrome though gained popularity came under criticism on a number of aspects.

Mason (1975) questioned the very 'generality' of the mode. He pointed out that a number of stressors do not trigger predictable response of three stages as explained by Selye.

The 'non-specific' characteristic of the theory was questioned. While Selye's theory is focused on universal physiological reactions, it has not given the due significance to psychological aspects. The theory assumes non-specificity. It also experimentally proved that the physiological response to a wide range of stressors such as extreme temperature, illness of a loved person, physical exercise, pain or noise is the same. Experiments by Mason (1975) proved that the physiological response to a strong emotion associated with sudden change in temperature was different from the milder emotion associated with a gradual change in temperature. Further, it was also found that the hormones released for different stressors were different. Certain stressful experience elicited adrenaline, nor-adrenaline and cortisol, while others released only two hormones. Studies indicated that a strong emotion triggered by a stress elicited three hormones in large amount. Thus, the physiological response was found to be associated with the severity of stress and the intensity of emotional reaction. Thus, the 'non-specificity' clause is disproved. Chrousos and Gold (1992) introduced modifications to Selye's doctrine of non-specificity. They proposed that the non-specific response applies to stressors that surpass a certain threshold level. Beyond this threshold, any stress elicits the syndrome universally. Stress cannot limit its explanation to physiological response. It is not a simple and direct relation between the stimulus (stressor) and a response (physiological changes).

A very significant factor called the 'organism' or the 'individual' is ignored in the model. This individual is a phenomenon with cognition, affect and behaviour. Cognition plays a vital role in determining the severity of stress. The degree of stress is determined based on the attribution the individual assigns to the situation. Two individuals may perceive the same situation with different intensity of stress.

The intensity of emotional reactions varies with the cognitive appraisal. Studies proved that the amount of hormonal secretion and physiological response depends upon the emotional reaction. Thus, the model seems to have underplayed or ignored a very significant psychological component called emotion in stress experience.

Thus, Selye's theory of GAS, though was tested and validated by many researchers, remains incomplete without taking the salient psychological components of cognition and emotion into consideration.

One significant aspect of GAS, which was universally accepted, is that prolonged exposure to stress impacts the health of the person due to the biochemical and physiological reactions and the wear and tear of various systems involved in the resistance and adaptation process.

Contemporary Physiological Model: Allostatic Load Theory

McEwen and Stellar (1993) picking up from Selye's model further expanded the phenomenon of the impact of stress on health and the resultant illnesses after prolonged exposure to stress. Their model helped in understanding the process of stress causing an illness. McEwen and Stellar (1993) coined the term 'allostasis', which means 'maintaining stability or homeostasis through change'. Allostasis is a process of adaptation to acute stress by releasing stress hormones in the body in the event of challenge with a goal of restoring homeostasis. In the words of McEwen (2005), "Allostasis refers to the adaptive processes that maintain homeostasis through the production of mediators such as adrenalin, cortisol and other chemical messengers".

The concept of allostasis is better explained with reference to the concept of 'homeostasis'. Homeostasis is defined as the tendency of a system, especially the physiological system to maintain internal stability, owing to coordinated response of its parts to any situation or stimulus that would tend to disturb its normal condition or function. Allostasis is the process that helps maintain homeostasis through the mediators such as HPA axis, autonomic nervous system, cardiovascular, metabolic and immune system. These mediators are known to be useful in promoting adaptation in post-acute stress. This is allostasis. However, if these systems are activated for a prolonged period, or repeatedly, one would experience allostatic load. Allostatic load is characterized by release of excess stress hormones, immune cells, and enhanced brain activity and cardiovascular response. A person who experiences allostatic load for a prolonged period is said to be at risk of developing disease because the allostatic load causes a drop in the effective functioning of the systems in the body.

To explain it further, normally when one encounters an acute stress, the allostasis through the mediating biochemical and physiological responses help one encounter the stress. This results in a number of bodily changes like increased heartbeat, breathing, sweating, blood pressure, blood sugar level. Once the stressful situation is passed, the allostatic response is shut off. In case the allostatic response fails to shut off because the stress situation continues, the body systems experience excessive pressure and subject themselves to wear and tear. According to McEwen, four situations are likely to give such allostatic load:

1 Multiple stressors hitting the person repeatedly
2 Lack of adaptation
3 Prolonged response
4 Inadequate response

Stress as a Stimulus—Engineering Model

If you remember the initial questions—related to your personal stress experience, there was a question related to 'who or what' is responsible for your stress. There are individuals who would identify an event, a situation or another person as the cause of their stress. In fact, they point out a 'stressor'. Researchers have been studying stress as an event or situation targeting a person, who responds to this situation. This approach is called 'stimulus' approach to stress. Research in this field studied stress as a major life event or the minor daily hassles.

Stress as a Stimulus—Life Events

Life events model of stress was put forth by two researchers, Holmes and Rahe (1967). The idea of their approach was that major life events whether positive or negative call for a change. These changes demand adjustments from the individual. Any adjustment to change is stressful because they disturb the set pattern of behaviour. Hence, stress refers to the degree and number of adjustments one has to make within a period of time in life. Holmes and Rahe (1967) intensively studied the major life events, the amount of stress each one produces, and standardized a scale called 'Social Readjustment Rating Scale' (SRRS). The scale is reproduced in Table 7.1.

Life events model of stress was easy to understand and simple to quantify and predict health risk. This was widely used by researchers. Hobson et al. (1998) revised the scale thoroughly and listed 51 items. Hobson and Delunas (2001) who used the scale on a large sample reiterated the scale's value as a diagnostic tool in identifying individuals at risk for health problems based on the scores.

With improved methodology, many longitudinal studies were conducted. The results were inconsistent.

Table 7.1 Social Readjustment Rating Scale (SRRS)

Rank	Life event	Mean value
1	Death of spouse	100
2	Divorce	73
3	Marital separation	65
4	Jail term	63
5	Death of close family member	63
6	Personal injury or illness	53
7	Marriage	50
8	Fired at work	47
9	Marital reconciliation	45
10	Retirement	45
11	Change in health of family member	44
12	Pregnancy	40
13	Sex difficulties	39
14	Gain of new family member	39
15	Business readjustment	39
16	Change in financial state	38
17	Death of close friend	37
18	Change to different line of work	36
19	Change in number of arguments with spouse	35
20	Mortgage over $10,000	31
21	Fore closer of mortgage or loan	30
22	Change in responsibilities at work	29
23	Son or daughter leaving home	29
24	Trouble with in-laws	29
25	Outstanding personal achievement	28
26	Wife begin or stop work	26
27	Begin or end school	26
28	Change in living conditions	25
29	Revision of personal habits	24
30	Trouble with boss	23
31	Change in work hours or conditions	20
32	Change in residence	20
33	Change in schools	20
34	Change in recreations	19
35	Change in church activities	19
36	Change in social activities	18
37	Mortgage or loan less than $10,000	17
38	Change in sleeping habits	16
39	Change in number of family get-togethers	15
40	Change in eating habits	15
41	Vacation	13
42	Christmas	12
43	Minor violation of the law	11

Source: Holmes and Rahe (1967). The Social Readjustment Rating Scale.

Criticism

1 The life events model ignores the role of organism. The individual in this model is conceptualized as a passive recipient of the stress from outside, and open and vulnerable, and takes the impact of it in the form of health risk or disease. This in fact is not true.

2 The model advocates that the life change units (LCU) for every event hold good for all individuals. In other words, the impact of adjustment is the same for all. This assumption can be challenged on the ground that each individual is unique in his/her cognition, personality,

past experience, emotional intelligence, apart from internal and external resources that help in coping.
3 The model is criticized severely on the basis of the scale that assumed prominence in quantifying stress and predicting illness. Life events model places equal value to all life events irrespective of their desirability. The assumption that all these events are quantified as units of stress in same direction ignores the residual affect states of these events as distress or positive stress.
4 The critics pointed out a number of items in the SRRS for their ambiguity. For example, change in financial status could mean both an improvement in status and depletion. Similarly, the change in responsibility at work may either be a burden or be a relief for a person determined by a number of internal and external factors.

Thus, the life events model was a good model that attributed psychosocial significant to the phenomenon of stress, which, until then, was viewed and studied only as a physiological process. However, it had some significant inherent limitations.

Daily Hassles

All of us experience minor, moderate and severe irritants on a daily basis: a cranky child at home, a nagging spouse or a demanding boss, disruption in water supply or electricity, delay in supply of gas cylinder, missing a bus, getting caught in traffic jam, misplacing important documents and so on. The list of it can fill hundreds of pages of this book. They are called daily hassles. These incidents are common and frequent in life. While major life events have the power of drawing good social support, the daily hassles do not attract significant social support. The impact of these daily hassles is cumulative in nature.

Lazarus and his colleagues argued that encountering these day-to-day unpleasant events has the potential to harm one's health and wellbeing. Kanner, Coyne, Schaefer and Lazarus (1981) developed an instrument that listed events such as 'not enough money for food', 'concerns about weight', 'concern about health of a family member'. The respondents had to tick those hassles they experienced in the past month and rated them on the perceived severity. They develop another scale called 'Uplift Scale' that consisted of items related to joy, peace or satisfaction. The purpose was to see whether 'uplift' experiences could mellow down the impact of hassles.

The basic flaw was the assumption of the individual's role as passive. The stimulus approach of stress almost negates the involvement of the individual's personal factors like cognition, past experience and personality disposition before responding to a stressful stimulus. Lazarus (1966) filled these with a more comprehensive theory.

Transactional Theory of Stress

The transactional theory of Lazarus is compete in the sense that it includes the response approach of the physiological changes, and the stimulus approach of stressors experienced through major life events and daily hassles. In addition, it explains the involvement of cognitive appraisal and the resultant coping behaviour to mitigate the stressful situation. According to Lazarus, stress is not the sole handiwork of either the environment or the individual, but it is in fact the transaction between the individual and the environment.

When the individual comes face to face with a stressful event or a situation, he/she makes a cognitive appraisal of the situation. To assess whether the situation involves a loss, threat or challenge, a number of factors influence the person and determine the overall situation. For example, when a family member is diagnosed with cancer and the medical advice is to go for immediate surgery followed by chemotherapy and radiation, the situation is highly stressful and invokes strong emotions and concomitant physiological arousal. However, the individual cannot remain passive. There is a need to decide on future course of action in terms of treatment. Here, the person first takes a cognitive appraisal about the disease, the stage in which the patient is (assessment of loss) and the prognosis of it following the treatment (assessment of threat). Once it is known that the patient is in initial stages (minimum loss) and the prognosis will be good provided the treatment is initiated immediately (potential threat is losing time), the individual makes an assessment of his/her resources—in terms of finances, and social support to manage hospitalization and post-surgery care, emotional support to the patient etc. When the person perceives that the resources can be managed with some effort, he/she perceives the situation as a challenge. On the contrary, if the person appraises that all the financial resources are dry and there is hardly any social support available and he/she himself/herself is shattered with the diagnosis and cannot think of managing the situation, there is perception of loss and threat, which increases the stress experience. Thus, the transactional model places a lot of emphasis on the cognitive appraisal.

The role of cognitive appraisal can be explained with a magical triangle.

Cognitive appraisal is central to the presence or absence of stress. Figure 7.4 depicts the triangle at the centre as cognitive appraisal. Stress is presented to the person as an event or situation characterized with a change, time line, ambiguity, conflict or criticism. None of these per se can be labelled as stressful. These situations /events as presented to the individual are subjected to cognitive appraisal. The process of cognitive appraisal takes into consideration the personal stakes involved in the demanding situation; resources available to meet these demands and locus of control. Based on this, the person moves either to the top triangle of eustress (positive stress) or to the right triangle (distress). The experience of emotions associated with distress, such as

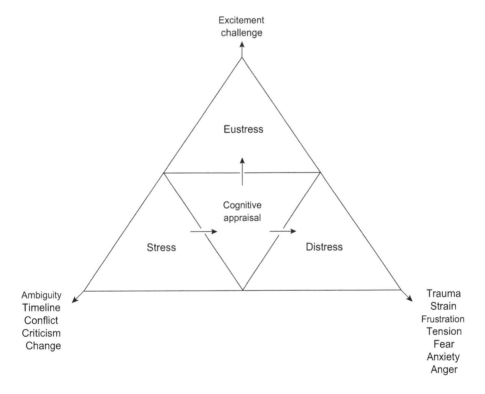

Figure 7.4 Cognitive Appraisal of Stress.

anxiety, fear, anger, trauma, is the consequence of an interpretation of an event as a threat, while the emotional reactions of excitement, and thrill are the consequences of perception of challenge by cognitive appraisal.

Primary Appraisal

Lazarus and Folkman (1984) explained that when individual confronts a new stressful situation, they operate what is called 'primary appraisal'. This evaluates whether the situation poses any danger to the person or block to any of the goals. The danger or block is assessed in terms of 'harm' (a loss or damage already occurred) or threat (having the potential to cause damage in future). Primary appraisal of the situation as threat or harm has a significant role in triggering the physiological responses and emotional distress. For example, a student while filling an online application for an attractive job realizes after pressing the 'send' button that the attachments enclosed to the application were wrong documents. To the question if this situation is harmful, the answer is 'yes' because in the absence of right attachments, the application would be rendered invalid. This triggers a perception of threat and emotional distress.

Secondary Appraisal

Simultaneously when the primary appraisal process is on, the secondary appraisal also is initiated. Secondary appraisal refers to the individual's assessment of one's own coping abilities based on the resources available. Resources refers to internal resources such as abilities, self-efficacy, determination, self-esteem, and external resources such as financial backup, material resources, social support network. Figure 7.5 depicts the process of cognitive appraisal and coping with stressful condition (Hariharan & Rath, 2008). When the individual endorses the presence of a danger to self or block to the goal in primary appraisal, and also endorses the non-availability of resources in the secondary appraisal, there is a clear threat perception.

This is accompanied by emotional ventilation in an attempt to adapt to the situation. On the contrary, when the primary appraisal acknowledges the presence of an immediate or potential danger, and also the availability of internal and external resources to adequately handle the stressor, then the individual is likely to perceive a challenge and experience thrill and excitement. The follow-up will be an attempt to cope with the situation successfully. Successful coping is that which results in minimizing or mitigating the stressor. If that happens, the stressful event gets terminated. On the contrary, if the attempts at coping fail to minimize the stress, then the process of appraisal starts all over again and the attempts are directed at reinterpretation of the stressful condition.

Cognitive responses to stress include one's beliefs about threat or harm, their causes and the extent of one's control over their occurrence or mitigation. Cognitive response to stress (particularly on perception of threat or harm) also includes problems in holding attention and concentration, disruption and distraction in performance of a cognitive task. Emotional response to stress includes any one or combination of a wide spectrum of emotions such as fear, anxiety, anger, frustration, excitement. Behavioural response to stress broadly triggers adaptation or coping. Adaptation refers to the individual's attempts to adjust to the situation by bringing in the necessary changes in self.

Thus, the transactional model of stress places significant emphasis on the organism or the individual and the cognitive, affective and behavioural dimensions of the individual. Rather than viewing stress just as a stimulus (stressor) or a response (physiological response), Lazarus' transactional model highlights the dynamic transaction between the environment and the individual.

Stress and Illness 253

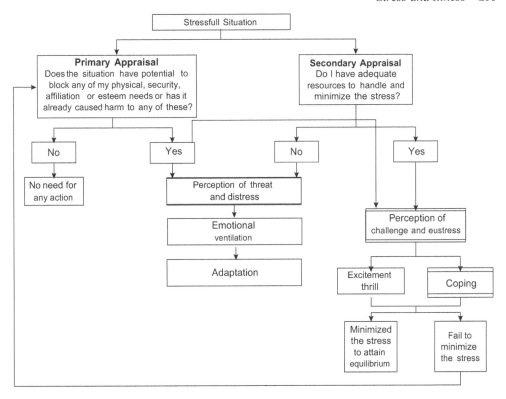

Figure 7.5 Cognitive Appraisal and Coping Process in Stress.

Box 7.1   Summary of Stress Theories

S. No.	Name of the theory	Proponent(s)	Salient features
1	Fight-or-flight	Walter Cannon (1932)	• Explains stress as a response • The individual perceives the stress • Sympathetic adrenomedullary system activates and secretes adrenaline and noradrenaline • Body goes into the arousal state and mobilizes additional energy • The person uses this additional energy whether to fight the stressor or flee from the situation
2	General Adaptation Syndrome	Hans Selye (1956, 1976, 1985)	• Response model • Physiological arousal on sighting stress • Stress response passes three stages, viz. alarm, resistance and exhaustion • Physiological arousal peaks during the alarm stage • Slight drop in physiological arousal but still above normal in resistance stage • Exhausts all resources, and energy is depleted if the stage continues. The result is acute health problem or death

(Continued)

S. No.	Name of the theory	Proponent(s)	Salient features
3	Major life events		• Stimulus model of stress • Major life events demand gross adjustments • The demand for adjustment is stressful • Stress causes illness • Every life event, positive or negative, has a potential to create stress • Stress induced by major life events is measurable in terms of life change units • Life change unit scores within a time frame can predict the health of the individual
4	Allostatic model of stress	Mc Ewen (1993)	• Response model • The physiological arousal in response to stress is useful in maintaining homeostasis. This is allostasis • If the physiological arousal does not shut off in time, it creates allostatic load • Continuation of allostasis results in overfunctioning and prolonged functioning of vital systems in body • The outcome of this allostatic load is wear and tear to the systems and illness
5	Transactional model	Lazarus and Folkman (1984)	• Apart from environment and physiological response, it is the transaction between the person and environment that is important • Cognitive appraisal of the stressors by the person decides whether there is stress or not • Primary and secondary appraisals determine the presence of loss threat, harm or challenge • The behavioural response in the form of coping, emotional response and cognitive response are explained in detail

Sources of Stress

Imagine a situation where you are experiencing stress after you have appeared in an examination. There are two broad possibilities for your stress. It may be because the question paper was very tough, or because you did not perform as good as you wanted to. The first reason relates your stress to an external source called the question paper, while the second reason cites an internal source of your 'expectation'. The sources of stress can be broadly classified into internal and external sources. We will discuss this source in detail.

Internal Sources

On a number of occasions, the source of stress is within the person. At the physical level, it could be an acute or chronic illness and the pain it causes. Physical illness has its psychosocial impact as it places significant demands on the person depending on the age, gender, social, professional obligations, personality disposition and health belief system.

It is observed that ageing and failing health have an association. Older people tend to have more health problems. Their perception of illness is found to be more stressful compared to the younger age group. Some of the reasons could their low self-efficacy, fear of disability, fear of death and low perceived support, besides the objective assessment of progressive decline in the speed of recovery. In a population-based Swedish study on non-dementia adults between the age groups of 66–97 years, Osmanovic-Thunström, Mossello, Åkerstedt, Fratiglioni and Wang (2015) found that perceived stress was associated with health-related stress. The results showed a significant relation between perceived health-related stress and age.

Higher stress perception among women was found in a study on patients suffering from atrial fibrillation. This refers to a cardiac condition with the symptom of an irregular and rapid heart rate, which causes poor blood flow in the person. Trovato, Pace, Cangemi, Martines, Trovato and Catalano (2012) studied 88 patients with atrial fibrillation. They measured psychological stress, illness perception, self-efficacy, hospital anxiety and depression in the subjects. The results examined the relationship of all the studied parameters with perceived stress. It was found that perceived stress was associated with gender, age, anxiety and depression. Women and older people perceived higher stress levels. Anxiety and illness perception explained 92.2% of variance in perceived stress. However, higher self-efficacy and adherence to diet were associated with lower hazards of perceived stress.

Thus, the internal source of stress is a complex phenomenon. A number of psychosocial factors interact among themselves and physical illness in determining the stress levels. Thus, while physical illness may be named as the major internal source of stress, given the mind-body relation all the other psychological factors play a significant role too.

Another source of stress from within the individual is internal conflict. It could be a conflict of aspiration and self-efficacy. When one's goals and aspiration are high but the individual has low self-efficacy, there is likelihood of experiencing high stress levels. Similarly, one may face a conflict between personal values. This normally happens in transition phases when an individual having one set of family values has to assimilate a new set of values that guide the institution or the culture.

This type of internal stress is something that is often resolved once the decision is made. However, the stress originates from low self-esteem, self-efficacy or inferior feelings may turn chronic, and has a negative impact on performance, health and wellbeing creating a vicious circle. Hence, it is advisable to seek professional help in such cases.

External Sources: This can also be termed as environmental stress. External sources of stress can be broadly classified into four, as depicted in Figure 7.6.

Family Environment: Ironically, while family is considered as a major source of support, it also is a major source of stress, particularly in the Indian culture. The logic is simple. Indian culture is highly affiliation-oriented (Hariharan & Rath, 2008). Marriage and family are considered strong institutions that presume lifelong affiliation. The cultural practices are such that the interpersonal attachments develop and strengthen with time. The bonding between the family members constitutes the basis for support and also mutual expectations. Failure in meeting the expectations is one of the major sources of interpersonal stress in the family. Similarly, when the children start growing into adolescents and come under the major peer influence and pressure, there may be a perceived variation between the family values and that of children. Illness and suffering by any family member either acute or chronic induce stress not only in the person concerned but also in others who have to become caretakers and support system. The physical strain, emotional experience, anxiety and concern drain them out, thus causing significant stress.

All major life events in life of any family member are a source of stress for the entire family.

Social Environment: Inequalities in the society create an environment that is a major stress for a number of people. In a diverse society like India, inequality is seen in multiple dimensions. Economic inequalities in society create various layers among people. More the distance in

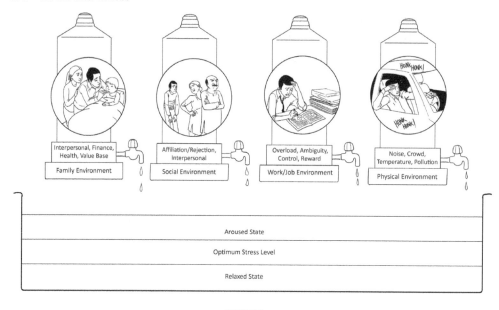

Figure 7.6 Sources of Stress.

layers, higher is the possibility of stress in interaction between the two groups. Gender inequality is yet another source of stress in social institutions such as workplace, political and religious places. There is a constant conflict arising out of fight for equality and fight against exploitation and oppression of women in society. Diversity in religion and caste is one of the politically created sources of stress in Indian society.

The other social inequalities giving rise to stress include discrimination due to skin colour, levels of education, occupational status, physical disabilities and scholastic achievement to name a few. Workplace, though constitutes a part of social environment, deserves discussion under a separate head owing to the multidimensionality.

Work Environment: According to WHO (1986), a healthy working environment is one in which there is not only an absence of harmful condition, but an abundance of health-promoting ones. Going by this, a number of organizations, particularly the multinational companies, have successfully designed their physical environment that includes a number of facilities that fulfil their need for food, physical exercise and relaxation. However, workplace stress originates from many other sources. The sources can be broadly explained under the following contexts:

- A mismatch between the work demands and pressures and personal knowledge, abilities, skills and competence
- Absence or very little control over the workplace
- Absence of support from the supervisors and colleagues
- Lack of clarity in the work one has to execute, the method to be followed, people to be involved and their hierarchical position (often known as 'role ambiguity')
- The work efficiency and output are not matched with recognition

It is necessary to distinguish between work pressure and work stress. Pressure at work in the moderate level is positive and functions as a propeller. It is considered a motivator. However, when the pressure is excessive and surpasses the capacity of the individual to handle, one experiences stress. Workplace stress can be discussed under two broad sources, viz. work content and work context.

Work Content: The meaningfulness attributed to a job one executes has a large influence on the satisfaction one derives from the work. For example, a farmer who toils in the field understands the purpose, process and the product for which he/she has been working. Therefore, the clarity of goal and the anticipation of antecedents to attain the goal in terms of amount of work, time lines and the intermittent signals of the success or failure of his/her efforts sustain the motivation until completion of the job and result in satisfaction if the outcome is positive. In contrast, an employee in an IT company recruited in a huge project is assigned a fragment of work from the huge project about which he may not have much comprehension. A number of teams work on the huge project, each team responsible for a fraction of the job. Only people coordinating the job of various teams positioned at higher levels in the hierarchy may have a comprehension of the project as a whole. The others at bottom levels of hierarchy find it difficult to perceive their role as meaningful. They just work against the time lines and the quantum of work to be completed. They may get stressed because of monotony, meaninglessness and heavy pressure.

While one understands the stress due to too much work, having too little work is equally stressful. When junior employees, in various IT sectors, are made to 'sit on the bench' due to lack of new projects, they suffer stress not only due to boredom but also because it lowers their self-esteem.

Working hours is yet another source of stress. Large population of Indian youth working in multinational companies and IT sector have odd timings. If these timings are not constant and they need to work in various shifts, the disturbance in the circadian system further adds to their stress. Apart from odd hours and shift in working hours, long hours of work are also stressful. Very often, executive-level employees shouldering the responsibility of project completion and coordination at various levels find themselves stretching their work for long hours. Fatigue, frustration and anxiety result from both the extended time and the type of job.

Very often, those working at the middle level in the hierarchy feel the stress because while they are assigned the responsibility of task completion, they are not empowered to control the situation. Lack of control and no participation in decision-making with regard to the method, pace and timings of work create stress. For example, the work hours of junior doctors is decided by a superior. The junior doctors in charge of the ward in the absence of the consultant have the responsibility of taking care of the patients but cannot take any major decision on the treatment process in the face of any exigency without consulting the senior consultant.

Work Context: This refers to the socioeconopolitical context in which one has to work. There is a sociopolitical factor and an economic factor or a combination of both that induces stress.

The sociopolitical context includes opportunities for developing career, and growth in the profession. Lack of promotions, unfair performance evaluation system and ambiguity in job roles give rise to stressful experience. Interpersonal relationships with colleagues, superiors and subordinates have a significant bearing on the stress levels of any employee.

Yet, another universal factor related to work context is the work-life balance. A person who is unable to organize his/her time, emotions and energy that is distributed between the work and home feels stymied. Career and work is only one dimension of life.

The ongoing progressive stress experienced by an employee due to responsibilities, working conditions, environment and pressures at workplace is normally termed as occupational stress. Occupational stress is not only detrimental to the health and wellbeing of the employee but also harms the organization. At a personal level, occupational stress results in accelerated ageing, illness and interpersonal problems outside the workplace.

Three contemporary studies related to workplace stress are discussed below. The causes of work stress were investigated in a sample of 51 employees from public, private and NGOs through interviews by Bhui, Dinos, Galant--Mieczniowska, de Jhong and Stansfeld (2016). The results found that the major causes of stress at work were adverse working conditions and management practices.

In a study on employees of Tehran University in Iran, Keshavarz and Mohammadi (2011) found the association between occupational stress and organizational performance. The results found an association between the work stress and the health condition of the employees on the one hand and a negative impact of it and their job satisfaction, commitment to work and performance at large on the other.

Hariharan, Prasad and Swain (2010) studied the stress and coping among the Indian pilots flying the commercial passenger flights. They included a sample of 122 pilots from four airlines that were managed by Government of India and private airlines.

The results showed a high level of occupational stress in the senior pilots, compared to those lower in hierarchy. Stress levels of pilots varied along the airlines they were affiliated to. This indicated that some airlines induced more stress. Coping styles varied with levels of stress. Majority of pilots showed a rigid coping style.

It is very evident that across the globe, the stressors related to work environment are by and large the same. Lack of human touch, objectivity in performance evaluation, fair treatment to employees and workload to match the ability of the employee are some simple measures to minimize the stress in them. This measure is beneficial to the organizations since it reflects on the increased productivity of the organization.

Physical Environment

As a student of psychology, you may have carried out several community-based projects. In case you have you can recall your experience in the following conditions, if not, you can just imagine the experience of being in such condition.

Environmental stress refers to the way humans and animals respond to the physical, chemical and biological features of environment, which are hazardous to health and wellbeing. It includes exposure to natural disasters, electromagnetic radiation, extreme climates, pollution in the air, water and food, noise and overcrowding in the place of living. Few types of environmental stress are discussed below. It is important to be mentioned that it is not an exhaustive list.

Natural Disaster

Natural disasters such as earthquake, tsunami, cyclone, floods or draught have a severe impact on those whose geographical proximity is closer to the disaster-prone area. The stress experienced in natural disaster is two-fold. The initial stress response to such intense disaster may be physiological that may be labelled as 'fight-or-flight' response. However, the long-term impact may be one of post-traumatic stress disorder (PTSD). Months and years after the disasters when the social and the political support is no more continuing, the people impacted by the disasters are found still handling their stress and rebuilding the natural loss and coping with the loss of their close family member or friends. People orphaned in the tsunami decades ago, and the victims of the great earthquake in Latur, and of super-cyclone in Orissa are still coping with their residual stress of loss of lives and property.

Climate Stress

Climate stressors constitute one of the major sources of environmental stress suffered across the globe. They are typically long-term stressors. The striking feature here is the absence of control by the individual, who is forced to adapt to the climate condition whether extreme heat or cold. In a classic study, Obradovich, Migliorini, Paulus and Rahwan (2018) established the relationship between climate change and mental health. The sample constituted two million residents of the US. They obtained the data of daily meteorological information for a decade between the years 2002 and 2012. This was combined with the data of nearly two million residents on the reported mental health difficulties. The results indicated that a change in temperature between 25°C and 30°C and above was clearly associated with difficulties in mental health aspect by 0.5% point. Further, more alarming is the finding of the study that 1°C of five-year warming associates with 2% point increase in prevalence of mental health problems. It also found that Hurricane Katrina was associated with an increase of 4% point in problems related to mental health. Their study inferred that stress due to climate change poses a serious threat to mental health.

Chemical Stress

We are exposed to chemicals in our natural home and working environment. The chemicals and pesticides used in food products, the daily use of disinfectants and cosmetic items do have chemical components in them. However, the toxic filtration that is done by the liver and kidney shields us from the impact of it. Yet, when the exposure to chemical inhalation, consumption and contact with skin crosses the capacity of liver and kidney's filtration, it impacts our health and wellbeing. One of the main entry points of chemical toxins entering the body is polluted air. A number of studies reiterated the association between air pollution and stress levels. In a significant study, Li et al. (2017) examined the health effects of air particulate matter (PM) less than 2.5 μm in diameter inhaled from industrial sources. The study was conducted on 55 healthy student volunteers. The results of blood and urine tests revealed that the participants who were exposed to PM had high levels of stress hormones such as cortisol, adrenaline and noradrenaline indicating a raised stress level. Apart from this, the levels of blood pressure were also found high among the participants.

Anthropogenic Stress

This refers to the stressors such as crowding and noise. People living in natural environmental setting close to railway track, airports or close to the heavy automobile traffic roads are exposed to the noise pollution. Research has continuously proved the stressful consequences of noise pollution. Westman and Walters (1981) provided a logical explanation to the association between noise and stress. According to them, the purpose of hearing is to alert and warn the person. Thus, sound has the potential to evoke emotions directly, leading to actions such as fight-or-flight. In such responses, the stimuli are translated into action with their concomitant physiological changes indicating stress.

WHO (2018) stated that noise pollution is one of the top environmental hazards impacting physical and mental wellbeing, particularly in the European region. Recent studies indicated that noise pollution, apart from causing hearing impairments, also has an impact on cardiac health, causing hypertension and ischaemic heart diseases, invokes negative emotions as annoyance and causes sleep disturbances (Münzel et al., 2018; Kerns et al., 2018).

Crowding is yet another source of environmental stress. At a global level, particularly in countries like India and China facing the consequences of population explosion and increasing density is a major cause of stress at the national level. Apart from the direct impact on individual's health and wellbeing, the harm it causes to the biodiversity is the major concern of environmentalists. As students of psychology, while we totally endorse the global concerns, we will examine the impact of crowding on stress.

Most of the studies on the association between crowding and stress have been conducted on rats. In one study by Lin et al. (2015), two groups of rats were studied—one exposed to social crowding (by placing eight rats in a standard cage) and the other constituting the control group (by placing four rats in a standard cage). The impact of crowding on affective behaviour and metabolic system was studied. Results revealed that the rats in the experimental group manifested modest anxiety-like behaviour. Metabolic changes included increased adiposity or fat deposits, and significant elevation in serum leptin.

Crowding stress casts a negative impact on health and emotional states of human beings also. Scientific research on human subjects is few in this field for two reasons. First, research ethics prevents experimental design on human subjects. Studies on natural settings have too many psychosocial confounding variables making it difficult to isolate the impact of crowding. Nevertheless, one can recall one's own experience of stress after being in a crowd or having to execute a work in a crowded environment. You might have experienced crowding stress interfering with the work efficiency, cognitive functioning and emotional state. The productivity is very likely to be suboptimal, and the emotional state is likely to be negative. When the exposure to crowding is temporary, the impact is short term. However, prolonged exposure to crowding results in slow and chronic stress.

Energetic Stress

This is technology-related stress. There are a number of electromagnetic radiations that are passed on the earth. They emit ionizing and non-ionizing radiation. The ionizing radiation originates from ultraviolet and X-rays and gamma rays, while the non-ionizing rays emit from microwaves, radio-frequency waves etc. Non-ionizing rays are found to be relatively safer, while ionizing rays are found to cause damage to the cells and DNA. The outcome of this is said to be 'geopathic stress'. This is relatively a new terminology. It can be defined as the study of earth energies and their effect on human wellbeing. The best way to cope with geopathic stress is to have intermittent technology holiday in a day when one has to switch off the mobile phones, computers, laptops and television sets and expose oneself either to a social environment or to a natural environment.

Ergonomic Stress

This refers to the stress induced by the efforts of the individual to fit oneself to the designs of man-made objects. Very often, the term is used in the context of workplace, referring to the work stations, the furniture, keyboard and computer screens, mouse etc. Ergonomic stress is the outcome of the stress experienced by the body due to prolonged hours of sitting or standing position at work, positioning oneself in a bad posture, restricting oneself to a limited physical space etc. Efforts put in to adapt oneself to the space and the ill-designed objects result in heavy stress at the physical and psychological level after long exposure. Very often, employees who have to work on the computers for long hours are found to experience chronic stress of this nature.

Though the sources of stress are discussed under different heads, they are not mutually exclusive. A stress from one source may also be connected to the stress from another source (e.g. physical illness is closely related to the problems of managing finances for the treatment). An individual accumulates stress from various sources. As described in Figure 7.6 as long as the total volume of stress is within the limit, it functions as a motivator. When it crosses the limit, it casts a negative impact on health and wellbeing. The outcome of stress accumulates from multiple sources can be explained with the analogy of a fuel tank in a car. Fuel is an essential ingredient to start the car and keep it moving. If the fuel level touches the rock bottom, the car fails to start. On the contrary, if the fuel overflows the tank capacity and the car continues to run, there is a risk of the car catching a fire. Stress is a very essential component to create and sustain the motivation of the individual to work. If there is no stress, the individual feels no motivation to do any work and still suffers from what is called 'boredom stress'. On the contrary, if there is excess accumulation of stress from single or multiple sources the individual may reach and remain in arousal state for long period, which is highly stressful and detrimental to one's health and wellbeing.

Optimum Stress Level (OSL)

Optimum stress level (OSL) is that degree of stress with which an individual is able to work happily and optimally (Hariharan & Rath, 2008). It relates to a condition where one is 'adequately stressed to be productive'. We have already discussed that the total absence of stress from any source leads to boredom. It can even be construed as only a concept that is hard to find in reality. We have also discussed that if the stress levels are very high, it is hazardous for the individual, rendering one ineffective in normal functioning. There comes the question of what is that 'desirable' level of stress that allows the individual to optimize the productivity? The answer to this is not that simple. While discussing the theories of stress, we endorsed that the cognitive appraisal of the situation plays a significant and determining role in the experience of stress. Here is where the individual differences come into picture. Cognitive appraisal is influenced by a number of factors such as age, gender, culture, past experience, available resources and a hoard of factors related to personality. There is some variance in the threshold level of stress among population. Further, this threshold level is dynamic in the same individual across time line. Taking into consideration all these factors, the optimum threshold level (OSL) is construed as a zone rather than a line that is known as stress threshold level (STL). Figure 7.7 depicts the OSL zone for an individual. When the stress levels are within the limits of this conceptual zone, one is expected to function optimally.

When one is found below this level, he/she is expected to be in a relaxed state. If the stress level shoots beyond the OSL, one goes into the arousal zone. Normally, during the life time, a person shifts to each of these positions. However, the effort of the person should be to optimize the time in the OSL zone. Staying in either above (arousal) or below (relaxed), the OSL for a prolonged period will be detrimental to one's health and wellbeing. Further, when one finds oneself in an arousal zone for a considerable period (normally trying to meet the time line in a job or due to sudden loss of a loved person), one needs to make conscious efforts to come down to a relaxed zone (by taking a short break or engaging in a hobby) to counterbalance the negative impact of the prolonged period in an arousal zone.

One can determine one's OSL by maintaining dairies for specific time periods of one month, six months or a year. Do you want to measure your OSL zone? Then respond to the exercise explained in Box 7.2.

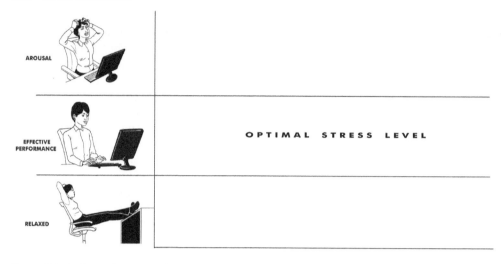

Figure 7.7 Optimum Stress Level (OSL).

Box 7.2   Know Your OSL

- Maintain a daily dairy of your significant events and activities and record the associated affect/emotion/feelings with each of these. Alternatively, you can recall the significant activities and events and the associated affect/feeling/emotion.
- Also record your performance at work, home and society during this period.
- Identify those events and activities where the associated affect/feeling/emotion was negative.
- Rate each of the emotions on a 10-point scale of stress that ranges from 'stressful = 1 to extremely stressful = 10'.
- Now, identify your performance in the corresponding periods. Rate each of this performance satisfaction/productivity on a 10-point scale of 'Not at all productive = 1 to extremely productive = 10'.
- Plot your stress scores for the time period, e.g. one year/one month as shown in the figure.
- Plot your corresponding scores of performances.
- Identify points of your highest performance.
- Look at your stress scores corresponding to them.
- The range between the stress scores that correspond to high performance constitutes your OSL.

Measuring Stress

Measurement of stress closely corroborates with the way stress is conceptualized. When stress is construed as a response, the method of measurement is physiological and biochemical changes using machines or chemical analysis of body fluids such as blood and urine. When stress is studied from the perspective of stimulus (stressors), the method used for measuring is standardized scales that call for objective identification of stressful life events demanding adjustments. When the study of stress focuses on cognitive appraisal of the event /situation, the method requires the use of standardized scales that involve subjective rating of the major stressful events or daily hassle or a combination of both. Each method has its own strengths and limitations.

Physiological Measure

There are two distinct and objective methods of recording physiological measures of arousal state that indicates stress.

Electrical and Mechanical Equipment

The sympathetic nervous system results in the activation of vital functioning leading the individual to a physiological state of arousal. The physiological arousal results in the increase in blood pressure, respiration and galvanic skin response (GSR). They are considered the prominent indices. One has the option of even choosing the equipment with a single parameter and measuring it in the individual. This equipment is available in a compact form to facilitate recording of the physiological changes in 24 hours so that the time of arousal states during the day is specific. They can be matched with the activities, emotional reactions, coinciding with arousal states. Alternatively, all the parameters can also be studied by using single equipment that records variations in all the parameters. This is called polygraph that indicates changes in respiration, GSR and blood pressure.

Biochemical Analysis

While the physiological arousal to stress due to the response of the sympathetic nervous system is measured by electrical and mechanical equipment, the biochemical changes due to endocrinal response to stress are measured by biochemical analysis. Due to the endocrine response to stress, the two hormones released into the blood stream are corticosteroids and catecholamines. Cortisol is the most important corticosteroid, while adrenaline and noradrenaline belong to the class of catecholamines. Sample of blood and urine indicates the levels of these chemicals in the body. The procedure of collecting blood and urine samples is simple. They are subjected to analysis in a pathology laboratory by a qualified technician.

These measures of stress are said to be objective and accurate. However, certain issues of these measures are debatable. For example, there may be other 'non-stress' reasons for changes in the heart rate, respiration or GSR. For some subjects, the very act of placing a sensor in some part of the body itself may cause anxiety and thereby an increase in heart rate, respiration and GSR. Further, the use of the equipment, and miniature forms of them involves considerable expenditure. The additional factor is the inconvenience caused to the subject in drawing blood, though minor factors need a mention here.

Psychological Scales

LIFE EVENTS

Measuring psychosocial parameters by using standardized scales is an accepted method in the field of psychology. The objectivity of quantification is optimized by the standardization procedure of the scale. This method of measurement is appropriate when stress is viewed as a stimulus. The first-ever attempt to measure stress from the psychosocial perspective was made by

Holmes and Rahe (1967). Following the steps in a standardization procedure, they constructed Social Readjustment Rating Scale (SRRS). The scale measures the stress units of various major life events, where death of a spouse measures the highest with 100 units. The participants are required to follow recall method and tick those major life events they encountered in the past year. The stress units are totalled indicating their level of stress. They correlated this measure of stress with the health status.

This method has the advantage of its simplicity in administration and measurement. The objectivity of the measure is optimized by including a wide range of life events such as stressors, which cover the experience of all adult age groups. Sarafino (1994a) reported that on administration of scale in a sample of 2800 adults, only 15% reported that they experienced none of the events listed in the scale. The items in the scale are well discriminated. However, the major weakness of the scale is the recall method it adopts. Further, certain items such as 'change in living condition' are ambiguous. This scale that measures stress as a stimulus does not consider the subjective assessment and its dependent subsequent emotions. Many researchers who consider stress as a transaction criticize the scale for not taking into consideration the significant aspect of individual differences based on the appraisal of the situation. Yet, another lacuna in the scale is the limited scope of its application in countries that have a culture different from Western nations. For example, 'being fired at work' may be very common in countries where employment opportunities are high, but encountering the same in a country that limits the opportunity may be much more stressful.

Nevertheless, based on its objectivity and other advantages, many scales were standardized in line with SRRS. Life Experience Scale (Sarason, Johnson, & Siegel, 1978), PERI Life Events Scale (Dohrenwend, Askenasy, Krasnoff, & Dohrenwend, 1978), Unpleasant Event Schedule (Lewinsohn, Mermelstein, Alexander, & McPhillamy, 1985) are a few to mention.

DAILY HASSLES

While major life events scales measured stress from the stimulus perspective, researcher who emphasized on the significance of cognitive appraisal and the related aspect of individual differences strongly felt the need of introducing cognitive-based subjectivity. Another observation on the SRRS is that very often, our major source of stress relates to the minor irritants of everyday life: incidents like an argument with the boss, getting caught in traffic jam, restricted water supply, night-time construction work in the neighbourhood to mention a few. Based on this, Lazarus and his team constructed what is called the 'Hassle Scale' (Kanner, Coyne, Schaefer, & Lazarus, 1981). The scale lists a number of items related to daily irritants ranging in magnitude. The respondent is asked to rate them in severity. This takes care of cognitive appraisal, and individual differences based on that. The same event has the scope of varying in severity as per the individual appraisal. The developers of Hassle Scale also wanted to check if the positive events have the characteristics of counterbalancing the impact of hassles. They constructed a scale to measure the positive experiences and called it 'Uplift Scale'. In a study where the Life Event Scale, Hassle Scale and Uplift Scale were administered on the same sample and the correlation of each of the scales with that of health status was verified, the results revealed a significant, but weak, correlation of health status with Life Event Scale and Hassle Scale. Hassle Scale had no correlation with Uplift Scale. Hassle Scale was found to have a stronger correlation with health status compared to Life Event Scale.

From all the studies, one can infer that while the standardized scales of life event or daily hassles are considered good measurement tools of stress, there still seems to be one piece of the puzzle missing.

LABORATORY EXPERIMENTS

Researchers have measured stress in laboratories by inducing stress in the subjects. This is done by creating a stressful situation such as a challenging cognitive task to be completed in the environment of loud noise, excessive light, or oppressive heat or cold. The task in the laboratory can also have a passive role for the subjects, such as watching a horror movie. The measurement of stress in laboratories can combine the physiological measurements (that includes changes in the function of vital organs and biochemical changes in blood and urine) and psychological measurement by administration of scale, intervention and observation and recording of behavioural changes during and immediately after the exposure to simulated stress.

The laboratory-based experiments have the advantage of controlled condition. Since the intervening variables are controlled, it is possible to identify the cause-and-effect relationship. However, the major constraint of laboratory setting is the problem of generalizability of it to real-life response in natural setting.

QUASI-EXPERIMENTS IN NATURAL SETTING

Quasi-experiments are planned in natural setting by simulating stress. This enables to overcome the limitations of artificiality in laboratory setting. The physiological or psychological parameters of stress or a combination of both is taken up to quantify stress in natural life situation. For example, stress in its physiological and psychological dimension is measured after or before a public performance, preceding a job interview or landmark examinations that involve high stakes.

In a quasi-experiment, Hariharan (1990) studied the impact of stress on children's cognitive problem solving in order to explore and compare coping behaviour of resilient and non-resilient children. The study was conducted in the month of April when the temperature was above 40°C, in the afternoon after the children completed their last examination of the academic year. The subjects were a subsample of a larger study. As part of the experiment, 25 children from classes 6, 7, 8 and 9 were asked by the school principal (who was the accomplice 1) to wait in a class room to take few psychological tests as a continuation of the study in which they were part of the large sample. The children were given a cognitive task. Once they finished, the researcher was interacting with the children and explaining the second cognitive task involving arithmetic problems they have to solve within a given time. At this point, two stern looking 'Medical Scientists' in long white lab coats carrying weird instruments (accomplice 2 and 3) entered the class room accompanied by the principal. The principal introduced them as scientists who wish to conduct some simple medical tests on these children as 'they were only students available in the campus as others had already left'. The 'scientists' told the children that their medical tests could be 'slightly painful', but their participation helps in the advancement in medical sciences. The researchers requested the 'scientists' to wait until she completed her job. In the meanwhile, the 'scientists' started arranging the table by spreading their 'equipment' that contained spirit lamps, 10cc syringes and other unknown tools.

The subjects were given a cognitive task similar to the earlier one. The two tasks were compared. The behaviour of children was observed and recorded. An introspective report was taken. At the end, the subjects were debriefed.

The findings on cognitive task showed a significant difference between pre- and post-simulated stress in all children. One non-resilient child from class 8 chose to run away from the class room without seeking permission. The coping behaviour of resilient and non-resilient children indicated differences in the coping techniques adopted.

The quasi-experiments have a combined advantage of controlling the intervening variables and avoidance of artificiality of the laboratory setting. It provides the scope for measuring the parameters of stress on physiological and psychological dimensions. Quasi-experiments would reap reliable results provided the planning is meticulous with all measures to control the intervening variables with a contingency plan of meeting immediate field-level challenges. The execution of quasi-experiments should be precise so that the control is optimum.

Stress and Illness

Have you ever observed individuals suffering from viral fevers, infections or cardiac problems after passing through a major crisis in life? Did it ever come to your notice that people meeting minor or major accidents also reporting about being in a difficult phase of life when they are encountering a life problem or being worried about something? Try to recollect events in the lives of people around you.

Stress, acute or chronic, is found to have close association with the health of the individual. Stress-illness link can be analysed and explained from two different points—direct or HPA axis stress response and indirect or the health risk behavioural response to stress.

Direct Impact of Stress on Health

The physiological and biochemical changes in the body in response to stress perception have been explained in earlier sections of the chapter. The activation of the sympathetic nervous system leading to excitement and enhanced functioning of cardiovascular and respiratory systems tax the major vital organs. The HPA axis activation triggers release of stress hormones into the blood, thus creating a biochemical imbalance in the body. These two reactions have their detrimental impact on normal physiological function of the systems in human body. The most affected systems as per research until now are the cardiovascular, respiratory, digestive, reproductive and immune system.

Indirect Impact of Stress on Health

The indirect impact of stress on health is mediated by biochemical response to stress. Exposure to stress is associated with significant changes in two dimensions, viz. emotion and cognition. The situation presents a concrete problem to the target individual who needs to apply his/her cognition in appraising and solving the concrete problem that is stressful. Simultaneously, the situation also stimulates some negative emotions such as fear, anger, anxiety and other emotions of the same family in varying intensity. Taking both the cognitive appraisal of problem and emotion into consideration, the individual, influenced by several other factors such as past experience, personality components and the availability of resources, chooses a coping strategy. The chosen coping strategy focuses either on the problem or on the emotion. On occasions when the stressful situation triggers intense emotions, it has an impact on routine health-related behaviour such as eating, sleeping and exercising. Very often, the adverse impact is seen in the individual's noticeable neglect of nutrition either due to loss of appetite or because of anxiety and preoccupation with the problem. The second casualty is sleep. The individual is likely to lose sleep while under severe stress. A decrease in nutrition and sleep, which is essential activities of tissue regeneration on regular basis, casts a negative impact on the health of the individual.

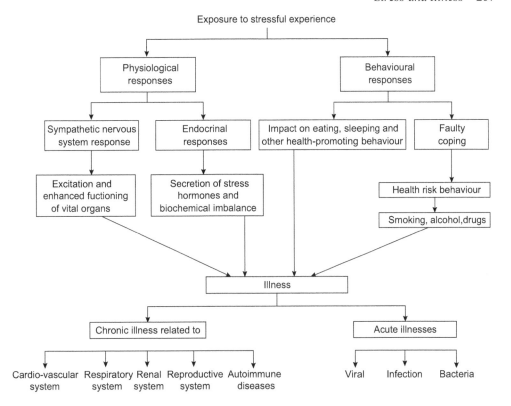

Figure 7.8 Stress-Illness Link.

The second indirect connection between stress and illness relates to health risk behaviour. The illness risks of stress from the physiological and behavioural factors are presented in Figure 7.8.

Though we discuss acute and chronic stress under separate heads for the sake of convenience, both are closely associated. For example, frequent exposure to acute stress places the physiological system under wear and tear due to strain. A person exposed to chronic stress already has his or her system vulnerable, which is triggered on the face of an acute stress resulting in a major health event such as a cardiac attack, cerebral stroke or an angina pain. The impact of stress on various body organs and their functioning is explained in Figure 7.9.

With the understanding of basic logic explained above about the link between stress and illness, let us now go into details of research that linked stress with illness, related to specific systems.

Impact of Stress on Immune System

Let us briefly recapitulate the functioning of the immune system. This is the first line of defence in the human body, which fights invaders, called antigens from entering the human body. The antibodies produced by bone marrow, lymph nodes, spleen and thymus prevent the antigens from invading our body fluids and cells. The antibodies are phagocytes and lymphocytes. Phagocytes attack any antigens in general and, hence, called non-specific immune cell. The

268 *Stress and Illness*

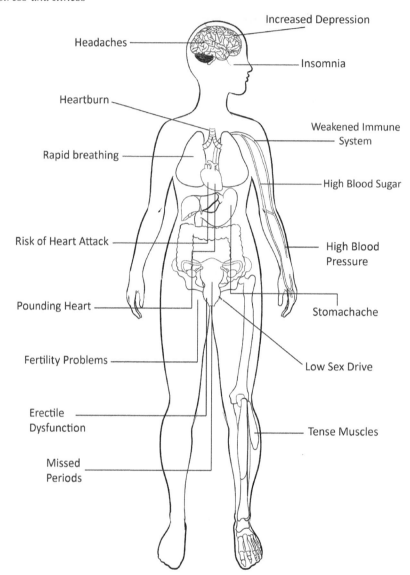

Figure 7.9 Impact of Stress on Body Organs.

'T' cells produced by thymus guard against antigens entering the cells. B cells put up a fight at the body fluid level even before the invaders attempt to enter the cells. The immune system in healthy condition has these cells functioning competently and prevents the viruses, bacteria or infection entering the body and thus preserves the health of the person. This is termed as 'immunocompetence'. When the immune system fails to prevent the antigens from their invasion and subsequent damage, it is known as 'immunocompromise'.

Exposure to stress is said to give rise to immunocompromise. The relationship between the stress and immune response was first discovered by Ader and Cohen (1975, 1981) who could condition lowered immune response to a neutral stimulus of sweetened water, which was initially introduced in combination with an immunosuppressant. This and subsequent studies identified the relationship between psychological state and immune system, giving rise to a new branch called psychoneuroimmunology. It is inferred that the cortisol secreted in response to stressful encounter inhibits the egress from the lymphoid tissues. The weakness causes the block in proliferation of T cells, thus reducing the total count of T lymphocytes responsible for memory, hypersensitivity and suppression, the consequence of which is a weaker immune system. This was suggested in a study by Dong, Zhi, Bhayana and Wu (2016). Their study was on brain-injured mice, to inquire into the mechanism in which the cortisol caused lowering of the number of T cells. They tried to track the T-cell outfit in lymph nodes by administering hydrocortisone. The results revealed a significant fall in the lymphocytes in general and T cells in particular. The decrease in the number of T cells negatively correlated with the increase in the cortisol level in the blood. Thus, it is evident that an increased level of cortisol functions as immunosuppressant, which weakens the immune system.

Maier, Watkins, and Fleshner (1994) had explained in further detail that the sympathetic nervous system is responsible for innervating the immune organs such as bone marrow, spleen, thymus and lymph nodes.

The link between stress, immunosuppression and illness has been proved by a number of studies. One of the classic studies was by Cohen et al. (1998). They studied 276 healthy volunteers. They were interviewed on the stressful experiences in the recent past. Following this, they had to inhale a common cold virus. The results revealed that the participants who encountered chronic stress related to job or relationships were more likely to develop cold compared to those who did not face such stress.

Wound healing is a condition that is influenced by the immune system. It may be a recovery from an injury or a surgical process. Infections and complications of the wound are indices of poor healing. Doering, Moser, Lemankiewicz, Luper and Khan (2005) studied a sample of 72 patients who underwent elective Coronary Artery Bypass Surgery (CABG). They found that those who manifested symptoms of depression at discharge suffered infections and poor healing compared to their counterparts who did not have depressive symptoms.

The relation between stress and wound healing was also studied experimentally. Kiecolt-Glaser et al. (2005) involved 42 married couple and experimentally induced blister wound. The objective of the study was to investigate into the impact of holistic marital interaction on wound healing by examining the pro-inflammatory cytokine production. The participants were measured on their hostile behaviours. First, the participants were involved in a discussion related to social support and their interpersonal relation. On the second occasion, they were interviewed on the conflicts involved in their relationship. Sample fluid from their wounds was collected at the intervals of 2, 7 and 22 hours after the blisters were administered. Results revealed that the healing was slower in post-conflict interview session, compared to social support discussion session. Secondly, those who measured high on hostile scores showed slower healing.

Another method of experientially studying the wound healing is to create a punch biopsy. This creates dermal and mucosal wounds that facilitate daily quantification of wounds by measuring their size. Kiecolt-Glaser, Marucha, Malarkey, Mercado and Glaser (1995) studied a sample of 13 female caregivers of dementia patients and another 13 non-caregiver women matched on sociodemographic dimensions. They were administered punch biopsy wounds that measured 3.5 mm in their non-active forearms. They were followed up to the wound healing. The findings showed a clear negative association between stress and wound healing. The caregiver group took 24% longer time to heal the wound. It should be reiterated here that the family caregivers of dementia patients encounter severe stress.

Errors in Immune System and Autoimmune Diseases

The evolution of psychoneuroimmunology as a branch can be tracked to the discovery of connection between the central nervous system, endocrinal system and immune system. The nervous system and immune system react to stressful encounters. Their connectivity thus also impacts the immune system.

The immune system sometimes is susceptible to erroneous functioning. In that process, it mistakes the body's own cells as an antigen or invader and starts attacking and destroying it. As a consequence of such self-inflicted harm, the individual suffers from what is known as 'autoimmune diseases'. The type of autoimmune disease depends upon the part of the body that is affected by the system. Rheumatoid arthritis is an autoimmune disease with the symptoms of stiffness, inflammation and pain in the joints. Grave's disease is another autoimmune disease that impacts the thyroid gland. The symptoms are often muscle aches, fatigue and gain in weight. Multiple sclerosis is another condition resulted due to the immune system attacking the nerve cells. The symptoms include weakness and poor coordination of muscles, pain due to muscular spasm. Type 1 diabetes mellitus is caused when the immune system harms the insulin-producing cells in the pancreas. The skin disease called psoriasis is caused because of the overactive immune system that leads to the collection of T cells in the skin. This makes the skin mistake that the cells in it are destroyed and reproduced rapidly. As a result, silvery plaques are formed on the skin.

All the above illness conditions are said to be associated with high levels of chronic stress.

People frequently suffering from infection and viral attacks need to be assessed on their psychological distress. The patients opting to go for major or minor surgeries too need to be assessed for their psychological affect state. Interventions aimed at minimizing the stress should constitute part of the treatment regimen. Various psychosocial interventions aimed at mitigating stress will be discussed in detail in later chapters.

Stress and Cardiovascular Disorders

The major physiological reaction to stress occurs in the cardiovascular system that consists of heart and blood vessels involved in blood circulation. The cardiovascular system gets impacted by activation of sympathetic nervous system, which triggers secretion of adrenaline and noradrenaline. The changes due to this in the cardiovascular system include the following:

- Increase in blood pressure
- Increase in heart rate
- Adipose deposits and plaque formation in blood vessels
- Formation of clots in the blood

A number of studies proved the relationship between the affect state and coronary heart disease (CHD). It may not be scientific to speak in terms of cause-and-effect relationship between these two, because the changes in various physiological systems are triggered by a stressful encounter. Hence, it is not logical to claim a direct link between stress/affect state and cardiovascular disease.

Hypertension a condition where the person's heart is forced to pump blood into the body more harder with greater force. One of the reasons is confronting a stressful condition. Repeated exposure to stress makes the individual vulnerable to hypertension. The impact of this is higher strain on heart. Left uncontrolled, hypertension results in heart attacks, strokes or heart failure.

This may subsequently lead to kidney failure or blindness. Stress arising from various sources such as workplace, marital conflict, natural disasters and continuous exposure to environmental stress such as traffic noise, oppressive heat, pungent smell and bright light is found to enhance the blood pressure and place one vulnerable to hypertension. A study on African Americans by Sims et al. (2012) established the relationship between hypertension and perceived social discrimination among African Americans. A social situation where one has to face evaluation by others causes tremendous anxiety and stress in some. Slater, Pertaub, Barker, and Clark (2006) conducted laboratory experiments to study the relationship between the simulated social performance like public speaking and the heart rate. They found elevated heart rates and anxiety accompanying public speaking task for people who had phobia for the task compared to others who did not have phobia.

If one applies the transactional analysis, the individuals differ in their cognitive assessment of stressful condition. Hence, the physiological arousal, consequent to attaching the label of 'stress' to a situation, is determined by one's appraisal. The research question related to this fact is, what are the characteristics of people who are more prone to coronary heart disease on encountering chronic stress?

The association between the risk of cardiac problems and certain personality type was a chance discovery by the cardiologists Friedman and Rosenman (1974). When Friedman decided to renovate the furniture in the waiting room of his clinic, the person repairing it disclosed his observation to him that there was a pattern in the worn-out chairs. The tip of the armrests and the outer edge of the cushions of the chair were the parts that typically suffered the wear and tear. This suggested that the cardiac patients were literally sitting on the edge of their chairs and tapping or squeezing the armrests. This casual observation led to the investigation and finding that cardiac patients are likely to have a typical personality called type A personality.

Friedman and Rosenman's research contributions revealed that people of type A personality have certain unique characteristics that place them continuously under stress. They are different in their thinking, feeling and behaviour. They are the people who continuously chase deadlines, have high achievement motivation, aggressively pursue their set goals, and are high in competitive spirit, impatience and urgency in accomplishing things, intolerant towards those who are slow, less efficient and hostile, particularly towards those who get in the way of the person.

A number of negative states such as anger, contempt, disgust, fear and guilt have been found to be associated with cardiac ailments, particularly hypertension. A study by Nabi, Kivimaki, De Volgi, Marmot and Singh-Manoux (2008) followed up 10,000 London-based civil servants for twelve and half years. They found that those whose scores on negative affect states were on the top one third of scores had 32% higher likelihood to experience cardiac disease over a period of time. Depressive state includes a number of negative affect. There is increasing evidence to prove relation between depression and heart ailment. Increased risk for cardiac diseases and death due to it was found by following up patients suffering from depression (Glassman, 2007). Ten longitudinal studies independently proved that on an average people with depression had about 64% higher risk for cardiac diseases compared to those who did not have depression (Wulsin & Singal, 2003).

Impact of Stress on Respiratory System

The sympathetic nervous system's activation during stressful situations causes shortness of breath as one of the reactions. This is the result of constriction of airway from the nose to the lungs. Stressful episodes are found to impact the normal breathings. The individual under stress over-breaths, leading to lowered end-tidal carbon dioxide. This is called hyperventilation.

272 *Stress and Illness*

Hyperventilation has a negative impact on the respiratory health of the individual. In an experiment, Suess, Alexander, Smith, Sweeney and Marion (1980) placed 29 normal subjects in a stress condition by posing a problem of perceptual judgement, where they have a threat of receiving electrical shock in the event of crossing the stipulated number of errors. The stress was induced in four phases, viz. initial request for participation, decision of the subject, pre-task and the task of perceptual judgement. Measurement of end-tidal CO_2, heart rate, respiration rate and state anxiety was recorded, during stress, and compared with baseline records. Results of comparison of several phases revealed significant changes in end-tidal CO_2. This had no correlation with changes in rate of respiration. Thus, changes in end-tidal CO_2 in the face of stress were confirmed by the study. On the contrary, the study suggested that changes in respiration alone cannot be taken as the criterion. In such eventuality, an individual with no respiratory disease will be able to cope and inhale adequate oxygen. However, those predisposed or already suffering from asthma or Chronic Obstructive Pulmonary Disease (COPD) experience exacerbated breathing problem. According to Forsythe, Ebeling, Gordon, Befus and Vliagoftis (2004), among the patients with asthma, 20%–35% in the face of stress experience trigger of asthma. Their experiments on rats exposed to short- and long-term stress indicated that repeated stress over long term can trigger chronic inflammatory responses of the airway. The mechanisms in operation are different from short-term stress.

Laboratory-based studies proved the relationship of asthma with interpersonal stress, anger and sadness (Isenberg, Lehrer, & Hochron, 1992; Sarafino, Gates, & Depaulo, 2001; Lehrer, Feldman, Giardino, Song, & Schmaling, 2002). This is also found to show a decrease in pulmonary function.

Thus, the restricted inhalation and limited pulmonary function, by themselves, have potential of experiencing strain and panic. Such diminished respiratory functions for prolonged period of chronic stress will have heavy adverse impact on the system.

Impact of Stress on Gastrointestinal System

Before we take up the explanation of the impact of stress on digestive system, if will be of help to briefly describe the link between the nervous system and the digestion.

The stress and gastrointestinal distress relationship is bidirectional and complex. Psychological stress causes disturbance in the digestive system and vice versa. This is because of the close connectivity between the nervous system and the digestive system. While being controlled by the nervous system, the gut has its own neural network known as the 'enteric or intrinsic nervous system'. This system is known to exercise so much impact that this is also called 'the second brain'. The enteric nervous system lines the entire gastrointestinal tract from oesophagus to rectum. It plays a role in regulating the digestive process starting with swallowing of food, release of enzymes in breaking down food and segregating nutrients and waste product of food.

The enteric nervous system also has neurotransmitters like serotonin that establishes bidirectional communication with the central nervous system. On encountering a stress and subsequent fight-or-flight response, because of coordination between the sympathetic and parasympathetic system, the digestion process slows down, or even halts so that the energy is diverted to respond to the perceived stress. When the situation poses a stress of lower intensity, the digestive process may get disrupted temporarily, which may manifest in symptoms like spasm in oesophagus, pain in the stomach due to increase in acid secretion and experience of nausea, diarrhoea or constipation. The bidirectionality of brain-gut connection is also endorsed by research that proved that persistent disturbances in the gastrointestinal system give rise to stress.

The impact of stress on the gastrointestinal system is both short term and long term. Changes in the gastrointestinal system as a result of stressful experience include one or more changes. These changes include the following:

1. Gastrointestinal motility
2. Gastrointestinal secretion
3. Increase in intestinal permeability (enhanced control of material passing through gastrointestinal tracts into rest of the body)
4. Negative impact on gastrointestinal mucosa's capacity for regeneration and mucosal blood flow
5. Negative effects on the microorganisms in the intestines

These changes result in an array of gastrointestinal disorders like Irritable Bowel Syndrome (IBS), Inflammatory Bowel Disease (IBD), acidity and heart burns, peptic ulcers or Gastrooesophageal Reflux Disease (GERD) (Konturek, Brzozowski, & Konturek, 2011).

The digestive system is the largest immune system in the body. It hosts about 60%–80% of body's immunity. Considering the fact that the entire digestive system that includes the small and large intestines is the longest one if spread on the surface, it houses some pounds of bacteria. Some of these bacteria are good. But while under stress, the biochemical reaction caused by the sympathetic system destroys a large portion of these good bacteria. Thus, in the long run, it is responsible for inflammation. There are researches that suggested that the IBS and IBD may not have caused by stress but are aggravated by stress.

Stress experience results in weakening the digestive metabolism. This happens because the blood flow during stressful encounters is decreased for digestive function and is redirected to brain and muscles. If one is stressed while eating, the metabolism slows down either because of too slow or too fast eating or because of the negative emotional state while eating.

The two hormones that secrete in response to stress are cortisol and insulin. They misguide the body to preserve weight and fat instead of strengthening muscles. This again is harmful for overall health.

It is not very clear whether stress worsens a pre-existing gastrointestinal disorder or causes the disorder. Nevertheless, there is absolute clarity on the fact that stress has a negative impact on the digestive system, which is very important in supplying nutrients to every cell in the body.

Impact of Stress on Reproductive System

The hypothalamic-pituitary-adrenal axis (HPA) activation during stress has a direct impact on reproductive system. Every hormonal component in this activated axis such as corticotrophin-releasing factor (CRF), adrenocorticotrophic hormone (ACTH), beta endorphin and glucocorticoids has an adverse impact on female reproductive system by exerting a strong inhibitory effect on hypothalamic-pituitary-ovarian axis. Similarly, the biochemical imbalance caused due to excessive cortisol in the blood affects the normal reproductive functioning in the male. Let us briefly discuss the various ways stress affects the female and male reproductive systems.

Chronic and acute stress results in disturbance in the menstrual cycles of women. They include irregularity or the absence of cycles, painful cycles or changes in the length of menstrual cycles. This is called functional hypothalamic amenorrhoea. Stress, anxiety and depression reduce the sexual desire in women. Further, chronic stress also impacts the process of ovulation and fertilization. This is known as functional hypothalamic anovulation. This stress in a way creates a barrier in the conception of a woman. Even though she conceives, the health

Box 7.3 Impact of Stress on Various Systems

Systems	Impact
Cardiovascular	Hypertension, heart attack, heart failure
Respiratory	COPD, asthma
Immune	Arthritis
Digestive	Peptic/gastric/duodenal ulcers, IBD, IBS
Reproductive	Menstruation-related problems, infertility, abnormal sperm count

of the foetus has the impact of stress, apart from posing problems of postpartal adjustment in the mother. The hormonal imbalance resulting from stress worsens the premenstrual syndrome manifested in cramps, fluid retention, bloating and mood swings.

There is a close association between feelings of distress and menopause. They seem to have a bidirectional relationship, each causing and resulting in the other. Highly stressed women experience higher degree of menopausal symptoms like hot flushes. High levels of stress exacerbate the symptoms of a number of diseases related to the reproductive system, such as Polycystic Ovarian Syndrome (PoS), Herpes Simplex Virus, endometriosis.

The impact of stress on the male reproductive system is as bad as that of the female reproductive system. Chronic stress adversely affects the production of testosterone. This brings a decline in libidinal drive in men. This may even cause erectile dysfunction or impotence in men. Stress has a negative impact on male fertility. Men who experience repeated exposure to stress are found to have sperms that are not of normal size and shape and lower ability of sperm to swim and propel. Stress is known to directly impact the sperm production that falls significantly. Such impact on sperm quality reduces the chances of fertilization. The weakening of the immune system leaves the male reproductive organs vulnerable to infections as a consequence of which one may suffer infections of testes, prostate gland and urethra.

While stress has a devastating negative impact on various body systems and causes a number of illnesses, the vulnerability to diseases due to stress is subject to a number of factors unique to the individual. Hence though one cannot predict the impact of stress on health with the precision of mathematical formula, and foresee and measure the damage, the fact that stress casts a negative impact on health, the extent of it varying in degree has been repeatedly proved by research.

Psychosocial Moderators of Stress

The impact of stress on individual's health has individual differences. The reason is that the extent of stress experienced by a person depends on the cognitive appraisal of stress where the severity is weighted against a number of cognitive, personality and environmental factors. Let us discuss these factors.

Locus of Control (LoC)

Locus of control is one of the major factors taken into account during cognitive appraisal. The degree of stress experienced depends upon perceived locus of control. "It refers to the extent to which individuals believe that they or others around them or unknown factors can control events that affect them" (Hariharan & Rath, 2008). If they perceive that they can exercise major control on events happening in their lives, they are known as having internal locus of control. If they believe that to a large extent the events of their lives are controlled by people other than themselves, they are known to have external locus of control—powerful others. Alternatively, there are also people who believe that the events in their lives are controlled by some unknown factors like God, Fate or Luck. They are known to have external locus of control—unknown others.

Those with internal locus of control are found to perceive lower stress (Elliott, Trief, & Stein, 1986; Matheny & Cupp, 1983). Given the same personal stake, perception of stress varies between a person with internal LoC and one with external LoC. This is explained with the help of Figure 7.10.

The X-axis in the figure measures perceived stress, while the Y-axis measures the stakes involved. Given that the stakes involved in a situation are constant, a person with external LoC (line EE) perceives a stress of OE^1, while another person with internal LoC (Line II) perceives relatively less stress (OI^1). Why does this happen? Cognitive appraisal involves secondary appraisal wherein the individual evaluates the availability of internal and external resources to handle the stressful situation successfully. Those who assess that they are in control of the situation do so by taking into account the resource availability. Thus, a person who is confident of having the events and their consequences under control does not perceive a threat but takes it as a challenge to be met. Hence, the perception of stress is lower. On the contrary, a person who believes that the events and consequences are controlled by others or unknown factors is likely to perceive a passive role in encountering the situation and feel helpless in mitigating or minimizing the impact of stress. Hence, there is a higher level of stress experienced.

Locus of control involves a sense of personal control over various aspects. Control over one's ability to act upon the stress is called behavioural control. The ability of the person to understand the problem in the stressful situation, and think about alternative strategies is cognitive control. A control one perceives in making decision about one's life, such as planning a child, and the type of hospital for delivering the child, treatment plan for a cardiac ailment or choice of life partner, the courses to choose in university are known as decisional control. Equipping oneself with all information about a life situation, the antecedents and consequences of a disease, the way a medication or a therapy helps, and the repercussion of non-adherence and so on refer to informational control. An individual who perceives a sense of personal control over these and many other aspects experiences less stress compared to the one who perceives low or no control on these dimensions.

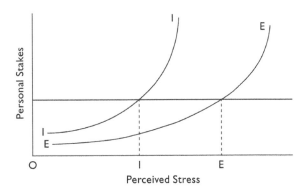

Figure 7.10 LoC as Moderator of Perceived Stress.

Self-efficacy

Self-efficacy is closely related to one's locus of control. It refers to one's judgement on one's own ability to execute courses of action required to deal with a situation. It plays a major role in coping with a stress situation, the perseverance one is likely to show in handling a situation, and the determination with which one circumvents the obstacles. Individuals with high self-efficacy are more likely to perceive lower stress and readily invest adequate efforts in overcoming a stressful situation. When an individual has trust in his ability to confront a situation and cope with it successfully, he/she is more likely to perceive lower stress compared to the one whose self-efficacy is low. For example, a student who believes that he/she can perform well in the forthcoming examinations, because of his/her capability in preparing well and performing well, experiences a sense of exhilaration and challenge compared to the one who is unsure of one's own ability in organizing and planning for a good preparation for the examinations and performance therein.

In a study by Vaezi and Fallah (2011) on English and Foreign Language (EFL) teachers, a negative correlation between stress and self-efficacy was found. In other wounds, higher the self-efficacy, lower the stress.

Hardiness

The concept of hardiness was coined by Kobasa (1979). It comprises of three components, viz. commitment, control and challenge. People who measure high on hardiness are found to have some protection from the impact of stress (Sarafino, 1994a). According to Kobasa, individuals who are committed find life and work more meaningful. This meaningfulness helps in valuing themselves and their work. Hence, they tend to put in efforts and influence social situations. People who have high control experience a sense of mastery over their lives. The characteristic of challenge disposes people to accept change as a normal pattern of life. Kobasa (1982) asserts that a person high on hardiness that is a composite of these three characteristics has higher resistance to stress.

The relationship between hardiness and stress may not be simple as assumed to be. If stress and illness are related, does hardiness play a moderating role on stress and illness? Does it play a significant role in perception of stress? Does hardiness itself provide a protective shield to the individual so that they keep themselves insulated from the life stress and experience higher levels of positive affect? Manning, Williams and Wolfe (1988) studied a sample of 468 participants from two different organizations. They studied the direct and moderating effect of hardiness on work and life stressors, and health-related outcomes. Results indicated a direct relationship between hardiness and emotional and psychological factors, which are assumed to play a crucial role in work performance and wellbeing. Individuals who were identified as hardy measured high on work satisfaction and low on job tension. They were found to be energized and less negative about life. They reported higher quality of life and positive affect state. In terms of physical health, they complained lesser somatic symptoms, depression and anxiety. The results also showed negative correlation between hardiness and four dimensions of work stress. The negative correlation indicating that higher the stress lowers the hardiness suggests that hardiness is not independent of demands of life. Maddi (2006) explained that hardiness has a combination of attributes that invoke the courage and motivation in the individual to work hard on the stressful situation in a way to redirect the situation from becoming disastrous to that of one that provides opportunity to grow. In other words, Maddi suggests the characteristic of resilience in hardy personalities so that encounter with stress helps them emerge as accomplished or successful individuals.

The fact that hardy people differ in their perception of impact of stress on them was studied by Chan (2000). A sample of 245 secondary school students of China constituted the sample.

The results did not find significant difference between the high hardy and low hardy children in appraising greater impact of positive events in life. Hardy students differed from the low hardy counterparts in perceiving lower impact of negative life events. Thus, many studies have their pointer, suggesting that hardy persons attribute lower negativity to stress and its impact on life.

Explanatory Style and Stress

The magnitude of stress experienced is to a large extent determined by one's appraisal and explanatory style. This refers to the attributional aspects related to three specific dimensions of stressful event. In a way, it can be called as a self-talk and perception.

The explanatory style covers three aspects related to the stressful situation, viz. the cause of stress, the impact it has on one's life and the outcome of it in terms of its longevity of time (Figure 7.11).

Causes

What or who is the cause of stress? If one points at one's own self or personal inability, incompetence or incapability or any other negative characteristic of self as the cause of the stress, the individual is likely to experience higher stress. On the contrary, if one identifies any individual or factors outside the self as the cause of the event, then the experience of stress is relatively lower. Attribution of the negative event to internal cause hurts more than when one perceives the cause an external, lying outside oneself. For example, a student who fails in an exam may attribute the cause to his low competence or a tough question paper. Attributing it to one's incompetence hurts more than when the cause is perceived as tough question paper.

Impact

The impact of a negative event may lie on one dimension of life (specific) and may have a spillover effect on many or all dimensions of life (global). For example, a student who fails in an exam may perceive that the impact of it is on his academic life. Here, the attribution is specific. But, if the student feels that his/her failure in exam not only jeopardizes the academic life but will impact the social life (the fiends deserting him/her), family relationships (parents and siblings feeling embarrassed), athletics (having to stop the practice to divert time to academics) etc., the impact is perceived and attributed as global. Perceived global impact is more stressful than the perceived specific impact.

Outcome

The severity of stress experienced also is determined by the perceived outcome of the negative event. The outcome can be perceived as stable or unstable. A stable outcome is one, which is perceived to be almost 'forever' or for a very long duration. An unstable outcome is one that is temporary and stays for a short duration. An individual who attributes that the outcome of a negative event is stable and is going to stay forever is likely to experience higher stress than one who attributes unstable outcome and feels that the negative outcome of the event would change for better over time. For example, a student failing in an exam, if feels that he would be branded as 'failure' for life, is more likely to perceive higher level of stress compared to the

278 *Stress and Illness*

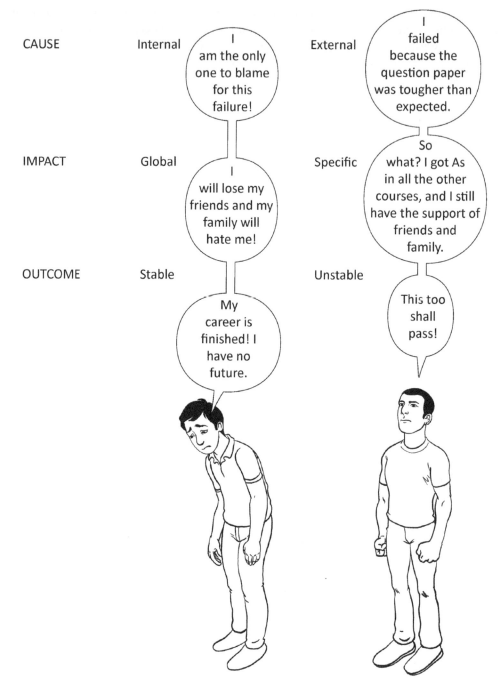

Figure 7.11 Explanatory Style of Stress.

one who feels that the label is temporary and will be forgotten once he/she clears the course subsequently.

An individual with the attribution of cause to internal factors, impact to global level and outcome to stable phenomena is said to have a pessimistic explanatory style. One who attributes the cause to external factors perceives specific impact and outcome as unstable is said to have an optimistic style. A person with a pessimistic style is more likely to perceive higher stress, while the one with optimistic style perceives lower stress. This in turn is likely to impact the health.

Stakes-Effort Balance & Stress

Stakes-effort balancing is a cognitive behavioural phenomenon. The cognitive appraisal of the negative event or situation includes the personal stakes under threat or harm. Based on the personal stakes involved, the individual invests his/her efforts to change the situation to protect what is at stake. The efforts invested should be worth the value of what is at stake. Thus, when the effort put in to encounter the stressful situation is equivalent to the stakes, the experience of stress is lower. However when the efforts invested are disproportionately higher than the stakes involved, the stress that is experienced in investing the efforts adds to the stress generated by the negative event itself and the overall stress experienced is likely to be higher. Similarly when the stressful event involves very high stakes but the effort invested is disproportionately lower, then the outcome in terms of changing the negative event is not likely to be positive. As a result, the frustration and helplessness of the individual add to the existing stress and the overall stress experienced is likely to be higher. Thus, in both the instances, the individual is likely to experience higher stress.

Figure 7.12 depicts the balance and imbalance between personal stakes involved and the efforts invested by one in encountering a stressful situation. The 'Y'-axis measures the efforts, while the 'X'-axis measures the personal stakes. Line SE-Se represents a situation where there is a good balance between the personal stakes involved and the efforts invested in encountering the stress. Here, one can see that at any point of the upward line, the efforts invested are almost equal to the stakes involved. In such situation, the experienced stress is relatively low. Line E-E is a condition where at any point the effort invested is higher than the stakes involved. In such situation, the individual is likely to feel exhausted, which adds to the stress. Contrastingly, line E^1-E^1 is a condition where the effort invested is less than the stakes involved at any point of the line. Thus, for want of efforts, the stressful event is likely to persist. Thus, a good integration of cognitive appraisal and the coping behaviour determines the degree of stress experienced in a situation.

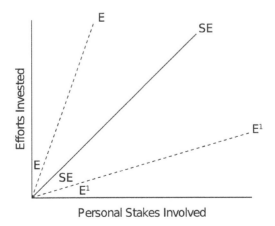

Figure 7.12 Stakes-Effort Balance and Stress.

Childhood Stress: An Alarming Phenomenon

Childhood stress is a phenomenon that is increasingly observed. Hence, it needs a special focus in this chapter. The impact of stress during childhood is much more harmful and long-lasting compared to that of adulthood. Hence, there is a need to understand various aspects of childhood stress and take remedial and preventive steps.

Just as the case of adults, children's stress also originates from internal and external sources. According to DeBord (1996), major life events that are stressful for children include parental death, divorce or remarriage, relocation, prolonged illness, being subjected for abuse, family or community violence, and natural disaster. While these categories of stress relate to the stress from home environment, children also face stress from school. Academic pressure and social pressure are two major dimensions of stress from school environment. Moksnes et al. (2010) specify that high expectations from school and pressure to be popular among peer groups are two significant sources of stress in school. Examination stress, fear of punishment from teachers and being a victim of bullying by others at school are named as stressful by children (Hesketh et al., 2010). Hariharan, Swain and Chivukula (2014) interviewed children between 5 and 15 years of age. They found that the most cited source of stress for children is school, followed by family and then peers. When asked to identify the places of their highly stressful experience, 50% of responses indicated the school, 46% indicated the family, while 16% of responses named the peers. It is alarming to note that what is assumed to be the major source of their support turns out to be their major source of stress (Figure 7.13).

Apart from stress from external sources, the children also face stress from certain feelings and attitudes of their own. Feelings of inferiority, jealously and guilt are the outcome of a mismatch between the external demands and the abilities of the child. Unable to cope with the demands, they end up with such negative affect. Besides these, certain experiences at the somatic level such as hunger, pain and fatigue have the potential to cause stress.

Figure 7.14 presents the various stressors for children classified into internal and external sources. The identified sources are not exhaustive, though. They vary with various factors such as age, gender, culture, nationality and socioeconomic status. However, one predominant source of stress particularly for Indian school children is academic life. Hariharan and Rath (2008) observed that the pressure for scholastic achievement for children resulted in alarming increase in the number of suicides in a single year that amounted to one per every two days.

Impact of Childhood Stress

Childhood is the stage when various organs in the physiological systems are developing into their full size and taking shape. Nurturance from the nutritional and psychological state is essential for healthy growth and functioning of these organs. Stressful experience during this critical phase of life causes disturbance and disruption in their healthy natural development. Hence, the impact of childhood stress is seen in the structural aspects of brain, as well as cognitive functioning and performance.

The physiological response to stress for a child is the same as that of an adult. The hypothalamus stimulates the pituitary gland that releases the adrenocorticotrophic hormone (ACTH). This in turn stimulates the adrenal gland to release catecholamine (adrenaline and noradrenaline) and cortisol. These stress hormones can travel through blood flow to the brain, because catecholamines are water-soluble and 50% bound to plasma proteins. When they circulate in the brain, they stick to the receptors located in various learning and memory regions of the brain. This influences their learning (Lupien et al., 2007) and memory (McClelland, 1996). The cortisol in

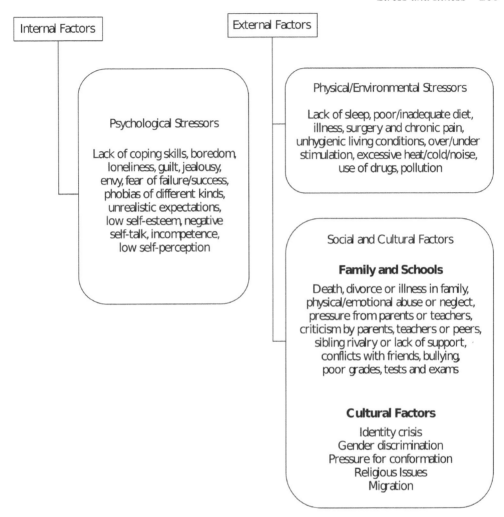

Figure 7.13 Sources of Stress for Children.

the blood negatively impacts the dendritic branching of the neurons, particularly the neurons in hippocampus resulting in deficit in any new learning (Woolley, Gould, & McEwen, 1990). The hippocampus is associated with the long-term memory (Bunsey & Eichenbaum, 1995). It sorts out the decoded information and transfers the same by creating associations. This function of transformation of information is disrupted by exposure to stress, and subsequent elevation of cortisol levels.

The prefrontal cortex is associated with higher order cognitive functioning. Just as the hippocampus, the prefrontal cortex has a number of glucocorticoid receptors that are sensitive to the corticosteroids in the body. Once these receptors are activated by elevated levels of corticosteroids, they cause disturbance in behavioural responses, mood and cognition (Roozendaal, 2002, 2003). Acute stress can result in rapid and dramatic exposure to cognitive functioning. But prolonged exposure to stress can cause architectural damage in the per-frontal cortex (Arnsten, 2009). The prefrontal cortex is also the seat of 'working memory'. This constitutes temporary storage of information that is needed for complex cognitive tasks like language comprehension,

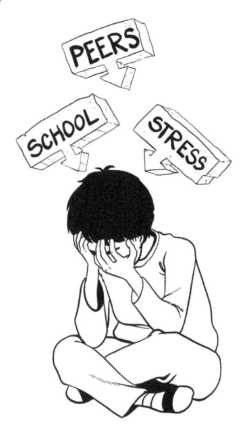

Figure 7.14 Childhood Stress.

learning and reasoning. Besides this, working memory is also required for the simultaneous storage and processing of information. When exposed to acute stress, children are found to face difficulties in recall and verbal memory. Children having post-traumatic stress disorders (PTSD) tested on neuropsychological aspects showed impaired performance on verbal learning tests compared to the normal children (Beers & De Bellis, 2002).

Very often, low academic performance and underachievement of children in school brand them as 'low achiever'. Lack of participation in classrooms and inability to answer questions are misconstrued as their lack of motivation or ability. Seldom do the teachers and parents examine their stress levels and damage it does to the nervous system and cognitive functioning. There is a need to screen these children on their stressful experience before planning any intervention that is limited to intensive academic inputs.

Children in their various developmental stages are differently equipped with their cognitive appraisal skills of the demanding situations. Further, depending upon their age experience and developmental stage their coping skills evolve. Hence, when the demands, particularly academic demands, match their cognitive development, they work under what is called optimum stress (OSL) by perceiving the task as challenging. When the demands are far above their cognitive abilities, they experience distress.

The severity and duration of exposure to stress are considered the major determinants of the impact on the child. On these criteria, Middlebrooks and Audage (2008) classified stress into positive stress, tolerable stress and toxic stress.

Positive Stress

Stress functions as a motivator when it is within a limited threshold in terms of degree and duration. This works as a propeller or a drive to push the child towards achievement and help in the development of the child. Situations that demand marginal adaptations to changes (e.g. having to speak in the school assembly after being successful speaker in the class room) cause mild physiological responses such as an increase in heart rate, hormonal levels and feeling of nervousness of speaking in the presence of the whole school that includes all teachers and seniors. This is positive stress. They are normal. They help the child in preparing for the event and cope with the new situation. Such positive stress contributes by helping the children avail an opportunity to perform, learn and grow further.

Tolerable Stress

This refers to acute stress that lasts for a short while. It could be any adverse event of high severity, such as the death of a loved one, witnessing a ghastly accident or a close friend being hospitalized for a serious disease. Such stressors certainly would have a serious impact. However, with the support of an adult, the child can overcome the negative impact. In the absence of adequate adult support, such events are more likely to have a negative impact on the health and performance of the child not only in the academic field but also in other dimensions of life such as social competence, self-confidence, self-esteem and a number of other psychosocial dimensions. However, there are major individual differences in identifying an adverse event such as 'tolerable stresses'. What is tolerable stress for one child could be a 'positive stress' for another and a 'toxic stress' for yet another child.

Toxic Stress

Stressful experiences that persist for long duration may have their impact on multiple dimensions of life and sometimes last for life. Hence, it is called toxic. Neglect, ill treatment, victimization, physical violence, assault or abuse or constant humiliation is some examples. Prolonged exposure to toxic stress is likely to result in exaggerated stress response. Tuakli-Williams and Carrillo (1995) conducted a study on African American and Latino pre-school children. The results revealed that exposure to severe psychosocial stressors such as poverty, violence, racism and environmental pollution in combination with poor health leads to low mood, problem with span of attention and stunted emotional development.

Behavioural Indicators of Stress in Children

The negative impact of stress is observed to be more pronounced in children below 10 years of age. The outcome of it is limited cognitive abilities, social competence and academic performance. Children who experienced prolonged deprivations in socioeconomic front, subjected to or witness of community violence, or victims of bullying in schools experience higher degrees of external stress (McLoyd, 1998). The manifestation of stress could be multifold. Aggressive outbursts, defensive behaviour, fear of school, refusal to go to school, reluctance in leaving home, apprehensions about the security of one or both the parents are some of the clear indicators. In such instance, there is a definite need for probing further and addressing the stress of the child. Similarly, a sudden drop in academic performance, preference for being alone, change in appetite or sleeping behaviour, change in affect state, irritability or spells of crying or weeping at the mildest stimulus warrant parental and school attention. A child may not manifest all the symptoms, but an observable change in any one of the areas of behaviour calls for effective handling.

Interventions for Childhood Stress

The intervention for childhood stress needs to include preventive steps, diagnostic tools and methods, and remedial measures for those who suffer the impact of childhood stress.

Preventive Steps

Small and simple but significant preventive steps can be planned by the adults in the lives of children in preparing the child for an impending minor stress. For example, simple readiness programmes can be designed for the child highlighting the positives and underlining the possible negative feelings of events such as the first days in the new school, the arrival of a sibling, taking a vaccination, possibility of the terminally ill and ailing grandparent dying. This can help the child prepare for the inevitable, which in turn soften the magnitude of the stress.

Helping the child in identifying and endorsing an emotion is a good preventive step. A child should know that all negative emotions such as anger, sorrow and frustration have an acceptable context. The expression of these emotions in the right context, in the right form and in right degree provides a scope for ventilation. Training children in appropriate emotion regulation is a positive step in helping children handle their stress appropriately. Suppressing the negative emotions is an unhealthy way of handling stress.

Diagnostic Methods and Tools

Prolonged stress experience has a devastating impact on behaviour and academic performance of children. In case children having underperformance fail to improve with academic intervention, there is a need for screening the child for stress level. Further, in view of the fact that stress causes major disruption in the structural and functional aspects of hippocampus and prefrontal cortex, a neuropsychological assessment and diagnosis will be very relevant.

A child manifesting problems in learning a new concept or skill or unable to recall the already learned material needs to be assessed on stress levels.

Those children in school having low attention span and negative mood states run the risk of being labelled as ADHD without proper diagnostic measures. Instead, they need to be properly assessed for their stress levels before being referred for neuropsychological assessment.

Remedial Measures

Children who are introvert are likely to suffer stress and suffer the suppression rather than actively seeking solution even to their external source of stress. In such instance, a sound remedial measure is to integrate play therapy into the school's routine. A therapist or a trained teacher assumes the role of an observer can carry forward their initial observations to further screening and diagnosis. Definite remedial measures should target either the source of stress or train the children in handling it effectively.

Children need to be equipped well with strategies of coping with school-related tasks and demands. In addition, a good remedial measure is to create opportunities for their free expression to teachers and peer groups. Close friendships with class fellows need explicit encouragement both by teachers and by parents so that the child develops the concept of a close, trusted confidante.

Box 7.4 Researcher's Box

- Standardization of stress scale with multidimensional source for Indian population would be a good value addition. This helps in identifying the major source of stress so that the target for therapeutic intervention is identified.
- Measuring childhood stress is a challenge. There is a huge gap in measurement tools for children's stress. Standardizing an Indian Sale for childhood stress provides a good diagnostic tool for paediatricians' child psychologists and educationists.
- Longitudinal studies on adolescents and young adults measuring high on stress and screening them on the status of health associated with various physiological systems can be a good study design establishing cause-and-effect relationship between stress and illness.
- Correlational studies can be designed to find out the relationship between stress levels and performance at work or academics. This calls for maintenance of records of stressful events and the work output on a daily basis. Measure both using identified tools and find a correlation.
- The OSL of employees of various work groups can be determined by designed studies that measures the stress assessment by the researcher and work assessment by the immediate supervisor at work. The data need to be thoroughly scrutinized and analysed to find out the peaks of work output and stress experienced. This, if combined with qualitative data, will be a very valuable addition to the theoretical basis of OSL.

Box 7.5 Practitioner's Box

- It is important to evaluate the stress levels of any client with any physical symptoms or common problems such as sleeplessness, loss of appetite.
- In case of very high stress, it may be a good practice to get physiological and biochemical analyses from a professional laboratory.
- Relaxation techniques using JPMR, Guided Imagery or *Yoga nidra* will be very appropriate.
- For patients with low motivation levels, using biofeedback is effective.
- Children referred for problems in academic performance or negative affect states need to be assessed for stress levels. Very often, high stress levels in children go undiagnosed. Once the source of stress is identified and addressed, the cognitive and behavioural symptoms reduce. If need be, when the source of stress is identified as parents or school, the source need to have sessions of counselling.
- Play therapy is effective in children who are introvert and suppress stress. This provides good opportunity to ventilate their emotions.
- Application of stress management techniques for patients with chronic illness helps in preventing aggravation of the condition.

All the above measures are very essential in contemporary national context where small family and working and busy parents are the norm and reality. Hence, handling childhood stress has to be taken up as a partnership programme of parents and schools.

References

Ader, R., & Cohen, N. (1975). Behaviorally conditioned immunosuppression. *Psychosomatic Medicine*, *37*, 333–340.

Ader, R., & Cohen, N. (1981). Conditioned immunopharmacological responses. In Ader, R. (Ed), *Psychoneuroimmunology* (2nd ed., pp. 611–626). New York: New York Academic.

Arnsten, A. F. (2009). Stress signalling pathways that impair prefrontal cortex structure and function. *Nature Reviews Neuroscience*, *10*(6), 410.

Baum, A. (1990). Stress, intrusive imagery, and chronic distress. *Health Psychology*, *9*(6), 653–675. doi: 10.1037/0278-6133.9.6.653

Beers, S. R., & De Bellis, M. D. (2002). Neuropsychological function in children with maltreatment-related posttraumatic stress disorder. *American Journal of Psychiatry*, *159*(3), 483–486.

Bhui, K., Dinos, S., Galant-Miecznikowska, M., de Jongh, B., & Stansfeld, S. (2016). Perceptions of work stress causes and effective interventions in employees working in public, private and non-governmental organisations: A qualitative study. *BJPsych Bulletin*, *40*(6), 318–325.

Bunsey, M., & Eichenbaum, H. (1995). Selective damage to the hippocampal region blocks long-term retention of a natural and nonspatial stimulus-stimulus association. *Hippocampus*, *5*(6), 546–556.

Cannon, W. B. (1932). *Effects of strong emotions*. Chicago: University of Chicago Press.

Chan, D. W. (2000). Dimensionality of hardiness and its role in the stress-distress relationship among Chinese adolescents in Hong Kong. *Journal of Youth and Adolescence*, *29*(2), 147–161.

Chrousos, G. P., & Gold, P. W. (1992). The concepts of stress and stress system disorders: Overview of physical and behavioral homeostasis. *Jama*, *267*(9), 1244–1252.

Cohen, S., Frank, E., Doyle, W. J., Skoner, D. P., Rabin, B. S., & Gwaltuey, J. M., Jr. (1998). Types of stressors that increase susceptibility to the common cold in healthy adults. *Health Psychology*, *17*, 214–223.

DeBord, K. (1996). *Helping children cope with stress*. https://www.researchgate.net/profile/Karen-Debord/publication/229025551_Helping_children_cope_with_stress/links/0a85e52f231261e7b6000000/Helping-children-cope-with-stress.pdf

Doering, L. V., Moser, D. K., Lemankiewicz, W., Luper, C., & Khan, S. (2005). Depression, healing, and recovery from coronary artery bypass surgery. *American Journal of Critical Care*, *14*(4), 316–324.

Dohrenwend, B. S., Askenasy, A. R., Krasnoff, L., & Dohrenwend, B. P. (1978). Exemplification of a method for scaling life events: The PERI Life Events Scale. *Journal of Health and Social Behavior*, *19*, 205–229.

Dong, T., Zhi, L., Bhayana, B., & Wu, M. X. (2016). Cortisol-induced immune suppression by a blockade of lymphocyte egress in traumatic brain injury. *Journal of Neuroinflammation*, *13*(1), 197.

Elliott, D. J., Trief, P. M., & Stein, N. (1986). Mastery, stress, and coping in marriage among chronic pain patients. *Journal of Behavioral Medicine*, *9*(6), 549–558.

Forsythe, P., Ebeling, C., Gordon, J. R., Befus, A. D., & Vliagoftis, H. (2004). Opposing effects of short- and long-term stress on airway inflammation. *American Journal of Respiratory and Critical Care Medicine*, *169*(2), 220–226.

Friedman, M., & Rosenman, R. H. (1974). *Type A behavior and your heart*. Greenwich, CT: Fawcett.

Glassman, A. H. (2007). Depression and cardiovascular comorbidity. *Dialogues in Clinical Neuroscience*, *9*(1), 9.

Hariharan, M. (1990). Invulnerable children some studies on disadvantaged childrens competence and coping style (Unpublished doctoral thesis).

Hariharan, M., Prasad, K., & Swain, S. (2010). Stress and coping styles of pilots in Indian civil aviation-An exploratory study. *Indian Journal of Clinical Psychology*, *37*(1), 60–68.

Hariharan, M., & Rath, R. (2008). *Coping with life stress: The Indian experience*. New Delhi: SAGE Publications India.

Hariharan, M., Swain, S., & Chivukula, U. (2014). Childhood stress and its impact on learning and academic performance. In: A. J. Holliman (Ed.), *Educational psychology* (pp. 127–139). London, New York: Routledge.

Hesketh, T., Zhen, Y., Lu, L., Dong, Z. X., Jun, Y. X., & Xing, Z. W. (2010). Stress and psychosomatic symptoms in Chinese school children: Cross-sectional survey. *Archives of Disease in Childhood*, *95*(2), 136–140.

Hobson, C. J., & Delunas, L. (2001). National norms and life-event frequencies for the revised social readjustment rating scale. *International Journal of Stress Management*, *8*(4), 299–314.

Hobson, C. J., Kamen, J., Szostek, J., Nethercut, C. M., Tiedmann, J. W., & Wojnarowicz, S. (1998). Stressful life events: A revision and update of the social readjustment rating scale. *International Journal of Stress Management*, *5*(1), 1–23.

Holmes, T. H., & Rahe, R. H. (1967). The social readjustment rating scale. *Journal of Psychosomatic Research*, *11*, 213–218.

Isenberg, S. A., Lehrer, P. M., & Hochron, S. M. (1992). The effects of suggestion and emotional arousal on pulmonary function in asthma: A review and a hypothesis regarding vagal mediation. *Psychosomatic Medicine*, *54*(2), 192–216

Kanner, A. D., Coyne, J. C., Schaefer, C., & Lazarus, R. S. (1981). Comparison of two modes of stress measurement: Daily hassles and uplifts versus major life events. *Journal of Behavioral Medicine*, *4*(1), 1–39.

Kerns, E., Masterson, E. A., Themann, C. L., & Calvert, G. M. (2018). Cardiovascular conditions, hearing difficulty, and occupational noise exposure within US industries and occupations. *American Journal of Industrial Medicine*, *61*(6), 477–491.

Keshavarz, M., & Mohammadi, R. (2011). Occupational stress and organizational performance, case study: Iran. *Procedia-Social and Behavioral Sciences*, *30*, 390–394.

Kiecolt-Glaser, J. K., Loving, T. J., Stowell, J. R., Malarkey, W. B., Lemeshow, S., Dickinson, S. L., & Glaser, R. (2005). Hostile marital interactions, proinflammatory cytokine production, and wound healing. *Archives of General Psychiatry*, *62*(12), 1377–1384.

Kiecolt-Glaser, J. K., Marucha, P. T., Mercado, A. M., Malarkey, W. B., & Glaser, R. (1995). Slowing of wound healing by psychological stress. *The Lancet*, *346*(8984), 1194–1196.

Kobasa, S. C. (1979). Stressful life events, personality, and health: An inquiry into hardiness. *Journal of Personality and Social Psychology*, *37*, 1–11.

Kobasa, S. C. (1982). The hardy personality: Toward a social psychology of stress and health. *Social Psychology of Health and Illness*, *4*, 3–32.

Konturek, P. C., Brzozowski, T., & Konturek, S. J. (2011). Stress and the gut: Pathophysiology, clinical consequences, diagnostic approach and treatment options. *Journal of Physiology and Pharmacology*, *62*(6), 591–599.

Lazarus, R. S. (1966). *Psychological stress and the coping process*. New York: McGraw-Hill.

Lazarus, R. S., & Folkman, S. (1984). Coping and adaptation. In: W. D. Gentry (Ed.), *The handbook of behavioral medicine* (pp. 282–325). New York: Guilford.

Lehrer, P., Feldman, J., Giardino, N., Song, H. S., & Schmaling, K. (2002). Psychological aspects of asthma. *Journal of Consulting and Clinical Psychology*, *70*(3), 691.

Lewinsohn, P. M., Mermelstein, R. M., Alexander, C., & MacPhillamy, D. J. (1985). The unpleasant events schedule: A scale for the measurement of aversive events. *Journal of Clinical Psychology*, *41*(4), 483–498.

Li, H., Cai, J., Chen, R., Zhao, Z., Ying, Z., Wang, L., ... & Kan, H. (2017). Particulate matter exposure and stress hormone levels: A randomized, double-blind, crossover trial of air purification. *Circulation*, *136*(7), 618–627.

Lin, E. J. D., Sun, M., Choi, E. Y., Magee, D., Stets, C. W., & During, M. J. (2015). Social overcrowding as a chronic stress model that increases adiposity in mice. *Psychoneuroendocrinology*, *51*, 318–330.

Lupien, S. J., Maheu, F., Tu, M., Fiocco, A., & Schramek, T. E. (2007). The effects of stress and stress hormones on human cognition: Implications for the field of brain and cognition. *Brain and Cognition*, *65*(3), 209–237.

Maddi, S. R. (2006). Hardiness: The courage to grow from stresses. *The Journal of Positive Psychology*, *1*(3), 160–168.

Maier, S. F., Watkins, L. R., & Fleshner, M. (1994). Psychoneuroimmunology: The interface between behavior, brain, and immunity. *American Psychologist, 49*(12), 1004.

Manning, M. R., Williams, R. F., & Wolfe, D. M. (1988). Hardiness and the relationship between stressors and outcomes. *Work & Stress, 2*(3), 205–216.

Mason, J. W. (1975). A historical view of the stress field. *Journal of Human Stress, 1*(2), 22–36.

Matheny, K. B., & Cupp, P. (1983). Control, desirability, and anticipation as moderating variables between life change and illness. *Journal of Human Stress, 9*(2), 14–23.

McClelland, J. L. (1996). Role of the hippocampus in learning and memory: A computational analysis. In: T. Ono, B. L. McNaughton, S. Molotchnikoff, E. T. Rolls, and H. Nishijo (Eds.), *Perception, memory and emotion: Frontiers in neuroscience* (pp. 601–613). Cambrige University Press.

McEwen, B. S. (2005). Stressed or stressed out: What is the difference? *Journal of Psychiatry and Neuroscience, 30*(5), 315.

McEwen, B. S., & Stellar, E. (1993). Stress and the individual: Mechanisms leading to disease. *Archives of Internal Medicine, 153*(18), 2093–2101.

McLoyd, V. C. (1998). Socioeconomic disadvantage and child development. *American Psychologist, 53*(2), 185.

Middlebrooks, J. S., & Audage, N. C. (2008). *The effects of childhood stress on health across the lifespan.* Atlanta, GA: US Department of Health and Human Services, Centers for Disease Control and Prevention..

Moksnes, U. K., Moljord, I. E., Espnes, G. A., & Byrne, D. G. (2010). The association between stress and emotional states in adolescents: The role of gender and self-esteem. *Personality and Individual Differences, 49*(5), 430–435.

Münzel, T., Schmidt, F. P., Steven, S., Herzog, J., Daiber, A., & Sørensen, M. (2018). Environmental noise and the cardiovascular system. *Journal of the American College of Cardiology, 71*(6), 688–697.

Nabi, H., Kivimaki, M., De Vogli, R., Marmot, M. G., & Singh-Manoux, A. (2008). Positive and negative affect and risk of coronary heart disease: Whitehall II prospective cohort study. *Bmj, 337*, a118.

Obradovich, N., Migliorini, R., Paulus, M. P., & Rahwan, I. (2018). Empirical evidence of mental health risks posed by climate change. *Proceedings of the National Academy of Sciences, 115*(43), 10953–10958.

Osmanovic-Thunström, A., Mossello, E., Åkerstedt, T., Fratiglioni, L., & Wang, H. X. (2015). Do levels of perceived stress increase with increasing age after age 65? A population-based study. *Age and Ageing, 44*(5), 828–834.

Roozendaal, B. (2002). Stress and memory: Opposing effects of glucocorticoids on memory consolidation and memory retrieval. *Neurobiology of Learning and Memory, 78*(3), 578–595.

Roozendaal, B. (2003). Systems mediating acute glucocorticoid effects on memory consolidation and retrieval. *Progress in Neuro-Psychopharmacology and Biological Psychiatry, 27*(8), 1213–1223.

Sarafino, E. P. (1994a). *Health psychology: Biopsychosocial interaction* (2nd ed.). Canada: John Wiley & Sons.

Sarafino, E. P. (1994b). Stress, biopsychosocial factors, and illness. In: E. P. Sarafino and T. Smith (Eds.), *Health Psychology: Biopsychosocial Interactions* (pp. 102–136). New York: Wiley.

Sarafino, E. P., Gates, M., & DePaulo, D. (2001). The role of age at asthma diagnosis in the development of triggers of asthma episodes. *Journal of Psychosomatic Research, 51*(5), 623–628.

Sarason, I. G., Johnson, J. H., & Siegel, J. M. (1978). Assessing the impact of life changes: Development of the life experiences survey. *Journal of Consulting and Clinical Psychology, 46*(5), 932.

Selye, H. (1956). *The stress of life.* New York: McGraw-Hill.

Selye, H. (1976). *Stress in health and disease.* Woburn, MA: Butterworth.

Selye, H. (1985). The nature of stress. *Basal Facts, 7*(1), 3–11.

Sims, M., Diez-Roux, A. V., Dudley, A., Gebreab, S., Wyatt, S. B., Bruce, M. A., ... & Taylor, H. A. (2012). Perceived discrimination and hypertension among African Americans in the Jackson Heart Study. *American Journal of Public Health, 102*(S2), S258–S265.

Slater, M., Pertaub, D. P., Barker, C., & Clark, D. M. (2006). An experimental study on fear of public speaking using a virtual environment. *Cyber Psychology & Behavior, 9*(5), 627–633.

Suess, W. M., Alexander, A. B., Smith, D. D., Sweeney, H. W., & Marion, R. J. (1980). The effects of psychological stress on respiration: A preliminary study of anxiety and hyperventilation. *Psychophysiology*, *17*(6), 535–540.

Taylor, S. E. (2006). *Health psychology*. New Delhi: Tata McGraw-Hill Education.

Taylor, S. E., Klein, L. C., Lewis, B. P., Gruenewald, T. L., Gurung, R. A. R., & Updegraff, J. A. (2000). Biobehavioral responses to stress in females: Tend-and-befriend, not fight-or-flight. *Psychological Review, 107*(3), 411–429. doi: 10.1037/0033-295X.107.3.411

Trovato, G. M., Pace, P., Cangemi, E., Martines, G. F., Trovato, F. M., & Catalano, D. (2012). Gender, lifestyles, illness perception and stress in stable atrial fibrillation. *La ClinicaTerapeutica*, *163*(4), 281–286.

Tuakli-Williams, J., & Carrillo, J. (1995). The impact of psychosocial stressors on African-American and Latino preschoolers. *Journal of the National Medical Association*, *87*(7), 473–478.

Vaezi, S., & Fallah, N. (2011). The relationship between self-efficacy and stress among Iranian EFL teachers. *Journal of Language Teaching and Research*, *5*(2), 1168–1174. doi: 10.4304/jltr.2.5.1168-1174

Westman, J. C., & Walters, J. R. (1981). Noise and stress: A comprehensive approach. *Environmental Health Perspectives*, *41*, 291–309.

WHO. (1986). *Work organisation and stress*. Institute of Work, Health and Organisations, UK

Woolley, C. S., Gould, E., & McEwen, B. S. (1990). Exposure to excess glucocorticoids alters dendritic morphology of adult hippocampal pyramidal neurons. *Brain Research*, *531*(1–2), 225–231.

Wulsin, L. R., & Singal, B. M. (2003). Do depressive symptoms increase the risk for the onset of coronary disease? A systematic quantitative review. *Psychosomatic Medicine*, *65*(2), 201–210.

8 Chronic Illness and Therapeutic Interventions

> It is highly frustrating! My blood sugar levels are found to be high. I have been majorly compliant with the medical advice—I have abstained from eating sweets, which is a big challenge for me. But, still, there is just a marginal change in my glucose levels.
>
> —fumed Rajeshwari

She is a branch manager in a nationalized bank. She is obese and engaged in a sedentary job with high levels of stress. On being diagnosed with type 2 diabetes, she took the advice of her physician to keep off sweets very seriously. However, she has not paid much attention to the other aspects of medical prescription on diet, exercise and stress management. She thought restraining from consumption of sweets is the major aspect that should take care of her sugar levels to supplement the medication. Ever since her diagnosis one year ago, she has been regularly monitoring her blood glucose first three months, but started to show erratic swings thereafter.

Rajesh was diagnosed with asthma when he was 13 years old. He is now 28 and is employed in a finance company. He says he has not had any episode of asthma for the past four months. This is the first time that he has such a long time with no flare-up of asthma.

Both diabetes and asthma are identified as chronic illnesses. Though they differ in their symptoms and the systems involved, both demand effective management.

What Is Chronic Illness?

Before defining the chronicity, it is appropriate to explain why we are referring to 'chronic illness' and not 'chronic disease'. What is the difference between disease and illness? 'Disease' refers to the pathophysiology of the condition that includes changes in the structure and function of a body's system. Contrarily, 'illness' connotes the perception of the condition, symptoms and experience of the suffering, coping with it and the responses of the family and health care providers. In other words, the term 'disease' is a biomedical concept, while 'illness' is a biopsychosocial concept. We will be explaining chronicity from a holistic perspective.

The term 'chronic illness' is widely used in several contexts such as clinical consultation, academic literature and discussion related to health policies. It is an umbrella term that connotes a number of characteristics and includes a number of diseases with those characteristics. However, the definition of chronic illness varies depending upon the focus on one or few characteristics.

Chronic illness is defined in terms of time line by some researchers. Warshaw (2006) defined it as "Conditions that last a year or more and require ongoing medical attention and/or limit activities of daily living". Chronic disease is referred to as "one lasting three months or more"

(Shiel, 2016). Even with those focusing on the time factor of the disease, there seems to be a difference. WHO (2016) defined chronic illness in detail. According to them, "chronic diseases are not passed from person to person. They are of long duration and generally slow progression". This definition focuses on the non-infection and non-contagious nature of the disease, as well as the pace of progression. Yet, it remains incomplete. Larsen (2016) argued that the definition of chronic illness should be from the perspective of the patient. According to her,

> chronic illness is the lived experience of the individual and family, diagnosed with chronic disease. The individual's and family's values impact their perceptions and beliefs of the condition and thus their illness and wellness behaviour. Their values are influenced by demographic, socioeconomic, technological, cultural and environmental variables. The lived experienced is 'known' only to the individual and family.

While the above argument is undisputable, this line of thinking may render the definition of chronic illness totally subjective.

What can be inferred from the above is that defining chronic illness has high complexity that involves a number of factors. It may be useful to first understand the essential characteristics of chronic illness and then derive a definition to include them all. Leventhal et al. (2004) stated that chronic diseases have five significant biological characteristics that categorically say that the diseases

1. Are systemic
2. Are life span problems, which do not manifest clinically up until middle age
3. Can be controlled (barring a few that can be cured)
4. Have the quality of impinging on a wide range of life activities
5. Are relatively quiet, punctuated by severe episodes of attacks

Chronic illnesses such as hypertension, type 2 diabetes involve more than one organ systems. Hypertension involves the heart and circulatory system, kidney functioning and the brain. In case of uncontrolled hypertension, the heart, kidney and the brain will be impacted. Similarly, in type 2 diabetes, the high level of blood glucose negatively impacts several organs and systems such as heart, kidneys, eyes and peripheral sensation.

These chronic illnesses have a longer history of their development in the body prior to their actual manifestation. Hypertension or type 2 diabetes starts developing in the body decades before the diagnosis is made. The development of these problems happens so silently that in majority of cases, hypertension because of the asymptomatic characteristic is diagnosed as a chance discovery when the blood pressure is routinely checked in the context of some other problems.

Be it hypertension, diabetes or asthma, it has long dormant periods interspersed by episodes of flare-ups. The blood pressure shoots up suddenly, the sugar levels spike up some days, and the wheezing attack knocks down a person with a severe episode. Very often, these episodes of attacks or flare-ups are considered periods of illness and the other periods as 'healthy'. This is typically because these periods attract the focus of cognitive and emotional dimensions. The illness management behaviour is actively involved during these episodes. The other quiet periods are ignored. The perceptual and experiential systems of the individuals are so designed to take into cognizance only the changes in conditions. Because of this, the flare-ups and episodes are treated just as an acute condition. Once it is managed effectively and the attack subsides, one is likely to ignore the dormant state of the disease once again. Thus, it is not uncommon for patients of chronic illness to treat the condition as sporadic episodes of acute attacks spaced across time periods.

Physiological Systems and Chronic Illness

Chronic illnesses are systematic. They are related to one or more systems of the human body. Each of the system has a number of diseases related to it. In most of the cases, the aetiology is genetic, hereditary, degeneration of cells/organs, exposure to high stress levels or health risk behaviour. The manifestation of symptoms is found to be either in adulthood or in late adulthood with a few exceptions of juvenile manifestations. It is believed that the diseases manifest after taking a long time to develop over a period of time. Until they manifest with symptoms, they remain dormant and silent. Depending on the system they are related to, the physical symptoms differ. Box 8.1 provides a list of chronic diseases related to various systems. However, this list is not exhaustive. A selected few are described in terms of aetiology, symptoms, treatment and prevention.

Box 8.1 Chronic Illness Related to the Systems

System	Diseases
I Cardiovascular system	1 Hypertension
	2 Arteriosclerosis
	3 Atherosclerosis
	4 Aneurysm
	5 Coronary artery/heart disease/coronary heart disease (CAD/CHD)
	6 Angina pectoris
	7 Myocardial infarction
	8 Rheumatic heart disease
	9 Congestive heart failure (CHF)
	10 Cardiomyopathy
	11 Valvular heart disease
	12 Arrhythmias
	13 Phlebitis
	14 Thrombophlebitis
	15 Deep vein thrombosis
	16 Varicose veins
II Pulmonary system	1 Chronic Obstructive Pulmonary Disease (COPD)
	2 Chronic bronchitis
	3 Emphysema
	4 Asthma
	5 Cystic fibrosis
	6 Adult Respiratory Distress Syndrome (ARDS)
	7 Lung cancer
III Endocrine system	1 Hyperpituitarism
	2 Hypopituitarism
	3 Hyperthyroidism
	4 Hypothyroidism
	5 Hyperparathyroidism
	6 Hypoparathyroidism
	7 Hypoadrenalism
	8 Diabetes mellitus
	9 Hypergonadism
	10 Hypogonadism

(*Continued*)

System	Diseases
IV Urinary system/renal system	1 Glomerulonephritis (chronic) 2 Renal failure 3 Adenocarcinoma of the kidney 4 Polycystic disease 5 Renal calculi 6 Urinary incontinence 7 Hydronephrosis
V Nervous system	1 Poliomyelitis 2 Degenerative disc disease 3 Headache 4 Epilepsy 5 Bell's palsy 6 Parkinson's disease 7 Dementias 8 Cerebrovascular accident
VI Digestive system	1 Gastritis 2 Peptic ulcer 3 Cancer of the stomach 4 Duodenal ulcer 5 Inflammatory Bowel Disease 6 Crohn's disease 7 Ulcerative colitis 8 Irritable Bowel Syndrome 9 Gastroenteritis 10 Carcinoma of the colon and rectum 11 Pancreatitis 12 Pancreatic cancer 13 Cirrhosis 14 Liver cancer 15 Hepatitis B, C 16 Cholecystitis 17 Cholelithiasis
VII Immune system	1 Rheumatic fever 2 Rheumatoid arthritis 3 Myasthenia gravis 4 Scleroderma 5 Lupus erythematosus
VIII Reproductive system	1 Premenstrual syndrome (PMDD) 2 Menopause 3 Endometriosis 4 Pelvic inflammatory disease 5 Vaginitis 6 Breast cancer 7 Prostatic cancer

The psychosocial aspects related to aetiology, symptoms and interventions are by and large common to many chronic illnesses. The discussion of the chronic illnesses has majorly focused on the biomedical aspects such as deviations in the functioning of the system/organ or the structure of the organs because of the glaring evidence produced by research in the field. However, the aetiology and interventions of various illnesses include the psychosocial factors without the mention of which the discussion is incomplete. Psychosocial interventions for chronic illnesses are discussed elaborately in general, while the interventions are suggested under each chronic disease. Some of the chronic illnesses are discussed by briefly explaining their symptoms, aetiology, treatment and prevention. The description is in simple non-technical language as done by Neighbors and Tannehill-Jones (2010).

Cardiovascular Diseases

This is an umbrella term that includes a number of diseases related to the heart (cardio) and the circulatory system or blood vessels (vascular). The most common symptoms of cardiovascular diseases are pain or tightness in the chest, shortness of breath, feeling of severe exhaustion, palpitation or irregular heartbeats. There are other symptoms that accompany the major symptoms. Profuse perspiration, blackout, fainting oedema in the limbs, nausea and vomiting are also experienced by many patients.

Some common diseases related to the cardiovascular system are discussed below.

Hypertension

This is a condition where the pressure of blood in the arteries is high creating tension in the blood vessels. This is a chronic condition that places the individual at risk for cardiovascular (blood vessels related to heart), cerebrovascular (blood vessels related to brain) and renal diseases.

Blood pressure (BP) that is considered to be normal is 120/80 mmHg (systolic/diastolic). If the systolic blood pressure ranges between 120 and 139 mmHg or the diastolic blood pressure ranges between 80 and 89 mmHg, the individual is diagnosed with pre-hypertension. When the BP is 140/90 mmHg or above, the person is diagnosed with hypertension. There are two major conditions where the arteries have high pressure of the blood flow:

a When the heart pumps more volume of blood.
b When the arteries narrow down.

The arteries have the characteristic of elasticity. They can accommodate the blood flow into their inner space. The inner space of the arteries is called lumen. The elasticity of the arteries is limited. When larger volume of blood is pumped into the arteries by the heart, the pressure of blood in the lumen is high.

The arteries narrow down because of reasons such as plaque formation in lumen or constriction of blood vessels due to high level of stress. When the inner surface of the lumen narrows down, the arteries experience the pressure of the blood flow.

Hypertension is of two types:

1 Primary hypertension or essential hypertension
2 Secondary hypertension

Aetiology

The aetiology of secondary hypertension is the disease to any organs such as kidneys, livers, lungs. Once the treatment to the diseased organ meets with good prognosis, the BP also drops down.

The cause of primary or essential hypertension is unknown. Some of the factors likely to contribute to primary hypertension are heredity, high salt/fat diet, obesity or high stress levels. Health risk behaviours such as smoking or having type 'A' personality are also considered to be contributing to primary hypertension.

Symptoms

Hypertension is known to be asymptomatic. The patient usually does not experience noticeable symptoms of the condition. Headaches, exhaustion, restlessness or sleep disturbance is normally misinterpreted and associated with various other reasons such as work pressure, heat, exposure to noise. If left untreated, hypertension damages the heart. This occurs because the heart while pumping larger volume of blood causes enlargement of the left ventricle, which is involved in pumping blood. This enlargement creating extra tissues does not have a proportionate increase in blood supply. It leads to a condition called ischaemia (reduced blood supply). Ischaemia causes episodes of angina (chest pain). The second consequence of untreated hypertension is a condition called arteriosclerosis (hardening of the arteries). This leads to lowering the arteries' power of elasticity. The chances of rupture of arteries are high.

Treatment

The treatment for hypertension is lifelong. The treatment package includes medication and lifestyle changes. The medication differs from person to person. Some medications are given for dilating the blood vessels to ease the blood flow. Some other medications include diuretics, which increase the urine output and thereby the volume of blood. Some patients are prescribed beta blockers, a class of medication that corrects abnormal heart rhythms. In view of this, it is advised to abide by the specific antihypertensive medication prescribed to a patient and not use the medication of another hypertensive patient as a temporary management measure.

Diets, low in fat and salt, are advocated for hypertension patients. Salt intake results in high sodium levels in the blood stream. Higher levels of salt result in water retention in body, which enhances the volume of blood. This leads to the overwork of kidneys that filter out the extra water. The kidneys gradually lose their ability to remove the water. Thus, the blood volume in the body is high. The heart is required to pump more blood into the arteries causing hypertension or high BP.

High intake of fat in diet causes cholesterol. High cholesterol in blood causes plaques in the arteries. Plaques and calcium (atherosclerosis) harden and narrow down the arteries. The heart has to exert much more strain to pump blood into them. For these reasons, patients with hypertension are advised low-fat and low-salt diet. Regular exercise helps in widening the artery pathways easing out the blood flow.

Prevention

Prevention of hypertension includes avoidance of health risk behaviours such as smoking sedentary lifestyle, and adopting health-promoting behaviour in diet, physical exercise and effective stress management. Maintaining the appropriate body weight is important prevention particularly for those who have family history of hypertension or cardiac-related illness.

Coronary Artery Disease (CAD)/Coronary Heart Disease (CHD)

This refers to a condition of the narrowing down of the arteries that supply blood to the heart muscle, called myocardium.

Aetiology

The cause of CAD is atherosclerosis as explained in detail under the aetiology and treatment of hypertension. The supplementary reason is psychological. People prone to type A personality, and those with inefficient management of anger and hostility are found to be at risk of CAD.

Symptoms

The main symptom is angina or pain in the chest due to ischaemia of heart muscle that is caused by overwork of the heart muscle in pumping blood into the hardened arteries.

The physiological symptoms include the following:

a One of the coronary arteries that supplies oxygenated blood to the heart muscle is blocked either due to the narrowing down of the artery or due to the formation of plaque, formation of blood clot or a blood clot travelling in the blood circulation and blocking the artery when the blood reaches there.
b This blockage deprives the heart muscle of the necessary oxygen.
c Lack of oxygen supply results in the gradual death of heart muscle.
d The process that causes death to the myocardium is called myocardial infarction, where 'infarct' means dead muscle. The infarction may either be a gradual process or be a sudden development.

Treatment

BIOMEDICAL INTERVENTION

Pharmacotherapy for angina involves medication for dilating the blood vessels. The other biomedical interventions are as follows:

a Angioplasty: This is a procedure where the narrowed blood vessel is opened by sending a catheter, which pushes the plaque and widens the lumen.
b Bypass Surgery or Coronary Artery Bypass Grafting (CABG): This is a surgical procedure. Here, the cardiothoracic surgeon creates an alternative path for supplying blood to heart by bypassing the blocked artery. Blood vessels from the breast area or the legs are chosen for alternative blood supply to myocardium.

PSYCHOSOCIAL INTERVENTIONS

a Type A Behaviour Modification Programme: Type 'A' behaviour is known to be highly stress-inducing. Research evidence indicates that type 'A' behaviour modification counselling to the patients who have suffered a myocardial infarction could successfully prevent 44% of second myocardial infarct (van den Akkar, 2012).
b Cognitive Behavioural Therapy is effective, particularly for patients who suffer infarction depression following myocardial infarction. It helps in reducing depression and social isolation.
c Psychological interventions with motivational interviewing, behavioural therapy of shaping to the patients for lifestyle changes and counselling for family for enhancing social support and planning appropriate reinforcement for healthy lifestyle behaviour of the patient help in introducing gradual change towards health-promoting behaviour.
d Stress management training in groups or tailor-made stress management programmes for the individual patients need to be designed for reducing stress levels through effective coping and adaptation.
e Standard physical exercise training in groups followed by motivational interventions helps in initiating and sustaining the behaviour.
f Psychoeducation in groups aimed at positive change in lifestyle is expected to provide a cognitive base. Mutual support and positive reinforcement from support group members are expected to function as a good motivator.

Angina Pectoris

This is otherwise known as chest pain or ischaemic chest pain. This is a symptom of coronary artery disease.

Aetiology

This is typically caused by prevention of oxygen supply to myocardium. Oxygen supply to heart muscle can be blocked either by a spasm in the muscle of the artery or due to atherosclerosis. In either case, the blood flow into the heart is restricted resulting in the lack of oxygen to the heart muscles.

Symptoms

The symptoms include a squeezing pain in the chest, tightness or heaviness in the chest accompanied by pain. The pain may radiate to left arm, neck and jaw. It may be a sudden onset or may recur. The main cause of this is overexertion of the heart. The heart overworks in many conditions such as physical strain, emotional upheaval or the need for digesting a huge meal. Many a time, angina is a signal for myocardial infarction in future.

Treatment

Pharmacotherapy involves vasodilators. When the patient suffers the angina pain, the medical advice normally is to place nitroglycerin under the tongue for immediate dilation of blood vessels that gives a quick relief.

Psychosocial interventions and prevention include all the measures discussed under coronary artery disease.

Myocardial Infarction

This translates to death of the tissues in heart muscle due to lack of oxygen.

Aetiology

What causes the lack of oxygen to the heart muscle? Activities that require more oxygen can be easily identified. They include physical exertion, shock, high level of stress. These situations demand the heart to function beyond its capacity. But, the volume of blood pumped is not adequate because of the condition of atherosclerosis. The consequence is the death of tissues in the heart muscles because of lack of or inadequate oxygen.

Symptoms

The symptoms normally include chest pain, with profuse sweating. The pain typically radiates to left arm, neck and jaw. There is uneasiness similar to indigestion. The symptoms vary in intensity depending upon the size of infarction.

Treatment

The first aid to myocardial infarction is to relieve the respiratory distress by making the air passage clear by making the patient lie down flat and loosening the clothes. The patient needs to be taken to the nearest hospital/nursing home for medical attention. Starting the oxygen line and pharmacotherapy is the immediate biomedical interventions.

The psychosocial intervention is the same as described under CAD.

Congestive Heart Failure (CHF)

This refers to a condition where the heart fails to pump the amount of blood required for the body parts. The blood vessels in the circulatory and respiratory system become congested. Heart failure can occur for two reasons:

a When the heart cannot pump adequate blood
b When the heart cannot fill adequately

The first condition is when the heart is at work (systolic) and the second when the heart is at rest (diastolic).

Aetiology

Development of congested heart failure is a slow process. It is normally preceded by a cardiac condition characterized by the exertion of heart. These could be myocardial infarction, coronary artery disease, rheumatic heart disease or even hypertension. In all these conditions, the heart muscle is found to overwork.

Symptoms

The prominent symptoms include shortness of breath, rapid heartbeat that is not explained by physical exertion, stress or anxiety. Such rapid heartbeat is known as tachycardia. Repeated tachycardia leads to a rapid decline in the function of left ventricle, slowly culminating in heart failure.

When the blood flow to body part is inadequate, the oxygen also will be inadequate. In order to compensate the loss of oxygen, one tries rapid breathing. Thus, the breathing is found to be short and fast. Progression of congestive heart failure is characterized by fluid build-up in the circulatory system. This can be seen in the form of oedema in the feet and ankle, distension of veins in the neck. Heart failure also results in congestion of liver and spleen or congestion of lungs.

Treatment

Pharmacotherapy aims at lowering the body fluids or slowing down and strengthening the heartbeat.

Psychosocial treatment aims at prevention of depression and social isolation because the CHF slows down the pace of patient. As a result, the patient may not be able to carry out regular activities one is used to including socializing. The severe exhaustion bears heavy on the patient. All these are likely to lead the patient to chronic depression. Psychosocial intervention has to be preventive in nature.

Cardiomyopathy

The term cardiomyopathy means cardiac muscle disease. In other words, it refers to a condition where the heart muscle deteriorates in its function of pumping blood, which happens due to contraction and expansion of cardiac muscle. The condition is found to lead to congestive heart failure and myocardial infarction, which are related to the weakening of cardiac muscle.

Aetiology & Types

There are two types of cardiomyopathy, viz. primary and secondary. The cause of primary cardiomyopathy is not established though an association between alcoholism and the condition is observed. The most common secondary type is dilated cardiomyopathy. In this, the heart muscle is found to lose the elasticity, which makes the heart enlarge. It is common experience that when a piece of elastic is continuously meddled by pulling from both ends, it tends to lose its elasticity and fails to contract and remains enlarged in size. The same logic applies to cardiac muscles. The enlarged heart muscle becomes weak in its function of pumping blood due to loss of elastic power. This leads to heart failure. Another type of cardiomyopathy characterized by enlargement of heart muscles is inherited. This enlargement is often found to cause leakage of heart valve. Yet, another type of secondary cardiomyopathy is normally found to be associated with ageing. In this type, the heart muscle is found to become rigid. The rigidity of the muscle also poses problems in contraction and expansion, thus making the pumping of blood difficult.

Symptoms

The symptoms are common with the congestive heart failure.

Treatment

This condition is treated with pharmacotherapy for maintaining the quality of life. The psychosocial interventions are the same as mentioned under CHF.

Varicose Veins

Varicose veins commonly appear in the lower extremities. They are the enlarged, swollen and twisted veins, blue or dark purple in appearance. In the leg region, blood is supposed to flow upwards against the gravity. This is facilitated by the leg muscles that contract and relax. The valves in the vein are supposed to close after the blood flows in a direction so that the retrograde of blood flow is prevented. The valves in varicose vein allow the blood to flow in wrong direction or cause a slow flow of blood and allow pooling of blood. Prolonged blood pooling in veins carries undue pressure on the walls of the vein and results in their stretching.

Aetiology

Activities that slow down the flow of blood in veins and increase in the pressure on the vein walls are responsible for varicose veins. Pressure of body weight on the lower part of the body is one of the reasons. Included under this category are conditions of obesity or pregnancy. Apart from this prolonged state of standing or sitting also causes the slowing down of blood flow. Hereditary is also a cause of this condition.

Symptoms

The prominent symptoms are cosmetic in nature. The veins get thick, hard and out of shape. The development of this condition is gradual. Very often, it is not painful. However, some patients do experience pain, swelling and heaviness around the veins that are enlarged. In severe cases, there can be significant bleeding in the vein or ulcer formation.

Treatment

More often, the medical advice for varicose veins is lifestyle changes. Lifestyle changes involve avoidance of prolonged standing posture, exercise for improving blood circulation, regulation of diet for losing weight. Positioning the legs elevatedly while in sitting or lying down also eases the blood flow. The patients are also advised to abstain from smoking. In short, inculcating health-promoting behaviour and avoidance of health risk behaviour is a good measure of treatment and prevention of varicose veins.

Stroke or Cerebrovascular Accident

This is a disorder that can be classified under the cardiovascular and nervous system. In simple terms, it refers to a condition where damage is caused to the brain from the interruption of blood supply to it. This has the potential to cause long-term disability. The severity of the consequences varies from mild to life-threatening. It could be a medical emergency.

Aetiology

Very often, the blood supply to the brain is interrupted because of arteriosclerosis. Due to inadequate supply of blood, some brain cells suffer lack of oxygen and die. The blood flow interruption can be caused due to two reasons:

a **Ischaemic Stroke:** Ischaemic stroke is a stroke to the brain caused due to the obstructions in the blood vessel that carries blood and oxygen from the heart. The main reasons for the obstruction are narrowing down of the vessels due to fatty deposits. These fatty deposits can lead to two types of blockages:

   i **Cerebral thrombosis:** A clot developed in the brain artery can plug and block the blood flow. Very often, the clot is formed where the blood vessel narrows down due to arteriosclerosis or thickening or hardening of the blood vessel.
   ii **Cerebral embolism:** This is a condition where the blood clot that forms at another location in the circulatory system due to plaques formed because of atherosclerosis breaks loose and travels in the blood stream. When it reaches the blood vessels in the brain and finds them too narrow, it plugs the path of blood flow.

   More often, the main cause for embolism is clots formed in the heart due to irregular heartbeats known as 'atrial fibrillation'. These clots get dislodged from heart and travel in the blood flow.

   In case of both thrombosis and embolism, the final outcome is blocking of the blood flow (known as ischaemia) and stroke. The difference between cerebral thrombosis and cerebral embolism is that in case of thrombosis, the clot is formed in the cerebral blood vessel, while in embolism, the clot is formed in other location.

b **Cerebral Haemorrhage:** This refers to the bleeding in the cerebral region. It happens because of uncontrolled hypertension and arteriosclerosis. The pressure on the blood vessels is high, and the elasticity of the vessels is lost because of arteriosclerosis that is characterized by hardening and thickening of the arterial walls. Unable to take the pressure of the flowing blood, the vessels rupture causing bleeding. The blood vessel rupture also takes place due to aneurism where the arteries become weak. The haemorrhage may occur in any blood vessel. This happens suddenly, and the symptoms are also sudden.

Symptoms

The symptoms of a cerebrovascular accident or stroke include one or more of the following:

a Dizziness
b Difficulty in walking
c Loss of motor balance or coordination
d Difficulty in speech
e Difficulty in comprehension and following instruction
f Numbness or paralysis in face, limbs or one side of the body
g Blurred vision
h A sudden severe headache
i Nausea or vomiting

Treatment

Medical attention given within the golden hour of onset of symptoms is highly recommended. If the patient suffers a paralysis, it takes very long for rehabilitation. Majority of patients with a severe stroke may not revive. Pharmacotherapy with anti-blood coagulants and antihypertension are aimed mainly at prevention of relapse.

Physical therapy and speech therapy are introduced when the stroke causes physical disability or speech problem. In many cases, depending upon the damaged tissues in area of brain, the patient loses certain faculties like hearing, speech, cognition, vision.

Prevention

Maintaining the normal blood pressure is the most important preventive measure. Those diagnosed with hypertension are the prime 'at-risk' group. High clinical adherence by hypertensive patient with adherence to medication, diet, exercise, stress management, regular monitoring and medical reviews is very essential in preventing cerebrovascular accidents. In addition, working on giving up the health risk behaviour such as smoking, sleep deprivation and managing the prescribed Body Mass Index (BMI) is also important precautions to be taken by a hypertensive patient.

Pulmonary Diseases

The pulmonary system is related to our breathing. It is also known as the respiratory system. This involves all the organs from the nose to lungs. Problems related to any of these organs or the process are brought under the category of illness related to pulmonary/respiratory system.

Cystic Fibrosis (CF)

Description: CF is characterized by mucous secretions, which are atypical and put the affected individual at risk for infections, particularly those affecting the pulmonary system.

302 Chronic Illness and Therapeutic Intervention

Complications could be often fatal for majority of the affected individuals. This is due to lung infections followed by problems related to sterility in men, issues related to puberty and insufficient functioning of the pancreas.

Aetiology: CF is a recessive monogenic disease. It is an autosomal recessive genetic condition affecting the respiratory and digestive systems. Two defective cystic fibrosis genes are inherited by the affected individual, one each from the two parents.

Symptoms: Symptoms are not generalized and may differ from individual to individual based on the severity of the condition. High levels of salt (sodium and chloride) in the sweat, pancreatitis and respiratory symptoms such as continuous cough with mucous productions, wheezing, dyspnoea (shortness of breath) and inflammation observed in the nasal passages characterize CF.

Treatment: The primary aim of any pharmacological treatment is to target the abnormal mucous production. Complicated biomedical treatment requiring adherence to a number of aspects places the patient and family in a difficult situation both physically and psychologically. Hence, the treatment plan should be inclusive of therapy addressing both these aspects (Figure 8.1).

Asthma

Description: Asthma, also known as bronchial asthma, is a chronic lung disease. It is a hypersensitivity disorder marked by difficulty in breathing due to inflammation and constriction of airways in lungs, often reversible voluntarily or with treatment. Severe asthmatic attack (asthmaticus) can be life-threatening.

Aetiology: Asthma is precipitated due to various factors (intrinsic or extrinsic). Psychosomatic explanations have also been provided to explain the aetiology. It is primarily attributed to either allergic or non-allergic causal factors. Chronic pulmonary infections may lead to an intrinsic attack. Allergens like dust, pollen and other irritants and changes in temperature are responsible for an extrinsic attack. Stress experienced by the individual is also one of the commonly studied aetiological factors. Asthma is also precipitated by neutral stimuli when they are conditioned to a stress-inducing stimulus. For example, a patient allergic to pollen may have an attack by the similar smelling incense stick.

Symptoms: Wheezing, severe dyspnoea, cough, chest tightness are all the hallmark symptoms experienced during an attack.

Treatment: Pharmacotherapy prescribes usage of bronchodilators and corticosteroids to provide relaxation to the muscles and control inflammation. Psychological therapies to provide relaxation, and develop desensitization to triggers and practising adherence to medical and exercise regimens are recommended to minimize and control the attacks. Psychoeducation about the disease and self-management skills play a key role in the treatment of asthma.

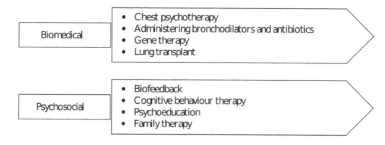

Figure 8.1 Comprehensive Treatment Plan for Cystic Fibrosis.

Prevention: The allergens causing the attack can be identified and managed/avoided. Relaxation therapy and avoidance of exposure to stress-inducing environment (e.g. visiting the terminally ill, participation in an agitation where emotions are high) constitute a good preventive measure.

Chronic Obstructive Pulmonary Disease (COPD)

Description: Chronic Obstructive Pulmonary Disease is characterized by airflow obstruction due to chronic bronchitis or emphysema. COPD is chronic and progressive in nature with no cure. Chronic bronchitis and emphysema are taken together under the umbrella term COPD as both the conditions share similar aetiology, pathophysiology and symptoms. Both the conditions coexist, with one of the conditions affecting the individual majorly. COPD is characterized by inflammation leading to obstruction of the lung tissue resulting in restricted or no airflow.

Aetiology: Cigarette or tobacco smoking is the leading cause of COPD diagnosis. Other risk factors include air pollution, exposure to hazardous occupational materials or experiencing any chronic respiratory conditions. A genetic abnormality α_1-anti-trypsin deficiency is known to cause about 1% of COPD cases.

Symptoms: Dyspnoea (shortness of breath), cyanosis (discolouration of skin, lips and nails), chronic cough, sputum production while coughing, pursed-lip breathing (resulting in sending air out of the lungs), weight loss, wheezing, obstructed airflow and haemoptysis (spitting blood while coughing) are some of the common symptoms of COPD.

Treatment: Pharmacotherapy inclusive of bronchodilators, inhalers, oral steroids and other medications primarily aims at symptom management. Treatment is provided to slow down the progression of the disease and enhance the individual's overall quality of life.

Pulmonary rehabilitation with a focus on smoking cessation needs attention from health psychologists to plan intervention modules in effective management of COPD. Motivational interviewing, cognitive therapy and aversion therapy for smoking cessation are some of the ways to stop the associated health risk behaviour.

Prevention: Preventive measures would include abstinence from smoking and avoiding respiratory irritants, ensuring that healthy dietary and exercise habits are incorporated in everyday schedule.

Abstinence from smoking calls for large-scale public awareness programmes. Such awareness programmes must target the institutions such as educational institutions, government institutions and private sector organizations. Workshops, symposia, booklets, video shows, flexes and banners, street plays, media shows, newspaper articles are the methods through which the campaign against smoking can spread across the countries. The pulmonary departments in hospitals can hold workshops for small groups of patients as part of the treatment package. The person who has successfully given up smoking sharing experience with patients would be a good measure to create cognition and provide a model.

Endocrine System–Related Diseases

The endocrine system refers to the number of glands and their hormonal secretion. These hormones are responsible for various functions in the body. Abnormality in the functioning of any glands in the body causes illnesses. They are classified as illnesses related to the endocrine system.

Thyroid Gland

The thyroid gland is responsible for managing the body's activity levels and growth. Excessive and inadequate amount of thyroid production results in hyperthyroidism and hypothyroidism respectively.

Hyperthyroidism (Overactive Thyroid)

Description: Hyperthyroidism is characterized by excessive production of the T_4 hormone by the thyroid gland.

Aetiology: The condition could be idiopathic in nature, i.e. where the cause is unknown. Otherwise, heredity, high intake of iodine in meals, excessive thyroid medication and tumours are some of the common causal factors for hyperthyroidism. Hyperthyroidism often results from an auto-immune condition called Grave's disease, which causes excessive secretion of the thyroid hormone.

Symptoms: There is a noticeable physical protrusion of the thyroid gland. The condition is called goitre. Commonly experienced symptoms include hyperactivity, tremors, weight loss, sleep troubles, intolerance to heat, bowel troubles, excessive thirst and sweating. Psychological consequences could include depression, anxiety, short attention span, nervousness and irritability.

Treatment: Treatment includes surgery to the thyroid gland, radioiodine therapy or medication to essentially treat the excessive levels of hormones secreted. Treatment should also focus on psychological rehabilitation to help individual's cope with changes resulting from hormone therapy. These issues can be addressed through Cognitive Behavioural Therapy to deal with negative psychological consequences and adapt to the recommended lifestyle changes.

The fact that a number of negative psychological reactions are associated with the hyperthyroid condition should be made known to the patient. Adherence to medication and its significance need to be explained to the patient.

Hypothyroidism (Underactive Thyroid)

Description: Hypothyroidism is characterized by inadequate secretion of the T_4 hormone by the thyroid gland. Congenitally acquired hypothyroidism is referred to as cretinism. Cretinism, if untreated, may result in physical and mental retardation.

Aetiology: Hypothyroidism might result from treatment undertaken for hyperthyroidism. An auto-immune condition called Hashimoto's disease or inadequate consumption of iodine can also cause hypothyroidism.

Symptoms: Symptoms associated with hypothyroidism are the converse of those associated with hyperthyroidism. Weight gain, low activity, fatigue, decreased sweating, constipation, skin dryness, intolerance for cold and pain are some of the commonly observed symptoms.

Treatment: The treatment primarily consists of hormone therapy to stimulate thyroid gland secretions. Psychological interventions are similar to hyperthyroid.

Diabetes Mellitus (DM)

Description: Diabetes mellitus is a chronic condition marked by a hike in the glucose level in the blood; it is known as hyperglycaemia. It primarily affects the body metabolism. There are two types of diabetes mellitus:

Type 1 Diabetes Mellitus

Type 1 diabetes was previously known as insulin-dependent diabetes mellitus (IDDM). The onset of this condition is usually seen in childhood; one is susceptible to this condition before the age of 25. This is attributed to genetic factors and due to the inability of the pancreatic glands to produce any amount of insulin. The other reason for it is a virus. In response to the virus, the immune system develops antibodies, which have the potential to kill the cells that produce insulin. This lack of insulin production affects the blood glucose levels in the body requiring the individual to depend on insulin injections.

Type 2 Diabetes Mellitus

Type 2 diabetes was previously known as non–insulin-dependent diabetes mellitus (NIDDM). The onset of this condition is usually seen in adulthood. This is attributed to lifestyle factors and due to the inability of the pancreatic glands to produce sufficient amounts of insulin. This insufficient insulin production affects the blood glucose levels in the body. Insulin injections are not recommended for type 2 diabetes.

Aetiology: It is caused due to pancreatic malfunction. Pancreatic islets of Langerhans do not produce any insulin in type 1 diabetes mellitus, while the pancreatic islets of Langerhans produce insufficient amount of insulin or cannot make use of the amount of insulin produced in type 2 diabetes. The risk factors for type 2 diabetes include obesity, large consumption of carbohydrates, atherosclerosis, high stress levels and sedentary lifestyle.

Symptoms: Excessive thirst, hunger and urination are characteristic symptoms of diabetes mellitus. Pain, problems in vision and fatigue are few of the other accompanying symptoms of the illness. Psychological factors to be considered in diabetes include non-compliance to healthy lifestyle and quality of life among patients. Non-compliance to diet, exercise and medication are attributed to the complexity of the prescribed regimens and the longer time period for which one is required to adhere. The patient's quality of life is adversely affected due to the physical disturbances interfering with one's everyday activities and interpersonal relationships.

Treatment: Treatment programmes include regimens for diet, medication and exercise to essentially keep in control one's blood sugar levels. Cognitive Behavioural Therapy, stress management techniques and psychoeducation are all recommended under psychological therapy.

Renal Diseases

The urinary or renal system does the job of cleaning. The renal system is responsible for filtering out the toxic particles and water from the blood. If this process is disrupted, the body fails to get purified blood. Problems with various parts involved in filtering function result in illnesses related to the renal system.

Chronic Glomerulonephritis

Description: Cluster of diseases affecting the kidney's glomeruli (filtering system) is referred to as glomerulonephritis. This condition is also known as nephritis, glomerular nephritis or nephrotic syndrome. When the glomeruli are affected, it impairs the filtering mechanism of the kidney resulting in the accumulation of bodily fluids and wastes. Glomeruli of the kidney play a crucial role in filtration. Chronic glomerulonephritis is usually asymptomatic for a long time before it is diagnosed. It progressively affects the functioning of the glomeruli in the kidney.

Chronic glomerulonephritis has the potential to cause complete kidney damage and may often result in chronic hypertension.

Aetiology: Chronic glomerulonephritis could have genetic cause in a few cases. Cause of the disease condition is often unknown. It is found to affect individuals with no prior history of any kidney problems. It could also be due to any abnormality related to the immune system, which is not diagnosed. Most often, recurring episodes of acute glomerulonephritis for a long time with exacerbation of the condition with each remission may affect the functioning of the kidneys fatally.

Symptoms: The symptoms include uraemia (waste products in blood), albuminuria (blood protein), oliguria (low levels of urine output) and haematuria (blood in urine), and oedema in various parts of the body, fever and lack of appetite reported during acute glomerulonephritis.

Treatment: Symptomatic treatment is recommended with emphasis on the treatment and management of blood pressure levels. Chronic glomerulonephritis has no specific treatment as such. Haemodialysis or kidney transplant is suggested for sustaining life. Dietary recommendations are advised for preventing further damage to kidneys or their failure and include limited intake or fluids, salt and proteins. When adherence to the prescribed diet becomes difficult, cognitive and behavioural interventions have to be given.

Renal Failure

Description: The incapacity of the kidneys to clear the blood of waste products is referred to as renal failure. The process of cleansing the blood involves formation of urea, which is filtered out of the body through kidneys during urination. The failure to filter out this urea leads to a high level of pent-up urea in the body known as uraemia or urine in blood. This finally leads to the urea getting converted to ammonia, which affects every other system and induces toxicity in the body.

Aetiology: The aetiology for acute and chronic renal failure is different. Chronic renal failure is gradually occurring and commonly due to chronic kidney diseases. Prolonged substance abuse, alcoholism and diabetes mellitus could also lead to renal failure.

Symptoms: Renal failure isn't significantly symptomatic until most of the kidney functioning is impaired. Common symptoms could be uraemia, issues related to fertility, indication of acute renal failure and bone weakness.

Treatment: Symptomatic treatment is suggested. Dietary regulations are emphasized by limiting sodium and protein intake, and medications such as antihypertensives, diuretics and related antibiotics are prescribed. Chronic failure is addressed through dialysis and transplantation of the kidneys. Often, as the frequency of dialysis increases, the day-to-day routine and social life of the individual are affected as everything has to be adjusted around the hospital visits for dialysis. This makes the individual feel constrained and dependent. Counselling from a health psychologist would be beneficial to the client in adjusting to the demands of this chronic condition. In case salt-free diet becomes difficult, the prescribed diet may be introduced following the behavioural techniques of shaping.

Prevention: Keeping the risk factors contributing to kidney failure under control is the way to prevent renal failure. Preventive measures could include abstinence from smoking, practising good dietary habits, indulging in regular physical activity and keeping one's weight under control. It is also important to ensure that both blood pressure and blood sugar levels are under control.

Nervous System and Diseases

The human nervous system is a complex controlling unit of the functioning of all the systems in the human body. It is related to physical sensation, motor action, affect, cognition and behaviour that encompasses simple behaviours like reading this part to solving a complex problem related to rocket sciences. Damage, degeneration or intrusion into this system results in a number of illnesses.

Epilepsy

Description: Epilepsy is a chronic disease resulting from an abnormality in the reticular system. The condition is marked by sporadic seizures resulting from abnormal electrical activity in the brain.
   Aetiology: The cause of epilepsy is unknown in most of the cases. Degenerative diseases, congenital conditions, tumours in the brain, alcoholism and other infectious diseases are some of the reasons why epilepsy is caused.
   Symptoms: People with epilepsy suffer from both physical and psychological symptoms. The individuals suffer from various types of seizures. They are petit mal, grand mal and status epilepticus. Unconsciousness, sensation and motor disturbances are characteristic features of the illness. Lack of control over one's physical condition, stigma associated with the condition, depression and anxiety are all commonly experienced.
   Treatment: The focus of treatment is to manage the epileptic seizures. Medication is prescribed for the same. Psychoeducation is recommended to help individuals deal with psychological consequences of the condition. Restoration and sustenance of a normal functioning of day-to-day life is the goal of psychotherapy.

Parkinson's Disease

Description: Parkinson's disease is a chronic neurodegenerative disease affecting areas in the midbrain.
   Aetiology: Although the cause is unknown in most cases, dopamine deficiency is thought to be responsible for acquiring this condition.
   Symptoms: Parkinson's disease is characterized by both motor (decelerated speech, tremors, rigidity in movement and crouched posture etc.) and non-motor (behavioural and sleep disorders, depression, urinary incontinence etc.) symptomology.
   Treatment: Symptomatic treatment is suggested for Parkinson's disease. While pharmacotherapy is recommended to treat symptoms, a more comprehensive approach inclusive of specialists to help deal with speech, behavioural and physical problems is suggested for better prognosis.
   Prevention: Supplementation of vitamin B_{12} is recommended as one of the preventive measures.

Spinal Cord Injury

Description: Spinal cord injury refers to neurological damage to the vertebral column protecting the spinal cord. It is characterized by disturbance or loss of motor control and sensation among other things. Based on the cause, location and severity of the damage, injury is determined. The injury might or might not result in paralysis based on the above-mentioned factors.
   Aetiology: Automobile accidents, falls, wounds, injuries resulting due to sports or occupational activities are some of the common causes leading to spinal cord damage.
   Symptoms: There are short-term and long-term consequences of spinal cord injury. Depending on the damage, partial or complete loss of movement is determined. Quadriplegia occurs

when there is complete damage to the cord in the neck region. Damage to the lower section of the cord results in paraplegia. Often, bladder and bowel movements and sexual dysfunction are experienced. Respiratory and cardiovascular troubles might also arise.

Treatment: Treatment focuses on arresting the damage caused and preventing further injury to the spine. Immediate treatment comprises of surgery and medication, while rehabilitation is suggested for sustained long-term care.

Dementia

Dementia is a syndrome with varied symptomology affecting the geriatric population. It is characterized by progressive loss of cognitive functions.

Alzheimer's Disease

Description: The most common type of dementia is Alzheimer's disease. Alzheimer's disease is a chronic brain disorder resulting from death of neurons. It is marked by cognitive deterioration affecting one's emotions, behaviour and personality. The behaviour of the person is highly unpredictable.

Aetiology: The exact cause for the condition is unknown. Heredity, infections and autoimmunity are thought to play a role in acquiring this condition.

Symptoms: Symptoms might range from mild cognitive impairments in the early stages to complete mental retardation in the later stages of the condition. Partial or complete loss of short-term memory, attention and communication problems, personality changes and inability to concentrate are some of the serious consequences of the condition. The individual is dependent on the caregiver for physical and emotional support. The emotional state of the patient has wide variations. The patient develops disorientation that progresses in time. Due to this, the behaviour of the patient is highly unpredictable. Loss of memory results in inability to recognize and interact with family members and friends. The conversations of the patient are marked by high irrelevance and incoherence.

Treatment: Treatment focuses on sustaining mobility and good physical health. Adequate care for ensuring a hygienic environment with emotional support is recommended.

Headache

Description: A very common problem resulting in pain could be due to some neurological pathology. Pain from a headache could range from mild to life-disabling based on the type of headache the individual suffers from.

Headaches are primarily classified into different types based on the frequency, severity and duration.

Headaches are commonly categorized into two types:

Primary Headache

These headaches are not attributed to any underlying medical conditions and could be due to any of the two reasons: tension or vascular changes affecting the vessels in brain. The common types of headache under this category include migraine and tension-type headaches among other types.

a **Migraine Headache:** Migraine headaches are thought to occur due to constriction and dilation of blood vessels. The individual essentially suffers from pain on the one side of the head near the temples. Migraines could be accompanied with aura (visual disturbances) or without aura. Nausea, vomiting and other bowel problems are also observed. Pain experienced from migraines could be incapacitating affecting the individual's overall quality of life.

b **Tension-Type Headache or muscle contraction headache:** This results from facial, neck and head responses to stressors. These headaches last long and induce a consistent throbbing pain.

Secondary Headache

These headaches stem from a secondary condition/illness such as fever, hypertension. In such cases, the headache is one of the symptoms of the conditions and not the primary illness affecting the individual.

Aetiology: Apart from the role of pathophysiology and heredity, headaches could be triggered due to a vast number of factors:

1 Environmental (fumes/smoke, changes in temperature, noises or allergies)
2 Dietary (consumption of certain food items, which are known to trigger particular headaches for few individuals, consumption of alcohol and not eating regular and timely meals)
3 Hormonal (headaches experienced during menstruation, headache induced by hormone therapy)
4 Emotional (experience of stress, personality disposition of the individual)
5 Lifestyle (irregular sleep patterns and lack of exercise)

Symptoms: Headache symptoms are experienced based on the nature of headache affecting the individual. Symptoms can range from mild to disturbing. They can be constant or intermittent in how they affect the individual. Dizziness, nausea and vomiting are some of the common symptoms of headaches.

Treatment: Treatment depends on the type of headache experienced. Pain management and symptom relief are the primary goals of treatment. Pharmacotherapy with relaxation and lifestyle modification are often suggested to control the frequency and intensity of the attacks. Biofeedback therapy is suggested across studies to treat headaches. Cognitive Behavioural Therapy for migraine headaches is found to be effective (Mehta & Dhal, 2010).

Prevention: Preventive measures include stress reduction, diet and lifestyle changes, abstaining from possible triggers and reducing anxiety to one's anxiety levels. Meditation and physical exercise are suggested to be incorporated in one's everyday life.

Gastrointestinal Diseases

It is the digestive system that is responsible for providing nutrition to the entire body. The digestive system involves a large number of organs starting with mouth to the rectum. A large number of chronic illnesses are associated with this system. We will discuss a selected few here.

Inflammatory Bowel Disease (IBD)

IBD constitutes two diseases: Crohn's disease and ulcerative colitis. Both the conditions are primarily the consequence of immune system dysfunction. They have an association with psychological distress in the diagnosis and prognosis. Distress and disease activity of both the conditions are interlinked and cause tremendous difficulty for the affected individuals. Treatment for these two conditions usually targets both the primary symptoms and the distress caused due to the periods of symptom flare-ups.

Crohn's Disease (CD)

Description: Crohn's disease is a chronic disease commonly grouped under Inflammatory Bowel Diseases (IBD). In Crohn's disease, there can be gradual and progressive inflammation observed in any part of the gastrointestinal tract.

Aetiology: There is no clarity yet on what specifically contributes to this disease. Genetic, immune system dysfunction, other infections and psychological factors are all suggested to be having a role in causing CD.

Symptoms: Frequently accompanying symptoms of the condition are abdominal pain, diarrhoea, fever and weight loss. Crohn's disease has periods of remission and exacerbation of the symptoms. It might lead to bowel cancer in severe cases. The psychosocial life of the individual is affected with disturbance in interpersonal relations at work and home. The patient is disturbed with dependency issues and concern over lack of control on one's bowel discharges. Patient is also preoccupied with constant anxiety about the prognosis.

Treatment: Symptomatic treatment is suggested, and surgical intervention is recommended to treat obstruction in severe cases. Treatment for CD includes anxiety measures through relaxation therapy. Rational Emotive Behavioural Therapy and cognitive interventions to reduce the anxiety and beliefs on interpersonal relations may help in reducing the symptoms.

Ulcerative Colitis (UC)

Description: Ulcerative colitis is an inflammatory bowel disease. It is characterized by chronic inflammation and ulceration of the colon and rectum. It does not include the inflammation of small intestine.

Aetiology: Causal factors are not known. Auto-immune triggers, role of hereditary factors and diet are all mentioned as causes. However, no substantial evidence in support of the suggestion is traced. Ulcerative colitis is observed to worsen during periods of increased stress. This suggests the condition to be psychosomatic.

Symptoms: Abdominal pain due to the ulcerations, anaemia, diarrhoea and bleeding is some of the commonly experienced symptoms. One of the severe complications is colon cancer.

Treatment: Pharmacotherapy with lifestyle modifications is suggested. Dietary changes and stress reduction are recommended. Guided Imagery, *Yoga nidra*, mindfulness, meditation are some of the relaxation exercises. Patients who have problems continuously in the relaxation technique may be recommended biofeedback.

Peptic Ulcer Disease (PUD)

Description: Ulcers are usually the resultant of overactivity of pepsin acting on the linings of the gastric tract. This happens when they fail to break down the proteins. Ulcers in the stomach are commonly referred to as gastric ulcers, while those affecting the duodenum are duodenal ulcers. The area acted upon by pepsin, when exposed to hydrochloric acid, exacerbates the condition.

Aetiology: The role of H pylori bacteria is suspected in causing the ulcers. Tobacco consumption, excess intake of alcohol and substance abuse are also factors thought to be contributing to the ulcers. Psychological stress experienced by the individual is often mentioned as a factor in worsening the condition of individuals with ulcers.

Symptoms: Intense pain in the stomach characterizes peptic ulcer. Acid reflux, nausea and weight loss are some of the common symptoms. Extremely complicated cases might result in bleeding and cause inadequate secretions or increased secretions of mucous in the stomach.

Treatment: The primary focus of treatment is to protect the stomach lining and ensure that the overacidic environment in the stomach is neutralized. This is achieved with the prescription of antibiotics and antacids. Surgical intervention is recommended in severe cases. Psychotherapy is suggested for acquiring stress management skills. Behavioural change in diet intake is effective. Changing the quality, quantity and frequency of diet needs to be attempted through cognitive intervention and stimulus control. Cultivating the habit of small quantity of intake at higher frequency may be tried through conditioning to the alarms and messages set to the mobile phone.

Irritable Bowel Syndrome (IBS)

Description: IBS is a chronic intestinal disorder of the large bowel with no lesions or inflammations. It is understood commonly as a motility disorder.

Aetiology: No specific factors are known to cause this condition. Gut infections, resistance to certain food products and psychogenic factors (stress) are all thought to be contributing to the condition. Alcohol and spicy foods are known to cause irritation resulting in the experience of IBS.

Symptoms: Commonly observed symptoms include diarrhoea and constipation. The individual might predominantly suffer from one of these or both.

Treatment: Pharmacotherapy is suggested to treat the accompanying symptoms. Cognitive Behavioural Therapy is recommended under psychological interventions for the clients. Stress reduction techniques (using biofeedback) are suggested. Cognitive affective interventions and stimulus control may have a positive effect on changing the diet and health risk behaviour.

Exposure to typical Indian therapeutic interventions that included *Yoga asanas*, practice of *pranayama*, meditation, adherence to *Sattvic* diet for 15 days was found to be effective for patients suffering from gastrointestinal disorders. They were found to have relief from anxiety and depression, associated with gastrointestinal problems (Mishra & Sinha, 2001).

Immune System–Related Diseases

The immune system protects the body from diseases. Ironically in certain conditions, they are found to cause diseases. They are called autoimmune disorders. When the immune system mistakes the healthy cells in the body for invading foreign bodies, they destroy the healthy cells, resulting in chronic conditions.

Rheumatoid Arthritis

Description: Rheumatoid arthritis is a chronic autoimmune disease affecting all age groups including children. It is referred to as juvenile arthritis (Still's disease) in children. The condition

312   *Chronic Illness and Therapeutic Intervention*

is characterized by inflammation caused primarily to the synovial tissue of the joints. Inflammation might affect any of the connective tissues in the body.

Aetiology: Causal factors contributing to this disabling condition are not known. In most cases, the condition is an outcome of autoimmune dysfunction.

Symptoms: Synovial tissue damage results in pain, swelling, stiffness and finally immobility. Characteristic symptom is the ulnar deviation observed in the fingers of hands. Many accompanying problems include other infections, anaemia and fatigue.

Treatment: There is no cure for arthritis. Periods of remission and exacerbation are commonly experienced by the individual with rheumatoid arthritis. Management includes pharmacotherapy to provide relief against symptoms. Psychological counselling, CBT, relaxation, self-efficacy training and coping skill training are helpful in preparing the patient to deal with the chronic condition. Interventions that include techniques for pain management would be highly helpful.

Pancreatitis

Description: Pancreatitis refers to inflammation of pancreas resulting in pain. There are two types of pancreatitis: acute and chronic.

Aetiology: Pancreatitis is idiopathic for majority of the diagnosed individuals. Heredity, alcoholism, autoimmune disease(s) and problems in pancreatic functioning (the presence of gallstones obstructing the pancreatic duct) are some of the commonly discussed causal factors of pancreatitis.

Symptoms: The symptoms for the acute and chronic pancreatitis are different. While the acute form is characterized by intense and sudden pain in the abdomen, severe back ache characterizes chronic pancreatitis. Vomiting and nausea are commonly reported. Gradually, pancreatic functioning is completely impaired and the individual might develop diabetes mellitus and other problems related to their digestive system.

Treatment: Treatment offered differs according to the cause and nature of pancreatitis. It could include anything from administering antioxidants to surgical interventions based on the severity of the condition. In case the patient develops anxiety over the condition, relaxation exercise helps in reducing the anxiety.

Reproductive System and Diseases

The reproductive system works in good coordination with the endocrinal system. This is responsible for the sexual behaviour. Disease to this system impacts the emotions, and behaviour directly and indirectly.

Premenstrual Syndrome (PMS) and Premenstrual Dysphoric Disorder (PMDD)

Description: Premenstrual syndrome (PMS) is a cluster of physical and psychological symptoms experienced by females prior to the onset of menstruation. 'Premenstrual tension' was the term coined in the very beginning to describe the clinical symptoms underlining the condition (Frank, 1931). Later, emotional tension was identified as only one of the many components of the condition. Greene and Dalton (1953) stated that all the other physical and emotional symptoms and fluctuations of these symptoms that have been associated with the menstrual cycle must be taken into account and proposed for the condition to be named as premenstrual syndrome.

Premenstrual syndrome is a very generic term, which is inclusive of an extensive range of physical, emotional, behavioural symptoms experienced by the women for several days to just a week before the onset of menses and recedes following the period of menstruation. These symptoms are interactional in nature (van den Akker, 2012). The severe form of PMS is premenstrual dysphoric disorder (PMDD).

Aetiology: The exact cause(s) underlining PMS/PMDD are still uncertain. The aetiology is assumed to be multifactorial and complex (Dickerson, Mazyck, Pharm, & Hunter, 2003). Figure 8.2 depicts the biological and psychological antecedents.

These factors are assumed to play a role in exacerbating the symptoms already experienced by the women, which are brought about by the hormonal activity before the onset of menses (van den Akker, 2012; Neighbors & Tannehill-Jones, 2010). Certain ingredients in diet such as caffeine, salt, chocolate, refined sugars and sedentary lifestyle contribute to aggravating the symptoms of PMS/PMDD though not responsible for causing the same (Swami, Narain, Kanwal, Mishra, & Singh, 2017).

Symptoms: Though more than 200 symptoms are considered to be associated with PMS, the most prominent and consistently discussed are irritability, tension and dysphoria (Steiner and Born, 2000). This refers to a state of general uneasiness, and unhappiness that lowers the feelings of wellbeing. The morbidity of the condition (PMS/PMDD) is often understood in terms of the severity and chronicity of the symptoms experienced by the women (Khajehei, 2015). Common somatic, behavioural and psychological symptoms are mentioned below (Figure 8.3).

Treatment: Elucidation of effective treatment of both PMS and PMDD has been problematic largely due to the difficulty in having accurate diagnostic criteria and measurement of the same (Steiner and Born, 2000). As there is no clarity regarding the causal factor(s) of PMS/PMDD, the goal of treatment is largely focused on symptom relief. Practice of yoga was found to be effective in relieving anxiety and depression in women having problems with menstrual cycle (Sridevi & Krishna Rao, 1996).

Approaches to treatment are broadly categorized into non-pharmacological and pharmacological as shown in Figure 8.4.

Chronic Illness and Psychological Factors

In a case study where the homemaker against the medical advice physically overexerted and encountered a flare-up of her arthritis, it disrupted almost every aspect of the lives of the patient, her husband and their relationship. This disrupts their plan for the long-awaited family reunion, stopped the husband from attending an important meeting outside the country, created a crisis even for meeting the daily needs since all household helpers were on leave. The husband while empathized with her condition was also annoyed with her for ignoring medical advice.

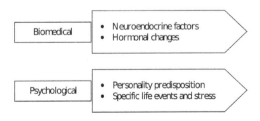

Figure 8.2 Aetiology of PMS (PMDD).

314 Chronic Illness and Therapeutic Intervention

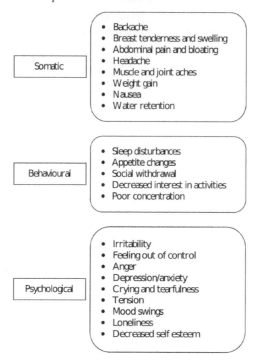

Figure 8.3 Biopsychosocial Symptoms of PMS/PMDD.

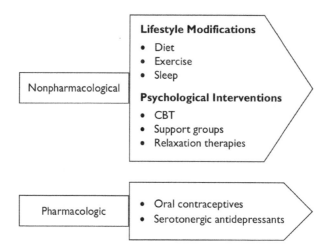

Figure 8.4 Treatment Approaches to PMS/PMDD.

The above example is a testimony to the fact that chronic illness has its impact on the physical status, and the changed physical status has its effect on multiple dimensions of life. The impact of a chronic condition is not only on the patient but also on the family.

The psychosocial factors associated with chronic conditions encompass the patient's and the family's

– Cognition of illness
– Emotions and
– Coping behaviour with the illness condition

Illness Cognition

Illness cognition refers to the person's own understanding of the disease. This comes not so much through reading, but a lot of it is contributed by one's own experience. A combination of learning from external sources and through experience constitutes one's illness cognition. Illness cognition is also known as illness perception or illness representation. According to Leventhal and Ian (2012), it refers to five dimensions related to patient's illness perception:

1 Identity of illness, where the symptoms are connected to a diagnosis that labels the disease
2 Time line or duration of the course of illness
3 Causes or aetiology of the disease
4 Consequences of the disease condition and
5 Cure/control of the disease through treatment

Individuals with the same chronic conditions are likely to differ in their perception of illness on these five dimensions. This is as natural as individual differences in perception of other aspects in life, such as education, marriage, an event, a gadget, a political party or even a simple aspect like a sunrise. Individual's past experience, sociodemographic aspects and cultural background contribute significantly to their perceptions, forming, developing and changing the schema. Illness perception is no exception to this. Experiences play a dominant role in illness perception. Such perceptions may not match the scientific facts, and may sometimes be irrational, or wrong; yet, they constitute the patient's unique perception on which the behaviour rests. Illness perceptions elicit the illness affect on the one hand and the behaviour on the other.

Individuals familiar with the labels of certain chronic diseases form a schema about it based on the information they have on it through reading, experience of others reported to them or witnessed. However, once they are diagnosed with a chronic disease, the schema is likely to undergo certain changes based on personal experience, direct advice from physician, and new information from medical research and so on. The mental schema of an illness is dynamic and is likely to change with every experience. These changes in the schema may sometimes be based on inaccurate information. But, in most of the cases, the treating physician does not make any efforts to assess the existing schema of the disease in their patients. Hence, there is high possibility that the patient's illness behaviour originates from an invalid schema rather than an unconvincing medical advice, and results in suboptimal prognosis. Hence, assessment and understanding of patients' illness perception/cognition/representation assumes significance for the physicians to make the necessary corrections if needed and enhance the adherence behaviour thereby as a measure of making the treatment effective.

As long as the schema of the disease is formulated on the basis of information from outside, the schema may be in line with the five factors delineated by Leventhal and Ian (2012). But once the individual experiences the illness, the schema may expand beyond these five objective dimensions. It includes the emotional dimensions associated with the suffering of the illness condition.

Symptom Perception

Perception of symptoms is part of illness cognition. Chronic illnesses typically have dormant phases punctuated by episodes of attacks, medical emergencies and flare-ups. The patients' health-seeking response depends upon their accuracy of perceiving the symptoms, classifying it as related or unrelated to the chronic condition, and, if related, the seriousness of it to warrant medical attention and if not 'manage' the same with self-medication or home remedies. Thus, the accuracy in perception of symptom determines the next course of action. Hence, it is important to understand the factors that influence the symptom perception. According to Broadbent and Petrie (2007), extreme symptoms are perceived accurately, followed by appropriate health behaviour. To elaborate this, we may take the example of severe pain in the chest accompanied by profuse sweating, which is perceived as signals of cardiac attack leading to immediate health-seeking behaviour.

The same is not true in perception of elevated blood pressure or heart rate because the symptoms are subtle and not perceivable by the patient. There is normally ambiguity of symptoms. A number of studies showed the inaccurate perception of symptoms by patients with chronic illness. People's perception of heart rate and blood pressure was found to be inaccurate and did not correlate with the actual readings taken in the laboratory (Pennebaker, 1984), and estimates of blood glucose levels manipulated in the laboratory settings (Cox et al., 1985). Though about 90% of hypertension patients claim that their close monitoring enables them to identify the escalation in their blood pressure indicated by their symptoms, there is evidence contrary to this (Brondolo et al., 1999; Meyer et al., 1985). The wrong perception of symptoms is associated with our readiness. Humans are attuned to perceive gross and obvious changes in our somatic systems and are not accustomed to notice the vague and subtle changes, unless one is trained well in doing so. In our day-to-day life, our attention is majorly focused on external factors rather than the physiological process within. Hence, unless there is a majorly observable deviation in the system it fails to catch the human attention.

Symptom perception relies on a combination of information from external and internal sources. The experiences of physical pain, discomfort or emotional state constitute the internal cues, while the expressed observations by others or one's own encounter with certain situations may contribute to external cues. To explain it better, we can use an example. A patient with primary hypertension may feel that his/her blood pressure is high when someone makes an observation that he/she looks very tired, or when one feels exhausted after a heavy schedule in the whole week. Thus, a normal feeling of exhaustion is likely to be misrepresented as an illness symptom.

Symptom perception normally coincides with the illness schema one has. Based on this schema, one indulges in the process of screening the cues or information and selects only those that fit into the existing schema. For example, the common idea about symptoms of heart attacks consists of pain in the chest, radiating to the left hand, profuse sweating and problem in breathing. Going by this schema, it is likely for a cardiac patient to ignore the symptom experiencing some tightness and discomfort in the chest followed by an urge to pass motion as a 'gastric attack', while it could be the alarm for a heart attack. Once this is experienced and the patient survives the attack, these symptoms change the previous schema of heart attack and include the other symptoms to it. Next time, when the patient really experiences a discomfort above the diaphragm combined with an urge to pass motion, he/she is likely to perceive it as a symptom of heart attack.

The schema of the illness changes continuously. The schema includes not only the label, cause, consequences, time line and controllability of the disease, but also the concerns and worries, apprehensions and hopes, the symptom-appropriate behaviour and their consequences and the impact of flare-ups on the family members. The changes in schema happen with every new experience. For example, if the patient experiences no relief in pain or discomfort with one medication, then the schema changes with regard to the outcome of medication. The schema may change because of one's own failure of outcome with a medicine or a report of the same by a significant other.

Affect State

The role of emotions or affect in chronic illness cannot be undermined for various reasons:

- The emotional state of the patient has a significant bearing on the health-seeking behaviour and adherence to medical advice.
- The affect state of the patient significantly contributes to the treatment outcome or prognosis.
- The positive or negative affect is closely associated with illness representation. Illness cognition contributes to the patient's affect state, and the affect state constitutes a significant part of illness cognition. Thus, there is a two-way relationship between the two.

Negative mood, trait and affect state are found to exacerbate the illness symptoms. An arthritis patient with high levels of anxiety is more likely to experience more severe pains than the one in the same condition maintaining a positive affect state. Negative moods in chronic patients also tend to restrict their activities. Patients with high negative affect are found to be hypervigilant. They normally indulge in increased scanning of even minor experiences, notice increased number of symptoms and attribute the same to their chronic illness (Broadbent & Petrie, 2007). When a wide range of symptoms are perceived and reported, there is a probability of confusing the physician and thereby misleading the line of the medical investigation process.

It is expected that patients with chronic illnesses such as cancer, cardiovascular disease, arthritis experience higher levels of negative affect compared to the normal. However, the research evidence disputes it as a misnomer. The findings failed to establish higher prevalence of depression, anxiety or psychological distress among patients with chronic illness. Nevertheless, the chronically ill do undergo episodes of emotional distress in the form of anxiety or depression.

Antoni et al. (2001) made a reference to the possibility of positive emotional reaction as an outcome of severe and life-threatening chronic illness. They argued that there may be instances when a chronic illness diagnosed in the patient makes an allowance to escape from a distressing life burden. There may also be occasion when the patient after a diagnosis of a chronic illness starts discovering in oneself the mastery, personal strength, competence and resilience. Such new insights about one's own positive characteristics are associated with positive emotions. This is possible only in cases of illnesses that can be effectively managed through high self-efficacy but not with those illness conditions, where the progression of the disease is irreversible and has a debilitating effect.

Association between Chronic Condition and Negative Emotions

There are two possible associations between chronic illness and negative affect:

1 **Direct association**: Here, the characteristics of the disease may induce or suppress certain hormones and cause depression.
2 **Indirect association**: Perception of several deprivations, restrictions and limitations enforced by the disease may lead to anxiety, depression and other negative emotions in the patient.

Direct Association

Chronic illnesses bring in certain physiological changes in the system. Sometimes, these physiological changes may be such that they have the potential to trigger depression or anxiety. Leventhal and Leventhal (2004) argued that direct association between the affect and disease-related physiological changes is found more in neurological diseases. In case of Parkinson's disease, one of the characteristics of the disease is the reduction in cerebrospinal fluid (CSF) levels of what is known as 5-hydroxyindoleacetic acid (5-HIAA). This is the major metabolite of serotonin. The reduction in this is found to be responsible for about 40% of prevalence of depression (Cummings, 1992).

We have already discussed about the hypothalamic-pituitary-adrenal (HPA) axis getting activated during stressful encounters. Dysregulation of this axis induces to generate pro-inflammatory cytokines, which is found to be implicated in inciting the depressive processes. In case of diabetes, the HPA dysregulation is identified. Further, the pro-inflammatory cytokines induced by the depression also positively contribute to maintaining the diabetic condition. The diabetic condition again causes HPA dysregulation. Thus, it forms a vicious circle, associating diabetes with depression.

Indirect Association

The indirect association between chronic illnesses can be explained through the link between body and mind. The chronic condition of the patient may give rise to a number of discomforts, pain and disability at the physical level. This experience has a bearing on the psychological state of the individual. Secondly, the chronic condition of the patient may demand a number of restrictions in the lifestyle. For example, restrictions in diet for a hypertensive and diabetic to minimize the intake of salt and sugar respectively create a feeling of being deprived of the enjoyable dish. Adherence to low-fat, low-carbohydrate diet, restriction in the quantity and frequency of food, having to self-inject insulin lead to impose checks during social eating. They may be cause for embarrassment at times when in a social function, due to diabetic condition, one cannot wait to join others until the dinner is formally announced because one's blood glucose level suddenly drops leading to fainting sensations drawing the attention of everybody in the function. Gradually, a patient with chronic diabetes may start avoiding social functions. Feelings of social isolation and deprivation of social participation are likely to lead to depression. While the example cited above relates to the diabetic condition, the consequences of social isolation and deprivation are true in case of other chronic conditions such as arthritis, hypertension, migraine, epilepsy or neurological conditions such as Parkinson's disease. The reasons may be many, such as social embarrassment, avoidance of inconvenience to others, unsuitability of the event to the illness condition.

In certain cases, the medication used for the chronic condition may give rise to negative emotions such as side effects. For example, the process of reducing blood sugar levels through insulin generates the feelings of fatigue and anxiety, which are also the feature of depression.

Depression, anxiety and anger are found to be related to chronic illness when there is activity restriction, physical disability or hospitalization. It is the functional impairment and loss of autonomy due to chronic illness that causes negative emotions than the chronicity of the disease itself. Early research has the evidence for the physical inactivity playing a significant mediating role in the association between chronic condition and depression (Aikens, Aikens, Wallander, & Hunt, 1997).

While the association between chronic illness and negative affect is evident, the path and process of relationship seem to be complex with a number of factors playing their role. However, it is important to emphasize on the existence of association between chronicity and negative affect so that screening for the affect state constitutes part of the diagnostic package followed by appropriate intervention forming a part of treatment package.

There have been a number of recent research investigating into the negative affect as comorbid condition among the chronic patients. Peltzer and Pengpid (2016) attempted to estimate anxiety and depressive features in various chronic diseases among patients in three South Asian countries like Cambodia, Myanmar and Vietnam. They administered HADS on a sample of 4803 adult patients. Results revealed that 17% of patients tested positive for anxiety disorders, while 39.1% were found to have depressive disorder. The highest rate of anxiety was found among cancer patients. The highest rate of depression was found in patients with Chronic Obstructive Pulmonary Disorder (COPD) followed by those with kidney diseases, Parkinson's disease and cardiovascular disease. Further, having more than one chronic condition and poor quality of life was associated with anxiety, as well as depression.

A study by Hariharan, Gadiraju, Kishore and Vemuganti (2014) attempted to estimate the prevalence of anxiety and depression in patients with chronic illness related to cardiovascular, pulmonary, gastrointestinal systems and skin diseases. The sample constituted 664 patients visiting the hospital for clinical consultation related to their ailments in any one of the four systems mentioned above. The patients were first screened by Patient Health Questionnaire 9 (PHQ 9), and then administered Hospital Anxiety and Depression Scale (HADS) and Beck's Depression Inventory (BDI). Projections were made for prevalence of depression and anxiety in patients with chronic problems in the four areas. Table 8.1 presents the prevalence rates among patients.

The prevalence of depression and anxiety as found from the table is alarming for all chronic conditions. The negative emotions in these cases were not diagnosed until the study administered them the relevant tests. Thus, the negative affect remained undiagnosed and untreated. The negative affect left with no intervention is not a desirable condition because the emotional state is closely associated with the illness behaviour and particularly clinical adherence.

Chronic patients with depression and anxiety are likely to have exaggerated perception of their symptoms, which further contributes to their negative affect. It is not uncommon for them to associate even the unrelated symptoms with their disease condition. Katon, Lin and Kroenke (2007) carried out a systematic review of research between 1966 and 2006 using the database related to chronic illness of diabetes, coronary artery disease, congestive heart failure, asthma, COPD, osteoarthritis, rheumatoid arthritis with associated symptoms of depression and anxiety. Their findings suggested a strong association between somatic symptoms and depression and anxiety. The association between them was found to be as strong as their association with objective physiological markers. In case of two studies, there was an indication that improvement in affect states was related to drop in somatic symptoms though there were no improvements in physiological levels. This suggests the close association between the cognition and affect. The negative affect and enhanced symptom perception are closely related.

Table 8.1 Prevalence of depression and anxiety among patients with chronic illness related to cardiovascular, pulmonary, gastrointestinal and dermatological diseases (prevalence per population of 1000)

	Depression		*Anxiety*	
	Moderate	*Severe*	*Borderline*	*Caseness*
Cardiovascular	236	133	140	321
Pulmonary	127	133	121	267
Gastrointestinal	136	82	153	306
Dermatological	61	79	134	171

While the negative affect is associated with illness cognition, it is also associated with the health/illness behaviour of the patient. As already discussed, the patients with chronic illness have disease-appropriate prohibitions in lifestyle. For example, smoking is prohibited for patients with cardiovascular and pulmonary diseases, and alcohol is restricted for patients with diabetes and cardiovascular disease and prohibited for patients with liver problems. However, alcohol and tobacco consumptions are addictive and closely related to the emotional states. This is a sufficient reason for screening the chronic patients for affect state and treating them with appropriate intervention for negative effects such as anxiety and depression.

Banhato et al. (2016) conducted a study on patients with multiple chronic conditions to identify the symptoms of depression and investigate the concomitant risk factors associated with it. The sample consisted of 1558 participants with more than one chronic condition that included hypertension, diabetes and chronic kidney disease. Results revealed that the largest percentage of patients (36.07%) with diabetes were found to have depression followed by those with hypertension (33.75%) and chronic kidney disease (30.56%). Large percentage (20.20%) of people with three chronic conditions suffered from depression compared to those with two (5.20%) and a single (4.60%) chronic condition. The larger percentage of women were found to have depression compared to men. Smokers among the patients were found to show depressive symptoms. The authors stated that about 70% of cigarettes smoked by the patients with depression were the ones with higher degree of nicotine dependence. This suggests the potential risk of perpetuation of smoking behaviour among those chronic patients with the comorbid condition of depression.

Chronic patients with negative affect are more likely to have non-adherence or low adherence to the prescribed lifestyle that constitutes part of the disease management package. Effective coping with the illness has the key for keeping the illness under control.

Illness-Stress Relationship

It is not appropriate to draw generalized inferences related to adjustment with chronic illnesses. Several factors have their significant influence. Coping behaviour with the illness depends on the answers to a series of questions. What is the personality make-up of the patient? Is the chronic condition treatable? Curable? Does it involve lot of pain and discomfort? Is it potentially life-threatening? Is the progression of the disease fast? Does it create disability? Does it shorten the life? The answers to every question posed here contribute to the coping behaviour of the patient. For example, coping with the diagnosis of hypertension cannot be the same as the diagnosis of duodenal cancer in the last stage. Such complexities involved in the implications of diagnosis make it impossible to group all chronic illnesses into one sample and draw generalized statements on coping behaviour with respect to one common aspect like the illness duration.

Coping refers to a dynamic process triggered by the cognitive appraisal of the situation that analyses whether the situations has a potential threat or harm to the individual, the availability of the resources to mitigate the threat and the possible outcome of action. The process of coping involves the person, the environment and the relation between the two. The cognitive assessment includes the personal stakes involved, locus of control, and internal and external resources necessary to encounter the situation so that the impact of the stress is minimized by changing the situation itself. Effective coping typically includes emotional management and problem solving as a dual process. Instances where the chronic disease diagnosed is life-threatening or has possible progressive increase in severity of pain or disability invoke psychological distress right at the point of communication of diagnosis. It can bring a flood of reactions such as shock, disbelief, denial, anger, sadness, guilt, grief, helplessness, hopelessness. One may experience a roller-coaster of emotions. In such cases, effective coping should first aim at managing the emotional reactions. Jensen, Moore, Bockow, Ehde and Engel (2011) reviewed 29 articles to come up with coping related treatment goals for chronic patients with two common factors—pain and disability. Their review included patients with spinal cord injury, muscular dystrophy, multiple sclerosis, acquired amputation and cerebral palsy. Results suggested three sets of major measures to be included in the treatment package:

1 Task persistence, acceptance of disability, behavioural activities, exercise, ignorance of pain
2 Augmenting the self-efficacy in controlling the pain and its outcome
3 Seeking and obtaining social support.

Acceptance of disability is related to emotional management through cognitive exercise. Augmenting self-efficacy works on the motivation. Ignorance of pain combined with task persistence and engagement in activities distracts the attention from pain. Seeking and obtaining social support is the concrete problem-solving measure. Thus, coping behaviour involves activating cognition, emotion and behavioural dimensions in realistic manner.

Coping (behaviour) with chronic illness refers not just to the observable overt behaviour of the patient, but a number of covert processes preceding it. Illness behaviour may be a very simple straightforward response like seeking a medical treatment or a complex set of behaviours that include the patient's perception and interpretation of symptoms, emotional response to the illness and treatment-seeking response. Illness behaviour is not necessarily a negative behaviour. It can be a health-seeking behaviour too. It is defined as "varying ways individuals respond to bodily indications, how they monitor internal states, define and interpret symptoms, make attributions, take remedial actions and utilize various sources of formal and informal care" (Mechanic, 1995). We can state that illness behaviour refers to the set of covert and overt behaviour that involves illness perception, emotional reactions to the illness experience and its multifaceted connotation, and the overt behavioural response such as treatment seeking, compliance to medical advice that includes lifestyle changes. This demands coping with a number of factors that are internal and external. Apart from coping with the illness condition, the following are some major factors arising out of the chronic condition with which one needs to adjust or cope.

– Uncertainty
– Affect state as a direct or indirect outcome of illness
– Social isolation
– Powerlessness and loss of control
– Vulnerability, loss of dignity and stigma
– Diverse social response to the illness condition

Emotions Due To Uncertainty

Uncertainty is an integral part of chronic illness. It starts from the time of noticing the symptoms and continues at every stage. Once the person perceives the basic symptoms of an illness, a doubt originates in the mind (based on the existing schema of a disease) if the symptoms are suggestive of a particular disease. This doubt or uncertainty continues until the formal diagnosis is pronounced by the physician. Once this stage is crossed, there is ambiguity related to a number of aspects related to the disease such as its progression, treatment line, outcome possibilities, aetiology, side effects of treatment, alarms for medical emergency, financial drain, the possible impact on professional efficiency. Thus, the uncertainty in chronic illness seems never ending.

The uncertainty adds cognitive stress to the patient who is already physically stressed by the pain and discomfort caused by the chronic condition. The perpetual uncertainty about various aspects leads to a feeling of loss of control and helplessness that disrupts advanced planning and coping. Many times, when the patient encounters sudden changes in the health condition, it causes emotional distress and diminishes the quality of life. Uncertainty and unpredictability related to the disease create lot of confusion and the patient feels at loss to comprehend the meaning and the process of the disease.

The fact that a patient with asthma has been active until five minutes before suffering an acute attack and now requires immediate hospitalization gives rise to a feeling of inconsistency in experiencing health or illness. A patient with diabetes experiencing giddiness and falling unconscious may realize that the last time that one experienced the same feeling was due to the extreme heat, and never attributed the present experience to hypoglycaemia, and feel a sense of ambiguity and unpredictability of the symptoms and their causes. A hypertensive patient who suddenly experiences a facial paralysis may not understand the reason or the experience of the facial muscles pulling towards one side, and may find this unfamiliar experience highly dreadful. Thus, unpredictability, unfamiliarity, inconsistency and ambiguity are embedded in the very experience of chronic disease (Penrod, 2001). The element of uncertainty is certainly an added burden on the patient and family.

The patient may experience uncertain about various dimensions related to the chronic condition. There may be

- Lack of clarity about the illness itself. In other words, patient may not be able to understand whether the illness relates to digestive system, respiratory or cardiac
- Lack of information regarding the complexity and seriousness of the condition
- Ignorance about the treatment line, the time line of the disease and logic related to lifestyle change
- Ambiguity about the symptoms related to the chronic condition
- Lack of comprehension about the significance of reviews with the physician

It may not be wrong to state that most of the uncertainties are related to lack of or inadequate information, which is avoidable with improving doctor-patient communication. While the prevention for uncertainty is a small step, the impact of it is so huge that adds to the stress levels of the patient. The multiple impact of uncertainty on the patients is presented in Figure 8.5.

The patient is likely to experience doubt and uncertainty when the prognosis is vague, or contrary to expected lines. There is confusion and uncertainty when the patient receives contradictory information from different sources.

Sometimes, the patients may not be able to distinguish whether certain symptoms are related to their chronic conditions or due to natural reasons such as overexertions, ageing or climatic changes. For a patient awaiting diagnosis, for the one awaiting the surgery or a procedure, for the one recovering after surgery, the common experience is uncertainty and apprehension. For a cancer patient, while there is uncertainty preceding diagnosis and procedure like surgery, chemotherapy or radiation, the same uncertainty continues even after a successful treatment, when the patient lives in apprehension of recurrence. Once there is recurrence, there is uncertainty about the disease progression, pain and death. Thus, there is no phase in the life of a chronic patient where there is the absence of uncertainty. Research evidence indicates that the waiting period has the highest uncertainty. It is described as "a gruelling experience of unsure stillness" (Bournes & Mitchell, 2002, p. 62), a limbo (Montgomery, 2010) and "physical condition would experience a setback" (Arber & Spencer, 2013). Sense of vulnerability and unpredictability of future causes anxiety in chronic patients (Fisher & Crawley, 2013).

Chronic Illness and Therapeutic Interventions 323

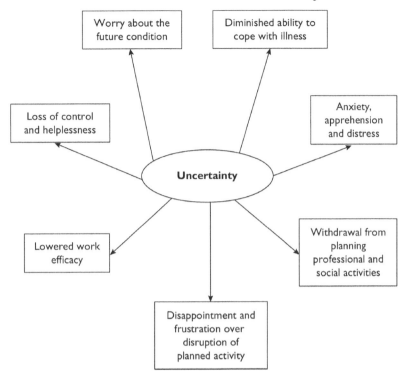

Figure 8.5 Impact of Uncertainty on Chronic Patients.

Prolonged hospitalization, bed rest or restricted activities limit socialization of patients leading to depression. Depression perpetuates inertia in chronic patients impacting adherence to medical advice. Anxiety and depression negatively contribute to prognosis. Hence, efforts need to be made in the direction of minimizing uncertainty.

Social Isolation

One of the positive contributions for good prognosis is the social support. Social isolation is a situation that deprives the patient of the advantage of social support. Social isolation can be voluntary or inadvertent. It happens when the individual withdraws not only physically but also psychologically from the highly desired social network resulting in a loss of place for oneself in the social group. As a result, the individual may deprive oneself from fulfilling the need for affiliation, fading out the activity of engagement with others, thus minimizing both the quantity and quality of social relationships.

Very often, social isolation among the chronic patients happens gradually but not suddenly. It is closely associated with the progression of the disease, onset of physical or mental disabilities, restriction on mobility or limitation in the ability to engage in social interaction. This is inadvertent. However, there is a possibility of voluntary social isolation in chronic patients. This happens when their body image is negatively impacted, or they perceive that the symptoms of their illness cause them social embarrassment. Nicholson and Shellman (2013) argued that individuals who are overweight may choose social isolation because of enhanced self-consciousness.

Research findings suggest that an increase in health problems leads to social isolation. Havens et al. (2004) found that older adults with multiple chronic conditions run increased risk of social isolation. Prevention of social isolation to a certain extent is under the control of the patients. Positive perception of one's condition as 'fit enough' to continue social engagement is a good preventive step. The patient's own perception and rating of health condition constitutes one of the determinants of social isolation. Those who have negative perceptions about their health and rate their health condition low are likely to experience more social isolation (Nicholson et al., 2013). Those chronic patients experiencing sleep deprivation during night find it difficult to engage in social relationship during the daytime. Passive participation may create mutual disinterest leading to social withdrawal.

Negative affect state like anxiety, depression or anger and irritability due to physical pain, discomfort or sleep deprivation may contribute to social distancing. Nicholson et al. (2013) found that people with depression have higher risk of social isolation.

Social isolation is a consequence of many factors related to chronic illness. Indian culture being highly affiliation-oriented, people experiencing illness require social support to a greater degree to enhance the healing process.

Powerlessness and Loss of Control

Internal locus of control, hope, physical activity, predictability, goal orientation and planning are some of the desirable integral part of life closely associated with wellbeing. There are the characteristics that the chronic condition of a patient may gradually forego owing to the illness condition. Perception of internal locus of control is self-reinforcing when the person attains control over situation in life. However, a chronic patient, originally oriented to internal locus of control, will gradually realize the loss of control over self with the progression of disease. Instances of symptom aggravation, poor prognosis of therapeutic intervention contrary to expectation, failing physical abilities associated with restrictions in activities, drug reactions, sleep disruptions, and diminishing productivity as the impact of chronic illnesses make the patient realize that his/her grip over the events in one's own life is now being loosened only to be lost gradually.

This loss of personal control over matters related to one's own life leads to loss of self-confidence and emotional turmoil, especially for a person who has been enjoying internal locus of control. Sometimes, the patient may experience a sense of personal loss, aggression and irritability over the loss of control, which in turn adversely contributes to a feeling of wellbeing. Failing physical health, placing restrictions on physical mobility or receding cognitive functioning as a part of disease progression forces the patient to accept the lack of internal locus of control and brings in with it a feeling of powerlessness. Thus, loss of internal control and feeling of powerlessness are closely interrelated.

'Power' refers to the ability of a person to act in order to produce the intended result. It is possible only when one possesses the control, authority and influence over the situation. 'Powerlessness' refers to the absence of all these resources. It leaves a person with the feeling of loss of resources to bring a desired result to enhance one's own wellbeing. A sense of powerlessness among the chronic patients has association of a self-image of worthlessness. The feelings of powerlessness may be real or perceived. A number of factors contribute to the feelings of powerlessness. They may be the direct outcome of chronic condition or the offshoot of the illness.

Failing physical health that is perceived as beyond one's personal control, pain, discomfort, suboptimal prognosis, events of flare-ups, resistance to medication, failure of a procedure or medical complications are some of the factors related to treatment issues. When the physiological system goes beyond the voluntary control of patient, it gives a severe sense of powerlessness. For example, experience of incontinence in patients was found to be associated with powerlessness (Hägglund & Ahlström, 2007).

There are a number of factors that are beyond the medical aspects and psychosocial in nature that subscribe to the feeling of powerlessness. Perception of physical disability or weakness may have an adverse impact on the patient's future plans and dreams. The realization that the progressive decline in quality of life leaves the cherished goal in life unattained gives a patient a severe sense of powerlessness in addition to depressive feelings. Increasing dependence on others for minor and major tasks adds to the feelings of compromise with one's own autonomy. This in turn also closely related to the loss of dignity apart from the sense of powerlessness.

In case the person, owing to chronic condition, has to lose the pay in the job due to prolonged absence or has to give up the job owing to health condition, one not just feels the economic loss, but also misses the long habituated daily routine, a sense of affiliation to the organization and a loss of social and professional identity. All these significantly contribute to the feelings of powerlessness. Walker (2010) found out how chronic patients who leave their job experience ruptured identities.

With the increasing complexity in chronic condition, the patient is likely to lose confidence and the ability to assess one's needs. Such situations attract intervention from others who coerce and convince the patient to initiate an activity or suspend one depending on the situation. Giving into such coercion by family caregivers or health care professionals reinforces the feelings of powerlessness and loss of control. It is very difficult to decide when a chronic patient should be relieved of self-management of illness. Self-management is something that positively contributes the sense of personal control, which is associated with the state of wellbeing. However, a patient with the progressive disease condition may be physically inefficient or cognitively not fit to continue self-management. Such patient is likely to compromise on adherence, which impacts prognosis. But relieving the patient of self-management may contribute to their feelings of loss of control and powerlessness. In such cases, mild admonitions from caregiver or health care professionals may cause a dent to their dignity. With the progressive decline in their condition, their day's activities may increasingly involve one or more of disease-oriented activities like hospital visit, laboratory visit for some investigation, doctor's visit for monitoring, timely medication, exercise, physiotherapy, diet, medication or injection. They increasingly realize that the illness has become the epicentre of their lives, replacing many the enjoyable activities. They are likely to start perceiving their loss of control over simple aspect like the activities of the day.

With progression of illness condition, increasing dependence and loss of autonomy may give rise to the feelings of being burden on others. This erodes the dignity of the patient.

Vulnerability, Loss of Dignity and Stigma

Dignity comes under threat in an uneven relationship where one has more power than the other. In patient-care provider relationship, the care provider assumes more power, compared to the patient who is at the receiving end. However, if the care provider invites more participation form the patient in decision-making, and the activities of daily living, it is perceived as a good measure of protecting the dignity of the patient. Protection of dignity comes with the importance given to the patient. Unfortunately, the elderly chronic patients in hospitals, particularly in India, have been feeling the loss of dignity as they perceive less importance given to them compared to other patients. This sense of being ignored or neglected was shared by a number of elderly patients with the author. Many felt discounted or neglected by health care professionals mainly because of their age. They experience loss of dignity with series of events such as having to wait for assistance, not being given a feedback, not involving them in decision-making, having no information or response to their question. Simple steps such as active listening, individual attention and explanation of the facts by health care professionals would go a long way in preventing the feelings of loss of dignity among them.

There are times when dignity comes under threat because of the stigma attached to certain types of chronic conditions. More often than not a disease is stigmatized because of lack of correct knowledge or wrong inputs about a disease. Patients with epilepsy, dementia, HIV/AIDS, hepatitis C or any visible disfigurement, such as severe psoriasis, rheumatoid arthritis, attract social attention. Hence, they avoid social contact due to the stigma attached to the disfigurement or a wrong notion about the disease itself. This constitutes external social pressure on the patient driving to social isolation, loss of control and powerlessness.

It is clear from the above discussion that the impact of chronic illness is just not medical but psychosocial too, with a close interlink between the two. The biomedical and psychosocial impacts of chronic illness are listed in Table 8.2. This helps in identifying the crucial aspects related to chronic illness, which enables to identify and plan appropriate interventions. Patient assessment helps in identifying the various impacts of chronic illnesses at the physical level and psychosocial level. Often, the impact is multilevel. Identification of specific aspects enables some to prioritize therapeutic intervention that is biopsychosocial in nature with a goal of enhancing the quality of life and optimizing prognosis.

The items in the box suggest that while the impact on physical pain is high, a larger impact is seen in psychosocial dimensions. The reason is the suffering at the physical level is selective depending upon the nature of illness. For example, physical mobility may not be impacted in certain types of cancers; similarly, change in gait and deformity may be seen only in few illnesses like rheumatoid arthritis. However, the psychosocial impacts are not as much illness-specific. A combination of some of the experiences listed in the box is likely to be present in every chronic disease.

Table 8.2 Biopsychosocial impact of chronic illness

Physical	*Psychosocial*
Pain	Difficulty in accepting the diagnosis
Discomfort	Denial
Weakness	Shock
Muscular rigidity	Adjustment with illness
Sluggishness/slowdown in movements	Coping with illness
Lowered physical activity	Anxiety
Impediment in mobility	Depression
Disruption in sleep	Loss of personal control
Incontinence	Loss of dignity
Fainting	Powerlessness
Deformity	Feelings of uncertainty
Changes in gait	Social isolation
Excessive loss or gain in weight	Diminished positive identity
Flare-ups/attacks of acute conditions	Feelings of insecurity
Sensitivity to weather conditions	Loss of life's goal orientation
Sensitivity to certain diet	Fear of pain
Need for exercise	Fear of death
Need for rest	Worries about finances
	Shame of stigma
	Dependence
	Feeling of guilt for dependence
	Loss of autonomy
	Helplessness
	Hopelessness
	Frustration

Coping with Chronic Illness

Adaptation and coping involve the processes of cognition, emotion and behaviour. In the context of chronic illness, adaptation and coping are responses to the illness condition, a setback in terms of the disease progression, side effects or resistance to medication, failure or suboptimal outcome of a therapy, onset of an illness-related disability, physical pain, discomfort or diminished mobility and increased dependence. All these situations are highly stress-inducing. The patient has only two options in such circumstances:

1. Adapt or adjust to the situation
2. Cope with the situation

Adaptation refers to the process where the individual changes his/her behaviour to suit the situation, while coping refers to the process where the individual attempts to change the situation to suit the individual's desires and goals (Hariharan & Rath, 2008). Adaptation or coping is preceded by a cognitive appraisal that takes into account, the stakes involved, and resource availability, which includes both internal and external resources. Internal resources refer to one's ability to change the situation. Ability includes one's cognitive resources such as knowledge level and comprehension, competence and a number of personal skills. External resources include the economic status, material possessions, social network, support system and social status. The cognitive appraisal involves primary and secondary appraisal. The decision to adapt/adjust or cope with the situation is determined by the cognitive appraisal. The cognitive appraisal process and the consequent adaptation/coping behaviour are depicted in Figure 8.6.

Harm refers to the damage already been done, while threat refers to the potential for harm. As depicted in Figure 8.6, the onset of chronic illness is the harm already done to the patient. In majority of cases, once a person is diagnosed with chronic illness, the possibility of cure is bleak, rendering one to the only choice to manage the condition with best interventions. In case of certain types of cancers that are 'cured', there is a constant apprehension of relapse of it, thus demanding regular medical consultancy and check-ups amounting to management. Once the primary appraisal confirms the harm (onset of chronic illness), the cognitive process triggers the secondary appraisal, which evaluates the availability of resources to mitigate the 'harm'. When the answer to this is 'No', the best course of option in restoring equilibrium is to accept the diagnosis and adapt to the situation. This calls for effective management of emotional reaction. Thus, the patient has to adapt or adjust to the chronic illness condition already diagnosed in the body.

On the contrary, the chronic illness is not one-time diagnosis with a static characteristic like amputation of a limb. It has the potential to deteriorate health condition with progression of the disease and its biological and psychosocial consequences. The secondary appraisal to this potential threat questions the availability of resources to challenge the threat. The answer to this is positive because in chronic illness, the disease progression and aggravations can be averted and minimized by certain health behaviour. In other words, by way of certain coping mechanisms through changes in lifestyle, such as committing to high adherence, utilizing social support to the optimum and managing the emotions effectively and sustaining positive affect state, one can effectively manage the illness so as to arrest its progression and prevent its psychosocial consequences. The above explanation leads to the inference that management of chronic illness involves a combination of adaptation and coping, for the best outcome. Adaptation or coping has to be applied purely on the realistic evaluation of controllability of the situation. While the onset of the disease has no control, the best course of action is to accept and adapt while prevention of progression is possible through exercise of control that needs to be coped by application of control through adherence and lifestyle changes.

328 *Chronic Illness and Therapeutic Intervention*

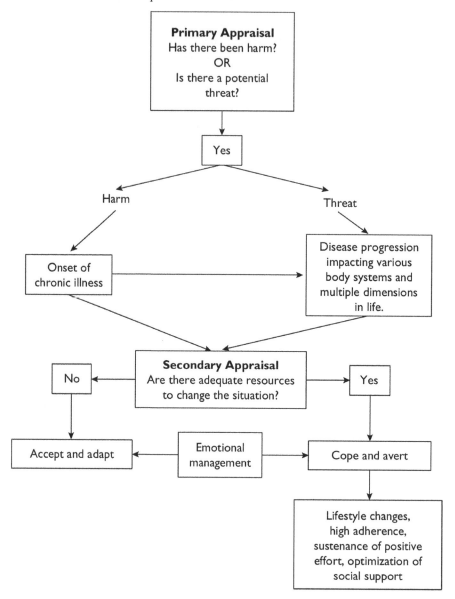

Figure 8.6 Cognitive Appraisal, Adaptation and Coping.

Adaptation

Adaptation refers to the changes in one's perception, emotion and behaviour to accommodate the changes in one's life situation. A person diagnosed with a chronic illness has to perceive it as a reality of lifelong condition, ventilate emotions in a chosen manner befitting one's own personality and circumstances, seek medical treatment to suit one's affordability, and incorporate changes in diet and activities, learn self-monitoring and create space for regular consultation with physician as directed by medical advice. Here, the individual in fact 'adjusts' one's life to match the new stressor in the form of diagnosis of chronic illness. Such adaptation resulting in keeping the chronic condition under control attains the goal of minimizing the stress and restoring the equilibrium. Successful adaptation is characterized by a number of functional indicators. De Ridder, Geenen, Kuijer, and vanMiddendorp (2008) named five indicators of successful adaptation with chronic illness:

1 Performing the adaptive tasks successfully
2 Not having psychological disorders
3 Maximizing positive affect and minimizing negative affect
4 Maintaining good functioning status
5 Satisfaction and high wellbeing in various domains of life

The factors mentioned above are in fact indicators of equilibrium. Davison and Jhangri (2013) found a positive relationship between adaptation, spirituality and health-related quality of life in patients diagnosed with stage 4 or 5 chronic kidney disease. Spirituality is found to be a unique factor in patients with health-related quality of life.

The response of adaptation is normally preceded by an active acceptance of the situation and fitting oneself into the frame placed by the situation. On the contrary, coping refers to a response that confronts the situation with a goal to prevent the situation from having a negative impact.

Coping

Coping with chronic illness refers to the active efforts of the patient following the cognitive assessment that the threat of disease progression involves high stakes and the resource availability warrants challenging the potential threat through activities that prevent, arrest or suppress the progression of the disease. In short, effective coping with chronic illness is efficient disease management. Two factors that are common between adaptation and coping with chronic illness are as follows:

1 Emotional management and
2 Active participation

When the diagnosed illness is life-threatening or apprehends severe pain in store, the natural reaction is one of emotional turmoil. Before a decision is made for planning the future course of medical treatment, which is a coping behaviour, it becomes imperative to first manage the emotions and bring it down to a stage that facilitates cognitive functioning to initiate coping behaviour in line of planful problem solving. Whether it is adaptation or coping, the patient's active involvement in terms of health behaviour is present. The ultimate purpose of both is to restore equilibrium in oneself. The equilibrium can be attained only when the cognitive appraisal triggers the right discretion for adaptation or coping, based on realistic assessment of controllability. Applying adaptation in situations of high controllability or coping in situations of low controllability would fail to reap optimum outcome.

Lazarus and Folkman (1984) have identified eight strategies of coping. Hariharan and Rath (2008) added the ninth type that is very relevant to Indian culture. These coping strategies are briefly described below.

CONFRONTIVE COPING

It refers to the efforts one takes to remove the obstacle in the way of goal attainment. This is possible when the person is able to identity either a person or a situation as an impediment to one's goal, thereby inducing stress. "It is explained as 'taking the bull by horns'" (Hariharan

& Rath, 2008) or statements such as "I stood my ground". "Made the other person change his/her mind" (p. 120). This type of coping may be relevant in certain situations where the chronic patient capable of certain activities of daily living is prevented by the overprotective caregiver, and the patient averts a possible situation of atrophy by standing his/her ground and proving to the other person that he/she can be autonomous to the optimum extent.

PLANFUL PROBLEM SOLVING

Planful problem solving is a problem-focused coping, conspicuous by the absence of emotion and pursuit of resolving the problem logically with adequate contingency plan.

Lifestyle changes in chronic illnesses can be coped applying planful problem solving, since it involves management of multiple factors demanding unlearning and learning processes. For example, a patient diagnosed with a cardiac condition is advised to quit smoking, reduce alcohol consumption, eat fibre-rich, low-fat, low-sodium diet, exercise regularly and manage the stress levels efficiently. All these required adequate and serious planning keeping in mind possibility of resistance, reluctance, relapse and procrastination. The action plan includes consulting a dietician, health psychologist and gym trainer.

SEEKING SOCIAL SUPPORT

Seeking social support as a coping strategy refers to the individual's active efforts to draw support from one's social network. The support sought can vary in its type. It can be material support, informational support, emotional support or support of services.

Social support can sometimes provide emotional blaming, break the monotony in a patient confined to bed, motivate a person to be adherent. Patients with higher social support measure higher on wellbeing. Overall wellbeing is found to be diminished in patients who are socially isolated (Golden et al., 2009). Social support has been found to reduce anxiety in patients. In a study by Chivukula, Swain Rana and Hariharan (2013), one hundred patients waiting for angiogram and CABG were tested on perceived social support, hospital anxiety and depression. The results of multiple regression analysis revealed that perceived social support had a significant negative contribution to anxiety and depression. In other words, those with high perceived social support were found to measure low on anxiety and depression.

Padhy, Lalnuntluangi, Chelli and Padiri (2016) studied the contribution of social support to enhancing adherence among patients with hypertension. They studied a sample of 75 men and 75 women. Results showed that a significant 16.3% of variance in adherence was predicted by social support. They concluded that significant social agents have a positive impact on the patient. They encourage health-enhancing behaviour, utilization of health care to the optimum and adherence to medication through social control.

While the positive impact of social support is undisputed, does the available support match the patient's expectation? Awasthi and Mishra (2008) studied a sample of 100 female patients with cervix cancer and 100 female patients with diabetes. They found that the available support for women was lower than the expected support.

POSITIVE REAPPRAISAL

This coping strategy can be termed as post-facto process that starts after the experience of stress. This process of coping involves ascribing positive attributes to the stressful experience. In the context of chronic illness, the patient goes through the stress when the diagnosis is communicated. After going through the emotional reaction, the intensity of which may vary depending on various factors, one is in the process of working towards the equilibrium. One method of reaching the equilibrium is to identify the positive factors in the stress situation (illness) itself. The patient tends to reappraise the conditions of illness in the light of the good outcomes arising out of it. For example, a patient diagnosed with arthritis may say "In a way, my illness is a boon to me. At least now my family thinks of having a household help and a cook. I am really exhausted managing all the work at home". Thus, the patient's process of identifying the desirable outcome of the illness is positive reappraisal.

This strategy of coping is similar to 'benefit-finding' or 'stress-related growth' or 'post-traumatic growth'. All these expressions refer to the positive life changes in the process of coping with negative or stressful events (Park, Lechner, Antoni, & Stanton, 2009). There have been a good number of research on benefit-finding with chronic illness. The findings indicate a positive relationship between benefit-finding and adjustment to illness. The range of illnesses found to use benefit-finding includes cancer (Danhauer et al., 2013), HIV (Milam, 2004) and spinal cord injury (January, Zebracki, Chlan, & Vogel, 2015).

DISTANCING

This refers to a strategy of coping where one attempts to make light of a serious situation, or manifest a casual attitude towards a stressful event. In the context of chronic illness, when the diagnosis is communicated to the patient, he or she either responds with a sense of humour or with a casual reaction. For example, when a patient is communicated that he/she has a cardiac condition that demands a bypass surgery, the patient responds saying "That's a news indeed! My subordinates in the office must know about it. They have been spreading a rumour that I am heartless". In one case that the author encountered a patient in her 80s, diagnosed with stage 4 cancer in intestines and reported her reaction to the diagnosis "No, I did not feel any severe negative emotions. I just thought, every other person is having cancer, and now I too have it". This patient underwent a surgery and chemotherapy and is a cancer survivor for the past five years with no relapse, aggravation or side effects.

When this strategy of coping is applied, illness conditions that are beyond one's control are best accepted as they are with least negative emotions.

SHIFTING THE BURDEN ON GOD/RELIGION/FAITH

When the primary appraisal ascertains that the harm caused is irreversible or the secondary appraisal reveals the absence of any resources leading to a perception of external locus of control, one of the techniques of coping that protects extreme damage due to psychological distress is coping through shifting the burden to something supernatural. This is something preached in the holy script of Srimad Bhagavad Gita, which advocates total surrender to God or the faith, after one put in his/her best efforts into the field. Shifting the burden on God in combination with any other active coping also brings positive results. There is research evidence that proved the positive outcome of spirituality, religion or faith.

Religion was found to be useful among cancer patients to improve their quality of life and adjustment to illness (Nairn & Merluzzi, 2003; Ross et al., 2009), provide meaning of illness and bring down distress (Kandasamy, Chaturvedi, & Desai, 2011) and reduce anxiety and depression (Kandasamy et al., 2011).

The other strategies like self-control, accepting responsibility and escape-avoidance are not effective in the context of coping with chronic illness.

Therapeutic Interventions

The primary intervention to any chronic illness is the medical intervention, and there is no dispute regarding this. However, the outcome of medical intervention will be optimum only when it is supported and supplemented with psychosocial intervention too. Medical and psychosocial interventions ideally have to be woven into single package, involving professionals from the relevant field of Medicine, Health Psychology, Nursing, Physiotherapy and Nutrition working as a team. The advocacy for changes in lifestyle that includes compliance to diet, exercise and abstinence from smoking, alcohol, certain type of food etc. cannot be handled with medication and needs cognitive restructuring, emotional management, behavioural changes and perhaps social/community involvement/participation. The relationship of chronic illness on the physical and psychosocial domain is listed separately in Table 8.2. Medical intervention takes care of the impact in physical/physiological levels. The psychosocial impacts can be grouped into the following major dimensions:

1 Incomplete or faulty schema about the illness
2 Emotional reactions originating from the schema related to illness (fear, anger, frustration, shock, anxiety, distress, depression, sadness etc.)
3 Depletion of motivation (hopelessness, helplessness etc.)
4 Situations created by inadequate /faulty schema and emotional state of the patient and family (ambiguity, mutual role expectations among patient, caregiver and professionals, communication gaps, social distancing, withdrawal, suppression etc.)
5 Behavioural responses to the diagnosis of illness, health/illness behaviour, interpersonal behaviour, adaptation and coping with illness.

The overall goal of psychosocial intervention to chronic patients is to optimize their quality of life. This involves keeping the intensity and frequency of physical and psychological symptoms at the lowest minimum level and maximizing the social and professional participation and performance levels, so as to enhance the life satisfaction, and quality of life. This process involved in achieving this is described in Figure 8.7.

The diagnosis of chronic illness comes with the experience of symptoms and information on the nature of the disease and potential threat. The experience is subjective. The information is either authentic or hearsay. Further, the subjective experience is open to personal interpretation. The illness schema forms and develops depending upon the source and nature of information and the meaning attributed to symptom experience. More often than not the schema is either incomplete, or faulty. Faulty schemas are results of either wrong information or information over flow majorly through internet sources. The diagnosis with the concomitant symptom experience and information gives rise to certain negative emotion. Negative emotions also originate from inadequate or faulty illness schema. Such negative emotions are responsible for lowering the motivation levels and trigger feelings of helplessness or hopelessness.

Further, more often than not the chronic illnesses are associated with certain existing lifestyle that must have contributed to the condition. Hence, they are known as lifestyle diseases.

The consequences of chronic illnesses cross the boundaries of physical suffering encompassing the cognitive, affective, motivational and behavioural domains of the individual and the family. Hence, the interventions must aim at attaining

1 Cognitive construction / restructuring
2 Emotional management / equilibrium
3 Motivational enhancement and
4 Behavioural change

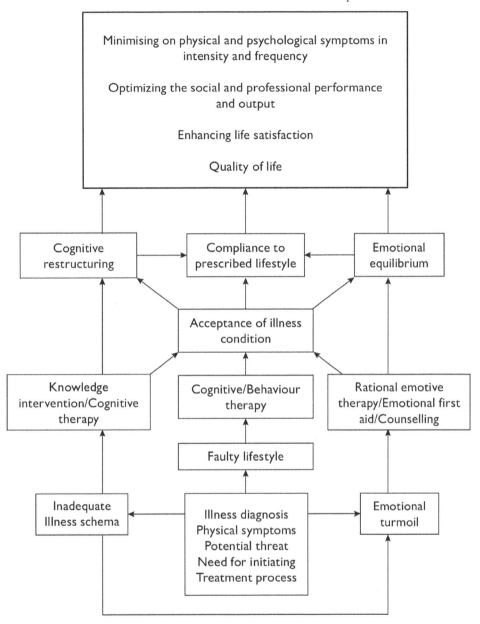

Figure 8.7 Psychosocial Intervention to Chronic Illness: Quality of Life.

The effective illness management comprises of the above besides the pain/symptom management of the disease. The psychosocial interventions for chronic illness thus should include

– Cognitive therapy
– Emotional (blaming) therapy
– Behavioural therapy and
– Motivational therapy

It is essential to clarify at this stage that the above therapies applied in the context of chronic illness should not be misconstrued as the ones in clinical setting but have to be ideally integrated into natural life setting so as to reap the optimum benefit. The persons receiving the interventions are not chronic patients with mental health issues but are those with chronic physical health problems with minor imbalance of equilibrium at emotional, cognitive and behavioural levels. With these basic foundations, we shall discuss various therapeutic interventions for chronic illnesses.

Baseline Assessment

Before deciding on the intervention, it is necessary to have a complete assessment of the patient's physical pain, affect state, motivational levels and lifestyle (health behaviour). This constitutes the baseline data. When this is compared with the scores in post-intervention phases, one can assess the effectiveness of the interventions and their sustainability.

Baseline assessment should include the physical, physiological, psychological status and existing functional level of social and professional parameters. The physical and physiological assessments are done by the medical professionals. Psychosocial assessments need to be done by a health psychologist. Based on the assessment reports, the psychosocial interventions need to be planned. The psychosocial therapies are planned based on some basic theoretical principles.

The primary objective of therapeutic intervention to chronic illness is for effective management of the illness condition on all dimensions. This targets the patients and their families. However, some of the interventions can also be part of public health measures targeting the population for prevention of chronic or non-communicable diseases through creating awareness and imposing restrictions on health risk behaviour and promotion of a healthy lifestyle. Let us first discuss psychosocial intervention for illness management.

Interventions for Chronic Illness Management

There is ample research evidence establishing the relationship between physical condition and overall wellness with various psychosocial interventions. Chivukula, Hariharan, Rana, Thomas and Andrew (2017) studied a sample of 250 CABG patients in intensive care units (ICU), following the surgery. The results indicated that psychosocial care was an effective predictor of hospital wellbeing and ICU trauma. Psychosocial care positively contributed to wellbeing and negatively contributed to ICU trauma. When psychosocial care was high, wellbeing was high and ICU trauma was low.

Seema, Thomas, Pienyu and Srinadh (2015) in their study on pregnant women showed a positive correlation between spirituality and wellbeing. Hariharan and Padhy (2008) highlighted the significance of spirituality and Hindu rituals in enhancing wellbeing.

The impact of stress, anxiety and depression on the illness and quality of life among chronic patients has been established by a number of studies. Chivukula, Swain, Rana and Hariharan (2013) have highlighted the mediating role of perceived social support in minimizing anxiety and depression among cardiac patients. Based on these findings and a number of other research that established a link between psychosocial factors and chronic illness, quality of life and wellbeing, it can be logically argued that deliberate attempts to introduce the positive psychosocial inputs would result in enhancing the prognosis of the chronic illness, wellbeing and quality of life in the patients.

Principles of Psychological Therapy

Therapeutic interventions can be conceived, planned and executed effectively with understanding of the basic principles. Some of the cognitive, affective and behavioural responses are embedded in the functioning of the nervous system. For example, the lack of memory, coordination and the behavioural responses associated with a dementia patient has its roots in nervous system functioning. Some other behaviours such as eating unhealthy food, not having adequate sleep, being irregular with medication can be traced back to learning. Yet, other behaviours like getting addicted to alcohol, smoking may have their origin in genetic factor or childhood experience or acquired behaviour.

The basic principles responsible for triggering covert and overt behavioural responses are as follows:

1 Conditioning
2 Reinforcement and
3 Observational or social learning

The responses get strength and turn into habits either because of their association with certain stimulus or because they receive a reward that satisfies a need in the person. For example, a person who has been in the habit of ordering junk food during the weekends may have the tendency to do so every weekend even after the diagnosis of obesity, a risk factor for many chronic illnesses that prohibits junk food. This happens due to the conditioning that has been associated with being at home on a holiday with the behaviour of ordering junk food.

The second principle is that of reinforcement. The behaviour that is followed by a reward, satisfying an existing need, is likely to be strengthened. Similarly, the behaviour that is followed by a punishment causing pain or discomfort is likely to be weakened. There is a third principle that is related to learning by observation, called observational learning, where an individual tends to emulate certain behaviour by observing others. In a way, this is also related to reinforcement, because only those behaviours are learned that are found to be rewarding in the original model.

Before discussing cognitive interventions, it is important to understand the problems in cognitions, starting from their formulation to the process.

Cognitive Schemas and Distortions

Cognitive schemas are the major feeders of the thoughts. The way the individual conceptualizes his/her world comprises of the significant beliefs about self, people, conditions, events and the environment. These structures of beliefs and assumptions related to various aspects of one's life are referred to as cognitive schemas. These schemas may be positive or negative. The experiences of the individual, and their interactions with others and the information from various sources constitute the basis for the schemas.

Schemas that relate to everyday occurring are called 'active schemas'. In a chronic condition of health, the changes and symptoms related to day-to-day life are active schema. Similarly, there may be schema related to affect, or feelings that may be either positive or negative. Some schemas are amenable to change, while others are not.

The schemas related to various aspects develop and change with significant additions of information and experience. Sometimes, wrong information or a freak experience may contribute to distort the cognition, event or environment. The thought process around the wrongly developed schemas reflects errors in the reasoning. This, in turn, leads to cognitive distortions. Cognitive distortions are normally identified in clinical populations such as depression patients (Beck, 1967) and in patients with other psychological disorders (Freeman, 1987; DeRubeis, Tang, & Beck, 2001). Some of them are found in milder intensity in patients with chronic illness.

1 **Dichotomous Thinking:** This refers to the thought process that something has to be exactly in line with one's expectations. If not, it is regarded as failure. For example, a patient diagnosed with hypertension believes that being highly adherent to medication must hold the blood pressure under control, all the time. When one sees the blood pressure shooting up on days filled with stress, one may feel that the medication is of no help, since it plays no role in controlling the blood pressure during the stressful period. Such thought process is 'all-or-none' thinking. They classify medication as extremely effective or absolutely not. Here, the natural physiological response to stress is not taken into cognizance. The fact that the blood pressure generally under control on other days is because of the medication is discounted. Such cognitive distortions need to be identified in the process of assessment through interviews.
2 **Selective Abstraction:** Sometimes, an isolated event or experience is used to draw a generalized inference. This is called selective abstraction. A patient with chronic arthritis who walks with an awkward gait, but socially very active, may take one single incident of one's inability to climb a few steps in a picnic spot, where one had to stay away from the venue of events and conclude that he/she is 'unfit to be amidst others'. This triggers that patient's decision from avoiding all social gatherings leading to social isolation and depression. All the other occasions where one enjoyed the company of others in various functions and outings are not included in drawing the inference of one's being 'unfit for social participation'.
3 **Mind-reading:** This relates to the individual's assertion that he/she knows the thinking and feelings of another person. Very often, this augments the negative thoughts. Chronic patients who have an acute phase that prolongs for a while or patients who are confined to bed and lose their autonomy even in simple activities of daily living feel a sense of frustration. They nurture the feeling that they are burdening the caregiver. Such thoughts can be depressing and also irritating. When under such situations, a mildest admonition by the caregiver or a slightest delay in attending to the needs of the patient can be a trigger to originate a thought that the caregiver considers him/her as a burden. Once triggered, one may look for the events and incidents that substantiate such thought. The patient may then start nurturing the thoughts such as 'he/she is disgusted with my dependence'. These thoughts may vary in their intensity.
4 **Catastrophizing:** This occurs when an individual takes a single event and exaggerates it so much that it turns fearful, generating anxiety, fear and thereby the physiological responses. For example, a cancer patient who has successfully gone through the treatment may apprehend a relapse or bad news every time he/she goes for the regular review consultation with the doctor. The patient may entertain negative thoughts such as 'the doctor may find a lump/growth in the adjacent place. I may have to go through the treatment all over again, what if it is a fast-growing cancer this time?' Such negative thoughts generate severe anxiety, impacting the physiological parameters, sleep, diet and general health. It may sometimes be so bad to impact the quality of life and wellness of the patient prior to the review consultation.
5 **Overgeneralization:** One of the fallacies in thinking originates from overgeneralization. This refers to chalking a rule based on one or few negative events. For example, a cardiac patient, who is a 58-year-old woman, refuses to undergo a bypass surgery. She believes that

women do not survive a Coronary Artery Bypass Grafting (CABG). Her argument is that she knows two cases where her 73-year-old aunt and another colleague of her age died soon after the surgery. Based on these two instances, she strongly believes that it is fatal for women to undergo CABG. Thus, these two negative events constitute the basis for her decision against undergoing the surgery depriving her of an enhanced quality of life that is envisaged after the surgery.

6 **Labelling and Mislabelling:** Attributing a negative connotation to self may lead to labelling or mislabelling oneself. This, in turn, may be responsible for an irrational behaviour. Applying this in the context of chronic patient is not farfetched. A patient diagnosed with primary hypertension may brand oneself as a 'cardiac patient' on the logic that the blood pressure measures the pumping of the blood by heart in its working and resting conditions. Therefore, hypertension classifies one as cardiac patient. By doing so, one may slow down the pace of activities, avoid certain postures like bending, certain activities like lifting, even normal weight, and even stop regular exercise in the gym. Thus, the patient may create an inaccurate or false identity of one self, and behave accordingly, which may be counterproductive to the chronic condition.

7 **Magnification/Minimization:** When individuals magnify imperfections/setbacks and minimize positives, they are cognitive distortions. Positives and negatives, be it experiences, outcomes or characteristics, are the realities of life. How one perceives them has an impact on one's thoughts, perspective and behaviour. A patient with any chronic illness who exaggerates a minor setback in his/her health condition or fails to endorse an improvement in condition or absence of a distressing symptom is said to be experiencing cognitive distortion. Such undermining of improvements or overemphasizing the setback or adverse event is likely to lead the patient to depression. Further, it distorts the symptom presentation to the doctor leading to confusion and incorrect line of medical investigation. If unattended, this may lead to self-perpetuation of depression, and deterioration in quality of life.

Interventions to Cognitive Distortions

There is a need to assess and determine whether the chronic patient's illness perception has cognitive distortion and irrational beliefs related to the diagnosis present condition and future course. If such distortions are discovered, then the patient needs to be exposed to cognitive interventions. The basic approach to this is called ABCDE approach. Here, the A, B and C constitute the assessment part, while D and E form the intervention part.

'A' refers to the activating event. The activating event is the incidence that triggers the cognition. It could be the diagnosis of the illness and its communication to the patient. B refers to the belief related to the activating event, e.g. the belief of the patient that diabetes is a dangerous disease with no cure. "It is difficult to control. I can not control my diet or lead a discipline life. I am finished". C refers to the consequences. For example, the diagnosis that one has diabetes may trigger a thought that one's health condition has started the irreversible downward slope. Since leading a disciplined life is impossible in the present profession, one is doomed. It may not be long before one touches the lowest point and die because that was exactly what happened to one of his/her parents.

The A, B and C cover the assessment part. The assessment can be done through interview with the patient. Exaggerating and catastrophizing the situation is one type of cognitive distortion, while totally discounting the seriousness and denial of one's diagnosis is another way of distorting facts. Both need to be handled by challenging with care and support in a rational way. This is the time to apply D and E.

338 *Chronic Illness and Therapeutic Intervention*

D refers to disrupting or challenging the dysfunctional thoughts and beliefs. Challenging is done through rational questions such as 'why is it not possible to control the disease?' What makes you think so? What is the basis on which it is concluded that one 'cannot' have a disciplined lifestyle? Under what circumstances did the parent die? What are the differences in the two conditions? These questions and the discussions in these lines should continue until logical thinking and demolition of irrational beliefs.

E refers to the effects of the new rational thoughts, action plan and behaviour. Actions get initiated by answering questions, disputing the irrational beliefs and replacing them with more logical and viable beliefs.

Cognitive Interventions

The type of intervention for a patient should be identified on the basis of the assessment report. The interventions are designed to target the cognition, affect, behaviour or the situation.

Cognitive Therapy: Assumptions

The basic assumption of cognitive therapy is that thoughts are significant determinants of behaviour on the one hand and affect state on the other. Both affect state and behaviour have a very high influence on the illness condition. Positive thoughts spring positive affect and constructive behaviour, while negative thoughts pave a path for negative affect. They cause either inaction, delayed action or destructive actions.

The goals of cognitive interventions in chronic illness should be:

1 To build adequate cognitive base about the chronic condition
2 To start the process of cognitive restructuring

Building Cognitive Base

If the assessment report of the patient diagnosed with chronic illness reveals a paucity of knowledge about the illness, there is a need to build a healthy and adequate cognitive base in the patient. This is done through appropriate knowledge intervention or psychoeducation. Knowledge intervention can be prescribed through various methods:

Enhancing the Quality of Doctor-Patient Communication

The most authentic source of communication for the patient is the treating doctor. The information provided by the doctor is considered valuable and taken seriously. However, owing to the poor doctor-patient ratio in India which is 1:1800 (Deo, 2013) of consultation time the doctor could allot to patient is dismally reduced. In a study by the author and her team, the mean consultation time for a cardiac patient was found to be seven minutes with the time ranging between 2 and 22 minutes. Given such constraints, the best way to enhance the quality of communication and include relevant knowledge component in the process of consultation is to introduce a checklist. The patient should be given a checklist prior to the consultation time. The checklist should have a number of aspects relevant to the diagnosed illness. It must assess the patient's knowledge about the normal physiological/biochemical process and the deviation in the illness, treatment options, time line of the illness, medication schedule, the way the medication works, diet and exercise (with the logic for the same), alarm signals indicating medical emergencies, need and frequency of review consultations. The patient should be asked to tick those aspects where he/she is confident about the current knowledge. Those items identified as 'not known' should be carefully highlighted and discussed with the doctor during consultation. This enables to optimize the consultation time, and also enhance patient satisfaction. Once this practice goes into the system, the knowledge intervention automatically gets integrated into the consultation process. With the highest authenticity of such knowledge input, the patient adherence is likely to increase.

Group Interventions

Knowledge intervention can be imparted in group settings. This can be done by the doctor or a health psychologist. The schedule of knowledge intervention programme can be drawn in every hospital taking the common chronic diseases, such as hypertension, diabetes, COPD, arthritis where the prevalence is shown as high. Knowledge intervention programmes can be planned for the patients in groups of 20–30. The content of knowledge interventions has to be carefully planned to focus on functional knowledge. The contents must include the following:

  i Essential facts about the illness
 ii Risks involved in the illness
iii The need for placing oneself under treatment
 iv Possible serious outcomes of not treating illness
  v The impact of illness on affect and cognitive functioning (where relevant, e.g. dementia, diabetes)
 vi Pain management techniques
vii Need for techniques of stress management
viii Role of the patient in managing illness through lifestyle changes and its impact
 ix Significance of social support in managing illness
  x Need for self-monitoring and alarm signals to seek emergency medical intervention

The contents of knowledge intervention have to be in simple, non-technical language. Transfer of knowledge can be done by a professional who directly addresses and interacts with the group of patients, or it can be an audiovisual presentation. However, direct interaction involving a professional is likely to be more effective than the audiovisual exposure.

In a study by Andrew (2018), both the methods of direct interaction and audiovisual exposure of knowledge intervention were found to be effective though the direct interaction method was found to be superior in its impact. This study recruited the patients diagnosed with primary hypertension and divided them into five groups. The five groups were found to be homogenous on all demographic variables including the duration of illness. The first and second groups received hypertension knowledge intervention of 30-minute duration through direct presentation by a medical professional. The only difference was that the first group received the intervention only once, while the second group received the intervention for the second time with a gap of two weeks. The third and fourth groups received the same knowledge intervention by the same physician, but through a 30-minute video clipping. The third group had a single exposure to the intervention, while the fourth group had a repeated exposure with a gap of two weeks. The fifth group was a control group that received no intervention but received the standard medical care. The participants were followed up for six weeks. The groups were compared on their scores on pre- and post-intervention scores on hypertension knowledge, adherence, B.P. readings, anxiety, depression, perceived social support and self-efficacy. The findings clearly indicated the positive impact of knowledge intervention by showing a significant difference between the control group and the four intervention groups. The positive impact was found in adherence, B.P. reading, self-efficacy, perceived social support, anxiety and depression. This indicated that by providing knowledge intervention in any form, the management of hypertension is enhanced. Results further showed that relative efficacy of the form and frequency of hypertension. The group that received knowledge input directly through the professional with a repeated session was found to have the highest impact in terms of higher adherence and lowered B.P. readings followed by the group that had direct intervention but only once, and then by the group that had audiovisual exposure but only once. The group that had repeated audiovisual exposure was found to be the one that though had the benefit, the impact was relatively lowest in the order that was found to be closer to the control group.

The results could track a pathway from knowledge intervention to hypertension management. It was found that knowledge intervention contributed to self-efficacy, which in turn positively impacted adherence. Enhanced adherence helped in improving hypertension management. It is important that the contents of knowledge intervention lay a special emphasis on the role of the patient in managing the illness effectively. It is not uncommon for the patients to assume that medication alone is responsible for controlling the chronic illness. The intervention that focuses on the significance of patients' participation in management of illness brings a new insight into the patient. When the intervention is direct interaction with the physician, it opens a scope for the patients to involve in an open interaction, bringing in specific issues or problems related to the concerned patient. Further, a group intervention with direct involvement of physician widens the scope of knowledge and shared experience from all the patients in the group.

How does knowledge intervention work? There is a strong logical connection between cognition, affect and behaviour. Knowledge intervention helps in two ways.

a In case of the absence of knowledge, it creates a knowledge base and creates an authentic cognitive foundation regarding the illness. Cognitive structuring takes place in such cases.
b In case of existing wrong schema, it replaces the wrong schema with the correct one, thus reorienting the patient on the illness. Cognitive restructuring occurs in such cases.

The strong cognitive foundation instils a conviction related to the illness and its management. The cognitive base related to the risks involved in deviating from medication or lifestyle triggers a negative affect. On the contrary, cognitive base related to the individual role in managing the disease triggers self-confidence and motivation to actively participate in illness management through lifestyle changes, close monitoring and regular review. Thus, knowledge interventions by facilitating cognitive restructuring trigger the appropriate and adequate affect and motivation culminating in illness appropriate behaviour to manage the condition effectively to prevent progression and minimize flare-ups.

Psychoeducation

Knowledge intervention is also referral as psychoeducation. Typically, psychoeducation is given to the patient, as well as the family. Thus, depending upon the nature of chronic illness the family can be involved where the caregivers' role assumes significance. Knowledge intervention has been proved effective in the context of chronic mental health problem. Bäuml et al. (2006) reported that psychoeducation brought down the cases of rehospitalization of schizophrenia patients from 58% to 41% in a two-year period.

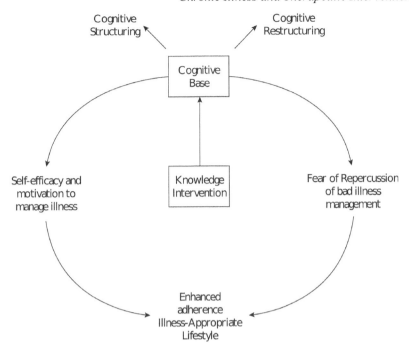

Figure 8.8 Impact of Knowledge Intervention.

Psychoeducation helps in building a strong and authentic cognitive base. This helps in dissipating the ambiguity and apprehension, which is the main cause of anxiety that adversely affects the immune system. It also helps in bringing out the effective coping with the illness.

The positive impact of psychoeducation on effective coping is studied by Chivukula and Nandinee (2018). They introduced psychoeducation as intervention for 150 elective surgery patients of CABG, knee replacement and visceral surgery. The patients were provided psychoeducation in the form of booklets that carried necessary information about the surgery. Results suggested that psychoeducation helped in lowering psychological distress, and post-operative pain and also enhanced their effective coping with the condition.

Knowledge intervention or psychoeducation while transferring knowledge also modulates emotional and motivational aspects to facilitate the patient to cope with the illness to reap the best outcome in terms of adherence and prognosis. By doing so, it minimizes the ambiguity and uncertainty, the two main ingredients to trigger negative affect. Such comprehensive intervention is more effective than the ones that aim for reducing negative affect like anxiety and distress.

Thomas (2016) compared the effect of two types of interventions on the patients who underwent CABG as elective surgery. She conducted the study on 300 patients equally divided into three groups. The first group received cognitive and affective intervention through a package called Programme for Affective and Cognitive Education (PACE). These patients were exposed to a 30-minute video programme involving a cardiothoracic surgeon, a health psychologist and a patient who has successfully undergone a CABG. The contents consisted of the surgical procedures involved as explained by the surgeon, the aftermath of it, precautions, rest, activities during recovery, time taken for recovery and the fundamental dos' and don'ts' imposed by the medical professional. The peer patient explained and addressed the normal apprehension, what to expect on regaining consciousness post-surgery, the pain, discomfort, and the ways to cope with it, factors that help in better coping, ways to optimize social support and the significance of self-efficacy. The health psychologist emphasized the role of positive thinking, self-efficacy and relaxed disposition in wound healing and pace of recovery.

The second group was exposed to the audio instructions on Guided Imagery, a standard relaxation therapy. The third group was not given any intervention but had the standard medical care. The intervention groups received the intervention the day before the surgery and the day before the discharge from the hospital. They were provided with the CDs on discharge with an instruction to use them as and when they felt the need.

The patients were measured for their anxiety, depression and psychological distress at pre-intervention, and then a month later. They were also assessed for their adherence and overall prognosis following the surgery. Results revealed that both the interventions were effective in reducing the psychological distress significantly and thereby contributed to the prognosis. However, the group that was exposed to PACE showed two paths. PACE was found to contribute to distress reduction on the one hand and also directly contribute to prognosis. A five-month follow-up on a subsample revealed that the PACE group was physically and mentally ready to resume normal schedule of work about four weeks earlier compared to others.

Positive Affect and Thought Induction

Research evidence clearly suggests the link between thoughts and affect state. Based on it, one can infer that by training one towards positive thoughts, positive affect state can be elicited. Positive affect contributes to wellbeing and triggers active and positive behaviour. Positive thought intervention is an effective cognitive intervention. Fredrickson (2001) who postulated broaden and build theory of positive emotions argues that positive emotions are helpful in broadening the thought-action repertoire and build personal resources leading to enhanced wellbeing. Positive emotions help in displacing negative emotions, and contribute to resilience (Fredrickson, 2002). Research in the field of psychoneuroimmunology has proved the impact of thoughts, emotions and immune functioning. Ayurveda principle also advocated the role of positivity in health and wellbeing. Positive thought induction as part of cognitive intervention is a good innovative measure to control and manage chronic illness.

Biswas (2011) used the hypnotherapeutic method in inducing positive thoughts as a package with relaxation in a sample of patients with HIV/AIDS. The results showed positive changes in coping strategies, and desirable changes in immunological parameters.

Positive thoughts do not coexist with anxiety and depression. They are mutually exclusive. Positive social support is a factor that helps in reducing negative affect and enhancing positive thoughts.

Social Support

Social support constitutes a very effective intervention for chronic patients, particularly in many of the Eastern cultures where the need for affiliation is a very strong. Visiting the sick, elderly, hospitalized or the patients who have undergone surgery is built into Indian culture. Taking some essential nutrients such as fruits, or extending financial or material support for the family, extending services such as taking care of the needs of children, providing transport, accompanying for medical consultations are spontaneously offered by the relatives, friends and community. This helps in reducing the anxiety levels of the patients related to certain dimensions like worrying about children school, food for the family. Further, social support also functions as a great absorber of negative emotion related to the illness condition. The presence of the well-wishers itself functions as a reassurance. The conversations distract the patient's attention from the symptoms. Discussion or topics other than the illness provides the needed relaxation, and induces positive thoughts. Sometimes, it triggers emotional relaxation in patients. In either case, the negative affect is minimized and positive thoughts are instilled and invoked.

Studies have suggested that perceived positive social support plays a significant role in reducing psychological distress and enhancing the pace of recovery, and illness experience. Awasthi and Mishra (2007) studied the relationship between social support and illness consequences in a sample of 100 women between the age group of 30 and 65 years diagnosed with diabetes. Illness consequences were measured on three dimensions. Psychological consequences related to illness experience such as aches, stomach upset, poor eyesight. Consequences on psychological dimension related to experience like problems with sleep, disinterest in work irritability. Interpersonal consequences refer to our feelings of disinterest to interact with others clearly reflected in behaviour related to interpersonal relationship. Results showing negative correlation between social support and illness consequences of all the three dimensions indicated that when the social support is perceived high, the illness experience on all the three dimensions tends to be low. Results further revealed that approach-coping strategies reduced illness consequences, while avoidance coping strategies increased illness consequences reported by the patients.

Social support contributes to health in two ways. First, it enhances the general wellbeing. Second, it functions as a buffer when the individual is under stress. This suggests that those who perceive high social support have relatively high levels of wellbeing. But those who are diagnosed with chronic illness and perceive lower levels of illness related pain, discomfort and negative affect.

Behavioural Interventions

Behavioural interventions are effective when the chronic patients have problem adhering to the prescribed lifestyle. The problem may relate to

a Giving up a behaviour identified as harmful for the chronic condition (e.g. abstinence from smoking for a cardiac or a liver patient)
b Initiate a new behaviour prescribed as a part of treatment to control and manage the pain or illness progression (e.g. regular physiotherapy sessions for a patient with spondylitis or arthritis. Start on a low fat, low carbohydrate, low salt and sugar diet for a patient diagnosed with hypertension and diabetes)

The two strong principles that guide human behaviour are conditioning and reinforcement. If an undesirable old behaviour persists, the probable reasons are either the presence of a strong conditioned behaviour or the old behaviour is receiving a positive reinforcement. Hence, the assessment procedure has to identify these factors. Once this is done, the attempt should be in the process of deconditioning or weakening the positive reinforcer in the natural set-up.

A number of techniques of behavioural therapy can be adopted in changing the behaviour of the chronic patients. What is important is applying the principles involved in behavioural therapy in natural setting to change the behaviour.

Use of Shaping to Develop New Behaviour

Shaping is a process through which the behavioural change is attempted in progressive marginal changes. Habits are formed over a long period across life span. Lifestyles are set by several such habits and preferences. The habits strengthen because of the presence of strong reinforcers.

Hence, the medical advice to change lifestyle because of the diagnosis of chronic illness is likely to encounter stiff resistance from within or the inability to switch over to a new set of lifestyle suddenly. In cases where there is strong resistance, the changes in lifestyle may be initiated systematically in doses of marginal changes.

Stimulus Shaping

The process involves introducing gradual modifications in specific property of the stimulus so that the transfer of response to a new stimulus is facilitated. Imagine a situation where the person is used to a specific stimulus and responds positively to that. But that stimulus is no more desirable to the person, and hence, a change in the stimulus is inevitable. But, this change in the stimulus is not accepted easily with the same response. Under such circumstances, it is desirable to use this technique. For example, if a patient diagnosed with diabetes is advised to change the staple food from white rice to broken wheat, this change is not palatable. The resistance for such change is so strong that the patient is unable to gulp more than two morsels of the meal. Starving is also not desirable for a diabetic. Hence, the change can be introduced through stimulus shaping. For this, at first a time target has to be set by the health psychologist in consultation and with the patient. During this time, a ratio of white rice and broken wheat should be decided with a very low proportion of broken rice at the beginning. This proportion should be changed very gradually, targeting the response of finishing the served portion of meal. The change in the proportion should be so gradual that the patient gives the desirable response of eating behaviour without much difficulty until the target of replacing rice with broken wheat is attained.

Response Shaping

This is a process by which responses that are close to the target are reinforced systematically and differentially (Jena, 2008). This procedure will be effective in strengthening the behaviour where a chronic patient is relearning a response, which was lost to the illness or learning a new skill that is relevant to the illness. For example, a patient who suffered a paralysis stroke and is in the process of recovering is advised physiotherapy. The paralytic condition poses a challenge to any meaningful movements, which are very clumsy at the initial stages of trial. This is the time when the responses anywhere near the direction of target motion need to be appropriately positively reinforced and those that are remote to the target moments are not.

Prompting and Fading

They are closely linked procedures. Prompting involves facilitating the persons with a cue or a discriminating stimulus to elicit a behaviour that is intended to be learned. Fading refers to gradual withdrawal of this stimulus so that the newly learned behaviour sustains independent of the cue and is established as a habit (in the context of chronic illness).

This technique can be used to enhance the behaviour of medication adherence in a chronic patient. A patient diagnosed with hypertension is expected to take antihypertensive medication daily at a time prescribed by physician. A diabetic patient is advised to inject insulin before breakfast. Unused to such schedule, the patients are likely to forget their medication. Very frequently, they forget to carry their medicines when they travel or have their breakfast or meal outside. A prompt by a family member, an automatic alarm set in the mobile phone, may contribute a goad cue for taking medication. The same is applied in keeping the schedule for consultation with the physician, checking the B.P. or blood sugar levels, exercise time etc. In order to reduce the patient's dependence on the prompt for their adherence behaviour, and set the behaviour as habit, the prompt should be designed to fade out gradually. After an observation that the patient has got used to the schedule, the alarm or human prompt timing may be gradually delayed and then withdrawn after the adherence behaviour gets integrated into daily routine.

Systematic Desensitization

This is a procedure where the patient is first trained to relax totally. When in relaxed state, the stimulus of fear, anxiety or phobia is gradually introduced to the patient. The introduction of anxiety-provoking stimulus has to be very systematic in a step-by-step manner. This enables the patient to associate the relaxation experience to the stimulus that is originally anxiety-provoking. The principle of classical conditioning and reciprocal inhibition operates. Reciprocal inhibition theory postulates that if an anxiety-provoking stimulus is introduced in the presence of a condition or experience that is antagonistic to anxiety, then the association between that stimulus and the response of anxiety weakens. This techniques in likely to be effective in situation where a chronic patient is found to dodge and defer an essential treatment procedure mainly due to the fear and apprehension. For example, a patient diagnosed with cancer in its preliminary stage avoids chemotherapy because of fear of the side effects that one has heard of. Delaying chemotherapy may not be desirable. In such cases, the patient can be trained in a relaxation technique. When one is in a totally relaxed state, the patient may be described the procedure of chemotherapy being administered. Gradually, the description may extend to having almost no reaction, except perhaps the discomforts of IV line. The description has to be synchronized with the real process. After observation of reactions and ensuring the absence of significant anxiety response, the next session may have a video clipping introduced when the patient is in the total relaxed state. The video may show an actual chemotherapy administered to a patient. Thus, progressively the patient may get desensitized to the idea of receiving chemotherapy. The actual chemotherapy can be administered after the patient attains total relaxation in the therapeutic setting.

Motivational and Behavioural Intervention

Behavioural change is one of the significant aspects in management of chronic illnesses. There are a number of reasons that contribute to prevention of behavioural change. Factors such as fear, anxiety, apprehension, lack of knowledge, misgivings, denial and lack of seriousness in perception of the condition or repercussions are a few to mention. However, more often than not, the reason for resistance to behavioural change is motivation. There is a close interlink between the motivational and behavioural aspects. Every human being would admit the significance of health in one's life and wishes to have the best health condition. But when it comes to performing and maintaining the behaviour for the best health condition, they face difficulties. How do we get people to adopt health-promoting behaviour in their best interest, yet bothersome or difficult to do so? Putting it straight, how do we motivate people to pursue the undisputed goal of attaining and sustaining the best management of chronic illness, which demands a set of adherence behaviour? Once this question is answered, ensuring behavioural change to manage the chronic illness becomes easy.

Factors Obstructing Behavioural Change

A number of factors influence the individual to continue the status quo and prevent behavioural change. They are briefly described below.

Self-regulation

One of the crucial influences in changing behaviour is self-regulation. In the context of health behaviour, it refers to a process whereby the individual consciously invests efforts at overriding the existing habits and behaviour that pose health risk, and overpower impulses that have repercussion on the health conditions, to attain the goal of positive health status. It involves a number of overt and covert actions. It calls for the capacity of the individual to project oneself into the future, adopt suitable attitudes, plan in a way to suit the future projection of self, use wisdom in choosing the behaviour from the alternatives and focus on the goal attainment. This is initiated detecting discrepancies between one's present state and the state envisaged by the set goal. Self-regulation in fact is a process that has an objective of pursuing a long-term goal. Ironically, though humans are bestowed with the capacity of delayed goal satisfaction, they are often found to give into impulses, face difficulties in perseverance and are defeated by procrastination.

Resistance to Change and Fear of Novelty

Resistance to change is a natural human tendency. Preference for continuing in comfort zone over treading an unknown path is in a way avoidance of threat. In a situation of chronic illness where the patient has an option between continuing the status quo that has high probability of aggravation of illness condition or treading the prescribed path of health adherence, which is unknown and therefore uncomfortable and unpalatable, one faces an avoidance-avoidance conflict. Given such circumstances, highlighting the health goals of the individual and the present condition that contrasts the set target may help in experiencing the 'need' for attaining the target and initiating the behaviour.

Difficulty in Initiating and Maintaining the Behaviour

Very often, there is an initial enthusiasm to adopt the lifestyle that is prescribed for a chronic condition. People tend to adopt a prescribed diet and exercise, give up on health risk behaviour such as smoking and alcohol consumption. The behaviour sustains as long as the new behaviour holds its novelty value. Once that is lost, the chances of retraction are high. Unless the individual develops an intrinsic motivation, and enjoys the new behaviour, the probability of relapsing remains high.

Social Facilitation and Barriers

For a chronic patient, the behavioural change is adopted and implemented in a social context. The social set-up in which the behaviour occurs has certain facilitators and barriers that are naturally set. For example, in the attempts of a diabetic patient advised to go for walk in the morning and evening, if a family member friend or colleague who makes it a point to accompany the patient and make the walks interesting, the patient may gradually shun the natural resistance and come to the stage of enjoying the walks. This constitutes natural facilitator for the exercise behaviour. From this point, the walking exercise gradually turns into a habit. On the contrary, the same walking exercise also may have barriers. The same walking companion may find one excuse a day for skipping the walk or enter into unpleasant arguments and discussions during the walks, making the experience unpleasant. This reinforces the resistance in the patient and demotivates. It may pay good dividends in helping the patient identify the facilitators and inhibitors in the social environment. Efforts should be at enhancing the facilitating forces and minimizing the forces that restrain the behavioural change.

Methods to Handle Obstructions

There are intervention techniques that help the chronic patient fight the inhibitors and trigger the drive for behavioural change.

Motivational Interviewing

This is a "client-centred directive style for enhancing intrinsic motivation to change by exploring and resolving ambivalence" (Miller & Rollnick, 2002). Motivational interviewing is a therapeutic technique built on the basis of Carl Rogers' optimistic humanistic theories. It activates the natural capabilities for a positive change in the patient with chronic illness. This natural capability for change to the positive is present in everyone, but is dormant in many. The role of the health psychologist is directive, and the goal is to elicit self-motivational statements aimed at behavioural change. The method is based on certain assumptions:

1. The best source of information related to the behaviour change lies with the patient.
2. Patient's vision of future and personal values has strong impact on setting goals.
3. The goals set by the patient are based on the individual motivation.
4. Focusing on the discrepancy between the set goals and the present position creates the need to drive the patient towards the goal.

The technique of motivational interviewing is based on four core principles. These principles guide the patient towards behavioural change triggered by self-motivation. The core principles are as follows:

1. Expressed empathy
2. Rolling with resistance
3. Supporting self-efficacy and
4. Developing discrepancy

Empathy is one of the core values of counselling. It is integrated into the interaction with a client. In case of chronic patients, their inability to adhere to the clinical prescription, the pain that they suffer, and the uncertainty and ambiguity they face or other problems need to be empathized and expressed. This lays the foundation for a trustful relationship between the patient and health psychologists. The success of motivational interviewing depends on a healthy relationship with mutual trust.

Resistance on the part of the client is a natural phenomenon in a counselling setting. It is manifested in the client in the form of arguing, interrupting, denying or ignoring. Manifestation of resistance is an indication to the health psychologist that the client is defiant, because the client's perspective of the situation is different. This calls for intensifying listening and changing the direction. For example, an obese patient with a cardiac problem may resist the medical advice of regular physical exercise because it is difficult, demands commitment of time and moving out of one's comfort zone. Hence, the patient may make statements such as "Regular walk for one hour in the morning time is just unthinkable for me". The health psychologist instead of falling into the trap and engaging in argument should encourage the client to elaborate further on the issue.

Self-efficacy is a phenomenon that may not clearly surface for everybody. In many instances, the individual lacks self-efficacy despite possessing the necessary capability of accomplishing the goal. By applying empathy and support, the attention of the client needs to be brought to his/her strengths. This helps in invoking hope and optimism and subsequently the trust that the behavioural change is feasible. Self-efficacy plays a pivotal role in bringing in behavioural change. Building self-efficacy in the chronic patient is a significant step in motivational interviewing. Only after developing self-efficacy can a patient endorse the discrepancy of preserve state and the aspired goal.

Developing discrepancy is skilfully integrated into the counselling process. Application of listening skills helps the health psychologist identify how the patient's personal values are in contradiction to the present behaviour. Bringing this to the notice of the patient motivates the change in behaviour. When the patient's attention is drawn to the consequences of the present behaviour which is not found to be in convergence with the values, triggers cognitive dissonance. The role of the health psychologist is to trigger thinking in the patient along these lines so that he/she comes up with appropriate arguments for the change. Thus, the patient, through motivational interviewing, is helped to identify the discrepancy, develop self-efficacy and thereby develop intrinsic motivation that would initiate and sustain behavioural change.

Motivational interviewing or motivational counselling as called by some has been found effective in enhancing adherence by showing behavioural change through medication adherence among patients with asthma (Borrelli et al., 2007), adherence to diet, exercise, smoking abstinence in hypertension patients (Anshel & Kang, 2008; Levensky et al., 2007) and losing weight in female patients diagnosed with diabetes. Motivational interviewing can be effective by applying the following skills:

1 Asking open-ended questions
2 Listening reflectively
3 Summarizing the client's arguments and statements
4 Affirming the patient's feelings and experiences
5 Eliciting self-motivational statements

These skills constitute the skills of counselling. A health psychologist with good training in counselling is normally skilled with the above techniques.

Biofeedback Intervention

The contemporary trend in health practices emphasizes on the evidence-based action, which in simple terms translates to 'seeing is believing'. Very much in line with this trend is biofeedback technique. As evidenced in the various health behaviour models, cognition plays a significant role in triggering behavioural role. By and large, many of the health behavioural changes have a long-term goal and the evidence of benefit is not witnessed until the behavioural change sustains for a long term. Unable to see any positive outcome from the behavioural change, the patient is likely to relapse to the comfort zone. Instead, if the patient has an evidence of beneficial outcome immediately after the new behaviour is adopted, the patient's motivation to sustain the behaviour may enhance. Biofeedback is equipment that facilitates this process.

Almost all the chronic illnesses have been proved to be related to the stress levels. But rarely, the treatment package includes interventions for stress management. The only reference to stress is found to be an advisory note to the patient to manage the stress efficiently. With no concrete input on the techniques of effective stress management, the patient has no clue to implement the medical advice. In short, though stress is a significant contributor to the aggravation or progress of chronic condition, it is not given the significance it deserves.

Chronic Illness and Therapeutic Interventions 349

The use of biofeedback provides an opportunity to the patient to witness the impact of various relaxation interventions such as Guided Imagery, 'Yoga nidra', music therapy. The principles and the process need to be understood first. The relationship between the stress and physiological arousal is well researched and documented. There is evidence that the stress message to brain triggers the HPA activation. The arousal state is associated with the activation of sympathetic nervous system, biochemical changes in the body and 'fight-or-flight' behavioural response, as well as a negative affect state. This causes a rise in blood pressure, a faster pace of respiration, an increase in skin temperature and changes in muscular tone. When the stress experience is at cognitive and affective levels, the physiological changes take place. So, the principle of relaxation is to consciously place the body parts and mind in relaxed state so the changes take place at physiological level that is contrary to the changes under stress. The pulse and heartbeat slow down, blood pressure drops, respiration slows down, and skin temperature drops. If only the patient gets an opportunity to have the evidence of these positive changes in the physiological system as a consequence of relaxation exercises, it would motivate the patient to practise it as part of the daily schedule that is in compliance with the medical advice. This is because the evidence witnessed works as a powerful cognitive base and creates a conviction that translates to positive behavioural change.

Biofeedback equipment is so designed to attach various sensors to measure pulse, respiration, galvanic skin response (GSR) and muscle tone in the subject. These sensors are also attached to the computer monitor that records the changes in these physiological parameters. The subject is comfortably positioned in front of the biofeedback machine. The health psychologist instructs appropriate relaxation steps. The patient follows the same. While following the instructions, the patient may view the changes visually either on the monitor or on the graph after the session. Having the evidence on the positive consequences of relaxation functions as a good motivator.

As correctly identified, if the human motivation is handled appropriately, behavioural change and maintenance become easy.

While planning interventions, it is appropriate for the health psychologist to take up the assessment and identify the correct factor that is a restraining force causing impediment to behavioural change. There may also be a need to plan interventions in combination for optimal outcome.

Box 8.2   Researcher's Box

- There is a dearth of assessment tools to determine the psychosocial state of chronic patient. Developing and standardizing the illness-related knowledge test, general assessment tool for assessing the affect state and general tool for measuring the health behaviour would be good value addition.
- Designing knowledge intervention programmes for specific disease would be a good research contribution. These interventions can aim at small groups or take the shape of public health awareness programmes.
- For chronic diseases where the prevalence is progressively on the rise and projections are alarming, interventions may be designed for younger age groups with the objective of arresting the progression in prevalence.
- Interventions may specially aim at enhancing quality of communication between the physician and the patient. Pre- and post-test for knowledge assessment, and illness management indicate the impact of doctor-patient communication on disease management.
- In case of life-threatening chronic illness like cancer, the impact of cognitive and affective intervention on quality of life and disease progression can be measured by adopting pre-test/post-test control group design.

Box 8.3 Practitioner's Box

- The practitioner would have the right biopsychosocial status of the chronic patient by assessing the cognitive, affective and behavioural status of the patient. Hence, it is advisable to assess the knowledge about the diagnosed illness, anxiety, depression, stress levels and the health risk behaviour and health-promoting behaviour that already exists in the patient.
- Based on the results of the assessment, the practitioner may plan appropriate intervention or combination of two or more interventions for the patients.
- Few interventions as mentioned in detail in the text may be adopted.
- In order to enhance adherence, simple interventions such as reminders set in the mobile phone, or automatic reminder messages from the office of the physician may be effective.
- For the patients emotionally shattered after the communication of diagnosis, the first intervention needs to necessarily address the emotions. The first target is to bring emotional equilibrium. The cognitive and behavioural interventions should be followed.

References

Aikens, K. S., Aikens, J. E., Wallander, J. L., & Hunt, S. (1997). Daily activity level buffers stress–glycemia associations in older sedentary NIDDM patients. *Journal of Behavioral Medicine, 20*(4), 379–390.

Andrew, A. (2018). *Form and frequency of cognitive intervention: Impact on adherence and management of primary hypertension* (Unpublished doctoral thesis). University of Hyderabad, Hyderabad, India.

Anshel, M. H., & Kang, M. (2008). Effectiveness of motivational interviewing on changes in fitness, blood lipids, and exercise adherence of police officers: An outcome-based action study. *Journal of Correctional Health Care, 14*(1), 48–62.

Antoni, M. H., Lehman, J. M., Kilbourn, K. M., Boyers, A. E., Culver, J. L., Alferi, S. M., ... & Carver, C. S. (2001). Cognitive-behavioral stress management intervention decreases the prevalence of depression and enhances benefit finding among women under treatment for early-stage breast cancer. *Health Psychology, 20*(1), 20–32. doi: 10.1037/0278-6133.20.1.20

Arber, A., & Spencer, L. (2013). 'It's all bad news': The first 3 months following a diagnosis of malignant pleural mesothelioma. *Psycho-Oncology, 22*(7), 1528–1533.

Awasthi, P., & Mishra, R. C. (2007). Role of coping strategies and social support in perceived illness consequences and controllability among diabetic women. *Psychology and Developing Societies, 19*(2), 179–197.

Awasthi, P., & Mishra, R. C. (2008). Expectation and availability of social support in cancer and diabetic women patients. *Indian Journal of Clinical Psychology, 35*(2), 127–137.

Banhato, E. F. C., Galil, A. G. D., Campos, T. D. S., Colugnati, F. A. D., Richter, K. P., Bastos, M. G., & Cupertino, A. P. (2016). Depression symptoms among patients with multiple chronic conditions. *Journal of Depression and Anxiety, 52*(3), 2167–1044.

Bäuml, J., Froböse, T., Kraemer, S., Rentrop, M., &Pitschel-Walz, G. (2006). Psychoeducation: A basic psychotherapeutic intervention for patients with schizophrenia and their families. *Schizophrenia Bulletin, 32*(suppl_1), S1–S9.

Beck, A. T. (1967). *Depression: Clinical, experimental, and theoretical aspects*. New York: Hoeber.

Biswas, U. N. (2011). Positive thought induction for arresting disease progression: A hypnotherapeutic application in HIV/AIDS. *Psychological Studies, 56*(2), 192–205.

Borrelli, B., Riekert, K. A., Weinstein, A., & Rathier, L. (2007). Brief motivational interviewing as a clinical strategy to promote asthma medication adherence. *Journal of Allergy and Clinical Immunology, 120*(5), 1023–1030.

Bournes, D. A., & Mitchell, G. J. (2002). Waiting: The experience of persons in a critical care waiting room. *Research in Nursing & Health*, 25(1), 58–67.

Broadbent, E., & Petrie, K. J. (2007). Symptom perception. In: S. Ayers, A. Baum, C. McManus, S. Newman, K. Wallston, J. Weinman and R. West (Eds.), *Cambridge handbook of psychology, health and medicine*. Cambridge: Cambridge University Press.

Brondolo, E., Rosen, R. C., Kostis, J. B., & Schwartz, J. E. (1999). Relationship of physical symptoms and mood to perceived and actual blood pressure in hypertensive men: A repeated-measures design. *Psychosomatic Medicine*, 61(3), 311–318.

Chivukula, U., Hariharan, M., Rana, S., Thomas, M., & Andrew, A. (2017). Enhancing hospital well-being and minimizing intensive care unit trauma: Cushioning effects of psychosocial care. *Indian Journal of Critical Care Medicine: Peer-Reviewed, Official Publication of Indian Society of Critical Care Medicine*, 21(10), 640–645.

Chivukula, U., & Nandinee, D. (2018). Coping, hospital anxiety and depression and pain experience in elective surgery patients: Role of psycho-educational interventions. *Paripex-Indian Journal of Research*, 7(5) 45–47.

Chivukula, U., Swain, S., Rana, S., & Hariharan, M. (2013). Perceived social support and type of cardiac procedures as modifiers of hospital anxiety and depression. *Psychological Studies*, 58(3), 242–247.

Cox, D. J., Clarke, W. L., Gonder-Frederick, L., Pohl, S., Hoover, C., Snyder, A., ... & Pennebaker, J. (1985). Accuracy of perceiving blood glucose in IDDM. *Diabetes Care*, 8(6), 529–536.

Cummings, J. L. (1992). Depression and Parkinson's disease: A review. *The American Journal of Psychiatry*, 149(4), 443.

Danhauer, S. C., Case, L. D., Tedeschi, R., Russell, G., Vishnevsky, T., Triplett, K., Ip, E. H., & Avis, N. E. (2013). Predictors of posttraumatic growth in women with breast cancer. *Psycho-Oncology*, 22(12), 2676–2683.

Davison, S. N., & Jhangri, G. S. (2013). The relationship between spirituality, psychosocial adjustment to illness, and health-related quality of life in patients with advanced chronic kidney disease. *Journal of Pain and Symptom Management*, 45(2), 170–178. doi: 10.1016/j.jpainsymman.2012.02.019

De Ridder, D., Geenen, R., Kuijer, R., & van Middendorp, H. (2008). Psychological adjustment to chronic disease. *The Lancet*, 372(9634), 246–255.

Deo, M. G. (2013). Doctor population ratio for India-The reality. *The Indian Journal of Medical Research*, 137(4), 632.

DeRubeis, R. J., Tang, T. Z., & Beck, A. T. (2001). Cognitive therapy. In: K. S. Dobson (Ed.), *Handbook of cognitive-behavioral therapies* (2nd ed., pp. 349–392). New York: Guilford.

Dickerson, L. M., Mazyck, P. J., & Hunter, M. H. (2003). Premenstrual syndrome. *American Family Physician*, 67(8), 1743–1752.

Fisher, H., & Crawley, E. (2013). Why do young people with CFS/ME feel anxious? A qualitative study. *Clinical Child Psychology and Psychiatry*, 18(4), 556–573.

Frank, R. T. (1931) The hormonal causes of premenstrual tension. *Archives of Neurology and Psychiatry*, 26, 1053–1057.

Fredrickson, B. L. (2001). The role of positive emotions in positive psychology: The broaden-and-build theory of positive emotions. *American Psychologist*, 56(3), 218–226.

Fredrickson, B. L. (2002). Positive emotions. In: C. R. Synder and S. J. Lopez (Eds.), *The handbook of positive psychology* (pp. 120–134). New York: Oxford University Press.

Freeman, A. (1987). Cognitive therapy: An overview. In: A. Freeman and V. Greenwood (Eds.), *Cognitive therapy: Applications in psychiatric and medical settings* (pp. 19–35). New York: Human Science Press.

Golden, J., Conroy, R. M., Bruce, I., Denihan, A., Greene, E., Kirby, M., & Lawlor, B. A. (2009). Loneliness, social support networks, mood and wellbeing in community-dwelling elderly. *International Journal of Geriatric Psychiatry: A Journal of the Psychiatry of Late Life and Allied Sciences*, 24(7), 694–700.

Greene, R., & Dalton, K. (1953) The premenstrual syndrome. *British Medical Journal*, 1, 1007–1014.

Hägglund, D., & Ahlström, G. (2007). The meaning of women's experience of living with long term urinary incontinence is powerlessness. *Journal of Clinical Nursing*, 16(10), 1946–1954.

Hariharan, M., & Padhy, M. (2008). Religion and rituals as aids to psychological wellbeing- A Hindu perspective. *Journal of Indian Health psychology*, 2(2), 138–145.

Hariharan, M., & Rath, R. (2008). *Coping with life stress: The Indian experience*. New Delhi: SAGE Publications India.

Havens, B., Hall, M., Sylvestre, G., & Jivan, T. (2004). Social isolation and loneliness: Differences between older rural and urban Manitobans. *Canadian Journal on Aging/la revue canadienne du vieillissement, 23*(2), 129–140.

January, A. M., Zebracki, K., Chlan, K. M., & Vogel, L. C. (2015). Understanding post-traumatic growth following pediatric-onset spinal cord injury: The critical role of coping strategies for facilitating positive psychological outcomes. *Developmental Medicine & Child Neurology, 57*(12), 1143–1149.

Jena, S. P. K. (2008). *Behaviour therapy: Techniques, research and applications*. New Delhi: SAGE Publications India.

Jensen, M. P., Moore, M. R., Bockow, T. B., Ehde, D. M., & Engel, J. M. (2011). Psychosocial factors and adjustment to chronic pain in persons with physical disabilities: A systematic review. *Archives of Physical Medicine and Rehabilitation, 92*(1), 146–160.

Kandasamy, A., Chaturvedi, S. K., & Desai, G. (2011). Spirituality, distress, depression, anxiety, and quality of life in patients with advanced cancer. *Indian Journal of Cancer, 48*(1), 55–59.

Katon, W., Lin, E. H., & Kroenke, K. (2007). The association of depression and anxiety with medical symptom burden in patients with chronic medical illness. *General Hospital Psychiatry, 29*(2), 147–155.

Khajehei, M. (2015). Aetiology, diagnosis and management of premenstrual syndrome. *Journal of Pain & Relief, 4*(4), 193.

Larsen, P. D. (2016) Chronicity. In P. D. Larsen (Ed.), Lubkin's Chronic illness: Impact and intervention (9th ed., pp. 5–6). Jones & Bartlett Publishers.

Lazarus, R. S., & Folkman, S. (1984). Coping and adaptation. In: W. D. Gentry (Ed.), *The handbook of behavioral medicine* (pp. 282–325). New York: Guilford.

Levensky, E. R., Forcehimes, A., O'Donohue, W. T., & Beitz, K. (2007). Motivational interviewing: An evidence-based approach to counseling helps patients follow treatment recommendations. *AJN The American Journal of Nursing, 107*(10), 50–58.

Leventhal, H., Halm, E., Horowitz, C., Leventhal, E. A., Ozakinci, G., Sutton, S., ... & Johnston, M. (2004). Living with chronic illness: A contextualized, self-regulation approach. (Eds) Stephen Sutton, Andrew Baum & Marie Johnston. *The SAGE handbook of health psychology* (pp. 197–240). London: Sage.

Leventhal, H. O. R., & Ian, B. (2012). The common-sense model of self-regulation of health and illness. In: L. D.Cameron and H. Leventhal (Eds.), *The self-regulation of health and illness behaviour* (pp. 56–79). London: Routledge.

Mechanic, D. (1995). Sociological dimensions of illness behavior. *Social Science & Medicine, 41*(9), 1207–1216.

Mehta, M., & Dhal, A. (2010). Cognitive behavioural management of chronic daily headaches. In: M. Hariharan, G. Padmaja and M. Padhy (Eds.), *Trauma and pain: Biopsychosocial perspectives* (pp. 31–44). New Delhi: Global Vision Publishing House.

Meyer, D., Leventhal, H., & Gutmann, M. (1985). Common-sense models of illness: The example of hypertension. *Health Psychology, 4*(2), 115.

Milam, J. E. (2004). Posttraumatic growth among HIV/AIDS patients 1. *Journal of Applied Social Psychology, 34*(11), 2353–2376.

Miller, W. R., & Rollnick, S. (2002). *Motivational interviewing: Preparing for change*: New York, NY: Guilford Press.

Mishra, M., & Sinha, R. K. (2001). Effects of yogic practices on depression and anxiety. *SIS Journal of Projective Psychology and Mental Health, 8*, 23–27.

Montgomery, M. (2010). Uncertainty during breast diagnostic evaluation: State of the science. *Oncology Nursing Forum, 37*(1), 77–83.

Nairn, R. C., & Merluzzi, T. V. (2003). The role of religious coping in adjustment to cancer. *Psycho-Oncology: Journal of the Psychological, Social and Behavioral Dimensions of Cancer, 12*(5), 428–441.

Neighbors, M., & Tannehill-Jones, R. (2010). *Human diseases* (3rd ed.). Delmar: Cengage Learning.

Nicholson, N. R., Dixon, J. K., & McCorkle, R. (2013). Predictors of diminished levels of social integration in older adults. *Research in Gerontological Nursing*, 7(1), 33–43.

Nicholson, N. R., & Shellman, J. (2013). Decreasing social isolation in older adults: Effects of an empowerment intervention offered through the CARELINK program. *Research in Gerontological Nursing*, 6(2), 89–97.

Padhy, M., Lalnuntluangi, R., Chelli, K., & Padiri, R. A. (2016). Social support and adherence among hypertensive patients. *AJHM*, 1, 33–40.

Park, C. L., Lechner, S. C., Antoni, M. H., & Stanton, A. L. (2009). *Medical illness and positive life change: Can crisis lead to personal transformation?*. Washington, DC: American Psychological Association.

Peltzer, K., & Pengpid, S. (2016). Anxiety and depressive features in chronic disease patients in Cambodia, Myanmar and Vietnam. *South African Journal of Psychiatry*, 22(1), 940. doi: 10.4102/sajpsychiatry.v22i1.940. PMID: 30263167; PMCID: PMC6138068.

Pennebaker, J. W. (1984). Accuracy of symptom perception. In: A. Baum, S. E. Taylor and J. E. Singer (Eds.), *Handbook of psychology and health: Social psychological aspects of health* (Vol. 4, pp. 219–252), Taylor Francis.

Penrod, J. (2001). Refinement of the concept of uncertainty. *Journal of Advanced Nursing*, 34(2), 238–245.

Ross, K., Handal, P. J., Clark, E. M., & Vander Wal, J. S. (2009). The relationship between religion and religious coping: Religious coping as a moderator between religion and adjustment. *Journal of Religion and Health*, 48(4), 454–467.

Seema, N. N., Thomas, S., Pienyu, R., & Srinadh, B. (2015). Spirituality and wellbeing among antenatal women. *Indian Journal of Health and Wellbeing*, 6(12), 1241–1243.

Shiel, W. C. (2016). Definition of chronic disease. *MedicineNet*.

Sridevi, K., & Krishna Rao, P. V. (1996). Yoga practice and menstrual distress. *Journal of Indian Academy of Applied Psychology*, 22, 47–53.

Steiner, M., & Born, L. (2000). Advances in the diagnosis and treatment of premenstrual dysphoria. *CNS Drugs*, 13(4), 287–304.

Swami, M., Narain, M., Kanwal, K., Mishra, M., & Singh, S. (2017). Premenstrual syndrome: Correlation and functional impairment. *Journal of Mahatma Gandhi University of Medical Sciences and Technology*, 2(1), 18–22.

Thomas, M. (2016). *Impact of psychosocial intervention on adherence and prognosis in patients undergoing coronary artery bypass grafting* (Unpublished doctoral thesis). University of Hyderabad, Hyderabad, India.

Van den Akker, O. B. (2012). *Reproductive health psychology*. London: John Wiley & Sons.

Walker, C. (2010). Ruptured identities: Leaving work because of chronic illness. *International Journal of Health Services*, 40(4), 629–643.

Warshaw, G. (2006). Introduction: Advances and challenges in care of older people with chronic illness. *Generations*, 30(3), 5–10.

WHO. (2016). Non-communicable diseases. Available from: http://www.who.int/topics/noncommunicable_diseases/en/

9 Psychology of the Caregiver and Careprovider

Patient care is a process. This involves a complex coordination between the family caregiver, professional care providers and the patient. The complexity of the process will be appreciated if one looks into the contextual dynamics of the three individuals involved. Let us examine the condition of the patient who is diagnosed with a chronic illness. The patient is the person, who experiences the pain, discomfort, disability of the disease and the side effects of treatment. The patient perceives this diagnosis against his/her health beliefs, the existing knowledge base with regard to the disease, fears, apprehension, anxiety, worries, hope and expectations from the health care professional and family caregiver. His/her illness/health behaviour is determined by the physical energy, motivation and outcome expectations. The physical pain, emotional turmoil, helplessness, frustration and perception of dependency may trigger a number of reactions that are often expressed or displaced on the primary or family caregiver. On the other extreme, there is also a possibility of efforts to suppress all feelings under a stoic exterior.

Let us now try to understand the condition of the caregiver. Most often than not in case of chronic and terminal illness the caregiver is the spouse, though there are caregivers who are the children, parents, siblings or relatives of the patient. What is significant to note is that the caregiver is a close family member, and in majority of cases, it is the spouse. When the spouse is the primary caregiver, he/she is very close to the age of the patient. In case the patient is elderly, the caregiver too is elderly. Thus, the physical energy levels that play a crucial role in caregiving need to be taken into consideration. The caregiver has to be viewed with his/her knowledge or cognitive base regarding the disease. Further, accepting the diagnosis of a loved one creates its own emotional reactions such as shock, denial, sadness, fears and anxiety about the suffering of the loved one. While handling one's own emotion, the caregiver also has the responsibility of handling the emotions of the patient efficiently. The primary responsibility of the caregiver is 'being there for the patient' physically and psychologically, administering medication, diet and nutrition, helping him/her with activities of daily life, responding to pain and discomforts even during night time, handling and setting medical equipment like nebulizer, oxygen, IV line to which one may be exposed for the first time, participate and play a decisive role in decision-making on the treatment. Besides such direct patient care, it is the caregiver who normally substitutes the normal family role of the person taken to illness now. Then, the additional responsibilities increase by two-fold—taking care of the patient and substituting the sick person's role for the other family members. It is the caregiver who has to manage the finances, coordinate with the health insurance or the employer, and identify resources to meet the treatment expenses. While discharging these responsibilities, the caregiver also needs to maintain his/her own health, career, social networking, and balance the time, energy and other resources between the patient and other dimensions of life.

The third but a most important angle in the patient care is health care professional—the physician or the surgeon. Among the many patients, one has to be identified with typical problems,

Psychology of the Caregiver and Careprovider 355

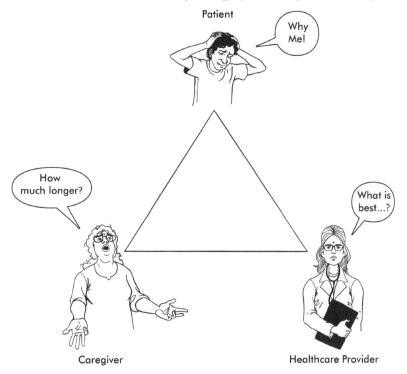

Figure 9.1 Patient, Caregiver, Health Care Provider Triangle.

diagnosis and medical advice. When the caregiver reports a medical emergency, it has to be given priority and be accommodated within the crowded schedule. The doctor has to ensure that the diagnosis is cent per cent correct and discuss the treatment options with patient and family in an objective manner. Further, the doctor has to understand and address various fears and apprehensions of the patient and the family members, and appraise the family about the disease, its progression, prognosis and possible adversities and medical emergencies and the associated course of action. Ideally, a doctor enriching his practice with biopsychosocial approach also has to address the psychosocial aspects of the patient and caregiver, which include addressing anxiety, dissipating fears, educating them on the disease course, treatment outcome and service availability. Thus, while the doctor's focus should continue to be the patient and the disease, the associated psychosocial factors need to be attended too.

As shown in Figure 9.1, these three individuals constitute a simple triangle that depicts the complex process of health care for the patient.

Psychology of the Caregiver

Case 1 Gayatri

Gayatri, a 73-year-old homemaker, has been a caregiver for the past 23 years. Her husband, Aryaman, who is eight years older than her suffered his first heart attack when he was 58 years old. Gayatri, 50 at that time, with their only son still in class 9 became the family caregiver. Following is the narrative about her role in her own words.

My husband suffered a heart attack weeks before his retirement from Government service. My son was young and still in School. We are just a middle-class family who depended on my husband's salary. I had to take a decision on meeting the hospital expenses. I called my relatives in our native place and requested them to put the house for sale. My husband recovered after having two stents.

A few years later, there was another medical emergency as he had a cardiac attack. The doctor advised a bypass surgery. I was extremely careful about his diet, medication and sleep after he was discharged and was under my care at home. Initial few days, he was in pain, had no appetite and was not eating well despite all my attempts to motivate him by changing the menu for each meal. I was tired and lacked energy as my sleep was very inadequate. There were times when I expressed my displeasure to his being uncooperative in taking adequate nutrition. However, when I sat alone, I used to regret for my outburst and understand that his lack of appetite could be because of the strong medication. After all he is the one who is in pain. These thoughts put me back to the right frame of mind to resume my role as the caregiver.

I frequently used to forget taking my B.P. tablets. My blood pressure used to be high when I was attending on him during the hospitalization phase.

With my son away, and being the sole caregiver, I had to stay alert all the time. He had sporadic episodes of pain in the chest. In initial days following his heart attack and bypass surgery, I would panic. Subsequently, I developed a kind of mental preparedness to meet the challenge of medical emergencies. A bag with a pair of clothes and the medical files of my husband was always kept handy to save time in moving to hospital. Experience in handling emergencies also taught me to broadly distinguish between the symptoms of cardiac problem and others.

While things set into a routine and both of us were engaged with our daily chores, in 2015, he suffered a new setback—this time it was not related to his heart but he was diagnosed with cancer in his urinary bladder. It shattered us. He was 77 and I was 69 years old. He had to undergo a surgery. Soon after the surgery he suffered a cardiac event in the ICU. I was informed that his condition was critical. I had to be alone in the hospital during this period until my extended family members could reach the hospital. I had faith in some power beyond the human. I waited outside the ICU until things were better. It is four years since this surgery and subsequent chemotherapy cured him.

But evaluating the series of episodes and the role I played, I feel a sense of satisfaction and peace that I have always given my best and that he could successfully fight every time. I certainly endorse the strong support from those who stood by me and then the divine power in which I have faith. One factor I need to suggest is that if only I had better information, I could have done a better job perhaps.

Case 2 Bhavana

Bhavana, a 62-year-old homemaker, narrated her experience as a caregiver to her husband who suffered and succumbed to cancer. She recollected her experience.

My husband has been a smoker and that used to be my only point of conflict with him. It was in 2013 August that he was diagnosed with oral cancer and had to undergo a surgery.

When I waited outside the operation theatre the surgeon sent words to me. He showed me a lump of flesh and said 'this is what we removed from his jaw. But we saw that the disease has spread to the surrounding areas. Shall we remove all that too?' With no second thoughts I gave my consent thinking that removing the entire cancer cells ensures the cure.

Late in the night I was called into the ICU to meet my husband. I was in fact not prepared to see him in a condition where there were staples all over his jaw. The doctor explained that they had to remove the jaw bone, take a piece from the rib and place it in the jaw. My role of caregiving started only after he was moved to the room in the hospital. I had to do the nasal feeding. The nurse taught me how to do it. I was a bit nervous doing it for the first time, but got used to it subsequently. My worry was his disfigured face.

While attending on my husband I had to meet the challenge of convincing his employer bank to reimburse medical expenses since my husband's speech was not clear. Never even once I entertained the thought that the treatment would be a failure. I felt a sort of boosted up inner strength that kept me going with the process of caring. I used to give him bath carefully, feed him liquids, sit and talk to him and sleep next to him with a hand on him to reassure my support. I also had a very unstinted support from my siblings.

There was a relapse that developed into a very bad wound that continuously oozed and emitted foul smell. I dressed it every day careful not to show any expression on my face. There were several occasions when I had to handle his emotions. There were days when I cried in front of him when he said his end was nearing. I tried to distract him playing cards with him, asking him to watch me work in the garden or take him for a short walk. Finally, he breathed his last in my lap on August 27th, 2014.

I do not know where from I got all the strength to stand strong.

Today, I live with a satisfaction that I did justice to my duty as a wife. There is not even a single instance of regret in providing him all the care and love that he deserved.

The striking difference between the experience of Gayatri and Bhavana is the prognosis of the disease. The striking similarities are the caregivers' multitasking such as managing finances, drawing support, and giving the total support by making caregiving as their total focus. Neither of them answered positively to the question if they missed socializing, having their leisure, personal time to their health care activities such as daily exercise etc. They categorically said that everything else could wait. Perhaps this is one striking difference in these two cases when we compare them with the available literature on Western research.

The two cases of caregivers discussed above provide us ample scope to understand the definition of caregiver, their characteristics, the impact of caregiving on them, the factors that influence caregiving and many more aspects elated to caregiving. When we discuss the various aspects related to caregiving in the subsequent pages, it will be more meaningful if you relate them to the two cases.

Often caregiving is discussed in the context of chronic illnesses such as cancer, stroke, Chronic Obstructive Pulmonary Disease (COPD) renal diseases, organ failure, dementia, physical disabilities, mental illness, intellectually challenged, cardiovascular disease, diabetes mellitus etc. However, majority of research on caregivers has been on the caregivers of cancer patients. With few variations, by and large, caregiving is the same for chronic patients. Hence it will be discussed in general while making specific reference to the disease where necessary. For example, the nature of caregiving varies for the patients with dementia and patients with mental illness as the challenges for the caregiver are different from assisting or helping a chronic patient with activities of daily life or as a part of treatment process.

Patient Care: Caregiver's Perspective

A caregiver is an unpaid member of a person's social network who helps the patients with their activities of daily life. Caregiving happens to a person with an acute or chronic disease needing assistance to manage a variety of tasks that may include day-to-day activities like bathing, dressing administration of medication, tube feeding and ventilator care. In addition to the direct health care of the patient, caregiving also includes the management of the patients' finances, emotions, coordination with the social environment including that of health services. While caregiving is undoubtedly an act of love and devotion, it is a tremendous drain on one's physical and psychological resources. Very often, caregiving is discussed with reference to the elderly population, besides those with chronic or terminal illness. In contemporary Indian Society where the proportion of elderly population is on the increase, and nuclear families as reality, where the employment of youth has a global spread, and there is progressive increase in the prevalence of non-communicable diseases, the need for focusing on the caregiving and caregivers becomes highly relevant. With these changes in the social mosaic, the youth will find caregiving an increasingly difficult activity, not because of lack of will or devotion, but because of shrunken social support system (due to small family norm), increasing demands in the highly competitive job market and difficulties in managing a balance between caregiving and career.

The present trend of treatment that requires surgery, acute or chronic illness is shorter hospital stay. Patients are normally discharged from hospitals after the emergency care, phase of observation and satisfactory risk minimization. This makes them as the base for long-term care, calling for home-based patient care.

Caregiving has become a reality of life that occupies a significant time in contemporary society. In 19th and 20th century, caregiving was a short-term requirement. But, with advancement in medical science and changing life styles the life expectancy has gone up without a matching rise in quality of life. As a result, disabilities related to old age, and complication of chronic illnesses place a significant demand for caregiving.

As per a survey of 2004, in the US, 21% of households marked the presence of caregivers, where 83% of them were family caregivers. Such statistics are not available in India. However, it can be presumed that the scenario is not much different in our country (Shaji & Reddy, 2012).

In India, it is a challenge to be a caregiver, because hired caregiving lacks the professionalism and devotion. It is just one more job for these 'employees'. Further, an increasing number of cases come to the limelight where the patients are abused and physically harmed by the hired caregivers. A family member enters the role of caregiver with no prior notice, preparation or support from medical professionals. Given such circumstances, it is necessary that the family caregivers are provided the required support to optimize their efficiency.

Nature of Caregiving

Caregivers can be broadly classified into three:

1 Primary caregivers: They are the one who routinely extend the daily care for the loved one who is ill. They assist in daily chores such as brushing, bathing, dressing, feeding and administering medication, and the necessary relief activities such as connecting the oxygen, providing steam inhalation, nebulizer. They are the ones who coordinate with the medical professionals/hospitals, keep record of temperature, urine output, fluid input, blood pressure, maintain the medical files of the patient, and accompany the patient for regular medical reviews. They are also the persons who actively participate in decision-making regarding the treatment process.
2 Secondary caregivers: They are the persons who typically provide a backup to the primary caregivers. They are the weekend visitors for caregiving, run errands or assist the primary caregiver in their responsibilities.
3 Crisis caregiver: They provide support to the primary caregivers in the event of any medical emergencies like a fall or a major adverse event when the health condition of the patient shows a sharp decline demanding medical attention.

The discussion in the chapter is with reference to the primary caregiver. Primary caregivers are the persons who live with the patient with a schedule that occupies their time the whole day. They are also referred to as family caregiver.

Caregiver Responsibilities

In terms of time, the responsibilities of caregiving range from short duration of post-acute care following hospitalization and discharge to few decades of continuous care for the person with chronic illness. According to the US data, an informal caregiver spends 4.3 years on an average in caregiving activities (Donelan et al., 2002). There is no Indian data to compare. However, the caregiver time may not be less than what is found in case of the US.

In terms of tasks, the responsibilities of caregiver include assisting the patient with activities of daily living (ADL) and instrumental activities of daily living (IADL). Assistance in ADL consists of helping the patient in bathing, dressing, grooming, mouth care, toiletting, transferring between bed and chair, walking, climbing stairs, administering medicine and eating. These activities may appear very simple and routine. However, the checklist of these activities does not explain the hardships involved in bathing a patient with surgical wounds, one who resists bath, or one with obese body. The activities by themselves do not account for administering medications to a patient (with cognitive impairment) who cannot follow the simple instruction of swallowing the tablet. When there are multiple medications at different timings, the caregiver has to handle the complexity of their timings, dosages and those to be administered based on certain symptoms.

Instrumental activities of daily living (IADL) are relatively complex activities involving management and maintenance of aspects related to life. They include communicating and keeping companionship, managing transportation, shopping and preparing meals, managing personal finances, household maintenance and managing medication.

Factors such as unpreparedness, limited knowledge, need for using discretion in administering symptoms-based medication or responding to patient panic place the caregiver in a situation of decision-making against high ambiguity. They are normally unsure of the correctness of the decision. Supervision on the side effects of new medications and detecting the early signs and deciding their urgency are responsibilities with unreliable personal abilities. They cause considerable amount of stress in the caregivers.

Impact of Patient Care on Caregiver

Caregiving, particularly in India, is considered a highly noble service. It is done for a loved one and can be profoundly satisfying, and leaves a sense of fulfilment. However, caregiving can also be overwhelming and cause extraordinary strain on the physical, emotional, cognitive, social and professional dimensions of the caregivers. As a consequence, the caregiver may feel a sense of burden. Caregiver burden is broadly defined by Buhse (2008) as "a multidimensional response to physical, psychological, emotional, social and financial stressors associated with the caregiving experience". Given et al. (2001) defined it more elaborately. According to them, caregiver burden refers to "multidimensional biopsychosocial reaction resulting from an imbalance of care demands relative to caregivers' personal time, social roles, physical and emotional states, financial resources and formal care resources given the other multiple roles they fulfil".

When a person in the family is sick and gets hospitalized, the life of the caregivers is almost dislocated. With the caregiving turning the epicentre of life, the other dimension lines move to the second line. Allocation of time, energy, emotions and cognition to one's job, needs of other family members and social participation progressively decline. This exhausts the caregiver and creates a feeling of being overwhelmed with the responsibility of caregiving. This is what is caregiver burden.

The extent of caregiver burden is determined by a number of factors such as the age, occupational status, physical health condition, personality type, responsibilities towards other family members, availability of support from family, social support outside the family, economic condition of family, economic burden due to the illness of the family member, type of illness, duration, patient's degrees of dependence on caregiver, progression of the disease, prognosis and knowledge and skill related to caregiving. In addition to all these, the interpersonal relationship between the patient and the caregiver, patient cooperation and empathy for caregiver also constitute the caregiver burden. In a study on caregivers of COPD patients, Cain and Wicks (2000) found that caregivers who belonged to Black community and those above 55 years of age experienced less burden compared to Whites and those below 55 years of age. There are no differences in gender and relationship with the patient. In a population-based study in Mumbai, Bhattacharjee, Vairale, Gawali and Dalal (2012) identified the factors affecting the burden of caregivers of stroke survivors. Among the patient factors, incontinence, morbidity, neurological deficits and being a woman contributed to caregiver stress. Among the caregiver factors, long hours of caregiving, anxiety, disrupted sleep, financial problems and younger age were the factors that contributed to caregiver burden.

Let us discuss the positive and negative impacts separately.

Positive Impacts

Recall the two cases of caregivers mentioned at the beginning of this chapter. Both the persons reiterated their positive feelings of 'sense of satisfaction and fulfilment' derived out of caregiving. The majority of caregivers have endorsed positive experiences of caregiving. The survey conducted by National Opinion Research Centre (2014) in America recorded that 83% of caregivers reported positive aspects of caregiving. Their feedback included the following:

- A sense of reciprocation to someone who cared for them
- A sense of satisfaction that their loved ones were getting the best care
- A sense of personal growth
- An enhanced meaning and purpose of life
- A feeling of fulfilment that by being good caregiver they were setting a good role model and passing on good tradition to their children

Many caregivers report that the activities they are engaged in their given new role benefited them. This normally is the product of coping through positive reappraisal where the individual under stress appraises the situation highlighting the positive aspects of the stressful circumstances. This enables the individual to review the stressful situation by attributing a new meaning, sometimes with a tinge of spirituality. Such perspective has the potential to enhance their wellbeing. Haley et al. (2003) found that the caregivers who perceive more benefits of their caregiving role reported lower levels of depression. Higher levels of wellbeing and the sense of satisfaction sustain their positive impact in lifelong after the role is terminated.

The positive attribution that serving the sick enjoys in Indian culture adds the positive value to the role. What follows this is an informal positive social audit of the role of caregiver, which enhances the image of the person in the community. In addition to this, the perception of comfort that the patient derives out of the caregiver's services also adds to the self-esteem of the caregivers. When the caregiver is able to perceive the positive values associated with his/her role, amidst the stressful experience the probability of enhancing wellbeing and minimizing the impact of stress is high.

While endorsing and experiencing the positive aspects of caregiving is present, one cannot deny the experience of stress that the role brings. Researchers have noted the coexistence of both the positive experiences and good amount of stress and strain in caregivers (Beach et al., 2000; Harmell et al., 2011). The two-factor model suggested by Lawton et al. (1991) argues that caregivers experience both the emotional distress and the sense of satisfaction and growth. Their coexistence is compatible.

Negative Impact

Caregiving is an activity performed with an objective of assisting, comforting and healing the loved one who is ill. By default, it is an activity performed under stress, the source of which is the illness of the loved one itself. Concerns and anxiety about the diagnosis and health condition of the loved one, worries about the prognosis of the disease, internalization of the pain suffered by the loved one, ambiguity related to the symptom manifestations and constant doubts about correctness of action while the patient is under homecare, distress related to the disease prognosis, uncertainties related to financial management related to treatment cost, difficulties in balancing the role as caregiver, homemaker and employee become part of life for the caregivers creating multiple sources of stress. In addition to this, the demands of the role may cause deprivation or disruption to the basic needs like sleep, rest, nutrition, physical exercise, mental relaxation—all of which are natural therapeutic ingredients of stress. Thus, the caregiver who faces severe stress on the one hand and is prevented from natural stress management measures on the other becomes vulnerable to the impact of stress manifesting in various dimensions of health. The negative impact can be seen in physical, emotional and social dimensions of the person. In other words, the stress related to caregiving is no different in its impact on the individual's health discussed in the chapter on stress and its impact on health and wellbeing.

Impact on Physical Health

Impact of caregiving on physical health can be traced back to three antecedents. First, the caregiver very often forgets to take their own medications (for blood pressure, diabetes, etc.). The second reason is neglect of their sleep and nutritional requirements. The third reason is the neurochemical changes associated with the role stress. However, the negative impact on physical health depends on a few factors such as the duration of caregiving, the stage in which the patient is, disease progression and the intensity of caregiving. When these factors are on higher side, the probability of the caregiver's physical health taking a toll is higher. In the context of caregiving for children with diabetes, Raina et al. (2004) identified five factors influencing caregiver's health. They are background and context, characteristics of the child, caregiver strain, intra-psychic factors, and coping and supporting factors. Raina et al. (2005) acknowledged the past research that associated caregiving demands and behaviour of the care recipients to the caregiver health. But while doing so, they also reiterated the need for more research to identify the determinants of caregiver health and wellbeing.

Murphy, Christian, Caplin and Young (2006) conducted a focus group discussion on the caregivers of children with disabilities. More than 50% of the participants reported that the role of caregiving negatively impacted their health. Almost all of them experienced chronic fatigue and sleep deprivation. Chronic pain in the back and shoulder was seen as the consequence of lifting the child frequently. Most of the caregivers reported one or more chronic ailments. This was attributed to caregiving. Many of them ranked their own health needs as the lowest priority. They confessed neglecting their diabetes or hypertension conditions by attaching lower priority to it over the needs of the child with disability or other family members' needs. Some of them reported burnout as they perceived their role as a tunnel with no end at sight.

One of the requirements of caregiving involves physically handling the patients. Caregivers may injure themselves during such tasks, but may not have time to seek medical intervention or scope to have someone substitute their role until their recuperation. When they set low priority to their injuries and health condition, it is obvious that they do not even think of their wellness measures such as setting time for their regular exercise or leisure.

Stenberg, Ruland, and Miaskowski (2010) reviewed 164 research publications related to the effect of caregiving for cancer patients. They identified a list of more than 200 problems spread over various dimensions of life related to caregiving. The problem-related physical health includes pains and aches in various locations, poor quality and quantity of sleep, extreme fatigue, low energy levels and feelings of physical drain out, loss of weight, loss of appetite and indigestion. The enlisted problems are clear indicators of overwork and disruption of sleep and timely food, which are integral part of the very demands of the role as caregiver. Unless the caregiver makes a conscious effort to replenish oneself with required rest and nutrition, the negative impact on physical health cannot be minimized.

Impact on Emotional Health

1 **Positive Emotions:** Caregiving is considered as a service. All services, when voluntary, lead to a positive emotional outcome. Going by that logic, caregiving must elicit some positive emotions. But the paradox is that while extending services are associated with a 'feel-good factor', the situation of a loved one diagnosed with a chronic illness that needs support service has the natural consequence of negative emotions. The balancing act between the positive and negative emotions and the final outcome in terms of emotional health depend upon the focus with which the caregiving is extended. When the focus is on the task one is involved in and the comfort and benefit of it to the patient, it is likely to weigh more towards the positive emotional health. On the contrary, when the focus is the pain and discomfort that the loved one is going through and the minimal impact the caregiver is able to make in reducing patient distress and trigger a perceivable improvement in the patient health condition, the caregiver is likely to experience more negative emotions.

Indian philosophy advocates what is termed as '*Nishkamakarma*', meaning 'doing with no expectation of reward'. This philosophical disposition helps in experiencing an intrinsic reward of caregiving. The two cases of caregivers discussed at the beginning of the chapter highlight the caregivers' satisfaction and positive feelings.

Among the positive experiences, some caregivers have expressed that illness and caregiving helped to bring the family together. This facilitated to spend quality time together with the patient. Such situations were positive both for the patient and for the caregiver. Caregivers reported that the role enriched their experience as a new learning and brought a new meaning to their life and purpose. Some others attributed caregiving experience to enhancing their self-esteem (Kim, Schulz, & Carver, 2007; Stenberg et al., 2010) identified a number of positive aspects reported by caregiver from more than 150 research articles. They are appreciation of the time together, awakening of own strength, opportunity to 'pay back', change of world view, greater sense of being connected, enjoying the role of caregiver, finding purpose

and meaning in life, gaining better intimacy, increased respect for each other and considering caregiving a moral responsibility.
2 **Negative Emotions:** Very often, the caregiver role springs up when one is not at all prepared for it. It comes almost blocking everything else for which one is engaged mentally and physically setting the phase of life. For example, when couple are preparing for a quiet and peaceful retirement, a holiday with the children living abroad, marriage of the children or a long pending religious activity etc., the diagnosis of chronic illness of one of them shatters their plans and binds them to the illness and caregiving for which there was least preparation. This results in foregoing something pleasant that was looked forward to and engaging in something painful that was unexpected. This combination is bound to result in negative emotional experience.

The multiple responsibilities that the role demands place a feeling of burden on the caregiver. The longer the period of caregiving, the greater would be the caregiver burden. Patient care is often perceived as difficult, time-consuming and disruptive to one's own care, grooming and nurturing. Caregivers perceive personal tasks as feeding, washing or moving the patient more burdensome than the peripheral tasks such as arranging transport, doing household chores, coordination with the hospital. Tasks such as monitoring symptoms, handling the medical equipment, providing emotional comfort to the patient are considered emotionally strenuous, because the lack of required skills in the task invokes negative emotions such as fear, anxiety, uncertainty about the outcome.

Caregiver burden is more a subjective experience than the actual amount of work involved or the length of time spent in caregiving. Studies have shown that with availability of support in the task, caregiving is not experienced as burdensome (Goldstein et al., 2004). Highly sensitive caregivers are likely to invoke high-intensity negative emotions when their loved ones suffer the pain. To put it in the words of a caregiver who attended on her father in terminal stages of cancer and the mother, a stroke patient in her last stages, "It is torture to see your parents suffer. You feel absolutely helpless absorbing the pain. It is like someone beating you ruthlessly with a strong hunter with your voice gagged". Such expressions contain a complex combination of negative emotions like distress, fear, anxiety, helplessness, anger, guilt and anxiety. Stenberg et al. (2010) identified a long list of emotional reactions reported by caregivers. They are summarized under the broad heads of anxiety, depression, uncertainty, guilt and sexual issues. In addition, they enlisted a number of positive emotions and challenging emotional reactions. Some of the challenging emotional reactions are highly context-bound and realistic. Accepting the diagnosis of a disease like cancer in the loved one is the first challenge. It is very difficult to see anything positive in such situation. When the diagnosis is announced, the prime responsibility of the caregiver is to provide reassurance and emotional support to the patient. Hence, one's own emotional expressions sometimes are suppressed. One has to deal with the reality of disease progression and subsequent permanent separation from the loved one. This could be emotionally draining and exhausting. Further, there is always the challenge of addressing the dilemma of disclosing or maintaining the secret of prognosis to the patient.

Anxiety and depression are found to be the predominant negative emotion among the caregivers. In a longitudinal study conducted by Grunfeld et al. (2004), it was found that 30% of caregivers of terminal patients with breast cancer suffered anxiety, while 35% suffered depression. Many a time, the anxiety and depression of caregivers were found to be higher than those of the patients (Mollasiotis et al., 2011). Caregivers are sometimes more engaged with illness than the patients themselves. They are found to be involved in providing practical and emotional support. What casts a greater burden on them is to conceal the negative information from the patients and provide safe and filtered information (Mollasiotis et al., 2011). This generates a tremendous amount of emotional pressure on the caregivers.

The emotional distress and caregiver burden are also associated with the severity of illness and probability of their cure and survival. When the caregiver has a hope that the care for the loved one is going to bring positive outcome, the feeling of satisfaction and positivity is likely to be higher than the burden. When the caregiver knows that the care is only palliative, the anxiety, fear and other negative emotions are higher, particularly when there is demand for constant care and heighted alertness in observing the symptoms and needs of the patient. Avsar et al. (2013) compared the caregivers of two types of End Stage Renal Disease (ESRD) patients. One group consisted of caregivers of kidney transplant patients, while the second group had the caregivers of Continuous Ambulatory Peritoneal Dialysis (CAPD). The kidney transplantation is considered gold standard treatment for ESRD where the prognosis is marked by better quality of life and possibility of longer survival. CAPD requires a homecare with a change of dialysis four times every 24 hours. This intervention brings changes in the behavioural health pattern of the patient. Further, with the increase in the treatment of CAPD, patients experience complications at physical and emotional levels. This calls for continuous attention and alertness on the part of caregivers who are expected to identify them in time. The caregivers were assessed on their sleep quality, anxiety, depression and caregiver burden. When the two groups were compared, the caregivers of CAPD patients showed higher levels of anxiety and depression and low sleep quality and experienced 2.61 times greater burden. This could be because of the differences in outcome expectations of health conditions of the two groups of patients, as well as the different intensity of caregiving demanded by the two patient groups.

Illness and caregiving happen in a social context. The nature of patients' illness, the perception of illness by relevant social groups, their attitude, and response to the illness, expressed emotions towards the patient and support extended to caregivers play a significant role in influencing the caregiver's emotional health. Social reactions vary with the types of illnesses. To a large extent, extending social support and responding to the needs of the family with a chronic patient depend upon understanding and perceiving the disease in right perspective. While the society views physical illness like cancer, stroke or renal diseases in one perspective, their understanding of mental illnesses, diseases, schizophrenia, cognitive degenerative disease like dementia is different. Hence, their participation in extending social support also varies.

The caregiver burden varies with the type of disease. Some typical symptoms and characteristics of certain diseases lay an emotional burden on the family and caregivers. Cognitive impairment and the behaviour associated with it, and the impulsive actions of the patients of dementia pose a challenge to the caregivers and cause high distress. While on the one hand, it is painful to see one's loved one behave erratically and irrationally the other cause of stress is the consequence of such behaviour that may either harm the patient or others. Caregiving of such patients demands constant alertness and quick reflexes to physically prevent some of the actions of the patient. One caregiver, daughter of a 95-year-old dementia patient, described the episodes of her mother who ripped apart a mobile phone and put the battery in her mouth. She narrated an instance when she went to use the washroom when her mother was sleeping. By the time she returned, the 'Amrutanjan' (a pain balm) container from the bedside table was opened and half of the contents was consumed by her. She found that her mother was very swift in certain actions like pouring water into the pickle jar, on the dining table, soaking the *rotis* (Indian bread) made for the family meal totally in water, hiding the foot ware in her pillow case. The caretaker said:

> while these acts are hilarious in one way, it used to pain me to see my once intelligent and commanding mother reduced to such behavior. The additional work in cleaning the mess, the worry about the consequences of her eating the unedible substances made me feel drained out.

Similar plight is also reported by caregivers of schizophrenia patients. Caregivers of schizophrenia patients found difficulty in distinguishing the meaning of symptoms and disability (Barrowclough, Tarrier, & Johnston, 1996).

There are a number of chronic diseases with high prevalence for which the data related to caregiver burden is inadequate. Cardiovascular diseases and bronchopulmonary diseases find themselves in the list of ten most frequent causes of Disability-Adjusted Life Years (DALY) (Murray & Lopez, 2000). They require long-term assistance from family members. The emotional strain of caregiver and family burden for these diseases need to be studied. In fact, there are fewer Indian studies on the caregiver burden itself.

The difficulties experienced by the caregiver in caring for the patient are termed as family burden. This has both objective and subjective dimensions. Objective burden refers to concrete, practical problems such as financial problems, disruption in personal, social activities, family relationships. They can be identified, worked upon and resolved in a problem-solving mode. Subjective burden refers to the psychological reactions experienced by the family members due to the illness of the loved one, and as the consequence of objective burden. They are affect states denoting depression, anxiety, feeling of loss, loneliness, embarrassment, anger, helplessness, hopelessness etc. Irrespective of the type of illness, the family burden could be the same. Some of the common affect states of the caregivers of both physically ill and mentally ill patients are anxiety, depression, economic burden and feelings of isolation.

In order to understand the differences of caregiver burden for patients with physical and mental illness, Magliano et al. (2005) conducted a classic study on a sample of 709 caregivers of patients with schizophrenia and 646 caregivers of patients with physical diseases. The physical diseases included cardiac, renal, brain, lung problems and diabetes. The results revealed that the most quoted consequences of caregiving were constraints in social activities, negative impact on family life and feelings of loss. Caregivers of patients with brain disease experienced both objective and subjective burdens. Subjective burden was found to be high in caregivers of schizophrenia and other physical ailments. Social support in emergencies was found to be lower for schizophrenia compared to the other physical diseases. Lower social support was found to be associated with objective and subjective burden in caregivers.

Impact of Caregiver's Emotional Health on Patients

There is constant association between the caregiver and the patient. This provides an opportunity for the patient to perceive and infer from various physical, emotional and behavioural cues of the caregiver in the process of caregiving. Further, there is a psychological bond between these two family members much prior to their roles as the patient and caregiver. Thus, they have a cognitive schema about each other. Given this context, there is a fair possibility of the patient perceiving the physical fatigue, negative emotionality, lack of energy levels in their caregiver. They do have their impact on the patient. There is an interdependent relationship between the patient and the caregiver (Padmaja et al., 2016). The psychological state of one affects the other. The positive association between patient and caregiver in their psychological distress is proved by a number of studies (Hodges, Humphris, & Macfarlane, 2005). In case of cancer patients, it was observed that as the disease progresses and reaches a stage of palliative care, the caregiver is likely to experience higher levels of distress sometimes to the extent of developing psychiatric morbidity (Pitceathly & Maguire, 2003).

High levels of stress and depression negatively affected the caregivers. Studies confirmed the mutuality of affect state between patients and caregivers. In the context of caregiving to cancer patients, it was found that disease progression, symptoms and increased immobility brought

366 *Psychology of the Caregiver and Careprovider*

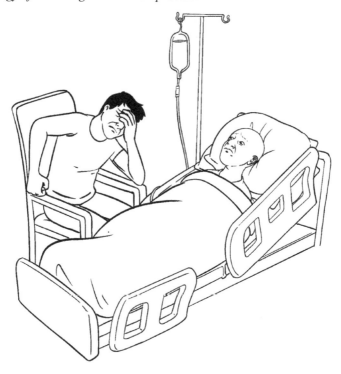

Figure 9.2 Reciprocal Relationship between Patient and Caregiver.

depression in patients. This is understandable because of mind-body relation in a human being. But it was also noticed that the depression in patients predicted the depression in the caregiver (Kurtz et al., 1995). The reasons could be many. First, the perception of pain and deterioration in the loved ones naturally causes negative affect. The second reason is an implicit attribution that the caregiving has not fetched desirable outcome also is highly unrewarding and contributes to depression (Figure 9.2).

Transmission of negative affect is also found from the caregiver to the patient. It was found that when negative affect transmitted from the caregiver to the patient, the impact of it was much more severe. The reason is simply the level of vulnerability of the patient. One who is already physically vulnerable, when takes the negative affect transferred from caregivers, feels much higher distress. Badger et al. (2007) studied the depression in cancer patients and their caregivers. They discovered that when transmission of anxiety followed the pathway from the caregivers to the patients, the impact was far greater than the pathway from the patient to the caregiver (Badger et al., 2007).

Padmaja et al. (2017) studied 100 cancer patients and their 100 caregivers on four affect dimensions, viz. depression, anxiety, distress and somatization. Results clearly indicated that caregivers' affect state transmitted to patients creating anxiety and depression in them. Depression, anxiety, distress and somatization in caregivers predicted anxiety and depression in patients. One may attribute this to several reasons:

– The patients internalize the anxiety and depression of caregivers
– The patient may start feeling guilty on perceiving depression anxiety and somatization in their caregivers and that in turn may make them anxious and depressed

- The negative affect state of caregiver may subtly communicate to the patients that the things are not really going well with the health condition
- The quality of caregiving may go down with the caregivers' negative affect causing a great concern, anxiety and depression in the patient

Affect states are closely associated with the quality of life, both for the patients and for their caregivers. Quality of life related to health in away is a measure of wellbeing that indicates the individual's perception about life with reference to set goals, expectations and standards in congruence with their culture and value system. This in turn is influenced by biopsychosocial factors. It includes a number of positive and negative perceptions of symptoms indicating the functioning at physical, mental, emotional, social and cognitive levels. The patient and caregiver have mutual dependence and reciprocity with regard to quality of life. Vanlalhruaii, Padmaja and Kopparty (2018) studied the mutuality of quality of life between the elderly cancer patients and their caregivers. The results suggested that when the patients' quality of life as cognitive functioning dimension is high, the caregiver's quality of life also is high. When the patient's quality of life is positive, the caregiver feels a sense of reward for the services in the form of patient's health outcome. This in turn enhances the wellbeing and quality of life of the caregiver. Padmaja et al. (2016) studied 206 cancer patients and their caregivers on their mutuality in quality of life. They found that a decline in quality of life in patients on few dimensions such as emotional and social functioning or general health status was marked by problem in caregiver's quality of life. Increase in symptoms such as pain, loss of appetite in the patient adversely contributed to caregiver's quality of life. Contrary to the expectations, the dependency of patients on the caregiver predicted higher quality of life of caregivers. Interpreting from cultural perspective, the authors explained it in terms of the caregivers' satisfaction in extending service to someone ill. That not only provides a sense of fulfilment, but also gives a feeling that the patient is under safe care where the possibilities of error are low compared to when the patient asserts self-reliance.

In view of the mutuality in the emotional health of the patient and the caregiver, there is a need to ensure healthy emotional state in the caregiver as an integral part of patient's treatment. This is because of the fact that in view of body-mind connection, attempts should be to protect and sustain the patients in positive affect state.

Impact on Caregiver's Social Life

The caregiver, while attending on the patient, also has to play other social roles and discharge responsibilities towards other family members, attend to the duties assigned to her job in the office, earn an income for running the family, maintain contact with the social network and sustain the personal space for recuperation from the role stress of caregivers. With an adult taken to chronic illness, the other adults are expected to compensate the sick person's role in the family, sometimes, pitching in for taking care of children's needs, attending to the household needs and social obligations. Playing multiple roles under stress is difficult. When the caregiver is a spouse, the burden is experienced in assuming multiple roles of two persons, familiarizing with the work in unknown fields. For example, the woman caregiver who was used to managing household responsibilities and the job responsibilities now has to manage the finances, transport, coordination with the sick spouse's office and peer group, contact with relatives and well-wishers each of which by itself is a demand on one's time and energy.

One of the major sources of stress is inability to balance the multiple roles. Those with flexibility in job try to manage work, household and patient care. Some who set very high standards

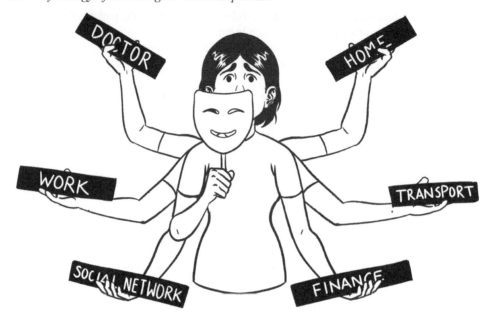

Figure 9.3 Multitasking of a Caregiver.

for themselves in all the dimensions are likely to experience a burnout or frustration for their inability to meet the standards. Some caregivers consider their time for professional work as a kind of relaxation, while some others feel that the entire time needs to be dedicated to caregiving, while rest of the things take a back seat. In this process, many start experiencing social isolation and disengagement from social life, which then becomes a source of stress (Bishop et al., 2007). Many report feelings lonely amidst a busy schedule because there is hardly any leisure or outlet of suppressed feelings (Figure 9.3).

One of the major impacts is on the socio-economic life. With one employed person taking to illness, source of family income is lost (unless the person's job is secured with provision for leave due to illness). Further, the treatment demands additional expenditure. If the spouse chooses to continue working, the patient care suffers. If the spouse decides to quit or change job to a part-time occupation, the finances will take a further toll. Thus, the family of the patient goes through a financial roller-coaster. Covinsky et al. (1994) in their study on a sample of 2661 patients investigated the impact of the illness on the families. The results brought to light the adjustments the family had to make owing to the illness of a person. In case of 20% of patients, a family member had to quit the job to assume the role of caretaker. In 29% of families, there was loss of major source of income, while 31% of family's life savings were drained out. The majority of such cases were from families of patients who were younger, poorer and functionally dependent.

Economic poverty is certainly a major source of stress for the caregiver. Simultaneously, the caregiver also faces informational poverty at the social level. Information is one aspect that strengthens the caregiver cognitively. This in turn brings a state of readiness to accept the realities on the one hand and equips the caregiver with necessary knowledge and skill to act appropriately to the growing needs associated with the patient and the disease on the other. It is lack of information that normally creates stress related to ambiguity and uncertainty. In the absence of information flowing from authentic sources such as hospitals and doctors, they tend to assume the role of a researcher and gather information from various sources, which need not necessarily be authentic. In the contemporary digital world, middle class population rely on internet sources for any information. When it comes to health-related information, the internet source is an easy access to an ocean of information. Unable to filter from there, the caregiver is likely to encounter more confusion than clarity. There is every possibility of ascribing to oneself what is convenient or ascribing everything that is negative. Both are harmful for failure in guiding towards the right caregiving behaviour.

Studies have highlighted the expressed need of the caregivers to have information related to diagnosis, treatment, symptom management, side effects and physical care after the patients' discharge from hospitals (Aslan et al., 2006). Very often, the caregivers did not know what information to seek until they encountered a crisis. Caregivers feel comfortable to have face-to-face communication with the doctors (Brown & Stetz, 1999). Further, they always wished that there is a contact person for the right advice at critical times (Wilkes, White, & O'Riordan, 2000).

The information deficit for the caregivers is very genuine across the globe and across social class in India. The majority of caregivers lose precious time in case of medical emergencies because they do not know how to respond. Very often, the treating doctors are unapproachable, or caregivers hesitate calling them because the rapport with the doctor has not been established to the degree that makes them feel comfortable to contact them.

The impact on caregiver's physical and emotional health is the realities to be identified and attended to. The disruption to the social life is an issue to be acknowledged and handled. Patient care can be optimized by endorsing these problems and planning intervention for caregivers. Apart from the direct impact on health, the caregiver burden also has an indirect effect on health. This was found to happen when caregivers were indulging in wrong strategies of coping that included smoking and alcohol consumption. An increase in use of alcohol and tobacco by the caregiver places their already fragile health under greater risk.

Psychosocial Interventions for Caregivers

Caregiving for chronic patients in India is by and large informal. Paid caregiving though has been picking up slowly, since the last one decade, is majorly unskilled or semiskilled personnel who are not 'chosen based on their aptitude' but are 'employed for an income'. This makes a huge difference in the quality of care. It is not uncommon to come across cases of abuse to the patient by the paid caregiver. The cost of such service is also high. In view of all, this informal caregiving by a family member is the priority. Even when the paid caregivers are employed, the person works under the close supervision of a family member. The employed caregiver's activities are often instructed by the family caregiver. Thus, the family caregiver continues to have the impact of caregiving, sometimes with the additional stress of managing the paid caregiver. In the whole process, the physical, emotional and social impact of caregiving turns the caregiver into a 'secondary patient', transmitting the negative repercussions of caregiving to the patient. Hence, the treatment process of the patient is incomplete unless the caregiver is provided the required intervention to optimize the outcome not only for the caregiver but also for the benefit of the patient.

The interventions for caregivers have to be psychosocial. They should be so designed that they address the identified needs of the caregivers. These need-based interventions range from simple strategies like psychoeducation to complex processes such as Cognitive Behavioural Therapy. The thumb rule for choosing the interventions has to be caregiver need. The objectivity of understanding the needs of the caregivers can be optimized by a formal assessment.

Caregiver Assessment

The major concerns related to the caregiver's hurdles are if he/she is

- equipped with everything (knowledge, skill, time, finance and social support) that is needed for efficient caregiving
- able to easily shift between the caregiver and other roles
- taking good self-care (that includes nutrition, sleep, exercise, time off from caregiving role, attending to health needs like regular medication and his/her appointment with the doctor)
- maintaining positive spirit (minimizing sadness, depression, hopelessness, helplessness etc.)

Caregiver needs can be assessed by taking a feedback on these four aspects with the necessary details under each of the categories. Such assessment can be made either through questionnaires or through interviews. If the answer to any of these questions is negative, the needs related to the question have to be addressed through appropriate intervention. If the response related to maintaining positive spirits is negative, the intensity of negative affect needs to be further assessed with standardized scales of stress, depression or anxiety as the case may be. This provides a sound assessment to decide on the intervention. Along the lines of the four areas discussed above, Northouse et al. (2012) have designed a precise tool called 'TASK' to assess the caregiver distress. The questions are whether the caregiver has the 'Tools' necessary to give the best care; has the 'Ability to juggle' the various responsibilities; has been taking 'self-care' and 'keeping the spirits up'.

There are also a number of standardized tools to assess the stress, anxiety, depression, social support and distress. The advantage with these standardized tools is the reliability and norm. These standardized tools can be used for further assessment on identifying on the four areas mentioned above. The type of intervention should be based on the identified needs.

Psychoeducation

Psychoeducation majorly targets the cognitive component of caregivers. When the caregivers have information need, psychoeducation is effective. The information needs of caregiver can be categorized under 11 types (Adams et al., 2009):

1. Treatment related
2. Disease related (diagnosis/prognosis)
3. Coping
4. Self-care and house care
5. Disease-specific (symptoms, progression)
6. Impact on the family
7. Support services
8. Relationship with spouse (particularly in case of mastectomy, hysterectomy or prostate cancer)
9. Hospital care
10. Follow-up and rehabilitation
11. Other practical issues

This can be termed as knowledge intervention. This empowers the caregiver in several ways. First of all, having adequate functional knowledge about the disease, symptoms and alarm signals creates a mental readiness and confidence of handling an adversity. Further, the preparedness created by psychoeducation prevents the caregiver from shock, inaction and confusion when found with sudden changes in patients' health condition. The information on homecare with good details equips the caregiver with the skills to handle a situation. Information support services strengthen the caregivers with alternatives when he/she needs a respite or when there is a specific need such as nursing care during nights, psychotherapy or household help. Information on the procedures and schedule during hospitalization is very important in dissipating ambiguity and uncertainty in the minds of caregivers. Further information on hospital care during emergencies or hospice centre for palliative care can constitute significant aids during crisis periods. All this information needs to be provided by the clinician or the nurse in the hospital.

The role of health psychologist assumes significance in preparing the caregiver with appropriate information on the probable impact of the disease, patient and caregiving on the family, the interpersonal relationship between the patient and the spouse, the expected caregiver burden, and the subsequent psychological reactions, need for self-care to minimize the caregivers' burden etc. The health psychologist must necessarily educate the caregiver on the need for taking breaks from the role so as to keep one's positive spirits. The caregiver may not have the right strategies of coping. For example, one may assume that the whole caregiving responsibility should solely be assumed by a single person. The skills of coping through seeking social support for such people may be helpful. Similarly seeking emotional support from other family members or close friends may provide great relief. The caregiver having information on such accepted strategies of coping will be able to practise the same at the time of need. Information on follow-up and rehabilitation is something that is of great importance. For example, when a diabetic patient with a developed gangrene is under treatment, it makes a huge difference to the caregiver to know the various possible ways of rehabilitating the patient after the limb is amputated. This information enables the caregiver to plan the future with minimum distress. Similarly, the caregiver of a patient with prostate cancer feels reassured when the doctor informs that the prognosis would be good and explains the importance of regular follow-up and assessment of prostate-specific antigen (PSA) level.

Very often, the psychoeducation intervention is delivered combined to the patient and the caregiver (Hoff & Haaga, 2005; Hudson et al., 2005; Budin et al., 2008). In majority of cases, psychoeducation is given face-to-face, sometimes with telephonic follow-ups. A number of studies recorded the positive impact of psychoeducation in terms of knowledge and skill related to care (Keefe et al., 2005; Hudson et al., 2008). Studies also reported that apart from changes in knowledge and skill, psychoeducation resulted in significant positive changes in psychological correlates of burden (Bultz et al., 2000). The impact of psychoeducation to the caregiver also benefited the patients who perceived improved functional support from the caregiver and better marital satisfaction (Bultz et al., 2000).

Psychoeducation creates a strong cognitive base. This has a positive impact in the affect state because the caregiver with the new knowledge base will be able to function more confidently with minimum mistakes. This benefits the patient in two ways. First, the quality of care will be better. Second, the positive affect state of the caregiver is likely to get transmitted to the patient.

Caregivers of patients with chronic kidney disease (CKD) were given psychoeducation through face-to-face communication/written information. Studies consistently showed improvement in knowledge. Some studies went to measure changes in domains other than knowledge. Gonzalez, Rivera, and Novoa (2005) studied 95 caregivers of patients requiring dialysis. Nurses provided them oral and written information relevant to the disease care. They assessed the difference in knowledge and caregiver burden before and after intervention. Results showed changes only in knowledge domains.

The positive impact of intervention can be seen in all caregivers irrespective of the disease in the patients. In a rural Indian study, Arjunan, Gopinath and Murthy (2011) provided knowledge intervention through structured training capsule to the caregivers of patients with diabetes. The training comprised of knowledge and skills of caregiving. There were significant improvements in knowledge and skills of caregivers cutting across the sociodemographic differences. Such structured training can satisfy the knowledge and information needs of caregivers of diabetes patients that enrich the quality of their care.

Tornay (2007) prepared an information handbook taking inputs from the patients and caregivers of chronic kidney disease (CKD) patients. With this, it becomes typically a need-based booklet to suit the caregivers. A sample of 135 caregivers of transplant patients were educated through these booklets. The results showed that apart from knowledge enhancement, the caregivers' fears and stress were diminished, and it helped them in better adaptation with the situation.

The caregivers of cancer patients undergo severe distress because of the progression of the disease and the pain the patient undergoes. Many of them are very cautious of avoiding any wrong action in the process of caregiving that enhances the patient distress. Information is an essential need for them. Pasacreta et al. (2000) structured a Family Caregiver Cancer Education Programme (FCCEP) and administered it face-to-face. The education was designed for six hours. This was successful in improving the caregiver's perception of health, as well as the confidence levels in their ability to provide patient care.

These studies suggest that the impact of knowledge intervention extended beyond the cognitive domain and brought positive changes in caregiver burden and quality of care.

Interventions for Psychological Distress

A chronic or terminal illness is just not limited to physical pain. Along with the disease come the fear of pain, fear of death, distress of the imminence of losing the loved one, the guilt of burdening the loved one and the loss of self-esteem in becoming dependent. The impact on the caregiver in terms of emotional distress has already been discussed. Though a repetition, it is relevant to summarize it here.

The caregiver experiences the distress similar to the patient about the apprehended pain, quality of life and the imminence of losing him/her. However, since the caregiver assumes the role of support provider for the patient, he/she is expected to put forth a 'strong disposition' to the patient pushing one's own emotional vulnerabilities under shield. This itself is highly distressing. The caregiver has to appear fairly confident about one's role to patient while experiencing ambiguity, uncertainty and confusion about several aspects; has to express hope and trust while feeling hopeless and helpless from within; has to conceal the lack of energy and physical stamina lest it impacts the patient; has to appear energetic and lively lest the low mood and spirit get transmitted to the patient. Many a time, such duality in the caretaker, though consciously practised, has a heavy adverse impact on the health and wellbeing. It is difficult to sustain a high standard of caregiving for a prolonged period. The psychosocial life of a caregiver sees many swings along the course of caregiving, as the patient transits from one phase to the other. The interventions should be so designed to match the psychosocial needs and intensity at different phases.

1 **Diagnosis Phase:** Shock, anxiety and need for support are high for the caregiver in this phase.
2 **Treatment Phase:** Worries about the loved one's ability to withstand and cooperate dominate this phase. This is the phase when the caregivers start gearing up for their role to meet

the challenges of patient response to treatment. The other aspects of concern during this phase relate to managing finances, and multitasking between the caregiver, employee and homecare roles.

3. **Survivorship Phase:** This phase is when the patient is showing good signs of recovery and 'cure'. The majority of caregivers tend to identify some positive aspects related to prognosis. But one area of negative affect is the caregiver's lurking fear that the disease (e.g. cancer) might recur, or the patient may experience a setback in health. The caregiver may have sporadic experiences of apprehension of various types, which is likely to impact the patient.

4. **Recurrent Phase:** Recurrence of the disease (e.g. cancer) or a major setback in the treatment outcome (e.g. the body showing signs of rejecting the implanted organ) is a source of devastating experience for the patient and the caregiver. It shatters the hope. The caregiver is likely to question his/her quality of care attributing the setback to self. A sense of hopelessness and pessimism may dominate. Anger, guilt and distress are likely to be highs.

5. **Advanced or End-of-Life Phase:** This is a phase where the caregiver encounters a situation with a cognition that all the caregiving is not going to culminate in reviving the patient. Understanding well that the care is not going to fetch the 'best' results, one is likely to settle down for the 'next best' where there is hope for providing the optimum comfort to the patient in the remaining time. But this is the time when the pain of the patient is also likely to be at the peak. Thus, the caregiver may experience that the care is almost fetching nothing. This leads to a state of helplessness, loss of confidence in self, leading to high level of distress. There is a chance of the caregiver drifting to severe depression—even of clinical levels.

Psychosocial intervention refers to either a package of interventions addressing the psychological and social issues or a predominant issue related to either psychological or social dimension. Since it includes an array of issues, it is important to design intervention to suit the right combination of issues the caregiver encounters. The issues can be identified by the phases of patients' disease trajectory, which is by and large universal or through interviews with the caregivers. Box 9.1 indicates the salient caregiver features of the phases of patient disease progression/phases and the need-based intervention for the phase.

More often than not the psychosocial interventions address a host of needs. Interventions of this type are also likely to be successful because the psychosocial needs are often intertwined. For example, the concern about managing the roles of caregiving and job is also linked to the concern about financial management, apprehension about recurrence or setback is linked to encouraging patient self-reliance. Hence, psychosocial intervention often addresses multiple issues. Chan et al. (2016) provided an integrated psychosocial intervention to the caregivers of patients diagnosed with chronic kidney failure opting out of dialysis and transplant treatment. In this randomized control group design, one group was introduced psychosocial care, while the control group received standard medical treatment. The intervention was provided through a palliative care nurse and a social worker. The package included a number of support components preceded by family need assessment, knowledge intervention that included besides the aspects of diseases, patient and caregivers' psychological factors and skills of patient care. It also included the service support of physiotherapist, psychologist and homecare visits. In addition, the caregivers were oriented on stress management and effective relaxation techniques. The family was provided skills for improved communication, counselling services and community service referral.

There was a follow-up at one, three and six months. The results clearly indicated the positive outcome of such intensive intervention. Caregiver burden in the study group showed a

Box 9.1 Psychosocial Intervention for the Caregiver along Patients' Phases of Disease Progression

Phase	Caregiver's dominant concerns	Intervention
Diagnosis	Shock, denial, anxiety, distress	1 Knowledge intervention 2 Cognitive intervention for acceptance of diagnosis 3 Intervention to enhance problem-focused coping so that the course of treatment is decided
Treatment	Worries about patient's ability to cope, organizing finances, planning for multitasking	1 Combined counselling of patient and caregiver to highlight patient's ability to cope 2 Family counselling for optimum participation by all members 3 Helping the caregiver set the priorities and chalk out an agenda accordingly 4 Facilitating peer interaction with caregivers of other patients 5 Skill training in major and critical aspects of caregiving like nasal feeding, nebulization as per the need. 6 Symptom identification training
Survivorship	Sporadic apprehensions about recurrence/setback	1 Knowledge input on the probability of recurrence 2 Symptom identification training
Recurrence or setback	Distress, hopelessness, helplessness, guilt and dejection	1 Cognitive therapy for acceptance of reality and the process involved in recurrence 2 Rational emotional therapy to identify reasons for recurrence and emotional management 3 Counselling for emotional ventilation and identification of positives 4 Family counselling to strengthen interpersonal relationship for mutual emotional support
Advanced or end-of-life phase	Hopelessness and dejection	1 Intervention to optimize formal and informal support 2 Spiritual therapy 3 Family counselling to optimize on the time with patient 4 Therapy to create readiness to accept the loss of patient

significant decline at one- and three-month interval compared to the baseline. There was a rebound at six months. Anxiety scores showed a significant decrease in one and three months of follow-up. These positive changes in caregivers' psychological state suggest their significance in patient's quality of life. In this study, there was a nominal change in patient quality of life though not statistically significant.

Very often, the biomedical orientation of treatment process does not take caregivers' psychosocial needs into cognizance. But with the increasing emphasis on holistic approach, it is time that patient care is revolutionized and includes the concerns of the caregivers.

Cognitive Behavioural Therapy

Caregiver burden is the outcome of a number of factors that includes patients' health condition, demands of caregiving in terms of physical work and time, need for juggling between roles, financial status, sleep disruptions and care for one's own health. Very often, while the fatigue and physical strain are the outcome of the heavy work demands, the psychological distress has a major contribution from two factors:

1. Appraisal of the situation by the caregiver (cognitive factor)
2. Ineffective/unproductive coping strategy adopted by caregiver (behavioural factor)

These factors are responsible in proliferation of stress. They can be addressed appropriately by Cognitive Behavioural Therapy. The objective of Cognitive Behavioural Therapy is to put a check on the thought process that enhances stress, and bring about a change in appraisal of the situation and ineffective coping strategies.

Very often, the caregiver finds it very difficult to accept the diagnosis and the progressive deterioration in the health condition of the loved one. In cases of neurocognitive diseases like Parkinson's or Alzheimer's disease, the behaviour associated with cognitive degeneration of patients brings a sense of disbelief in the caregiver that the patient, once known for the 'Sharp brain', could lose all the 'grit' and behave weirdly. Similarly, in cancer patients with metastasis, sometimes the behaviour turns violent, sometimes melancholy; the physical condition also may deteriorate very fast with conspicuous weight loss, episodes of epileptic attack, severe bleeding, breathlessness, unbearable pain etc. Every episode can be a source of shock and stress.

Secondly, the caregiver may sometimes have certain irrational beliefs that he/she should be the sole caregiver for the person, and that it is very selfish on the part of him/her to pay attention to one's own basic needs when the loved one is under so much suffering. Some of them may also entertain thoughts like the others in the family or community may not wish to allocate time and energy to share the caregiving responsibilities with the same degree of efficiency and devotion that he/she gives. One more irrational negative thought was often expressed by caregiver in attributing any negativity in patient condition to one's own suboptimal care. None of such thought processes positively contribute to enhancing the quality of care. If any, they may have a negative impact.

Many of the faulty thought processes contribute to ineffective coping strategies. For example, the belief that caring for the sick husband/wife is the sole responsibility of the spouse has the potential to overburden the caregiver and leave a number of social resources untapped. Then, the caregiving is likely to decline in quality with progress in time.

Cognitive Behaviour Therapy aims at bringing a cognitive restructuring and a behavioural change in the caregiver. The intervention works in the following ways:

- It is of great significance to work on the irrational thoughts that constitute the premise for various behaviours related to caregiving.
- It helps the caregiver have functional knowledge about the disease, its progression and symptoms. This in turn makes the person attribute any adversity to the nature of the disease rather than inadequacies in caregiving.
- Orientation about aetiology, prevalence and incidence provided in the right manner may aid restructuring the thought process in terms of probability leading to acceptance of the diagnosis.

- Cognitive restructuring in terms of human limitations in physical and psychological energy is sometimes useful in accepting one's own limitations leading to endorsing the need for self-care and attending to basic needs.
- Helping the caregiver identify the untapped resources and an evaluation of the same may change the appraisal of the available social resources and the need for seeking social support in the interest of the patient.

A few sessions of Cognitive Behavioural Therapy with adequate follow-up may be useful in reducing caregiver distress, enhancing the quality of caregiver behaviour and finally benefitting the patient.

There is research evidence in support of CBT as effective interventions for caregivers of patients with different chronic illnesses.

Secker and Brown (2005) conducted a randomized controlled study on the caregivers of patients with Parkinson's disease. The study included 30 caregivers whose score in General Health Questionnaire (GHQ-28) indicated a caseness. They were randomly distributed into two groups. The study group received 12–14 sessions of CBT, while the control group was not given any interventions. The two groups were compared before the intervention and three months after the intervention on GHQ 28 scores and their dimensions, as well as caregiver burden. At the base levels, the two groups showed no difference on GHQ or its dimensions. However, the two groups significantly differed on GHQ, as well as caregiver burden. The intervention group showed a significant decrease in somatic symptoms, anxiety, insomnia and social dysfunction. They also showed a significant decrease in caregiver burden and caregiver strain. These differences were stable at three and six months of follow-up.

A meta-analysis taken up by Kwon et al. (2017) identified the benefits of CBT for caregivers of patients with dementia. Arango-Lasprilla et al. (2014) provided CBT to caregivers of patients with dementia and followed them up until three months. They found that the caregivers benefitted with satisfaction with life and control of depressive symptoms.

Au et al. (2010) reported that the CBT could enhance the caregivers' self-efficacy for controlling upsetting thoughts, handling disruptive behaviours and using both problem-focused and emotion-focused coping strategies. Losada et al. (2011) found that their caregivers in the post-intervention phase could bring down their dysfunctional thoughts and depressive symptoms, and have a behavioural activation.

The caregivers of cancer patients often suffer from severe anxiety and distress. Given et al. (2006) exposed a sample of 263 patients and caregivers to ten sessions of CBT in a face-to-face mode in a randomized control group trial. The results showed a significant reduction in caregiver distress related to assisting the patient with symptoms. In addition, this also showed reduction in severity of symptoms in patients.

CBT on caregivers of cancer patients showed contradictory impacts. Studies also showed that CBT had minimal effect on the caregivers. O'Toole et al. (2017) reviewed the literature and conducted meta-analysis. They found that the impact of CBT on caregivers was very small and negligible. Hence, it may be desirable to have an integrated intervention module for caregivers of cancer patients.

The acknowledgement of the caregiver as the secondary patient, and identification of the caregivers' biopsychosocial factors subjected to the impact of the role demands and the designing of interventions for the caregivers are positive steps towards application of biopsychosocial approach to illness, health and wellbeing. However, the practice of including the caregiver in the health care process is not in practice in India. It is time that the health care system takes this need into cognizance and integrates it into the system to be the world leaders in the area.

Health Care Professionals—The Care Providers

The doctor assumes a key position patient health care. There cannot be two opinions in this regard. The role of the doctor is so significant that many cultures equate doctor to God. Indian culture has a popular Sanskrit line '*VaidyoNaraayanoHarih*'—meaning the doctor is 'God Himself'. This is understandable given the position of the patient, patients' family vis-a vis the doctor. The patient, taken to illness, realizing that the symptoms and the disability caused by it and the disruption to the activities are beyond one's management approaches the doctor. This is because the doctor is believed to be knowledgeable in the field of body system and diseases, and skilled in diagnosing, treating and restoring the health and wellbeing or minimizing the pain and disability. Thus, the patient and the family in a position of being vulnerable perceive the doctor as superior, powerful and capable of relieving him/her of the pain. Thus, from the patient's perspective it is a combination of vulnerability and trust that strongly comets to the doctor. The stronger these threads are, the more positive their impact on patient's response to treatment. This is based on the functional integration of body-mind that facilitates movement from the illness to wellness on the continuum. Thus, the doctor has a great impact on the patient's understanding of the disease, cooperation with the treatment with committed participation, the affect state and the health behaviour of the patient. Hence, a healthy relationship between the doctor and the patient is the first prescription of treatment for an optimal outcome.

This crucial relationship between the doctor and patients is an unwritten note of mutual acceptance and agreement of each other's role. Chipidza et al. (2015) stated that

> At its core, the doctor-patient relationship represents a fiduciary relationship in which, by entering into the relationship, the physician agrees to respect the patient's autonomy, maintain confidentiality, explain treatment options, obtain informed consent, provide the highest standard of care and commit not to abandon the patient without giving him or her adequate time to find a new doctor.
>
> (p. 3)

However, the sanctity of doctor-patient relationship often goes beyond such formal objective contractual level. Very often, patients choose to confide in the doctor their fears, worries and problems not only of their health but also factors associated with health.

The relationship between the doctor and patient is built of four pillars, viz. mutual knowledge, trust, loyalty and regards (Ridd et al., 2009). For each of these elements, there is a reciprocal relation. This is explained in Box 9.2.

Among the four components, knowledge about each other can be acquired through secondary source; loyalty is associated with the integral value system of the person. Trust is something that has to build over a period of time, through interaction and mutual assessment. Regard and trust are closely interrelated.

Trust connotes a belief that the person has no intent to harm, and is good and honest. In the context of doctor-patient relationship, the patients trust in doctor encompasses some typical behavioural characteristics reflecting a combination of professionalism and human qualities. The trust of the patient rests on his/her perception of doctor's competence, compassion, empathy, honesty, reliability. They perceive a sense of good will in the doctors, and expect a positive outcome of their visit. This implies that building a trust in the patient rests in the personality disposition, behaviour with patient, and feelings and concern for the patient besides the professional competence.

The determinants of trust between patient and doctor were identified by some studies. Pearson and Raeke (2000) reviewed about 200 articles and concluded that patient's trust in the

Box 9.2 Reciprocal Relationship between Doctor and Patient

Four pillars	Patient's commitment	Doctor's commitment
Knowledge	Knowledge about doctor's reputation, skill and competence	Knowledge about patient's health, affect state, family background, socioeconomic background, emotional state, strengths and weaknesses
Trust	Faith in doctor's competence, care and best intensions	Faith in patient's motivation, reported symptoms and participation in treatment process
Loyalty	Willingness to forgive the doctor for small inconveniences and pain in the treatment process	Commitment to treat but not to abandon the patient
Regard	Feeling and belief that the doctor likes and respects him/her as an individual and is always supportive towards him/her	Feeling that the patient's choice has to be considered, doubts clarified and autonomy protected

doctor positively correlated with physician's communication, level of interpersonal treatment and knowledge of the patient.

In another study, concordance between doctor and patient emerged as a major determinant of patient's trust in physician. This had a positive impact on improving the patients' enablement (Banerjee & Sanyal, 2012).

Development of trust is a process but not instantaneous. Trust between the doctor and patient evolves over continuous interaction between them in more than one session where the perceptual process carriers out the mutual assessment based on one's experience, 'feel-good factor' and the treatment outcome.

Models of Doctor-Patient Relationship

Based on the role played by the doctor and the patient, their relationship is explained in terms of three models by Szasz and Hollender (1956).

Active-Passive Model

In this model, the doctor is active and the patient is passive recipient of the decision on intervention and treatment regimen. Here, the patient is not treated as a 'thinking, feeling organism'. The focus is on the health condition as assessed by the doctor, and the goal is to revive the patient and relieve the pain. Very often, such relationship is seen when the patients' condition is critical, the patient is either unconscious or not in a position to respond meaningfully. In such instances, the ethics of informed consent from the patient is waived in the interest of preventing harm to the patient. Quick decision and initiating immediate intervention is the primary need. The informed consent in such cases is obtained from the family caregiver.

When this model is adopted with a fully conscious and communicative patient, it triggers fear, apprehension and anxiety in the patient, even though the doctor is highly competent and correct in his diagnosis and decision on treatment regimen. The patient goes to the doctor not just with the disease and its symptoms, but also he/she as a few fears, and questions related to the symptoms, desires to know relevant aspects related to the disruption or dysfunction of the system in the body, the prospects of correcting it and the probable time line for the treatment. The patient also has expectation of guidance regarding the diet, and activities to be complied. In other words, the patient would not feel satisfied if his/her participation is reduced to nil. Hence, this model is effective only when the patient's condition blocks any scope of communication.

Guidance—Cooperation Model

This model places the doctor on a higher pedestal, and the patient assumes a position lower. By virtue of professional knowledge, skill and experience, the doctor assumes the power to decide the course of action in the best interest of the patient. The patients' role is that of complying and cooperating in the process of treatment. In this model, the focus is the disease but not the patient. The treatment targets the disease, and the patient complies with the recommendations of the doctor because he/she also wants to be relieved from the disease.

This model is in total violation of biopsychosocial approach. There is every possibility of the patient assuming that the onus of cure or pain relief is totally on the doctor. Secondly, if the recommendations include changes in the lifestyle, the possibility of compliance is low. The reasons for low compliance are because the patient with little explanation or understanding about the benefits of lifestyle change will have no motivation to adopt behavioural change.

Further, the patient who perceives that the doctor is in control of his health condition is unlikely to see any personal role in the process of treatment. This model is seldom adopted.

Mutual Participation Model

This model places the doctor and the patient on equal plane, giving opportunity for participation from both ends. The model is based on endorsing expertise in both partners. While the doctor's expertise is in the field of medicine with due competence in diagnosis and treatment, the patients' expertise is endorsed in the experience of the disease, against his/her life situation, setting the goals for oneself and deciding on whether the treatment suggested by the doctor is feasible or not. The model preconceives interdependence of the two partners in attaining the health goals. Unless the patient shares disease experience and symptoms, the doctor's thinking in appropriate line of diagnosis is not possible. Similarly, unless the patient is properly oriented about the diseases condition, prognosis, lifestyle changes and expenditure involved, the decision of choosing the treatment course from the alternatives offered is not possible.

In this model, both the doctor and the patient have equal power. They engage in communication- and treatment-related activities that are mutually satisfying. Optimizing the outcome of this model depends upon the enrichment of communication between the doctor and the patient. Endorsing this as the most preferred model also acknowledges that the communication between the doctor and the patient plays a crucial role in determining the doctor-patient relationship.

Doctor-Patient Communication

Biopsychosocial approach to health and illness gives communication a vital role. The success of holistic approach to a large extent lies on the healthy doctor-patient communication. In case of chronic diseases, the patient has to manage the disease and the doctor should manage the patient. This concept originates from the wise saying "A good physician treats the disease and a great physician treats the patient who has the disease".

The medium of treating the patient is communication. Communication between the doctor and patient goes beyond exchange of information and knowledge. It is expected to have the basic ingredients of counselling skills like attention, listening to verbal and non-verbal communication of the patient and intensity of patient's expression. This is the role of the doctor when the patient is explaining the problem and symptoms. When the doctor assumes the active role, he/she would be effective when the expression of empathy, respect and support is integrated into the communication. In a study by Butalid et al. (2012), the quality of doctor-patient communication was compared between two periods spaced by two decades (1982 and 2001). The findings identified listening, respect and providing support as consistent themes in both the periods. The study identified changes in certain areas. A shift was noticed in the way the doctors explained things to patient, which was focused on clarity of explanation earlier and clarity on reasoning and advice in later period. In the 1980s, the communication was focused on obtaining patient's consent, while in the 2000s, the focus was on patient's choice. In the 1980s, the doctors owned the responsibility, while two decades later, the emphasis shifted to shared responsibility.

The communication revolved around the problem in the first phase, while it shifted to solution-based communication in the second. Overall, the patients were found to value the evidence-based medicine and participatory decision-making. What a patient values has its influence on a number of factors such as the patient's continuing with the physician, participation in treatment and a number of factors that include health outcomes. It may not be wrong to state that the quality of doctor-patient communication directly and indirectly impacts a variety of factors.

Impact of Doctor-Patient Communication

The first thing that the doctor-patient communication influences is the relationship between the two. Besides this, there is an array of factors it impacts.

Impact on Health and Wellbeing

It is not uncommon to hear from the patients that 'seeing the doctor' itself has a therapeutic impact on them. This is particularly true about patients who receive a sense of support and unconditional positive regard to address the negative emotional state in the patients. Thus, visiting the doctor brings in a therapeutic impact to patients with anxiety, fears and apprehensions.

Interaction with the doctor involves a good amount of information exchange. In a quality communication, the doctor is likely to explain relevant information on the disease, constituting a strong cognitive component. Explanation on hazards of violating prescribed lifestyle also associates a negative emotion of fear for non-adherence to medical advice. These two together help in bringing in the desirable behavioural change leading to better participation in the treatment process. All these are likely to culminate in better prognosis and positive outcome (Figure 9.4).

Physicians play a crucial role in enhancing the quality of communication. Some of the steps they need to follow include the following:

- Explain the disease condition in simple non-technical language suitable to the patient
- Encourage the patient to ask questions and give enough time to reflect on the information and come up with questions
- Ensure that the patient has the right comprehension about the disease by verifying with questions.
- Explain the need for changing lifestyle and caution the patient about the existing health risk behaviour that contributed to the disease condition

Psychology of the Caregiver and Careprovider 381

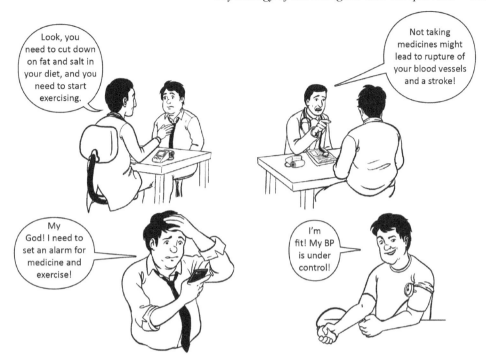

Figure 9.4 Impact of Quality of Communication on Prognosis.

- Educate on the symptoms and signs indicating medical emergencies and SOS steps
- Orient about the possible side effects of medication
- Explain about the need for monitoring and periodic consultation with the doctor
- Help the patient draw a chart for medication in case there are many medicines to be taken in a day

When the focus of communication is the patient, it is called patient-centred communication. There is research evidence to suggest the positive impact of patient-centred communication. Stewart et al. (2000) found that patient-centred communication is associated with higher well-being and less discomfort and health concerns. Effective communication has the potential to manage post-operative pain in surgical patients. In a study by Sugai et al. (2013), patients in one group were educated through oral communication and written material explaining the body's response to pain and the role of endorphin functioning as body's natural analgesic. Patients were also explained the negative impact of narcotics on production of endorphins in the body. The second group of patients did not receive this communication and was treated as the control group. Results showed that while 90% of patients in the experimental group avoided taking narcotics, contrastingly all the patients in the control group used the complete prescription of pain killers. Despite this, the control group patients recorded average pain scores than the pain scores of the experimental group. This is a glaring evidence of impact of effective communication on the patients' health behaviour and health management.

In a study by Swain (2013), the quality of doctor-patient communication was measured in a sample of 30 doctors and 300 patients with primary hypertension (the ratio of doctor and patients being 1:10). Based on the quality of communication, the patients were divided into high, medium and low quality of communication. The patients were followed up for six weeks. The results showed that the patients in high-quality communication showed high adherence and there was a significant drop in their systolic and diastolic blood pressure. The pathway analysis showed that the quality of communication had a trajectory to good prognosis via enhanced clinical adherence. The results indicated that quality of communication explained 6% of variance in adherence and 4% of variance in prognosis, which is small but statistically significant. Effective communication by itself cannot cure the disease. However, it significantly contributes to boosting the disease management.

The trajectory is simple. The information from the doctor impacts the adherence, which in turn impacts the treatment outcome. Friedman et al. (2008) studied a group of 300 patients undergoing ocular hypotensive therapy and 103 physicians. They enlisted the determinants of adherence. The results showed that those who received limited information from their doctors showed lower adherence. Wilson et al. (2007) found non-adherence and the subsequent poor health status in patients where the physicians had inadequate knowledge about patients, and made unilateral decisions without the participation of patients. These are indications of poor quality of communication.

Quality of communication suffers when the crucial information fails to flow either from the patient or from the doctor. However, the onus of enhancing the quality of communication lies on the doctor. In Wilson et al. (2007) study of chronically ill elderly patients, they observed that 27% of patients who skipped their medications either for side effects or because they found them ineffective did not report this to their doctors. Among the 39% of patients who skipped their medication due to the cost of it, 38% switched to low priced medication without the concurrence of the doctor. Such actions not only will have poor prognosis but also are likely to be associated with low patient satisfaction.

Impact on Patient Satisfaction

Patient satisfaction is an important component in the treatment process for two reasons—first, the patient's continuing with the doctor depends on patient satisfaction. Secondly, the sense of satisfaction contributes to reduce anxiety and fear and thus contributes to speedy recovery or minimizing the pain and trauma. Biopsychosocial perspective of treatment emphasizes on healing, in addition to the cure. As distinguished by Dalal (2016), "curing is removal of the disease whereas healing implies recovery of the patients from some trauma" (p. 33). The patient, approaching the doctor, looks forward to both cure and healing. While cure comes from the medical competence of the doctor in the correctness of his diagnosis and the choice of right medication or procedure, the healing experience is derived from the communication between the doctor and the patient. It may be inferred that the quality of communication contributes to the healing experience and manifests in the patient satisfaction. Patient satisfaction depends on a number of factors:

– Time given by the doctor
– Attention of the doctor when the patient speaks
– Attitude of the doctor towards the patient and caregiver
– Empathy of the doctor in matters related to the health problem (e.g. job pressure, financial constraints as constraints for treatment)
– Doctor's skills in explaining the disease-related aspects
– Scope given to the patient in expressing fears, seeking clarification
– Respect for the patient in expression of choice and preference

The list is not exhaustive. There may be few other factors on which the doctor's behaviour is judged and evaluated. By and large, when the communication is patient-centred, the satisfaction derived is normally high. Research evidence suggests the close association between the doctor's communication skills and patient's satisfaction. Biglu et al. (2017) studied patient satisfaction in eight specialized clinics in Iran. They found a strong correlation between the communication skills of the doctors and patient satisfaction. Flocke, Miller and Crabtree (2002) included 2881 patients and their 138 family physicians in their study. They concluded that the physicians who had person-centred style of communication were rated as having highest quality doctor-patient relationship and were found to elicit highest patient satisfaction.

Patient satisfaction is the outcome of both quality of service and the trust in the doctor. Quality of service includes both the biomedical services and the psychosocial care. Psychosocial care involves care services that are non-verbal (e.g. assisting a weak patient to the washrooms) and verbal (e.g. asking the patient by looking at the facial expression if he/she was experiencing any discomfort sitting in the chair). The patient perceives a number of psychosocial care components like empathy, respect and concern for the patient in the process of communication.

Chang et al. (2013) conducted a cross-sectional study on patients from seven medical centres in Taiwan who volunteered to participate in the study by responding to a questionnaire. The objective was to find the relation between service quality, patient trust and patient satisfaction. Results found that the perception of service quality influenced the patient trust, which positively contributed to patient satisfaction. Service quality includes the biomedical treatment and psychosocial skills that form an integral part of professional skills. Besides competence in the field of medicine, professional skills include communication and attitude that reflects transparently in the behaviour.

Communication as a determinant of patient satisfaction was endorsed by research across the globe. Chandra, Mohammadnezhad and Ward (2018) conducted an extensive review of literature to examine the association between trust, doctor-patient communication and relationship. They arrived at a conclusion that patient-centred communication, and trust are associated with patient satisfaction. This in turn is related to perception of better quality of health care services, better adherence behaviour from patient and better outcomes of treatment.

Patient satisfaction by itself is important for the health care providers to sustain their business of service. But patient satisfaction assumes significance for its contribution to patients' response to treatment and its outcome. Research across globe suggests that doctor's communication skills are a major determinant in this. Hence, it is essential to focus on the aspect of doctor-patient communication.

Despite the empirical evidence that emphasizes the need for communication skills in doctors as a constituent part of their professional skill, the medical curriculum in India has totally ignored this. These skills are expected to be acquired by the physician with practice and experience. This remains a challenge for the medical professionals starting their career. In a study by Agarwal et al. (2011), the surgical residents from the departments of surgery from various Indian hospitals were included. A survey was conducted to explore communication skills of residents. Results revealed that 81.7% of the sample reported that they never received any orientation on communication skills from their seniors. The results revealed that when the patients came in for emergency surgery, 31.7% residents spent 10–30 seconds and 68.2% spent about one minute with the patients. In case of elective surgery, 88.5% residents spent more than one minute in communicating with patients. None of them had any knowledge regarding the percentage of incidence of complications that should be explained to the patients. Residency is the time; the doctor is exposed to on-hand experience and training from the seniors. However, their observation of their seniors at work failed to lay emphasis on doctor-patient communication or building relationship. They observed that in emergency only 26.9% of operating surgeons interacted with the patient or the caregiver. The majority of them entrusted this responsibility to the juniors. Even in elective surgery only 50% of operating surgeons communicated with the patients. It is alarming to note that in elective surgery, only 71.43% of residents communicated to the patient about the diagnosis, 89.43% explained about the treatment, 45.24% informed about the option of alternative treatment, and 29.36% explained to the patients about the probable outcome. Only 50% of residents explained about the complications. All the residents admitted to have had arguments with their patients at some point. The study recorded an expressed need by residents for including the communication skills in their curriculum, which should cover various aspects of communication across medical situations including bedside manners. More than half of the participants expressed the need for including the communication skills in the final evaluation of their professional skill.

This lack of training reflects in the practice of the physician culminating in patient dissatisfaction, non-adherence and suboptimal treatment outcomes. The communication during consultation was often found to be poor. Sebastian et al. (2016) studied a sample of 105 patients who had consulted the doctors in the preceding 15 days, to find out various factors related to their satisfaction. The factors on which the patient judgement and evaluation were obtained included the patients' satisfaction with the doctor's behaviour, information volunteered by the doctor and the additional information sought by the patient. Results indicated that 39% of the respondents were not satisfied with their doctors. Patients identified inadequate consultation time, need for a friendly disposition, need for the use of simpler language in conversation, need for addressing the patients' worries and fears, and provision for better patient privacy.

A physician who is emotionally distant, technology-oriented and disease-focused can hardly reach the patient and reap the benefits of psychosocial approach to treatment.

Impact on Doctor's Satisfaction

Communication is a two-way process. The quality of communication should have similar impact on the dyads involved in it. Effective communication has a positive impact on the doctors too. Following are the benefits of quality communication on the doctor:

– Facilitates the doctor to know their patients well
– Contributes to the correct line of investigation for diagnosis
– Leads to higher job satisfaction, increased efficiency, productivity and wellbeing
– Helps in enhancing the reputation
– A good doctor-patient interaction sometime may function as a significant lead to a perplexing problem in medical field leading to a ground-breaking innovation

Patient satisfaction is found to be closely associated with doctor's satisfaction. Haas et al. (2000) found that the patients' satisfaction with health care and their global health status are closely associated with the doctor's job satisfaction. In an earlier study, Suchman et al. (1993) attempted to identify the correlates of physician satisfaction. The findings pointed at the patient satisfaction and doctor-patient relationship.

The impact of doctor-patient relationship can be seen on four major health outcome dimensions encompassing objective health measures (e.g. blood pressure), subjective illness experience, affect state and behaviour. When the relationship suffers an impairment and the patient

Box 9.3 Doctor-Patient Relationship: Impact on Health Outcome Variables

Dimension	Outcome variables
Objective health measure	Blood pressure
	Serum glucose level
	Serum triglyceride level
	Survival
	Frequency of visit of doctor
Subjective illness experience	Global health status
	Pain
	Satisfaction
	Knowledge and understanding of disease
Affect state	Emotional state (positive or negative)
Behavioural aspect	Adherence to treatment
	Coping
	Functional status
	Recovery

Source: Chipidza, Wallwork and Stern (2015). doi: 10.4088/pcc.15fO1840

feels dissatisfied, it leads to poor outcomes on the four dimensions (Gordon & Beresin, 2016). The impact on the health outcome dimensions is summarized in Box 9.3.

When the quality of doctor-patient communication is high, there is likely to be a positive impact on all these dimensions. The quality is high when there is a match between the intended communication and received communication (Swain et al., 2015). In other words, the objective measure of quality of communication is the similarity index between the intended and received information, i.e. when the patient understands what the doctor wanted to communicate.

The quality of relationship is likely to suffer because of one or more factors such as the patient, the doctor, the system or the mismatch between the patient and provider. They are explained in Box 9.4.

The doctor's endeavour is to strengthen the relationship with the patients and do full justice to the profession. However, the reality of the profession, particularly the Indian medical field, is different. The senior consultant and specialists are caught in a busy schedule where they are coping with doctor-patient ratio of 1:2000 against the WHO norms of 1:250. The junior residents on the contrary are struggling with their inadequate communication skills, which limit the outcome for their competence in the biomedical field, because with limited communication skills they cannot express their empathy, make the consultation patient-centred, elicit relevant information, address the fears and apprehensions of the patient. Then, they leave the patients unsatisfied. In a study by Hariharan and Padhy (2011), it was found that the junior doctors had lower emotional intelligence compared to their senior counterparts. This is not a congenial environment for establishing a healthy doctor-patient relationship.

The field reality in the Indian health system is that the majority of cases neither the senior doctors nor the resident are able to focus on factors that strengthen the doctor-patient relationship. The doctors are found to function under lot of pressure while trying their best to provide service to the patient.

Box 9.4 Factors Negatively Impacting Doctor-Patient Relationship

1	Patient factors	Explanation
	New patient	Rapport is yet to establish. It takes little time for this.
	Bad prognosis	1. When everything possible as per medical knowledge is done, without desirable outcome 2. The patient attributes the bad prognosis to doctor's competence
	Low health literacy	The doctor is unable to explain things to the patient because of low health literacy level. The patient feels overwhelmed when the doctor explains things because of cultural gap.
	Patient is judged as 'difficult'	The patient may exhibit the half knowledge he/she has about the disease. The patient may use resistance by using phrases like 'Yes----- but' indicating that he/she has no inclination to follow medical advice due to reasons one may cite. There may be mutual dislike between the doctor and patient.
	Family pressure	There may be distrust between the doctor and caregiver
2	Doctor factors	Explanation
	Burnout	Burnout on the part of the doctor manifests in lack of attention, poor communication, emotional exhaustion, tendency to be indifferent and detached. The patient feels unattended.
	Early phase of career	The lack of communication skills may fail to elicit relevant information from patient, or underplay the concerns and needs expressed by the patient, making the interaction appear disease-centred rather than patient-centred.
	Conflict with the treatment team	When the patient receives conflicting messages from different members of the team, the trust in the doctor is lost.
	Extremely busy doctor	When the patient, after making appointment, has to wait long hours for consultation, or when the doctor gives very little time for consultation and goes by what is recorded in case sheet by the junior doctors or nurses paying very little importance to the face-to-face communication with patient
3	Doctor-patient mismatch	Explanation
	Language barriers	The language spoken by the doctor and patient may be different owing to regional origins. Communication takes the heavy brunt in such cases.
	Cultural barriers	If there are huge class differences between the doctor and patient, the interaction may suffer. The patient may not feel comfortable if the doctor's interaction operates from a different cultural background.
	Locus of control	If the patient perceives that everything related to the health, treatment and time is out of one's own control, one may assume a totally passive role that is detrimental to doctor-patient relationship.
4	Systemic factors	Explanation
	Space/privacy	When the physical space provided for consultation has no provision for privacy, the communication may be inhibited from the either side. Such physical environment may have ample scope for distracting the attention of doctor or patient.

(Continued)

4	Systemic factors	Explanation
	High patient-doctor ratio	When there are fewer doctors to attend on a large number of patient, time and energy invested in each become limited. Patients are likely to feel that the doctor's focus is not on them and they feel like being treated as objects of disease.
	Documentation obligation	When the system/organization lays emphasis on documenting, lot of time goes into compiling the data. Even in the review meetings, the doctors may rely on the data available on the system at one click. This minimizes the scope for interaction.
	Cost	When the health care cost is very high, the patient may associate the doctor with the cost. The element of dissatisfaction may have a spillover to the doctor, thus negatively impacting the relationship with the doctor.

Source: Chipidza, Wallwork and Stern (2015), modified to suit Indian context.

Patient Care and Impact on Doctors

A senior physician working in emergency medicine recalled his experience:

I found my role highly challenging. I was always alert and ready to receive a patient wheeled in by an ambulance, take the case and comprehend the patient condition using my pan continental experience and expertise, spring into action. My sole goal was always to save the patient. In my career I received elderly people, youth, children, women with a variety of medical conditions like fracture of bones, severe head injuries, epilepsy, cardiac arrest, pulmonary problems, hypoglycaemia, allergic reaction etc. The hospital relied on my expertise and I enjoyed a good reputation. The sense of satisfaction that I experienced when my colleagues or the hospital referred to me as an efficient doctor assured me of my job satisfaction. I never knew when I gradually increased my work to a level that I had no time for other activities and shifted my entire focus on work. It happened very gradually so that the marginal increments of workload was not conspicuous, until one day when I found myself in a weird action of throwing things from my office table when I heard the siren of an ambulance coming into the hospital premises indicating that there is one more emergency case for me to attend. I caught myself in this action, and soon introspected and decided to reschedule my job commitment.

Another doctor narrated:

I had this young child, an automobile accident victim brought to the hospital bleeding profusely. The hospital followed the medical protocol. She was to be given blood transfusion. This was done. The team of doctors did their best. Then, I was told that more blood was needed. I volunteered to donate my blood because of the compatibility. The hospital team worked relentlessly for 48 hours. But finally, we failed to save the child. I am normally very objective. But this particular case upset me a lot. Could not get over the experience for several days.

The third doctor spoke in a tone of disgust and despair:

> At least a thousand times during my career I must have contemplated quitting my job in the hospital. It was disgusting to adapt to the culture of corporate hospital and its commercial face. But every time I had to pacify myself and continue as I could not afford to quit my job. I continued to work in an atmosphere where my values were constantly in conflict with my job requirements.

The case of first doctor is clearly a manifestation of burnout; the second doctor, occupational stress; and the third, a case of constant stress originating from the systemic factor in conflict with personal values.

These cases of doctors give an insight. It is true that the doctors face public expectations for the best treatment of patients. Sometimes, when the doctor fails to meet these expectations there is a quick public outburst and aggression. In such instances, it is important to have an empathetic analysis from the doctor's perspective. It is necessary to understand the psychosocial impact of patient care on the doctor.

The health care sector in every country and particularly in India is going through continuous changes since the early 2000s. Corporatization of health care, ever-changing technological invasion into medical field, continuous inflow of information on diseases and interventions across the globe, fragmentization of specialization and super-specializations, increased public awareness and consumerized doctor-patient relationship and advancement of chronic illnesses, such as hypertension and diabetes to youth and children, have placed the doctors on the mode of adaptation and coping with these changes. The doctor attends his basic responsibility of patient care while keeping himself/herself up to date on all the aspects as part of change management.

Some of the adverse situations under which the doctor functions need to be made explicit in order to get the doctors perspectives.

1. The expertise and experience of the doctor do not warrant a positive outcome in every case. Failures despite best efforts have their negative impact on doctors.
2. When patients get admitted in the hospital, the doctor works on the patient in the backdrop of knowledge that the family has pinned all hopes on the doctor. This itself is a pressure.
3. The doctor trying to handle a patient in critical condition has to work under several pairs of eyes and ears watching the process. This is a component that contributes to stress.
4. In the era of consumerism, though the doctor's competence and skill guide him in diagnosis and treatment, one goes by evidence-based practice to protect oneself.
5. Matching the variety of patient's cognitive level in communication is a great challenge for the doctor. Swift shifts in levels of communication in a day is a task that requires informal assessment of the patient's cognitive level, and designing impromptu communication package is a difficult task.
6. Patients returning with complications because of errors in following medical advice are highly frustrating and annoying. It calls for enormous frustration, tolerance, anger management and emotional intelligence in handling such patients without violating the clause of respect and acceptance for the patients.
7. Occupational stress and work overload piles up on the doctor in such marginal incremental way that one may not realize its burden into the symptoms of burnout until they start manifesting conspicuously.

8. In India, doctors have to choose between working in corporate hospitals or government hospitals if not in their own nursing homes. The corporate environment demands participation in their commercial-driven functioning, and the government sector requires their optimum efficiency in an environment that lacks even the basic infrastructure. Neither of the options are stress-free.
9. Balancing between the professional and family life, though is true in all professions, the doctor's profession many times demands deferring the family priorities in favour of attending professional emergencies and obligations.
10. Juggling between patient care, clinical trials, administrative responsibilities, procurement of equipment is something that requires high skills of time management, and has the potential to cause distraction of attention in every role.

Banerjee (2019) pointed out the asymmetry between workload and human resource in government hospitals forcing the work overload on doctors and paramedical staff. Contrastingly, the doctors in corporate hospitals see less number of patients. However, in corporate set-up the pressure to generate revenue is high on the doctors. Working in such set-up amounts to loss of autonomy. Physicians working in either of the sectors experience huge stress and their vulnerability to being 'burned out' is high.

Physician Burnout Symptoms

Burnout is a syndrome characterized by physical and psychological exhaustion, emotional detachment with the work and people at workplace, and decline in the adaptability to job demands. These initial symptoms may not be glaring and detectable. Gradually, the exhaustion, depersonalizations and increasing perception of lack of personal achievement start manifesting and become evident. It is not uncommon to see the psychosomatic manifestations gradually unfolding themselves. Progressively, the symptoms of burnout start manifesting in physical, psychological and behavioural dimensions of the doctor.

Shetty (2016) narrated how the doctors suppress their emotions. In the workshops he conducted for doctors in the hospitals, he usually asked them to discuss near-death experiences or the death of their loved ones. He stated that it always takes time for them to share it in the group. He cited the case of a gynaecologist who confided that he always felt that he did not do the best to save his father. Another broke into tears and accused the resource person for discussing such sensitive issues. Such feelings of guilt and pent-up emotions harm the doctors' wellbeing.

Doctors experiencing burnout cannot fulfil their professional obligations efficiently. They are less likely to be attentive, listening actively, connecting the various information into a theme, thinking and deciding on the correct line of investigation and diagnosis followed by accurate treatment.

The symptoms of burnout seen on physical, emotional and behaviour domains are list in Box 9.5. It is not necessary that the doctor experiencing burnout has all the symptoms. Secondly, the list is not exhaustive since there is always a scope for individual differences.

The symptoms don't appear suddenly. It is a gradual process, which pervades the professional life incrementally and likely to jolt one out if proper attention is not paid at earlier stages. One simple way to identify the onset and progress of burnout is by checking the energy levels. When one sets into work every day, one starts with a certain amount of physical energy, emotional energy and spiritual energy. If one experiences a subnormal level of energy in any of the three fields consecutively that may be taken as an early symptom.

Box 9.5 Doctor Burnout and the General Symptoms

Physical	Emotional	Behavioural
• Feeling exhausted most of the time • Lowered immunity and increased susceptibility to illness • Pains and aches in different locations of body • Change in appetite • Change in sleep pattern	• Emotional fatigue • Detachment from patients • Sense of defeat and loss of confidence in self • Experience of helplessness • Absence of motivation • Cynicism • Feeling of depression and disinterest	• Distancing from responsibilities • Avoidance of social and professional company • Procrastination • Displaced emotions • Taking to alcohol, drugs, as a means of coping • Errors of judgement in patient care • Frequent absenteeism from work

Prevalence

According to a survey on medical practitioners in India, Langade et al. (2016) found that the prevalence is high among Indian doctors. A large percentage of 45.02% reported high emotional exhaustion, while 65.98% of doctors scored high on depersonalization, and 87.14% recorded low scores on personal achievement. The high prevalence of burnout in Indian doctors may be attributed to typical situational factors such as high doctor patient ratio, infrastructural deficit, low patient literacy, long working hours, lack of autonomy, political and bureaucratic pressure and interference in work. More often than not the doctor experiences an external locus of control in discharging the patient services and meeting the organizational obligations.

Even in developed countries like the US, where the working conditions of the doctors are assumed to be highly congenial, the prevalence of burnout is found to be almost the same. The survey on a huge sample of 7288 physicians revealed that 45% of them experienced at least one symptoms of burnout (Shanafelt et al., 2012).

Based on the systematic review of publications, the estimation of burnout among doctors in China is placed somewhere between 66.5% and 87.8%.

The prevalence of burnout among doctors in various countries ranged between 30% and 76% (Shanafelt, 2009; Cohen et al., 2008; Legassie, Zibrowski, & Goldszmidt 2008; Ashkar et al., 2010).

The prevalence rates in various countries suggest the presence of it all over the world, indicating that burnout among doctors perhaps is an occupational hazard. Though burnout is a common phenomenon in all jobs, it is found to be high in those jobs that requires continuous interaction with a number of people. By virtue of this, the probability of burnout among practising and teaching doctors is likely to be high.

Onset and Progress of Physician Burnout

Burnout is another name for energy deficit in one or more of physical, emotional or spiritual domains. The problem is that draining out of this energy occurs so marginally and progressively

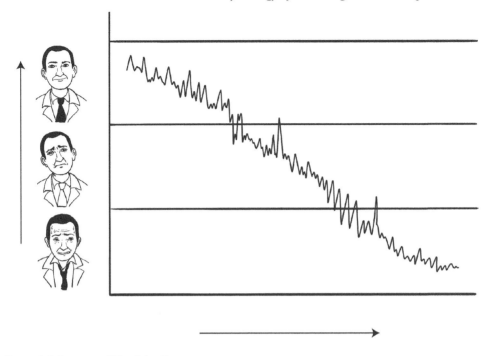

Figure 9.5 Progress of Physician Burnout.

that the decline is hardly noticeable on a day-to-day basis. We can depict the progress of it through a graph. The 'X'-axis measures the time, while the Y-axis measures the energy levels (Figure 9.5).

In phase 1, the physician has good resource of energy in all three domains. The functioning is by and large efficient. The stress levels fluctuate yet remain within manageable limits. Gradually, the frequency and intensity of exhaustion increases. Yet, one feels energetic more often and the intermittent fatigue is not really taken into cognizance. Swinging within the healthy zone, the doctor incrementally slides to phase 2. It is not noticed when the physician who has been functioning with optimum energy level has gradually sloped down, and touched the burnout zone. As the time progresses, the doctor experiences more frequent occasions of feeling energy loss and exhaustion, with occasional experience of efficient work and energetic feelings, and the 'normal energetic compassionate self'. The feelings of being 'drained out' now become more consistent. In every probability, the doctor attributes it to the natural experience of a physician, tries to stretch a little further and expand the working hours and try to give the best. During this phase, the doctor is likely to touch down the danger zone on few occasions manifested within increased irritability, disinterest to work and feeling of fatigue and other symptoms. They are likely to be interpreted as the outcome of busy schedule or age factor. There may be several defences that reason out though the doctor realizes that it has been very long since he/she enjoyed the work. Before one realizes, one is into the chronic physical burnout syndrome, occasionally slipping into the danger zone. This almost impairs the chances of the doctor recovering to the healthy zone.

When the doctor goes into the chronic symptoms of burnout, undiagnosed and unattained, there is every chance of entering the third phase, which is marked as 'danger zone'. Here, the doctor experiences high physical and emotional exhaustion, and feels dispassionate about the patients, work etc. The negative emotions start to get displaced. There is a significant decline in relationships with family members. Unable to handle the situations effectively, the doctor may adopt unhealthy coping techniques involving health risk behaviour such as consuming alcohol, drugs. The sleep is likely to be affected. All these may show a negative impact on the physical and mental health of the doctor. In case of severe morbidity, the depression may also trigger suicidal ideation in the doctor.

Causes of Physician Burnout

A number of factors contribute to physician burnout. There are personality factors of the doctor concerned, workload and organizational factors. Some of the factors contributing to doctor's burnout are as follows:

- Long hours of work
- Pressure to see more patients
- Non-conducive physical environment
- Pressure to generate more income for organization
- Demand for acquainting one with developing technology
- Need for spending time in non-medical factors such as building documentation
- Frequent interference in work
- Need to keep oneself abreast of the new developments in the field
- Conflicts in the team workers
- Threat of violence from patient's family and unsupportive management
- Medicolegal cases and legal battles
- Uncooperative colleagues and inefficient subordinates
- Continuously working with terminally ill and counselling the family

The causes of burnout can be one or many. It is not so much a factor of number of causes than the intensity of the cause. For example, continuous pressure to see more patients can stretch the working hours and lead to burnout over a period of time. As per research reports, burnout does not seem to be a universal phenomenon among doctors. This indicates that despite having a number of conditions potential to induce burnout, some physicians emerge resilient, and continue to work with optimum efficiency. However, the impact of burnout can be seen on the doctor, patient and the organization, finally resulting in the health care system of the nation.

Impact of Burnout

Impact on the Physician

Prolonged exposure to stress and the burnout adversely impacts the physical and mental health of the physician. It is found to be associated with psychiatric morbidity (Imo, 2017). Burnout involves continuous experience of high levels of stress. Due to the activation of hypothalamus-pituitary-adrenal axis, the cardiovascular system remains at high arousal for prolonged periods. Burnout is found to be associated with high risk of cardiovascular diseases (Melamed, Kushnir, & Shirom, 1992). The evidence of risk for cardiovascular diseases is seen in abnormal levels of cholesterol, triglycerides, glucose and uric acid in blood (Langade et al., 2016).

Findings of studies suggest that burnout has the potential to lead to post-traumatic stress disorder (PTSD) (Dyrbye et al., 2008). The impact of burnout may manifest in psychosomatic diseases, sleep disorders, alcoholism, substance abuse, loss of appetite and weight loss.

Impact on the Patients

The most devastating impact on patient is misdiagnosis. This will be followed by wrong line of investigations (in case the practitioner cares for evidence-based treatment) or wrong line of treatment. Precious time is lost in this process. In case the problem is serious, then there is a threat to the wellbeing or life of the patient. A patient scheduled for a laser surgery of her retina of the right eye recalled her experience—"I was diagnosed having holes in my retina of my right eye during a routine eye check-up. I was told that this doctor was a very senior retina specialist, and that his expertise is known all over the country. On the day of my surgery I waited in the hospital lounge and was feeling a bit tensed. When my turn came, I entered in, kept the hand bag I carried on a table in the room. I was asked to lie down on the operation table by the nurse who was preparing for the laser surgery. As soon as the doctor entered the room, he ordered me. 'Madam, is this your bag on the table? Please remove. This is not the place for your bag'. I felt humiliated, got up and silently removed the bag and placed it on the floor. I could not get over this harsh treatment. He was silent and started examining my left eye. I thought it was routine protocol to check the other eye that was healthy. I did not think he was going to do the laser surgery on my left eye until he brought the syringe close to my left eye. The moment I realised what was happening, I mustered courage to speak out 'Doctor, it is my right eye that has problem'. He stopped at once. Few seconds later my right eye received the treatment by the doctor. Even to this day, I shudder at the very thought that my left eye would have got the unwarranted surgery though I don't know the consequence of it".

Burnout in doctors will finally impact the patients, sometimes irreversibly. Inattentiveness, impaired memory, poor decision-making disregard for bedside manners, and lowered empathy levels cause great inconvenience to the patients. They feel confused, and their self-esteem is impacted by the doctor's lack of respect and concern for the patient. Welp, Meier and Manser (2015) stated that emotional exhaustions among physicians predicted higher mortality rates in their patients in ICU. Doctor's burnout is associated with quality care of patients related to safety care.

Impact on Health Care System

Burnout makes the doctor less productive and sometimes counterproductive to the health care system. When the burnout is severe and undiagnosed and not intervened, there is high probability of his/her quitting. All these impacts the system by enhancing the costs. Replacing a physician and training one to suit the dynamics of the hospital are both time- and cost-consuming. The negative impact of the burnout of physician on the patients has the potential hazard of bringing disrepute to the hospital. Hospital management in their interest must take initiative to assess and intervene for enhancing physician wellbeing from time to time. Measures will have to be taken to prevent burnout in doctors.

Interventions for Physician Burnout

Interventions for burnout can be taken up at individual level by the doctors, institutional level by the hospitals or policy level by the government.

Handling Burnout at Individual Level

The doctors need to handle burnout in two ways, viz. preventive measures to keep away from it and coping measures in case one detects the sign of burnout.

The very first step towards prevention is building a resistance for burnout. This is like building a strong immune system that resists illness. We had discussed earlier that burnout is associated with depletion of energy levels at physical, emotional and spiritual levels. Building resistance is possible by replenishing the energy levels from time to time, because every single day's activities draw from this reserve energy. Continuously drawing from the reserve energy is likely to empty the reserve. Hence, attempts have to be made to engage are such activities that energize the doctors on all the three dimensions to build the required resistance and block the drain.

Mindfulness has been found to be effective in preventing the burnout syndrome setting in. Practice of mindfulness helps one to be aware of one's own attention and intention from moment to moment in every activity one is engaged in. It is useful in identifying the frequency with which one reacts to a situation rather than responding. Frequent instances of reactions to situation should be considered as indications of burnout. That is a signal for the doctor to do one of the following:

- Take time off the work and engage in some enjoyable activity
- Practice relaxation exercise such as progressive muscular relations, *Yoga nidra*, Guided Imagery
- Set some personal boundaries at work and follow manageable timings. Avoid extending oneself beyond the set limits of work and time
- Rediscover the decision for the career in the field of medical sciences. It is time that the doctor reconnects to the original goal that directed one into the career, and reorient oneself to achieve this goal by reinventing one's strengths and getting directed by them
- The best method of maintaining the energy levels is by integrating physical exercise, emotional relaxation and spiritual inclination into the daily routine. They help in filling the energy reservoir on a daily basis.

Coping with the Burnout

When the doctor is found to have already entered the burnout zone and has been showing the symptoms of exhaustion, emotional instability disengagement and disinterest in patients and work, it is time that one takes a break for a while. A sabbatical that engages the physician in a different academic activity or research proves productive. Such symptoms may also need few sessions of Cognitive Behavioural Therapy. This enables the doctor to return to work with cognitive restructuring so that one is able to view situations from a different perspective and respond to it with a sense of professional detachment rather than reacting to it. Engaging in activities totally outside the job such as learning music, going on trekking or getting busy with gardening etc. helps in restoring the energy levels.

Yet another way of coping is to reduce the exposure to the stressful environment. The workplace is what is inducing stress, reducing the work timings, or reducing the responsibilities that cause stress works similar to good stimulus control. In addition to this, ensuring adequate nutrition, sleep and meaningful engagement is a good measure of damage control because the basic psychological need fulfilment ensures regenerative process, be it at physical or psychological level.

Intervention at Institutional Level

Enhancing the wellbeing of the employees and protecting them against burnout is one of the organizational responsibilities. It has to be taken up on priority in the interest of the organization. Following are some of the measures that can be practised by hospitals:

- Ensuring and protecting the autonomy of the physician
- Minimizing the documentation job for doctors and providing secretarial assistance for such jobs
- Putting an upper ceiling on the number of patients the doctor can see in a day (the number can vary for various specializations)

Psychology of the Caregiver and Careprovider 395

- Ensuring that the doctors have their days off in a week and respecting their time during the period
- Organizing periodical workshops to train the doctors in various relaxation techniques
- Making a health psychologist available in the hospital to assess the doctor's wellbeing at regular intervals
- Providing privacy in consultation rooms
- Providing protection to doctors from political interference and public threat
- Making annual vacation mandatory for all doctors

Intervention at Policy Level

The best preventive measure for physician burnout can come from policy level. There have been several studies reiterating the absence of appropriate training of skills of communication and coping in the curriculum of medical education. These are normally learned by doctors through on-hand experience, which is the hard way. Incorporating the skills of communication, time management and stress management and coping as part of medical curriculum equips the doctors to meet the challenges of the profession successfully. This would be a long-term measure.

Improving the infrastructure in Primary Health Centres and area hospitals would reduce the burden on doctors in urban areas.

Regular assessment of doctors on wellbeing should be made mandatory in every hospital. This helps in detection of burnout at the initial stages so that the intervention is cost-effective.

Intervention studies on burnout of doctors have suggested the effectiveness of various types. However, combination of intervention at all levels would be far more effective than the isolated ones at one level.

Box 9.6   Researcher's Box

- Studies can be planned to examine caregiver's resilience. The resilient caregivers can be identified by first assessing for caregiver burden. Wherever the burden is low, they can be identified and screened in for further tests for caregiver resilience. It will be of great value to assess and identify factors contributing to their resilience.
- The impact of interventions on caregivers and the patients can be studied. Caregivers can be divided randomly into different groups. Specifically, designed intervention in the form of social support to one group, spiritual practice to one and relaxation therapy to the third can be introduced and the impact on caregiver wellbeing and subsequent impact on patient wellbeing or distress reduction can be studied by following up for four to six weeks. The same study can be conducted with just one intervention group and a control group.
- Comparison of intervention for caregivers at different stages of illness can be planned. Relative impact of various interventions at various stages of patient illness can throw good insight on the patient stage-specific intervention for caregivers.
- Doctor-patient communication and its impact on patient adherence can be studied by participant observation method during consultation process. Themes of the communication can be evolved. The quality of communication can be inferred based on a number of factors such as the directionality of communication, meaningfulness, patient response etc. Few other criteria can also be evolved.
- Doctor-patient communication quality can be measured using similarity index. The impact of it on patient adherence and disease management can be studied by short-term follow-up.

- Doctors can be trained through interventions for high-quality communication. The quality of communication in trained doctors can be compared with untrained. The impact on patient can be measured.
- Longitudinal intervention studies can be designed to measure their preventive efficacy in physicians' burnout. The interns can be trained in communication skills, mindfulness, relaxation techniques, time management techniques and methods of identifying early symptoms of burnout. This group of interns can be followed up for ten years, assessing their wellbeing, burnout and coping at regular intervals. This group can be compared with an untrained group.
- Survey designs to assess physician burnout in different groups of doctors in various specializations give an insight into the prevalence of burnout in various specialities. This helps in planning and recommending appropriate interventions at systemic and policy levels.

Box 9.7 Practitioner's Box

- As a mandate, whenever a chronic patient goes for clinical consultation, the caregiver has to be recommended for psychosocial assessment along with the patient.
- Assessment of stress, caregiver burden and physical, emotional health of caregiver needs to be taken.
- Caregivers of patients at various stages require different interventions. Those where the patient's diagnosis is revealed need knowledge intervention, and those with patient in terminal state need spiritual intervention and coping strategies. Those exhausted with patient care for prolonged period need relaxation therapy and self-management techniques. Similarly, those feeling social isolation need to be given skills of seeking social support.
- Family counselling is very useful when the patient under palliative care is in constant pain.
- Cognitive Behavioural Therapy for caregivers who are irrational in their beliefs, suffer guilt or stretch themselves too much provides them a cognitive restructuring enabling them to view the problem from different perspectives.
- Health psychologists employed in hospitals may initiate workshops for management and doctors to orient them in identifying early symptoms of burnout, and various techniques of preventing it.
- The consultation for physician burnout as an institutional arrangement involving a practising health psychologist calls for equipping the department with good assessment tools. Assessment for measuring wellbeing, interaction style, emotional quotient, job satisfaction, occupational stress, etc. should be used on the doctors depending on the symptoms reported.
- The middle-level workers such as nurses, ward boys and front office managers also need to be assessed on parameters associated with stress or burnout.
- Interventions like CBT, mindfulness, Guided Imagery may be administered based on the need.

References

Adams, E., Boulton, M., & Watson, E. (2009). The information needs of partners and family members of cancer patients: A systematic literature review. *Patient Education and Counseling*, *77*(2), 179–186.

Agarwal, A., Agarwal, A., Nag, K., Chakraborty, S., & Ali, K. (2011). Doctor patient communication—A vital yet neglected entity in Indian medical education system. *Indian Journal of Surgery*, *73*(3), 184–186.

Arango-Lasprilla, J. C., Panyavin, I., Merchán, E. J. H., Perrin, P. B., Arroyo-Anlló, E. M., Snipes, D. J., & Arabia, J. (2014). Evaluation of a group cognitive–behavioral dementia caregiver intervention in Latin America. *American Journal of Alzheimer's Disease& Other Dementias®*, *29*(6), 548–555.

Arjunan, I., Gopinath, D., & Murthy, N. S. (2011). Role of informal care providers in home based long term care in diabetes mellitus at Kaiwara Primary Health Center area, Karnataka, India. *Asian Pacific Journal of Tropical Disease*, *1*(2), 127–130.

Ashkar, K., Romani, M., Musharrafieh, U., & Chaaya, M. (2010). Prevalence of burnout syndrome among medical residents: Experience of a developing country. *Postgraduate Medical Journal*, *86*(1015), 266–271.

Aslan, Ö., Kav, S., Meral, C., Tekin, F., Yesil, H., Ozturk, U., ... & Yazar, B. (2006). Needs of lay caregivers of bone marrow transplant patients in Turkey: A multicenter study. *Cancer Nursing*, *29*(6), E1–E7.

Au, A., Li, S., Lee, K., Leung, P., Pan, P. C., Thompson, L., & Gallagher-Thompson, D. (2010). The Coping with Caregiving Group Program for Chinese caregivers of patients with Alzheimer's disease in Hong Kong. *Patient Education and Counseling*, *78*(2), 256–260.

Avsar, U., Avsar, U. Z., Cansever, Z., Set, T., Cankaya, E., Kaya, A., ... & Keles, M. (2013, April). Psychological and emotional status, and caregiver burden in caregivers of patients with peritoneal dialysis compared with caregivers of patients with renal transplantation. *Transplantation Proceedings*, *45*(3), 883–886.

Badger, T., Segrin, C., Dorros, S. M., Meek, P., & Lopez, A. M. (2007). Depression and anxiety in women with breast cancer and their partners. *Nursing Research*, *56*(1), 44–53.

Banerjee, A. (2019). Physician heal thyself: Perspectives on burnout among doctors. *Perspectives in Medical Research*, *7*(1), 3–9.

Banerjee, A., & Sanyal, D. (2012). Dynamics of doctor–patient relationship: A cross-sectional study on concordance, trust, and patient enablement. *Journal of Family and Community Medicine*, *19*(1), 12.

Barrowclough, C., Tarrier, N., & Johnston, M. (1996). Distress, expressed emotion, and attributions in relatives of schizophrenia patients. *Schizophrenia Bulletin*, *22*(4), 691–701.

Beach, S. R., Schulz, R., Yee, J. L., & Jackson, S. (2000). Negative and positive health effects of caring for a disabled spouse: Longitudinal findings from the caregiver health effects study. *Psychology and Aging*, *15*(2), 259. doi: 10.1037//0882–7974.15.2.259

Bhattacharjee, M., Vairale, J., Gawali, K., & Dalal, P. M. (2012). Factors affecting burden on caregivers of stroke survivors: Population-based study in Mumbai (India). *Annals of Indian Academy of Neurology*, *15*(2), 113.

Biglu, M. H., Nateq, F., Ghojazadeh, M., & Asgharzadeh, A. (2017). Communication skills of physicians and patients' satisfaction. *Materia Socio-Medica*, *29*(3), 192.

Bishop, M. M., Beaumont, J. L., Hahn, E. A., Cella, D., Andrykowski, M. A., Brady, M. J., ... & Wingard, J. R. (2007). Late effects of cancer and hematopoietic stem-cell transplantation on spouses or partners compared with survivors and survivor-matched controls. *Journal of Clinical Oncology*, *25*(11), 1403–1411.

Brown, M. A., & Stetz, K. (1999). The labor of caregiving: A theoretical model of caregiving during potentially fatal illness. *Qualitative Health Research*, *9*(2), 182–197.

Budin, W. C., Hoskins, C. N., Haber, J., Sherman, D. W., Maislin, G., Cater, J. R., ... & Shukla, S. (2008). Breast cancer: Education, counseling, and adjustment among patients and partners: a randomized clinical trial. *Nursing Research*, *57*(3), 199–213.

Buhse, M. (2008). Assessment of caregiver burden in families of persons with multiple sclerosis. *Journal of Neuroscience Nursing*, *40*(1), 25–31.

Bultz, B. D., Speca, M., Brasher, P. M., Geggie, P. H., & Page, S. A. (2000). A randomized controlled trial of a brief psychoeducational support group for partners of early stage breast cancer patients. *Psycho-Oncology: Journal of the Psychological, Social and Behavioral Dimensions of Cancer, 9*(4), 303–313.

Butalid, L., Verhaak, P. F., Boeije, H. R., & Bensing, J. M. (2012). Patients' views on changes in doctor-patient communication between 1982 and 2001: A mixed-methods study. *BMC Family Practice, 13*(1), 80.

Cain, C. J., & Wicks, M. N. (2000). Caregiver attributes as correlates of burden in family caregivers coping with chronic obstructive pulmonary disease. *Journal of Family Nursing, 6*(1), 46–68.

Chan, K. Y., Yip, T., Yap, D. Y., Sham, M. K., Wong, Y. C., Lau, V. W. K., … & Chan, T. M. (2016). Enhanced psychosocial support for caregiver burden for patients with chronic kidney failure choosing not to be treated by dialysis or transplantation: A pilot randomized controlled trial. *American Journal of Kidney Diseases, 67*(4), 585–592.

Chandra, S., Mohammadnezhad, M., & Ward, P. (2018). Trust and communication in a doctor-patient relationship: A literature review. *Journal of Health Communication, 3*, 36. doi: 10.4172/2472-1654.100146

Chang, C. S., Chen, S. Y., & Lan, Y. T. (2013). Service quality, trust, and patient satisfaction in interpersonal-based medical service encounters. *BMC Health Services Research, 13*(1), 22.

Chipidza, F. E., Wallwork, R. S., & Stern, T. A. (2015). Impact of the doctor-patient relationship. *The Primary Care Companion for CNS Disorders, 17*(5), 10.

Cohen, J. S., Leung, Y., Fahey, M., Hoyt, L., Sinha, R., Cailler, L., … & Patten, S. (2008). The happy docs study: A Canadian Association of Internes and Residents well-being survey examining resident physician health and satisfaction within and outside of residency training in Canada. *BMC Research Notes, 1*(1), 105.

Covinsky, K. E., Goldman, L., Cook, E. F., Oye, R., Desbiens, N., Reding, D., … & Baker, R. (1994). The impact of serious illness on patients' families. *Jama, 272*(23), 1839–1844.

Dalal, A. K. (2016). *Cultural psychology of health in India: Well-being, medicine and traditional health care*. New Delhi: SAGE Publications India.

Donelan, K., Hill, C. A., Hoffman, C., Scoles, K., Feldman, P. H., Levine, C., & Gould, D. (2002). Challenged to care: Informal caregivers in a changing health system. *Health Affairs, 21*(4), 222–231.

Dyrbye, L. N., Thomas, M. R., Massie, F. S., Power, D. V., Eacker, A., Harper, W., … & Sloan, J. A. (2008). Burnout and suicidal ideation among US medical students. *Annals of Internal Medicine, 149*(5), 334–341.

Flocke, S. A., Miller, W. L., & Crabtree, B. F. (2002). Relationships between physician practice style, patient satisfaction, and attributes of primary care. *Journal of Family Practice, 51*(10), 835–841.

Friedman, D. S., Hahn, S. R., Gelb, L., Tan, J., Shah, S. N., Kim, E. E., … & Quigley, H. A. (2008). Doctor–patient communication, health-related beliefs, and adherence in glaucoma: Results from the glaucoma adherence and persistency study. *Ophthalmology, 115*(8), 1320–1327.

Given, B., Given, C. W., Sikorskii, A., Jeon, S., Sherwood, P., & Rahbar, M. (2006). The impact of providing symptom management assistance on caregiver reaction: Results of a randomized trial. *Journal of Pain and Symptom Management, 32*(5), 433–443.

Given, C. W., Given, B., Azzouz, F., Kozachik, S., & Stommel, M. (2001). Predictors of pain and fatigue in the year following diagnosis among elderly cancer patients. *Journal of Pain and Symptom Management, 21*(6), 456–466.

Goldstein, N. E., Concato, J., Fried, T. R., Kasl, S. V., Johnson-Hurzeler, R., & Bradley, E. H. (2004). Factors associated with caregiver burden among caregivers of terminally ill patients with cancer. *Journal of Palliative Care, 20*(1), 38–43.

Gonzalez, A. B., Rivera, J. V., & Novoa, S. O. (2005). The effectiveness of educational intervention in carers of patients in dialysis and evaluation of the load. *Rev Soc EspEnfermNefrol, 8*, 156–165.

Gordon, C., & Beresin, E. V. (2016). The doctor-patient relationship. In: T. A. Stern, M. Fava, T. E. Wilens, et al. (Eds.), *Massachusetts general hospital comprehensive clinical psychiatry* (2nd ed., pp. 1–7). Philadelphia, PA: Elsevier Health Sciences.

Grunfeld, E., Coyle, D., Whelan, T., Clinch, J., Reyno, L., Earle, C. C., … & Glossop, R. (2004). Family caregiver burden: Results of a longitudinal study of breast cancer patients and their principal caregivers. *Cmaj, 170*(12), 1795–1801.

Haas, J. S., Cook, E. F., Puopolo, A. L., Burstin, H. R., Cleary, P. D., & Brennan, T. A. (2000). Is the professional satisfaction of general internists associated with patient satisfaction? *Journal of General Internal Medicine, 15*(2), 122–128.

Haley, W. E., LaMonde, L. A., Han, B., Burton, A. M., & Schonwetter, R. (2003). Predictors of depression and life satisfaction among spousal caregivers in hospice: Application of a stress process model. *Journal of Palliative Medicine, 6*(2), 215–224.

Hariharan, Meena, & Padhy, Meera. (2011). Emotional intelligence of doctors. *Social Science International, 27,* 15.

Harmell, A. L., Chattillion, E. A., Roepke, S. K., & Mausbach, B. T. (2011). A review of the psychobiology of dementia caregiving: A focus on resilience factors. *Current Psychiatry Reports, 13*(3), 219–224.

Hodges, L. J., Humphris, G. M., & Macfarlane, G. (2005). A meta-analytic investigation of the relationship between the psychological distress of cancer patients and their carers. *Social Science & Medicine, 60*(1), 1–12.

Hoff, A. C., & Haaga, D. A. (2005). Effects of an education program on radiation oncology patients and families. *Journal of Psychosocial Oncology, 23*(4), 61–79.

Hudson, P. L., Aranda, S., & Hayman-White, K. (2005). A psycho-educational intervention for family caregivers of patients receiving palliative care: A randomized controlled trial. *Journal of Pain and Symptom Management, 30*(4), 329–341.

Hudson, P., Quinn, K., Kristjanson, L., Thomas, T., Braithwaite, M., Fisher, J., & Cockayne, M. (2008). Evaluation of a psycho-educational group programme for family caregivers in home-based palliative care. *Palliative Medicine, 22*(3), 270–280.

Imo, U. O. (2017). Burnout and psychiatric morbidity among doctors in the UK: A systematic literature review of prevalence and associated factors. *BJPsych Bulletin, 41*(4), 197–204.

Keefe, F. J., Ahles, T. A., Sutton, L., Dalton, J., Baucom, D., Pope, M. S., ... & Waters, S. J. (2005). Partner-guided cancer pain management at the end of life: A preliminary study. *Journal of Pain and Symptom Management, 29*(3), 263–272.

Kim, Y., Schulz, R., & Carver, C. S. (2007). Benefit finding in the cancer caregiving experience. *Psychosomatic Medicine, 69*(3), 283–291.

Kurtz, M. E., Kurtz, J. C., Given, C. W., & Given, B. (1995). Relationship of caregiver reactions and depression to cancer patients' symptoms, functional states and depression—A longitudinal view. *Social Science & Medicine, 40*(6), 837–846.

Kwon, O. Y., Ahn, H. S., Kim, H. J., & Park, K. W. (2017). Effectiveness of cognitive behavioral therapy for caregivers of people with dementia: A systematic review and meta-analysis. *Journal of Clinical Neurology, 13*(4), 394–404. doi: 10.3988/jcn.2017.13.4.394

Langade, D., Modi, P. D., Sidhwa, Y. F., Hishikar, N. A., Gharpure, A. S., Wankhade, K., ... & Joshi, K. (2016). Burnout syndrome among medical practitioners across India: A questionnaire-based survey. *Cureus, 8*(9), e771. doi: 10.7759/cureus.771

Lawton, M. P., Moss, M., Kleban, M. H., Glicksman, A., & Rovine, M. (1991). A two-factor model of caregiving appraisal and psychological well-being. *Journal of Gerontology, 46*(4), P181–P189.

Legassie, J., Zibrowski, E. M., & Goldszmidt, M. A. (2008). Measuring resident well-being: Impostorism and burnout syndrome in residency. *Journal of General Internal Medicine, 23*(7), 1090–1094.

Losada, A., Márquez-González, M., & Romero-Moreno, R. (2011). Mechanisms of action of a psychological intervention for dementia caregivers: Effects of behavioral activation and modification of dysfunctional thoughts. *International Journal of Geriatric Psychiatry, 26*(11), 1119–1127.

Magliano, L., Fiorillo, A., De Rosa, C., Malangone, C., Maj, M., & National Mental Health Project Working Group. (2005). Family burden in long-term diseases: A comparative study in schizophrenia vs. physical disorders. *Social Science & Medicine, 61*(2), 313–322.

Melamed, S., Kushnir, T., & Shirom, A. (1992). Burnout and risk factors for cardiovascular diseases. *Behavioral Medicine, 18*(2), 53–60.

Mollasiotis, A., Wilson, B., Blairs, S., Howe, T., & Cavet, J. (2011). Unmet supportive care needs, psychological wellbeing and quality of life in patients living with multiple myeloma and their partners. *Psychology, 20*(1), 88–97.

Murphy, N. A., Christian, B., Caplin, D. A., & Young, P. C. (2006). The health of caregivers for children with disabilities: Caregiver perspectives. *Child: Care, Health and Development, 33*(2), 180–187. doi: 10.1111/j.1365-2214.2006.00644.x

Murray, C. J., & Lopez, A. D. (2000). Progress and directions in refining the global burden of disease approach: A response to Williams. *Health Economics, 9*(1), 69–82.

National Opinion Research Center. (2014, May). Long term care in America: Expectations and realities. Retrieved from http://www.longtermcarepoll.org/PDFs/LTC%202014/AP-NORC-Long-Term%20Care%20in%20America_FINAL%20WEB.pdf

Northouse, L. L., Katapodi, M. C., Schafenacker, A. M., & Weiss, D. (2012, November). The impact of caregiving on the psychological well-being of family caregivers and cancer patients. *Seminars in Oncology Nursing, 28*(4), 236–245.

O'Toole, M. S., Zachariae, R., Renna, M. E., Mennin, D. S., & Applebaum, A. (2017). Cognitive behavioral therapies for informal caregivers of patients with cancer and cancer survivors: A systematic review and meta-analysis. *Psycho-Oncology, 26*(4), 428–437. doi: 10.1002/pon.4144

Padmaja, G., Vanlalhruaii, C., Rana, S., & Kopparty, S. (2017). Quality of life of patients with cancer: A determinant of the quality of life of their family caregivers. *Journal of Cancer Education, 32*(3), 655–661.

Padmaja, G., Vanlalhruaii, C., Rana, S., Nandinee, D., & Hariharan, M. (2016). Care givers' depression, anxiety, distress, and somatization as predictors of identical symptoms in cancer patients. *Journal of Cancer Research and Therapeutics, 12*(1), 53.

Pasacreta, J. V., Barg, F., Nuamah, I., & McCorkle, R. (2000). Participant characteristics before and 4 months after attendance at a family caregiver cancer education program. *Cancer Nursing, 23*(4), 295–303.

Pearson, S. D., & Raeke, L. H. (2000). Patients' trust in physicians: many theories, few measures, and little data. *Journal of General Internal Medicine, 15*(7), 509–513.

Pitceathly, C., & Maguire, P. (2003). The psychological impact of cancer on patients' partners and other key relatives: A review. *European Journal of Cancer, 39*(11), 1517–1524.

Raina, P., O'Donnell, M., Rosenbaum, P., Brehaut, J., Walter, S. D., Russell, D., ... & Wood, E. (2005). The health and well-being of caregivers of children with cerebral palsy. *Pediatrics, 115*(6), e626–e636.

Raina, P., O'Donnell, M., Schwellnus, H., Rosenbaum, P., King, G., Brehaut, J., ... & Walter, S. D. (2004). Caregiving process and caregiver burden: conceptual models to guide research and practice. *BMC Pediatrics, 4*(1), 1.

Ridd, M., Shaw, A., Lewis, G., & Salisbury, C. (2009). The patient–doctor relationship: A synthesis of the qualitative literature on patients' perspectives. *British Journal of General Practice, 59*(561), e116–e133.

Sebastian, N. M., Jesha, M. M., Haveri, S. P., & Nath, A. S. (2016). Gaps in doctor patient communication: A community based study. *International Journal of Community Medicine and Public Health, 3*(1), 264–269.

Secker, D. L., & Brown, R. G. (2005). Cognitive behavioural therapy (CBT) for carers of patients with Parkinson's disease: A preliminary randomised controlled trial. *Journal of Neurology, Neurosurgery, and Psychiatry, 76*(4), 491–497. doi: 10.1136/jnnp.2004.042291

Shaji, K. S., & Reddy, M. S. (2012). Caregiving: A public health priority. *Indian Journal of Psychological Medicine, 34*(4), 303.

Shanafelt, T. D. (2009). Enhancing meaning in work: A prescription for preventing physician burnout and promoting patient-centered care. *Jama, 302*(12), 1338–1340.

Shanafelt, T. D., Boone, S., Tan, L., Dyrbye, L. N., Sotile, W., Satele, D., ... & Oreskovich, M. R. (2012). Burnout and satisfaction with work-life balance among US physicians relative to the general US population. *Archives of Internal Medicine, 172*(18), 1377–1385.

Shetty, H. (2016). A challenge for the medical profession. *Indian Journal of Medical Ethics, 11*(4), 111.

Stenberg, U., Ruland, C. M., & Miaskowski, C. (2010). Review of the literature on the effects of caring for a patient with cancer. *Psycho-Oncology, 19*(10), 1013–1025. doi: 10.1002/pon.1670

Stewart, M., Brown, J. B., Donner, A., McWhinney, I. R., Oates, J., Weston, W. W., & Jordan, J. (2000). The impact of patient centered care on outcomes. *The Journal of Family Practice, 49*(9), 796–804.

Suchman, A. L., Roter, D., Green, M., Lipkin Jr, M., & The Collaborative Study Group of the American Academy on Physician and Patient. (1993). Physician satisfaction with primary care office visits. *Medical Care, 31*(12), 1083–1092.

Sugai, D. Y., Deptula, P. L., Parsa, A. A., & Don Parsa, F. (2013). The importance of communication in the management of postoperative pain. *Hawai'i Journal of Medicine & Public Health: A Journal of Asia Pacific Medicine & Public Health, 72*(6), 180–184.

Swain, S. (2013). Health communication between doctors and patients: Impact on patient adherence and disease prognosis (Ph.D Thesis) submitted to University of Hyderabad, India.

Swain, S., Hariharan, M., Rana, S., Chivukula, U., & Thomas, M. (2015). Doctor-patient communication: Impact on adherence and prognosis among patients with primary hypertension. *Psychological Studies, 60*(1), 25–32.

Szasz, T. S., & Hollender, M. H. (1956). A contribution to the philosophy of medicine: The basic models of the doctor-patient relationship. *AMA Archives of Internal Medicine, 97*(5), 585–592.

Tornay, E. (2007). Educational Information for patients and caregivers in Paediatric Kidney transplant. *Journal of Renal Care, 33*, 115–118.

Vanlalhruaii, C., Padmaja, G., & Kopparty, S. (2018). Quality of life of elderly cancer patients as predictor of their caregivers' quality of life. *Indian Journal of Gerontology, 32*(3), 273–281.

Welp, A., Meier, L. L., & Manser, T. (2015). Emotional exhaustion and workload predict clinician-rated and objective patient safety. *Frontiers in Psychology, 5*, 1573.

Wilkes, L., White, K., & O'Riordan, L. (2000). Empowerment through information: Supporting rural families of oncology patients in palliative care. *Australian Journal of Rural Health, 8*(1), 41–46.

Wilson, I. B., Schoen, C., Neuman, P., Strollo, M. K., Rogers, W. H., Chang, H., & Safran, D. G. (2007). Physician–patient communication about prescription medication nonadherence: A 50-state study of America's seniors. *Journal of General Internal Medicine, 22*(1), 6–12.

10 Health Resilience

The Story of Sindhu Tai—The Resilient Woman

Sindhu Sapkal was born on 14 November 1948 in Pipri Meghe village of Wardha district, Maharashtra, in a family of cowherds. She dropped out of school after 4th standard, married and gave birth to three sons by the age of 20. When she was pregnant for the fourth time, she was subjected to severe physical violence by her husband during her full-term pregnancy and was driven out of home. With no assistance, she gave birth to a girl child in the cattle shed. Rejected by her husband and parents, she took to begging to satisfy her hunger and made the burial ground her residence. She used her natural talent for music for begging.

She supported other beggars with her earnings. She saw a male abandoned child at the railway track and gave shelter to him. Gradually, she started adopting many orphans and turned it into her mission. As per records, she has taken about 1200 homeless under her wing. She is affectionately called '*Mai*' (Mother) by the inmates. She did not hesitate to provide shelter to her husband when he approached her as a destitute and looked after him as one of the inmates till his death. Her children joined her in her work along with a number of volunteers. Sindhu Tai is the recipient of more than 750 from national and international agencies including *NarishaktiPuraskar* from the President of India.

Going by majority of theories in psychology such as developmental theories, cognitive theories or health risk factors, Sindhu Tai should have succumbed to her continuous harsh environmental adversities at various stages. Four pregnancies between 12 and 20 years could have made her reproductive system highly vulnerable to severe problems. The physical violence on her during her full-term pregnancy could have been fatal. Delivering her fourth child in a cow shed all by herself with no assistance even to cut the umbilical cord could have had devastating effect on her physical and mental health. Making the cremation ground her home along with the infant could have caused her lose her mental balance. However, all these experiences failed to demolish her completely.

Not that they would have had no negative impact on her but despite all the devastating experiences, she emerged and evolved, finally to gain the spotlight at national level for her achievements. How do we describe Sindhu Tai in one word? 'Resilient'.

The concept of resilience essentially encompasses two major characteristics, viz. exposure to severe adversities in life, and significant achievements or adaptation indicating healthy functioning despite major assaults on the developmental process. Resilience connotes sustaining health and wellbeing despite high exposure to risk factors. If health is defined as complete physical mental and social wellbeing, then resilience refers to sustenance of physical mental and social wellbeing even in the face of severe or multiple risk factors that are normally expected to disrupt this state of health. Thus, resilience indicates a healthy functioning of the individual at physical, cognitive, emotional and social dimensions circumventing the obstacles, pains, trauma, disabilities and deprivations that pose a threat to such functioning. Discussing resilience in the context of Health Psychology is highly relevant because it helps in understanding the biopsychosocial processes that contribute to preserving health and wellbeing in the face of risks and adversities.

History and Development of the Concept of Resilience

The word 'resilience' has its origin in the Latin word 'resilive' that described 'leap back'. Explaining it in simple term, an elastic stretched to the maximum extent has the capacity to revert to its original shape and form. The roots of the concept thus can be traced back to physics, which defined resilience as 'ability of the strained body, by virtue of high yield strength and low elastic modulus to recover its size and form following deformations'. Thus, it suggests that the ability to leap back is 'innate' in the object. The earlier definitions of resilience logically followed this and related it to a 'trait' or a cluster of traits. Garmezy, a clinical psychologist by profession, observed the striking difference in the children of schizophrenic patients. He raised an inquisitive research question as to why some children of patients of schizophrenia with a genetic risk of developing mental illness succumbed to stress and life adversities, while others encountering the same risks flourished.

Garmezy's observation was on children of mothers with severe mental illness. Theoretically, children of such background were at risk of negative developmental outcomes such as low competence, disruptive behaviour compared to those coming from normal and healthy parentage. However, the school records, teacher ratings and peer feedbacks adjudged a number of such at-risk children developing normally and manifesting competence. Garmezy (1971) stated these children "bear the visible indices that are hallmarks of competence—good peer relation, academic achievement, commitment to education and to purposive life goal, early and successful work histories" (p. 114). This prompted him to shift his research from risk factors to survival and adaptation factors. This set the beginning of resilience research.

Anthony (1974) called these children 'invulnerable', because they were not vulnerable and perished owing to circumstance. Werner and Smith (1982) called them 'invincible'. However, these labels were later replaced with the term 'resilient' because the term invulnerable connotes that the individual is 'unscathed' by the life adversities, whereas the later research suggested that there is active process in operation that enables the individual to evolve with normal healthy adaptation (Masten, 1994) or excel in life in the face of adversities (Luther, 1990; Luther, Doernberger, & Zigler, 1993).

Resilience or Resiliency?

The initial research in the field identified children, adolescents and adults who faced adversities and emerged with no pathology in their performance and functioning. The focus of the research was to identify the characteristics of resilient individuals. A number of traits were identified by different researchers. They include traits reflecting general resourcefulness, flexibility in functioning and sturdiness of character, all together called ego resiliency (Block & Block, 1980), commitment, control and challenge in combination called 'Hardiness' (Kobasa, 1982), comprehensibility, manageability and meaningfulness, together called sense of coherence (SoC) (Antonovsky, 1979), need prioritization, readiness to cope with stress (Hariharan, 1990), high IQ, problem-solving competence and personal characteristics such as high self-efficacy, autonomy, agility, warmth and outgoing (Keyes, 2004).

Theoretical models of resilience such as Antonovsky's Salutogenic model describing sense of coherence (SoC) and Kobasa's hardiness model with its three c's (commitment, control and challenge) were in line with this concept. This wave of research involved an element of judgement in terms of performance functioning and achievement where the observed outcome was different from the expected one. Masten, Best and Garmezy (1990) and Masten (1994) described the phenomenon of resilience with its three unique distinguishable features:

1. The first type referred to individuals at risk whose outcomes are better than what is expected
2. Individuals with sustained positive adaptation in the face of continued adversities and stressful experience
3. Those who show a good recovery from trauma

However, in each of the above there existed an ambiguity related to the definition and measurement of 'risk', 'positive adaptation' and 'good recovery'. Is a single severe adversity considered a risk? In that case how to account for the multiple adversities and what should be the criteria to label something as adversity? Similarly, what is considered a 'positive adaptation' or a 'good recovery' from trauma? All these called for some performance indicators to be identified or similar set of personal traits to label one as resilient.

As evident, the personal traits and characteristics identified by various researchers failed to have any convergence. One of the reasons for it is the variance in the sample used for studies. The samples varied widely by including those with physical disability, children who are orphaned, homeless, sexually abused, those with chronic diseases, those who were victims of natural disaster and those who encountered any major trauma to name a few. Further viewing resilience as 'resiliency' connoting personal traits has the inherent disadvantage of limiting it to the unchangeable personal traits. Hence, Masten (1994) rightly cautioned that such connotation may indicate that a person does not possess 'what it takes' to circumvent the adversity. In such instances, the research is likely to lose its social value.

Subsequent research increasingly endorsed the presence of certain factors external to the individual that are likely to play a significant role in their resilience. They referred to effective schools, presence of a supportive significant adult, relationship with persons of high competence or those with pro-social behaviour, community support, or strong family or maternal support. The factors associated with resilience were called 'protective factors'. Research in this direction where the focus was on identifying the resilient persons and the associated factors was known as the first wave of resilience research.

Resilience as a Process

Three factors related to resilience have been discussed until now, viz. adversity or the risk factor, factors internal to the individual and factors external to the person. This raised a research question regarding the interaction among these factors. Could there be an interaction among these factors in a particular way that resulted in the individual's resilience or vulnerability? Anthony (1974) described the phenomenon with an interesting analogy that explained the variation in the impact of adversity on three dolls made of different raw materials. He said, when a doll made of glass is hit with a hammer, it breaks into small pieces. The same hammer if hits a plastic doll permanently disfigures it. On the contrary, if the hammer hits a doll made of steel emits a beautiful metallic sound but remains the same. The first one loses its existence, the second loses its original shape, while the third resists any damage while eliciting a metallic sound unlike the breaking glass. Though Anthony used this analogy to highlight the characteristic of the target doll as a determinant of its reaction to stress, the characteristics of a hammer should not escape our attention. The three dolls would retain their existence and shape if the hammer is made of paper or soft rubber. Thus, while the basic 'mettle' is of high significances, the intensity of stress or adversity also plays a major role. More important is the process behind evolving as a glass, plastic or steel dolls. The idea that exposure to adversity either enhances vulnerabilities or has a 'steeling effect' and decreases the vulnerability was accepted. Thus, if researchers looked for process whereby the internal and external factors interacted in a way to make one either vulnerable or resilient, the internal and external factors such as personal characteristics like autonomy, resourcefulness and the external factors like healthy relationships, good schooling or strong social support (called as 'protective factors') were construed as acting a buffer or even preventing the risk factors harming the person (Rutter, 1987). The buffering or preventing act is a process. This process does not happen automatically, but it happens with the individual's choice. The process may have its own pace. Thus, resilience refers to a continuous process but not a single event. This was used to explain the 'process of resilience'. Just as the adversities, resilience also has a cumulative effect. Achievement or positive adaptation in one instance boosts the achievement in future instance and in other areas.

Describing the process, Richardson (2002) propounded his simple linear model. He called it the meta-theory of resilience and resiliency. He described the process as a force that drives an individual to grow and emerge through adversities. Following are the key points of his meta-theory:

1 It is normal for an individual to encounter challenges to one's homeostasis through changes and disruption
2 These disruptions have the potential to push an individual out of one's comfort zone, which may help one to develop the characteristics of resilience and emotional growth
3 The individual, through adaptation, acquires biopsychospiritual homeostasis
4 Not leaving the comfort zone and achieving homeostasis results in stagnation

According to Richardson, everyone by default is in the biopsychospiritual homeostasis at biological, psychological and spiritual plane. Whether good or bad, one is used to this state and hence it is comfort zone. Changes in life are bound to occur. Such changes in the form of trauma, illness, abuse or accident disrupt the homeostasis. Once the homeostasis is disrupted, the person is forced to integrate. Individuals differ in this process of reintegration. Some may perish, some may adapt to the disruption, some others may bounce back to their original state, while yet others may bounce forward.

As the model describes (Figure 10.1), the individual is in a basic zone of biopsychospiritual homeostasis. A major life event, a severe stress or an adversity hits this person causing disruption. Now, the natural tendency is to restore homeostasis and reintegrate oneself. Depending on the choice of the individual in operating the protective factors, the integration may happen at different levels. One of the possibilities is that the individual either does not exercise the option of applying force to operate the protective factors or does not have the ability to do so. This person reintegrates himself/herself at a dysfunctional level. Another person may be slightly better than the first and reintegrate with a loss. However, both these individuals failed to return to their original level of homeostasis. The third person makes a better use of the protective forces and manages to 'bounce back' to the original level of homeostasis. The fourth one is different from all the other three. Here, the protective factors are used as a buffer against the adversities and help the individual boom up and attain what is called resilient reintegration. As shown in the

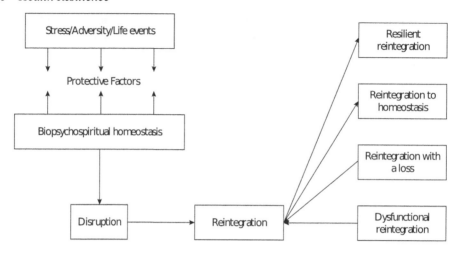

Figure 10.1 Richardson's Resilience Model.

model, resilient reintegration positions the individual at a performance and functioning higher than the original. Those who reintegrate back to homeostasis revert back to their original level of functioning, while the other two succumb to the adversities.

Thus, the model suggests that the protective factors are present in every individual. It is up to the person's personal motivation, efforts and skills in opting to activate these forces successfully to restore equilibrium or to spring up with vitality and vigour. Hence, Masten (2001) calls it the 'ordinary magic', indicating that it is a common phenomenon by operation of the adaptational system.

The attempts to study resilience as a process are called the second wave of research in the field. This process approach is widely accepted, though there have been few attempts to standardize and measure the process.

Following this were studies that attempted to foster resilience through interventions. This constituted the third wave. The ongoing fourth wave of research refers to discovering resilience at the biological level in cells and neurons (Masten, 2007; Wright, Masten, & Narayan, 2013).

Hariharan-Rajendran Synergy Model of Resilience

The subsequent research in resilience could convince the fact that resilience is not trait, but a process culminating in the product. It established the facts that three are essential factors in resilience such as adversities (that included life events, stress and risks), normal or above-normal performance and functioning (that referred to achievements and flourishing) and the operation of protective factors (that referred to internal characteristics of the individual and external factors from the psychosocial environment). Richardson's model delineated the buffering function of protective factor.

With the above field of knowledge, Hariharan and Rana (2016) postulated their model of resilience. It is called the 'Hariharan-Rana Synergy Model' because it explains the synergetic functioning of various factors in the process of resilience. Subsequently, the Hariharan-Rana model was replaced by the Hariharan-Rajendran Synergy Model (2019). The following are the basic constructs in the model.

Adversity

Adversity refers to multidimensional life conditions. Very often, adversities are interrelated. For example, the diagnosis of a terminal illness in a member of family is related to multiple factors apart from the biological illness. It has an impact on the psychological state of the patient, as well as the family members, financial state, treatment procedure sometimes causing relocation from home, professional life and incomplete task, public image. Thus, it was thought that resilience studies on homogenous groups are incomplete if the adversities other than the major factor are not taken into consideration. More important in resilient studies is to take into consideration the subject's perception of adversities than the adversity itself. There are three important aspects related to adversity, which determine its magnitude, viz. the severity of it in the perception of the person suffering it (subjective measure), frequency and duration of the same (objective measure).

Protective and Promoting Factors

What the earlier research called the 'protective factors' comprised of both internal characteristics of the individual and the external factors that are considered positive. The synergy model separated these two factors. The inherent characteristics of the person called 'intra-individual' factors are referred as 'protective' factors because they tend to protect the person from triggering adversities. The external factors identified by the person as positive experience are identified as 'promotive factors' because they are helpful in boosting or promoting the achievements of the person. The protective factors and promotive factors operate against the negative impact that the adversities are normally expected to have. Hence, together, they are called 'operating factors'.

Resistance

The research in resilience has been discussing resilience as a process. Richardson in his meta-theory referred to the 'buffer provided by the protective factors' so as to help in attaining resilient reintegration for a few whose homeostasis is disturbed by adversities. The synergy model took one step ahead in identifying this as 'resistance'. It is not the mere presence of certain personal characteristics and external support. There should be an effort by choice to set these operating factors in action, to resist the negative impact from the life stress. This resistance is initiated by the individual. It helps the individual in one of the two ways:

1. Insulates the individual in a way to minimize the impact of adversities
2. Restructures the life (sometimes including the adversities) in a way that the individual's functioning, performance and achievement spring up above the average level

Outcome Indicators

The index of resilience is the individual's performance, functioning and achievements in life. Performance and functioning are not mechanical indices in terms of hours of work per day. They comprise of qualitative factors such as happiness, contentment and positive affect. Hence, 'flourishing' is identified as one of the outcome indices, while 'achievement' in concrete term is the second index of outcome.

Thus, Hariharan-Rana Synergy Model postulates a synergy of adversity, operating factors and resistance, culminating in resilience. Figure 10.2 shows that while adversities, operating factors and resistance may be present in many independently, only when there is overlapping of the three does the resilience evolve.

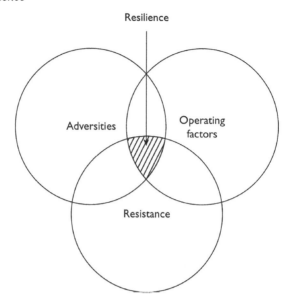

Figure 10.2 Synergy Point.

The path from adversity to resilience is through resistance and outcome. Figure 10.3 explains the path.

Figure 10.3 depicts the synergy model of Hariharan and Rajendran, which replaced the Hariharan-Rana Synergy Model. It explains that the protective and promotive factors help in resisting the impact of adversity on the one hand and lead to the positive use of the energy in accomplishing achievements and flourishing in life on the other. This happens despite the individual encountering adversities. The outcome of achievement and flourishing is made possible due to two possibilities: (1) the resistance helps in insulating the individual from the negative impacts of adversities; (2) resistance helps the individual to convert the adversity into advantage and restructure its characteristics into positive. In either case, undeterred by the adversity, the individual proceeds to perform and achieve. In cases where the individual manages to insulate oneself, he/she ends up surviving the adversity by not perishing under pressure. These individuals can be called the 'survivors' or borderline resilients. The second category who turn adversity into advantage and restructure the negative into positive are more likely to excel and emerge resilients. The magnitude of resistance combined with the level of excellence determines the product of resilience of different degrees.

The synergy model of resilience has a formula for measuring resilience:

$$\text{Resilience Index} = \frac{\text{Outcome Index}}{\text{Resistance Index}} \times 100$$

Outcome Index = Achievement + Flourishing

$$\text{Resistance Index} = \frac{\text{Operating Factor Index}}{\text{Adversity Index}} \times 100$$

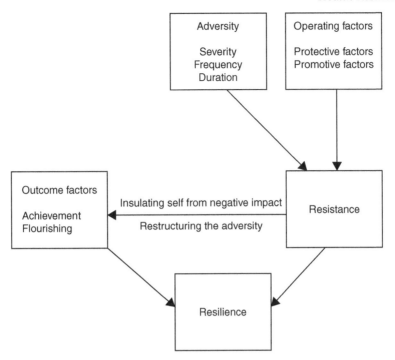

Figure 10.3 Hariharan-Rajendran Synergy Model: Pathway.

Rajendran, Hariharan and Rao (2019) developed and validated a Resilience Test Battery with the constructs adversity, protective factors, promotive factors, achievement, and applied the formula to derive the Resilience Index. The battery was found to be high on reliability and validity.

However, there are several steps to arrive at each 'index'. The model and the formula open the scope for measuring resilience in every person since it assumes its presence in everyone in varying degrees. This resilience manifests in the individual when one chooses to respond to a stressful situation by consciously activating the operating factors. An individual in whom the presence of operating factors is strong, and activated to resist the impact of adversity with optimum vigour, the resilience measure is high (with a value of 100 or more). With a weak presence of operating factors or a weak/incomplete activation of the same (which happens with the reluctance of the individual to quit the 'comfort zone'), there will be a weak manifestation of resilience. Thus, the model and the formula enable one to identify those labelled as resilient, borderline resilience and low resilience. This measurement and classification creates an opportunity to train those in borderline in exercising resistance by activating the operating factors.

This can be done in any area of adversity such as socioeconomic field, disabilities or health.

Factors Impacting Health and Health Resilience

As per the World Health Organization (WHO), the concept of health includes wellbeing. That refers to a positive state of physical, mental and social dimensions of the individual. It implies not only the absence of disease but also the ability to recover and bounce back from illness and other problems. One may infer from this that health and wellbeing can be construed as the frequency of falling ill, the duration of staying ill, the speed of recovery from illness and the strength of bouncing back to normal functioning. It can be further extended to include the way in which acute and chronic stress from various sources are handled in order to sustain one's cognitive emotional and social functioning intact, or the capacity of one to bounce back from the negative impact of the same in terms of time and energy reflected in resuming equilibrium.

The WHO identifies three broad areas with their potential influence on health and wellbeing:

- Social and economic environment
- Physical environment and
- The individual's personal characteristics and behaviour

Higher income, social status and education are identified as determinants of positive health and wellbeing, while poverty, illiteracy and lower educational levels are identified as determinants of negative health. Strong social support from family, friends and community is associated with better health and wellbeing, while weak social support is linked to poor health and wellbeing. Availability of safe basic amenities like fresh air, water, housing, roads and healthy working place is linked to positive health. In addition to this, healthy genetic inheritance plays a crucial role in determining the health and wellness. An individual with a healthy genetic endowment is likely to acquire and sustain good health compared to the one with an unhealthy gene. Besides all these, the individual's personality factors, and health practices in terms of health-promoting or health risk behaviour also constitute a major determinant of sustenance or losing health and wellbeing.

In principle, all the factors discussed above result in good health and wellbeing if positively disposed. In case these factors are negatively disposed, the individual is expected to have poor health and low wellbeing.

Having understood the connotation of health and the factors contributing to positive health, it is easy to conceptualize resilience in the context of health and wellbeing. Putting it in simple terms, an individual towards whom one or more of the determinants of health and wellbeing are not positively disposed, in spite of that one is able to sustain health and wellbeing, in case of any setback to health in terms of acute or chronic illness, is able to bounce back to health at a fast pace and resume functioning at a normal level or above that. Thus, a clear deviation from the expected lines of conditions of health and wellbeing is resilience.

Among the factors determining health are personality aspects. One of the factors named by a number of theories of health behaviour is self-efficacy. The individual's belief that he/she has the ability to do things such as adopting a health behaviour or quitting the health risk behaviour to attain the goal of positive health and wellbeing is one of the major protective factors for resilience. The other factors as identified by a number of theories are perception of severity and susceptibility to illness. A realistic perception in these aspects calls for adequate knowledge levels. It may be inferred that resilient persons possess the correct knowledge base about health and illness and adopt appropriate behaviour that promotes and sustains health or aids in bouncing back.

The other factors mentioned as promoting health behaviour by various theories are perceived control, perceived benefits, protection motivation, action planning, coping planning and so on.

Resilience in the Context of Health

Research on health-related resilience is picking the moments gradually. Noticing the few 'miracle cases' where the patient either survives a fatal medical event, shows faster pace of recovery or does not suffer the apprehended serious adversity in the form of disease progression perhaps has opened the research interest in the field of health resilience.

As already mentioned, one essential component of resilience is the presence of adversity. The presence of adversity is possible varying its severity as perceived by the person, frequency of it in terms of its occurrence and duration in terms of time. These three factors determine the 'experience' of stress caused by the adversity. It is highly possible that an individual encounters multiple adversities as an offspring of the main adversity. For example, diagnosis of failure of kidney functioning in the young adolescent in the family calling for periodical dialysis is causing a financial drain out, hospitalization leading to interruption in the college attendance, and a need for relocation of the family to a capital city where one has to adapt to various changes related to everyday life. It is also possible that an individual faces adversity from various independent sources at the same time. For example, when one is attending on a senior member of the family hospitalized with massive cardiac attack, there is call from the daughter's college that she is caught using drugs. That may be the same time when the long drawn legal dispute over ancestral property is judged by the court against the person, thus bringing a threat of losing the entire property.

Physiology of Resilience

HPA Activation and Resilience

The stress experienced during such circumstances has a physiological response having a direct impact on the health of the individual. To recapitulate, the physiological response to stress starts with the hypothalamus stimulating the pituitary gland to secrete corticotrophin-releasing hormone (CRH), which travels down to the adrenal gland and triggers the secretion of adrenaline, noradrenaline and cortisol. While cortisol helps in short-term adaptation to the stress, prolonged exposure to stress and continuously having higher levels of cortisol lead to a number of adverse health condition such as hypertension, cardiovascular diseases and lowered immune levels.

Feder, Nestler and Charney (2009) postulate that resilience may be associated with exercising control in release of CRH, and adaptive changes in CRH receptors. According to deKloet, Joels and Holsboer (2005), a quick onset of stress response along with its adaptive processes at biological level delineates resilience. Exercising control over CRH and cortisol levels leads to optimizing the function of glucocorticoid. Active response to stress is associated with lesser glucocorticoid responses. This was found in animal studies (Charney, 2004; deKloet, Joels, & Holsboer, 2005). Glucocorticoids are hormones secreted by the adrenal gland. They help maintain the equilibrium of blood glucose and blood pressure and have the anti-inflammatory quality. The negative effects are lowering of immunity. By regulation of CRH and glucocorticoid function, the positive impacts are optimized.

Dehydroepiandrosterone (DHEA) Level and Resilience

Studies found that those who give active stress response are different in certain hormonal levels in the body. Stress induces the release of a hormone called dehydroepiandrosterone (DHEA). It is produced by the adrenal cortex. It is circulated in the body along with sulphur that prevents it from being broken down. It gets converted into sex hormone and is useful in that way. High levels of DHEA are found to be associated with reducing the risk of cardiovascular diseases, age-related degenerative diseases, depression and even death as suggested by few studies.

Soldiers found resilient based on their best performance on encountering stress were found to have high levels of DHEA sulphate/cortisol ratio (Morgan et al., 2004). Higher DHEA levels were found to be associated with anti-glucocorticoids effectively on the brain.

Association between active response to stress and DHEA has to be underlined. The individual's active and conscious efforts to encounter stress or adversity are also a salient feature of resilience. Richardson implied that those who do not wish to leave their comfort zone when their biopsychospiritual homeostasis is disturbed cannot attain resilient reintegration. Those who choose to actively operate their protective factors to constitute a buffer against adversity are the ones who respond actively to stress. Thus, it can be inferred that it is the individual' active response to stress that is related on the one hand to resilience while on the other to high level of DHEA.

Regular exercise and a diet regimen with restricted calories are found to be associated with increase in DHEA in rhesus monkeys (Mattison, Lave, Roth, & Ingram, 2003; Copeland, Consitt, & Tremblay, 2002).

Neurobiological Response and Resilience

What is inferred by the discussion so far is that active and efficient response to stress is what is manifested in biochemical levels, as well as resilience, indicated by positive affect state and achievement or accomplishments in life. In that case, a host of physiological functioning is activated by a stressful encounter. All of them may be associated with resilience. This includes the hormones adrenaline and noradrenaline triggered by sympathetic nervous system and cortisol produced by the HPA axis, which after rapidly responding to stress shut off soon after. It includes the dopamine reward system, which helps in sustaining positive affect state during the phase of chronic stress or adversity. It also includes the hippocampus that is intact and well protected so that the new memories are formed as part of healthy cognitive functioning. The other neurobiological factor to be mentioned here is the well developed and efficiently functioning prefrontal cortex that regulates the emotional reactions and its subsequent behavioural reaction to stress by inhibiting amygdala, which is responsible for processing raw emotions.

It is found that people with high activity of left prefrontal cortex recover faster from negative emotions like anger, fear or disgust. Davidson (2000) proposed that when the left prefrontal cortex is optimally activated, it helps in inhibiting amygdala, calms down the associated negative emotions such as anxiety, fear or anger and helps the prefrontal cortex to facilitate behaviour based on rational planning.

Hippocampus is the part of the brain that is susceptible to damage in the face of prolonged exposure to stress, because elevated levels of cortisol cause damage to its neurons. Animal studies suggested that vigorous aerobic exercise helps in enhancing the levels of nerve growth factors, and helps in growth of cells in the region. This comes in handy to protect the impact of stress on the hippocampus.

The common thread between the meta-theory of Richardson, synergy model of Hariharan and Rana and neuroplasticity of Davisson is 'activation', suggesting a conscious, informed and involved role of the individual in response to adversity.

Genetic Influence on Resilience

After exploring the neurobiological factors associated with resilience, researchers also investigated into the role of genetic factors in resilience and its development. DNA studies have proved that variations in genes have a role in regulating the sympathetic system, HPA axis, serotonin system, which determine the strength and level of biological response to stress. Prakash, Archana and Kumar (2017) stated that genetic factors have a role in the HPA axis response to stress and the regulation of the same. It is associated with the functional variants in mineral corticoid and glucocorticoid receptor (GR) genes. It was identified in human beings as stated by deKloet, Joels and Holsboer (2005). Different researchers have identified different genes, playing a moderator role.

Though there is enough evidence on the role of genes in resilience, research has not yet converged and concurred in identifying specific genes.

Positive Factors Suggested by Theories

Positive health behaviour or health-promoting behaviour plays a crucial role in mitigating or minimizing the adversities and sustaining health and wellbeing. A cursory look at the theories of health behaviour enables us to identify positive factors related to health behaviour. Self-efficacy is identified as a positive factor by the Health Behaviour Model (Becker & Rosenstock, 1974), Protection Motivation Theory (Rogers, 1975), Health Action Process Approach (HAPA) (Schwarzer, 1999), Transtheoretical Model (Prochaska & DiClemente, 1982) and Social Cognitive Theory (Bandura, 1986). Self-efficacy is one factor that has been endorsed by majority of theories. Apart from this, factors such as motivation to protect oneself from illness (Protection Motivation Theory), positive attitudes towards health behaviour and the support of significant others (Theory of Reasoned Action), perceived behavioural control (Theory of Planned Action), awareness about the health and illness (Precaution Adaption Process Model, PAPM) (Weinstein, Rothman, & Stutton, 1998) and Self-Regulation Model (Leventhal, 1997, 2003) are also the positive factors that may contribute to resilience.

In summary, it may be stated that it is the strength of motivation and the belief in one's own ability to embrace health-promoting behaviour that sustains health in an individual.

Research on specific homogeneous groups has been taken up to explore the association between resilience and health. It is of interest to verify if the factors proposed by various theories play a significant role in providing, sustaining and restoring positive health among various resilient groups.

Chronic Diseases and Resilience

According to World Health Organization (WHO), chronic diseases refer to

> conditions of ill health that accompany the individual for a long period of time, produce incapacity, or residual disability caused by irreversible pathological alterations, demand rehabilitation and follow up over a long time and may present periods of improvement and periods of worsening in acute stages.
>
> (Barros, César, Carandina, & Torre, 2006)

This, as characterized by Subramanyan (1989), is a major stress event, followed by a series of minor events with negative consequences. A chronic disease has no permanent cure, and hence needs to be managed efficiently in order to reap the optimum outcome. Very often, chronic diseases are accompanied by anxiety and depression, thus negatively contributing to one's quality of life and wellbeing. The impact of negative emotions, state of anxiety and depression on prognosis of treatment is a well-researched area. The impact of stress on various physiological systems, the lowered immune levels and their contributions to perpetuation of symptoms triggering of medical episodes and delayed recovery from setbacks from time to time are aspects that have proved the association between negative psychological state and illness. This suggests that the association between resilience and chronic diseases may have to follow the pathway of cognition related to the disease, affect as a reaction to the disease and coping behaviour as a strategy to handle the disease. In other words, optimizing wellbeing in the face of chronic illness may be possible by adopting positive psychological response to the disease. This was beautifully summed up by Sharma and Misra (2010) who stated "Living with chronic illness makes demands on the capacity of the individual to adapt preserving a reasonable emotional balance, sustaining relationships with family and friends, and dealing with suffering (pain and other debilitating symptoms etc.)" (p. 284). Basic and functional knowledge about the disease helps in accepting the inevitability of its presence in one's system, and understanding the treatment regimen that includes lifestyle changes and the behavioural risk factors helps in invoking the motivation for clinical adherence and efficient management. Kohli and Dalal (1998) argued that the first step towards cognitive reconstruction is acceptance of suffering. This sets the process of healing. The assessment of the disease condition and cognition related to susceptibility for disease progression are basic important elements. Once the acceptance of diagnosis sets in, efforts to optimize the positive thinking and positive reappraisal of the disease condition help the individual of the disease condition, and help the individual to move out of negative emotions to neutral and then to positive. The motivation to stay healthy with all limitations of conditions caused by the disease helps one to assess one's own ability to strive for it. A strong self-efficacy, perception of internal control on disease management, strong social support positively contribute towards resilience. Characteristics like spirituality, gratitude, forgiveness are associated with effective coping in general. They are found to have a positive impact on prognosis (Priti, Yadava, & Sharma, 2012).

Working through one's pain of chronic disease may help one emerge as resilient with self-transformation. Perhaps this is what is associated with positive reappraisal of the disease itself. Anand, Srivastava and Dalal (2001) and Anand (2004) through his narratives brought the focus on how people with chronic diseases bring in psychological healing by effectively working through their pain and suffering and pave a path of transforming themselves.

Agarwal et al. (1995) named factors such as positive life orientation, sense of personal control and maintenance of positive affect state despite adversities as contributing towards expectation for recovery. According to them, such predisposition constitutes essential conditions in patients to mobilize internal resources, which in turn play a significant role in recovery. Future orientation, optimism, perceived control, relationship with family are associated with faster recovery and sense of wellbeing. These internal protective factors alone are not sufficient for fostering resilience. Alongside these, certain external factors that promote resilience interact with the protective internal resources for the best outcome in the form of recovery, effective management or arrest of disease progression. Upadhyay (2002) asserted that economic status alongside the internal resources has a role in predicting recovery.

Studies have been carried out on a number of samples of specific chronic diseases to explore their association with resilience. We will examine and report studies related to cardiovascular disease, diabetes mellitus, cancer, arthritis and few other diseases.

Cardiovascular Disease and Resilience

Diseases related to heart and blood circulation are called cardiovascular diseases. Conditions of the heart are related to the heart muscle, valves and the rhythm. Condition of blood circulation is associated with the blood vessels. Narrowing down of vessels and blocks in them may lead to problems such as hypertension, pain in the chest (angina), heart attack or stroke. Cardiovascular diseases include coronary artery disease (narrowing of arteries), heart attack, abnormal heart rhythm (arrhythmias), heart failure, heart valve disease, heart muscle disease (cardiomyopathy), to name a few.

Health Resilience 415

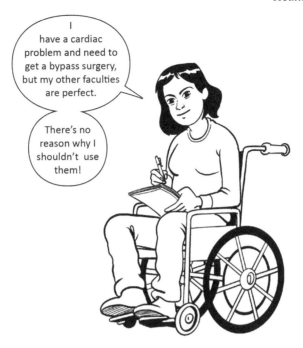

Figure 10.4 Utilizing the 'Non-sick' Faculties for Flourishing.

Cardiovascular disease calls for efficient management of the disease. Cardiovascular system and stress and negative affect are closely related. Hence, while bringing in lifestyle changes and being adherent to medication, it is important to regulate one's emotions and residual affect state directing it towards positive disposition. This helps in maintaining the normal levels of blood pressure and cardiac rhythm. Research in the field indicates good prognosis associated with positivity (Figure 10.4).

Affleck et al. (1987) conducted a longitudinal study on a sample of 287 patients who suffered a heart attack. The eight-year follow-up on the patients revealed that those who identified and reported the benefits of a cardiac attack showed lower levels of morbidity and are less likely to suffer another attack. Counting the benefits of a suffered attack in fact indicates positive reappraisal strategy of coping, where the person recounts the adverse event and analyses it in a positive perspective. This strategy of coping arrests the negative thoughts, brooding and subsequent stress from the already occurred adverse event and restores the positive disposition leading to optimizing wellbeing in the person.

Agarwal et al. (1995) in their longitudinal study on 70 cardiovascular patients found a correlation between positive life orientation and recovery. The other internal resources related to positive life orientation were personal control and affect state. Though no cause-effect relationship can be inferred between them, it is generally found that good recovery and these positive characteristics coexist.

Perceived personal control enables a person to initiate behaviour for faster recovery and prevention of progression of disease or future cardiac events. Helgeson (1992), Moser and Dracup (1995) found a positive association between perceived personal control and psychological adjustment three months and six months after the cardiac event. Moser and Dracup (1995) also found that those with personal control were less depressed. Sullivan et al. (1998) in their cohort study found that those with high self-efficacy demonstrated better physical functioning, and active at family and social levels at six months of follow-up. Higher self-efficacy that asserts one's belief in one's own ability functions as a positive booster for restoring effective functioning at every level. Robinson-Smith et al. (2000) studied a sample of 63 stroke patients. The results suggested that self-efficacy related to self-care positively correlated with quality of life. It was found that those patients who measured high on self-care and self-efficacy had higher quality of life and no depression at one-month and six-month gap.

By and large, the characteristics identified in the research are positive orientation that includes cognition, affect and motivational disposition of the patients that enhanced the wellbeing and reduced the risk of recurrence of cardiac event.

Diabetes Mellitus and Resilience

Diabetes mellitus is of two types, viz. type 1 and type 2. Type 2 is very common. This refers to a condition where one's body fails to metabolize glucose, which is the source of energy for the body. This can occur either because one's body resists the effects of insulin or fails to produce adequate insulin to maintain the glucose levels at normal range. India is one of the countries where the prevalence of diabetes is high and is progressively on the rise.

Once diagnosed with diabetes, the patient has to follow strict adherence to diet, exercise, self-monitoring in addition to medication. Low or non-adherence may lead to serious health adversities such as diabetes retinopathy, diabetes neuropathy, developing gangrene failures of kidney functioning, hypoglycaemia and coma—most often irreversible in nature. In view of the irreversible nature of disease progression, patients with adequate knowledge are careful and adherent.

It is important that the patients protect themselves from stress and negative affect, and maintaining good level of physical activity. The research on diabetes and psychological parameters started as a new field of interest for researchers. Let us examine some findings that suggest relationship between diabetes and resilience as indicated by effective disease management and positive psychological parameters (Figure 10.5).

Johnston-Brooks et al. (2002) in an interesting study included 110 diabetes patients in the sample. The findings indicated that self-efficacy was related to effective self-care. Self-care is a very significant component in effective management of diabetes. The HbA1c levels of those with better self-care were good. Further analysis revealed that self-care played a mediating role between self-efficacy and HbA1c level. It needs no great explanation to infer that a person who believes in the ability of oneself to manage the disease efficiently is likely to be good in self-care, which is an essential prerequisite for maintaining normal levels of HbA1c.

In another study, Yi et al. (2008) included a sample of 111 diabetes patients. They measured the resilience and HbA1c levels in the patients. The results revealed that resilience predicted the HbA1c levels for future. It was also found that resilience functioned as an effective buffer in the face of adversity and distress and prevented a declining self-care and worsening of HbA1c levels. A resilient person seems to have the capacity to insulate one's health condition from the adversities of life. As suggested by physiological changes during adversities in resilience, which is discussed earlier in the chapter, insulation of health from adversities is possible. When the adversities are handled without strong negative emotions, and even when the negative emotions are involved, a quick restoration of positive affect state and physiological homeostasis prevents or minimizes the system from suffering the impact of stress caused by adversities.

Health Resilience 417

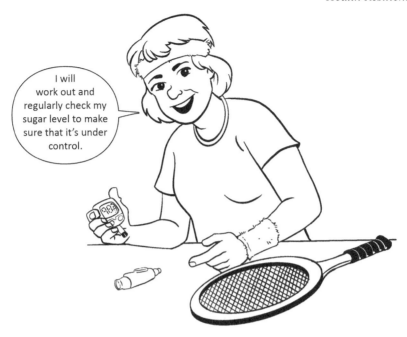

Figure 10.5 Resilience and Self-Efficacy.

DeNisco (2011) carried out a cross-sectional study on 71 diabetes patients. The results found an association between resilience and HbA1c levels. The correlation between them was negative where the higher the resilience level, the lower the HbA1c readings.

Diabetes calls for effective self-management for maintenance of blood glucose levels. A person emotionally reacting to the diagnosis of the disease is likely to contribute negatively to wellbeing. However, one who optimizes on the positive aspects and applies these strengths in coping with the disease is likely to enhance the wellbeing. Padhy, Chelli, and Lalnuntlunagi (2017) studied a sample of 78 patients between 30 and 70 years of age diagnosed with type 2 diabetes. They identified the factors contributing to self-management of diabetes. Results identified that self-efficacy and outcome expectancy significantly contributed to self-management of the disease. Individual's faith in one's ability to manage the disease when combined with a belief on positive outcome triggers one's active involvement in coping with the disease. A good self-management of the disease is successful in reducing the disease-related distress and protecting wellbeing in the individual.

In another study, Padhy, Chottai and Lalnuntluangi (2017) studied 150 patients with type 2 diabetes in the age group of 34–75 years. The objective of the study was to explore the role of self-efficacy and outcome expectancy on wellbeing. Results revealed that it was only outcome expectancy, which contributed to psychological wellbeing. Outcome expectancy calls for a strong cognitive base related to the disease. A person who has a sound knowledge about the disease is likely to know the outcome of changing the lifestyle and adopting appropriate health behaviour to cope with the disease. Hence, one of the factors for resilience in diabetes is knowledge about the disease and outcome expectancy of a behaviour. A person diagnosed with a chronic illness, seeking and acquiring knowledge about the diseases, is likely to have higher wellbeing and resilience, which follows the trajectory of appropriate health behaviour and outcome expectancy.

Disease management among diabetes calls for high motivational levels and perseverance in following the prescribed lifestyle. Self-care, more than the medical care, is the essential factor. Only when self-care fails and there is an adverse event or medical emergency, the medical care becomes crucial. A positive disposition is very essential for good self-care among the diabetes patients. Resilience has positive disposition as its integral part.

Cancer and Resilience

Cancer is of many types. The disease progression depends on its location and the type. The common characteristic of cancer is abnormal multiplication of cells. Though not factually true, the diagnosis of cancer is often considered as irreversible. Hence, it is associated with strong negative affect not only for the patient but for the family as well. This negative affect further contributes to the disease progression and recurrence. Thus, treatment of cancer often calls for biopsychosocial approach that provides healing alongside treatment for arrest of disease and cure.

With the emergence of psych oncology as a specialized field of research, there have been several studies associating psychological factors with the disease. Gotay et al. (2004) studied a sample of 320 patients who had cancer in different locations. They measured various psychological parameters. Result revealed that sense of coherence (manageability, meaningfulness and control) predicted mental health, quality of life and resilience in the patients. Morille et al. (2008) also found that sense of coherence improved resilience in patients with breast cancer.

Cancer survivors can be considered resilient. In their study, Costanzo et al. (2011) compared cancer survivors to non-cancer group of aged population. They found that cancer survivors exhibited relatively higher levels of positive psychological characteristics such as social wellbeing, spirituality and personal growth compared to the non-cancer group.

Resilience and the associated positive factors among the cancer patients are by and large similar across cultures. Studies conducted on Indian sample revealed the results not drastically different from the Western studies. Saraf et al. (2013) studied the patients who are cervical survivors of cancer. Their findings revealed that faith in God and religiosity were associated with meaning-making, and fostered resilience that helped the individuals to adapt to the illness. It suggests that religiosity and spirituality may help in reorienting the person to life. Adaptation to the disease is more likely to be successful with the new found meaning of life.

Indian culture, with their high affiliation orientation, draws good amount of positive resources from social support. It is an interaction between the positive internal factors and the positive external factors that protect or minimize the adverse impact of the disease and promote optimal quality of life and resilience. This was the findings by Somasundaram and Devamani (2016) on a sample of 60 cancer patients. They explored the relationship between resilience, social support and hopelessness. Resilience was found to be associated positively with social support and negatively with hopelessness.

A number of studies on patients with different diseases identified benefit-finding as a significant characteristic associated with wellbeing. Benefit-finding is a composite of three qualities, viz. resilience, self-reliance and appreciation of life. In a study of patients with breast cancer, Daugherty et al. (2005) found that benefit-finders showed higher spiritual wellbeing and significant decline in distress levels during the period of their treatment for cancer compared to non-benefit-finders.

Cancer among children is a well-researched phenomenon. While some children cope with cancer effectively and maintain high quality of life, others fail to do it. Some studies identified the factors associated with resilience. Orbuch et al. (2005) studied a sample of 190 children who suffered from various types of cancer. They found that children's relationship with parents contributed significantly to wellbeing. The relationship with factors was associated with psychological and spiritual wellbeing, while relationship with mother was found to be associated with psychological wellbeing. Both were beneficial in increasing resilience in them.

Parry (2003) studied a sample of 23 children suffering from cancer. He found that the uncertainties of cancer and coping with it evolved a new outlook on life for them. This helped in developing confidence, optimism and resilience in them. In another study, Parry and Chesler (2005) studied a sample of 50 children with cancer. They found that the two aspects associated with wellbeing and resilience are meaning-making and psychospiritual growth (Figure 10.6).

Resilience helps in bringing better quality of life among cancer patients. The response to treatment also is likely to be better among resilient because with its characteristic positivity, the negative affect state is minimized or mitigated. This is a significant contribution in bringing homeostasis at biochemical and physiological levels.

Arthritis and Resilience

Arthritis refers to a condition of inflammation of joints. The term describes about 200 conditions. The two most common types of arthritis are osteoarthritis and rheumatoid arthritis. Osteoarthritis refers to a condition where the flexible tissues called cartilage located at the end of bones get worn out over time. Rheumatoid arthritis is an autoimmune disease. Here, the immune system attacks the joints of the body. Rheumatoid arthritis is accompanied by pain, ache, stiffness and swelling in and around the joints. Sometimes, it may affect the immune system and other body organs. The main problem with arthritis is the pain that limits the physical mobility

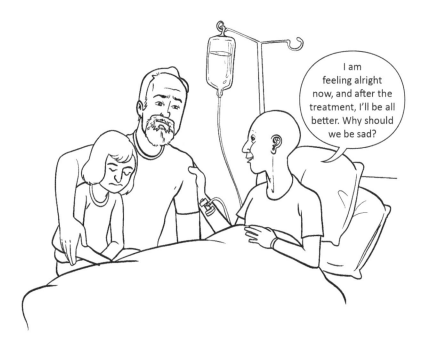

Figure 10.6 'Hope' in Chronic Patients with Resilience.

420 *Health Resilience*

of the individual disrupting the lifestyle. The challenge is to maintain fitness and sustain the ability to maintain daily activities, by managing the pain effectively. Resilient patients are more likely to be successful in effective pain management and carry out the normal activities.

Wright, Zautra and Going (2008) tried to identify the predictors of pain and physical functioning in a sample of 275 osteoarthritis patients. They found that two factors, risk and resilience, were important predictors of pain and physical functioning. Self-efficacy was found to play a mediating role between resilience and pain.

Smith and Zautra (2008) studied a sample of 263 patients with osteoarthritis and rheumatoid arthritis. They tested the sample on resilience pain and other psychological parameters. The results found that resilience could predict positive social interaction, as well as the affect state in the forthcoming week (Figure 10.7).

Abraído-Lanza, Guier, and Colón (1998) included patients with different types of arthritis in their sample. The results of their quantitative and qualitative analysis identified a number of positive factors. Patients who had the characteristics like hope, optimism and appreciation for life thrived the disease. Protective factors such as self-efficacy, self-esteem and positive affect positively correlated with wellbeing and thriving.

The findings of Narváez et al. (2010) on their study on a sample of 36 rheumatoid arthritis patients pointed that large-scale social support network and self-care were related to higher benefit-finding, which in turn predicted mental health. Having a wide circle of social network is useful in enhancing one's own involvement in self-care instead of developing dependence on the social resources.

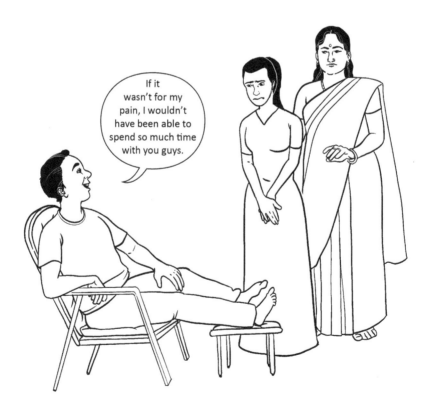

Figure 10.7 Benefit-Finding.

Other Chronic Diseases and Resilience

There are a number of other chronic diseases related to various systems of the body. Irrespective of the type of disease, all chronic illnesses that demand long-term management are likely to optimize wellbeing and sustain quality of life when resilience is present. Illnesses relate to renal system, nervous system, skeletal muscular system, digestive system, respiratory and other systems are included in this. Research findings that connect resilience to few chronic diseases are mentioned below.

Symister and Friend (2003) studied a sample of 86 patients of renal diseases. They identified both internal and external factors that helped sustain the wellbeing. The study found a positive relation between social support and self-esteem. This relation helped enhance optimism and minimize depression. Thus, the positive affect state is helped to sustain, which is very significant in thwarting the disease progression and episodes of medical emergencies. In another study by Ma et al. (2013) on 152 patients with chronic kidney disease (CKD), a positive correlation was found between resilience and health-promoting behaviour.

Parkinson's disease is a central nervous system disorder. The damage of nerve cells in the brain leads to drop in dopamine levels. This results in symptoms of Parkinson's disease that includes problems in movements and causes tremors, stiffness and loss of balance. The individual may live for 10–20 years after the diagnosis of the disease around 60 years of age. Thus, it requires very long-term management and care. Resilience helps in better management of the disease. Robottom et al. (2012) studied resilience in a sample of 83 patients with Parkinson's disease. They found that the higher the resilience, the lower the disability and better the quality of life both in physical and in mental health dimensions.

Multiple sclerosis is a degenerative disease. It is caused because the immune system destroys the protective covering of the nerves. Because of this, the communication between the brain and body is disrupted. This may result in a number of adversities such as pain, fatigue, loss of coordination, loss of vision. Medication and treatment can slow down the progression of disease. However, coping with the disease on a day-to-day basis is the biggest challenge. The individual's reorientation to life pays in coping with the disease. Pakenham and Cox (2009) in their study on 388 patients subscribed to the fact that resilience, self-reliance and appreciation of life, together expressed as benefit-finding, predicted positive adjustment at 12 months. Over a period of time, benefit-finding gained in strength.

Disabilities and Resilience

Disabilities vary in their type. It may be locomotive disability restricting the mobility of the person or disability of sense organs shutting down the sensory inputs of the concerned faculty, or intellectual disability that limits the cognitive function of the person. The disabilities could be congenital or acquired, reversible or irreversible. We limit our discussion here to the irreversible disabilities with which the individual has to cope throughout the life span. Some may consider it a limitation for achieving life goals and limit themselves to suboptimal goal attainment, while others may not be deterred by their disability in pursuing their life goals. The second category belongs to the resilient group. Lisha (2012) interviewed six persons with locomotive disability and applied interpretive phenomenological analysis in identifying the unique positive factors that helped them perform and achieve well despite their physical adversity. The study identified protective factors such as assertiveness, optimism, social interaction pattern, individual relationship and family support as contributing factors for their performance and success. Besides these, the promotive factors such as connectedness with others and the presence of social support were found equally significant. Logically, one can argue that the positive disposition towards life and society enables them to accept the imminence of the disability while endorsing the positivity in other dimensions of life. This helps in preventing the negative emotions taking the lead and substitutes with positive ones. There could be a mutually contributing relationship between the positive emotions and their wide social network and support system. This is true in case of any type of disability. Annalakshmi and Ragitha (2012) compared a group of students with hearing impairment with normals. The positive disposition is very evident in the findings. Those who were found to be highly resilient used less of emotionally impoverished experience compared to their counterparts who are low on resilience.

Hariharan, Karimi and Kishore (2014) studied a sample of 100 persons with locomotor disability, comprising 50 resilient and 50 vulnerable in the age group of 13–25 years. They were assessed on emotional intelligence and perceived environment (physical and social). Results indicated that resilient measured higher on emotional intelligence and were positive in perception of their environment compared to the vulnerable. The study suggests that positive perception and emotional strengths are important predictors of successful outcomes.

Thus, a positive perception of the disability affective and behavioural disposition is found to play a significant role in motivating the persons towards effective coping and better achievement in life. While resilience among the physically disabled occupies an important place in resilience research, the resilience among patients of mentally challenged deserves a special mention. Rajan and John (2016) studied a sample of 121 parents living with their mentally challenged children. They found a positive relationship between positive perception of disability and resilience. Thus, attributing a negative connotation to disability may function as a hurdle from moving ahead, while a positive perception helps accept the reality and make the best out of what is given.

Ageing and Resilience

The definition of successful ageing about half a century ago was 'the ability to detach oneself from the activities of the midlife as a kind of preparation for death' (Cumming, 1968). This definition was not accepted by the older adults because of its negative orientation. In contrast to this, Havighurst's (1961) definition identified successful ageing. It refers to a condition of staying actively involved in activities enjoyed in early-life. Thus, it emanates lot of positivity. However, this was also perceived as far from reality (Figure 10.8).

Ageing is a natural process of progressive slowdown of all systems. But successful ageing or healthy ageing requires high level of functioning in all domains of life, despite the natural phenomenon of slowing, degeneration and impairments. If we place healthy ageing alongside resilience, the striking resemblance is that resilience calls for high performance or achievement despite adversities, just as healthy ageing refers to high level of functioning on multiple domains despite the natural process of slowing down. Thus, when applied to the ageing population, maintenance of high levels of functioning refers to both resilience and healthy ageing.

Healthy ageing is possible among those who plan for the active functioning in later years. Just as the way one saves the resources to be of use in future, the one who saves the cognitive reserves can build up the cognitive abilities. A person engaged in further education continues to build the cognitive faculties. Brayne et al. (2010) stated that this can accommodate physiological insults such as plaques and tangles often seen in patients with dementia. The resource saving can be done in all the three dimensions that foster resilience, viz. internal, social and environmental. Building a strong social network, creating a physical and social environment that keeps one active, and sustaining positive affect can add to including personal resources such as

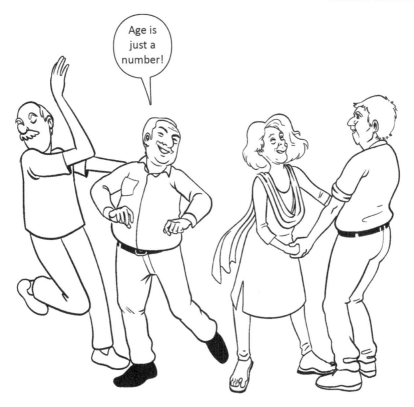

Figure 10.8 Optimizing on Abilities.

keeping oneself cognitively active and emotionally positive. This enables a person to compress the morbidity years and multiplying the functioning trajectory through the process of healthy ageing. This facilitates 'adding life to years' than adding 'years to life', which is a strong index quality of life.

Perna et al. (2015) studied a sample of 3942 elderly people who participated in a population-based cohort study. They found that resilient persons among the elderly were able to consume good servings of fruits and vegetables and perform moderate to high physical activities compared to the non-resilient elderly. This was irrespective of their socioeconomic background.

There have been pointers at economic aspects related to wellbeing. Lower economic burden and enhanced economic contribution are found to be associated with higher levels of wellbeing. Those with higher levels of wellbeing reported greater productivity, fewer absence from work and lower costs on health care. They showed higher employment outcomes (Shi et al., 2013). These findings were true even in case of people with chronic illnesses like fibromyalgia (which has the symptoms of widespread muscle pain, sleep and mood alterations), chronic pain in lower back and ankylosing spondylitis (an inflammatory arthritis affecting the spine and large joints). Lower wellbeing in these patients increased the overall costs in people with these chronic diseases.

While slowing down, progressive degeneration and gradual withdrawal from activities involving physical psychological and social dimensions are the natural expected process, a good proportion of the elderly stand distinct in deviation of the expected lines. What are the protective and promotive factors that help these people to encounter the natural adversities successfully?

Ramamurti and Jamuna (2010) have enumerated a number of concepts such as successful ageing, active ageing and productive ageing that contradict the natural process of progressive negativity related to ageing. According to them, 'graceful acceptance' of ageing is associated with positivity such as happiness and contentment. Well-exercised body and mind helps in slowing down the natural process of ageing. Kumar (1998), Ramamurti (1989) and Sachdev (1998) advocated engagement in activities involving physical and mental faculties to experience active ageing.

Research in India has identified a number of positive correlates of successful ageing. They include self-acceptance of changes related to ageing, self-acceptance of one's physical health, faith in the concept 'karma' (which connotes the philosophy of 'doing with no expectation of return' and 'events being predetermined' based on previous deeds) being flexible, faith in afterlife and presence of social support (Jamuna, 1988, 1994; Ramamurti, 1987, 1989).

Productive ageing refers to one's activities that are useful to self and others, useful to self and be self-dependent (Bhatia, 2002b; Kumar, 2002) and contributes voluntarily to community (Ramamurti, 2003).

While genetic predisposition plays a significant role, a number of psychosocial and behavioural factors assume equal importance in ensuring successful ageing and longevity. Jamuna and Ramamurti (2000b) and Jamuna and Ramamurti (2000a) in their study of longevity identified spiritualty, behavioural flexibility, high physical and mental activity levels, availability of strong social support and a psychological disposition to maintain calm in the face of stress, having association with life satisfaction and longevity. The explanation for this is that spirituality and religiosity provide emotional blaming in old age. Relating one's woes to God constitutes a good catharsis, while chanting of prayers has the therapeutic effects of lowering anxiety and stress.

Productive life by rendering service to the needy in the community has a good value in adding purpose to life. Benerjee (2000), Leder (1996) and Sharma (1994) in their independent studies found that those elderly extending service to the community found a harmony between the material and spiritual values to match their life. They lead a joyful and purposive life. This very well coincides with the philosophy of 'giving back to the society' and the positivities related to it. Social support has an element of mutuality. One who is involved in community service inadvertently builds a strong social network that constitutes a good source of support. Social support alleviates stress while fulfilling the need for affiliation and security (Rao, 2000; Singh, 1993; Sinha, 1999) and enhances wellbeing (Umadevi, 1991).

While the factors discussed above contribute to enhancing general wellbeing in the elderly, the health and wellbeing are also strongly influenced by health behaviour integrated into their lifestyle. A general awareness about health and hygiene and a strong motivation to translate it to their life is a major determinant of health and wellbeing in the elderly (Devi & Bagga, 1997; Savita & Darshan, 1999).

It is very evident from various studies that helping the people enrich their personal, social and environmental resources helps them in healthy ageing by developing resilience, and increases their general wellbeing.

Box 10.1 summarizes the positive factors associated with various chronic illnesses, disability and ageing that contribute to quality of life in the patients.

Interventions to Foster Resilience

Studies associating resilience to health have identified a number of positive factors internal to the individual (protective factors) and those in the environment (promotive factors). Internal factors such as hope, faith, spirituality, religiosity, forgiveness, optimism, self-efficacy,

Box 10.1 Resilience and Chronic Diseases

S. No.	Type of disease	Associated positive factors
1	Cardiovascular	1. Perceived personal control. 2. Self-efficacy 3. Positive reappraisal coping 4. Positive affect state
2	Diabetes mellitus	1. Self-efficacy 2. Self-care 3. Resilience
3	Cancer (adults)	1. Sense of coherence 2. Social wellbeing 3. Spirituality 4. Benefit-finding 5. Social support
4	Cancer (children)	1. Relationship with parents 2. Optimism 3. Confidence 4. Resilience 5. Meaning-making 6. Psychospiritual growth
5	Arthritis	1. Resilience 2. Self-efficacy 3. Optimism 4. Appreciation for life 5. Benefit-finding
6	Renal diseases	1. Optimism 2. Social support 3. Self-esteem
7	Parkinson's disease	1. Resilience
8	Multiple Sclerosis	1. Benefit-finding
9	Disabilities	1. Assertiveness 2. Optimism 3. Social connectedness 4. Family support 5. Positive perception, emotion and behaviour 6. Social connectedness
10	Ageing	1. Resilience 2. Continuation of cognitive activities 3. Physical and cognitive activities 4. Spirituality 5. Flexibility in behaviour

self-esteem, positive effect, benefit-finding, appreciation of life, sense of coherence and hardiness are found to mitigate or minimize stress and help the person cope with the disease effectively so that the disease progression/relapse or medical emergencies are decreased. Similarly, behavioural factors such as maintaining health promotive behaviour, having positive relationship with others, reappraising the diagnosis from positive perspective are also found to be equally significant in enhancing wellbeing and optimizing quality of life despite the presence of the diseases. Promotive factors such as strong social support and socioeconomic status are identified as positive contributors to resilience and sustenance of wellbeing in the face of disease.

An important factor to be endorsed is that the list of positive factors identified are not the inherent traits, but the characteristics that can be acquired, developed and nurtured in an individual. This sets the ground for proposing intervention for fostering resilience among people diagnosed with various acute and chronic diseases as an integral part of treatment plan. Such treatment plan very well fits into the much advocated biopsychosocial approach. Interventions can be planned at different stages. Clinical interventions, family interventions, intervention in educational institutions and community-level interventions may be effective in fostering resilience.

Clinical Intervention

The intervention provided after the diagnosis of a chronic illness is clinical intervention. This intervention should form an integral part of treatment regimen.

Studies have proved the significance of awareness about the disease and its association with management of the disease. Andrew and Hariharan (2017) have found the trajectory from knowledge intervention, self-efficacy, adherence behaviour, and effective disease management among patients with primary hypertension. Similar results were found in patients of cardiac by-pass surgery where the cognitive and affective intervention helped lower psychological distress, and enhance adherence and prognosis (Thomas, Hariharan, & Rana, 2016).

Taking a leaf from these findings, hospitals and physicians may plan knowledge intervention related to the specific disease at the time of diagnosis. The content of intervention may include the basic functional knowledge about the disease in its context with added emphasis on the internal control and the involvement and participation of the patient in disease management. This helps in boosting the personal control, self-efficacy and realistic illness perception and outcome expectancy, all of which contribute to health resilience.

In addition, the knowledge intervention should necessarily include inputs with respect to the role of negative emotions in hastening the disease progression, and the need for developing positive affect state.

Interventions involving the necessary skills to face any adversity with specific action points will be highly relevant for patients with chronic illness. Developing, appreciating and practising humour and optimism help in enhancing outcome expectancy.

Family Intervention

The major promoting factor in resilience is found to be social support. Intervention in the form of family counselling with a focus on the skills of explicit expression of support to the person diagnosed with a chronic disease will contribute positively in strengthening the wellbeing in the patient. The family intervention must focus on the role the family members can play in enhancing the self-efficacy of the patient in disease management rather than encouraging dependence and non-adherence. The support of the family should aim at helping the patient to be more self-reliant and be sensitive to the manifestation of symptoms. This boosts the self-confidence and self-efficacy in the patient and helps enhance resilience. Ungar (2013) states that young people's resilience is the outcome of quality engagement with adults. Families need to be counselled and trained on quality communication and interaction ingrained into child-rearing.

Interventions in Educational Institutions

Resilience interventions can be initiated at very early life. Childhood is a critical age for personality development. Intervention at early age helps the individual build the essential resources such as development of positive traits, emotions and cognitive functioning, which are found to be in resilient person. Positive emotions play a determining role in developing meaning and purpose of life.

Schools initiating conscious efforts towards invoking and nurturing positive emotions in students in fact help development of resilience in children. Intervention such as regular practice of Yoga, meditation, lifestyle changes (Kapur, 2013) and relaxation as group activities needs to be introduced right from early childhood education.

Helping the children endorses a negative emotion, and training them in their right expression also is an essential component. Very often, expression of negative emotions is discouraged as a manifestation of weakness. Negative emotion ventilated appropriately is more desirable than suppressing the same. Negative emotions are part of life and hence need to be ventilated before rekindling the positivity like optimism, perseverance and goal directedness.

On 7 September 2019, the scientists in Indian Space Research Organisation (ISRO) along with the entire country anxiously awaited to witness the success of Chandrayaan 2. The Prime Minister of India was present with the huge team of scientists. However, about 100 seconds prior to the landing on the moon the Lander lost communication with the Centre. This was a huge disappointment for the whole country and particularly to the scientists who had put in their years of knowledge and skill into the mission. The Chief of ISRO, Dr. Sivan, who is considered highly resilient, was devastated and totally shattered with this setback. Hours later, he could no more control his distress and allowed the tears to well up in the presence of the Prime Minister. The Prime Minister of India, himself a resilient person, gave a warm hug to Dr. Sivan and encouraged him to cry resting his head on his shoulder. This expression and consolation was very essential for resuming the challenges lying ahead for ISRO. This can be a very good example for expression of negative emotions appropriately.

Training the children to identify endorse and communicate the positivities in others helps in two ways. First, it encourages children to focus on the positives in others. Secondly, those whose positivities are endorsed by others feel encouraged to strengthen the same in oneself.

Knowledge intervention on health, diseases, lifestyle and health-promoting behaviour helps in realistic perception of illness and developing optimism regarding the treatment and prognosis. Helping the children count their blessings, forgiveness and expression of gratitude lays a good foundation for resilience in general.

Community-Level Interventions

Community-level interventions will be useful mainly to reap on building a good social support resource. In affiliation-oriented societies, the healing of the disease requires good social support system that is naturally built into the culture. However, this strength of Indian culture faces the threat of fading away in contemporary society where the emphasis of the youth is observed to have been gradually shifting to achievement. Thus, where there is a signal of the culture moving from collectivistic to individualistic orientation, attempts at reviving the affiliation need and its fulfilment lie in the hands of behavioural research. Cao, Yand and Wang (2018) in their study of parents who lost their only child identified the role of social support and resilience. They compared a group of bereaved parents with non-bereaved parents. While the bereaved group showed higher anxiety and depression compared to non-bereaved group, it was found that presence of strong support from family and resilience played a protective role in preserving their mental health. Thus, support from family and community constitutes good buffer against stress and adversities. Creating public awareness about the value of support and its contribution to healing can be first step for large-scale awareness. Educational institutions, community centres, workplaces can be the venue for fostering support system and reviving the practice of mutual aid, group support and support seeking behaviour in general. Though the support system in case of illness still continues in the form of seeking and donating blood to persons in need, the voluntary and spontaneous support at micro level calls for a revival.

Indian Perspective of Resilience Intervention

Though resilience studies were initiated in India in 1990s, they were sporadic. The research gained visibility in the early millennium of the 2000s. The contribution of Kapur (2013) highlighted the very Indian roots of resilience. She referred to the '*Sattva guna*' among the '*trigunas*' (consisting of *Sattva*, *Rajas* and *Tamas*) as a unique component of personality. Cabeza et al. (1997) compared pre-school children with and without psychiatric disturbances on '*trigunas*'. The results revealed that those without psychiatric disturbances had a '*Sattvik*' disposition. *Ayurveda* also claims that *Sattva guna* constitutes a major protective factor against psychopathology. What is very important to note is that according to *Kapur*, *Sattva guna* is not limited as an inherent characteristic but can be acquired and developed consciously.

Bethell et al. (2014) studied the role of resilience in mitigating the impact of childhood adversities on health and school engagement. Their findings indicated that resilient children who stayed calm and composed in the face of adversities in childhood had minimal negative impact on school engagement 'staying calm and in control' is the essential feature of *Sattva guna*. Taylor (2019) refers to the resilience skill that resembles the digestive fire where we take in, absorb and assimilate what is useful and discard the rest. The same treatment needs to be given to adversities. Positive outlook is found to be a natural outcome of *Sattva*. According to *Ayurveda*, inculcating and developing *Sattva* is possible through right diet, physical purification, control senses and mind chanting of *mantra* (prayer) and devotion. The third aspect relates to attention or focus. The mind can be trained to remain focused through meditation and *Yoga*. This helps in strengthening the mind and preventing its wandering in the face of adversities.

The fourth factor is generosity. Altruism or caring for others is assumed to stimulate the centres in brain associated with wellbeing. In *Ayurveda*, '*AshtangaHrdayam*' associates health with generosity. It identifies health behaviour such as eating wholesome food, enjoying a healthy lifestyle with a routine, practising detachment to objects, giving, forgiving, and serving others associated with practices that prevent diseases. This, in fact, was practised by the sages who stayed healthy.

Narayanan (2015) studied a sample of 1451 adolescent from lower socioeconomic background. He found a positive association between *trigunas* and resilience, where *trigunas* were significant predictors of resilience.

Strengthening in *Sattva guna* right from the childhood and enhancing the positive state of mind help in gradually building resilience right from early stage of life. Promotion of activities in schools that demand application of *Sattva* can constitute a good early intervention to promote resilience and health. Activities of *Yoga* and meditation, activities that require encouraging altruism (e.g. identify three good deeds of the week) and promoting a culture of forgiving friends can be easily incorporated and integrated into school activities.

Among the external promotive factors, the strongest of it being social support is very much ingrained into Indian culture. All that needs to be done is to revive it in society. Help-seeking behaviour is as much a skill as the help-providing behaviour. Identifying the needs of others and offering aid and the skill of seeking help and using the skill judiciously are the skills that can be taught to the students in school through stories such as '*Panchatantra*', as well as team games that constitute mutual support.

Indian history and culture projects ample examples of resilience and wellbeing among protagonist who successfully circumvented multiple adversities and yet performed well and attained the goal. The character of *Karna* in *Mahabharata* portrays resilience at various levels starting from survival after abandonment at birth by the mother, to rejection of disciple hood because of the social background, yet excelling in the skills of archery. *Karna's* character is an epitome of loyalty to social support (received from *Kauravas*) and goal directedness. Similarly, the struggles and adversities found by *Pandavas* on exile for 13 long years could not lower their wellbeing or determination to achieve their goal of their right to the kingdom. *Prahlada* was not a child to be deterred by continuous life-threatening attacks by his own father. In all these examples, faith, spirituality, steadfastness and optimism are seen as salient features.

History of Indian independence has several examples of resilience. Mahatma Gandhi, Sardar Patel, Jawaharlal Nehru, Lal Bahadur Shastri continuously faced multiple adversities in their struggle for freedom for the country. Their goal orientation, conviction in their struggle and faith in religion and a very strong social support sustained their struggle until they achieved independence in 1947.

Indians, by their very cultural roots, have the orientation towards resilience. Natural disasters, communal riots, epidemics, terror attacks, inadequate health and educational facilities are part of adversities of life. Yet, there is restoration of homeostasis. Hence, interventions in resilience are expected to bring effective outcome on Indian population.

Box 10.2 Researcher's Box

- Research attempts should focus on composite measurement of resilience, by taking into consideration the essential components like risk/adversity, positive factors and performance. This calls for brainstorming among psychologists, statisticians and software experts.
- Taking all the positive factors (internal and external) into account, a scale can be constructed and standardized. This scale administered on various resilient persons in homogenous groups will identify the most common factors across the homogenous groups. This may help in throwing light on the most essential positive factors associated with resilience.
- Research in the area of health resilience is scanty. Measuring resilience and its protective and promotive components in patients who survived a major illness will be a good value addition in identifying the components of resilience among those who successfully fought a health adversity.
- Very less research has been done in the Ayurvedic equivalents of resilience components. Apart from *trigunas*, the personality components mentioned in *Ayurveda* call for extensive study.
- Longitudinal study design would bring reliable insights. Identifying the resilient children and following them up until their adulthood will constitute good information on their additional adversities and protective and promotive factors, as well as their life accomplishments.
- Intervention studies on children or adults at health risk will be of good value. Assess resilience in adolescents identifying those who are resilient, borderline and non-resilient. Provide comprehensive intervention to all. Re-assess periodically and find out the relative impact of intervention on various groups.

> **Box 10.3 Practitioner's Box**
>
> - One of the fundamental skills the practitioners must have when the client approaches them is to help the client identify the positive aspects in oneself and the environment. This would be a good initiative to counterbalance the negatives with positives.
> - Clients with chronic illnesses need to be assessed on their levels of resilience and its various components, particularly self-efficacy, personal control, optimism, gratitude social support and life appreciation.
> - A session of knowledge intervention on the disease goes a long way in building a cognitive base. This should be followed by training in self-help.
> - An orientation of support seeking skills enables many chronic patients to get the right type of help from a right source.
> - Support groups among the similar chronic patients and group education and follow-up on its impact in terms of it being translated into practice may work effectively with homogenous groups.
> - Strengthening the family support through family counselling is a good strategy.
> - Helping the clients with disability or chronic illness by reconstructing their cognition about life in the context of illness or disability by focusing on the positivities and what is possible to achieve with the limitations set by their adversities helps them in developing optimism and enhancing hope.
> - Emphasizing on the activity levels for elderly clients is important. Optimizing on their physical and psychological aspects and remaining active by various chosen means need to be stressed.
> - Strengthening the value of spirituality or religiosity in those showing mild inclination towards the same will enhance their relaxation.

References

Abraído-Lanza, A. F., Guier, C., & Colón, R. M. (1998). Psychological thriving among latinas with chronic illness. *Journal of Social Issues, 54*(2), 405–424.

Affleck, G., Tennen, H., Croog, S., & Levine, S. (1987). Causal attribution, perceived benefits, and morbidity after a heart attack: An 8-year study. *Journal of Consulting and Clinical Psychology, 55*(1), 29.

Agarwal, M., Dalal, A. K., Agarwal, D. K., & Agarwal, R. K. (1995). Positive life orientation and recovery from myocardial infarction. *Social Sciences Medicine, 40*, 125–130.

Anand, J. (2004). Working through emotional pain: A narrative study of healing process. *Psychological Studies, 49*, 185–192.

Anand, J., Srivastava, A., & Dalal, A. K. (2001). Where suffering ends and healing begins. *Psychological Studies, 46*, 114–126.

Andrew, A., & Hariharan, M. (2017). Hypertension knowledge test: Development and validation. *The International Journal of Indian Psychology, 5*, 44–55.

Annalakshmi, N., & Ragitha, R. (2012). General well-being and emotional expressivity among hearing impaired and non-hearing impaired adolescents. *Journal of the Indian Academy of Applied Psychology, 38*(1), 134–137.

Anthony, E. J. (1974). The syndrome of the psychologically invulnerable child. In: E. J. Anthony and C. Koupernik (Eds.), *The child in his family: Children at psychiatric risk* (Vol. 3, pp. 529–544). New York: John Wiley & Sons.

Antonovsky, A. (1979). *Health, stress, and coping*. San Francisco: Jossey Bass.

Bandura, A. (1986). The explanatory and predictive scope of self-efficacy theory. *Journal of Social and Clinical Psychology, 4*(3), 359–373.

Barros, M. A., César, C. G., Carandina, L., & Torres, G. D. (2006). Desigualdadessociaisnaprevalência de doençascrônicas no Brasil PNAD-2003 [Social inequalities in the prevalence of chronic diseases in Brazil, PNAD-2003]. *Ciência&SaúdeColetiva, 11*, 911–926. doi: 10.1590/S1413-81232006000400014

Becker, M. H., & Rosenstock, I. M. (1974). Social-psychological research on determinants of preventive health behavior. *Behavioral Sciences and Preventive Medicine, 4*, 25–35.

Benerjee, S. P. (2000). Ageing, death and religion. In: A. P. Bali (Ed.), *Bio-social dimension of ageing* (pp. 145–154). Shimla: IIAS.

Bethell, C. D., Newacheck, P., Hawes, E., & Halfon, N. (2014). Adverse childhood experiences: Assessing the impact on health and school engagement and the mitigating role of resilience. *Health Affairs, 33*(12), 2106–2115.

Bhatia, S. (2002b). Participation of older persons. *Research and Developmental Journal* (Help age India), *8*, 8–15.

Block, J., & Block, J. (1980). *California child Q-set*. Palo Alto, CA: Consulting Psychologists Press.

Brayne, C., Ince, P. G., Keage, H. A., McKeith, I. G., Matthews, F. E., Polvikoski, T., & Sulkava, R. (2010). Education, the brain and dementia: Neuroprotection or compensation? EClipSE collaborative members. *Brain, 133*(8), 2210–2216.

Cabeza, R., Kapur, S., Craik, F. I., McIntosh, A. R., Houle, S., & Tulving, E. (1997). Functional neuroanatomy of recall and recognition: A PET study of episodic memory. *Journal of Cognitive Neuroscience, 9*(2), 254–265.

Cao, X., Yang, C., & Wang, D. (2018). The impact on mental health of losing an only child and the influence of social support and resilience. *OMEG-Journal of Death and Dying*. doi: 10.1177/0030222818755284

Charney, D. S. (2004). Psychobiological mechanisms of resilience and vulnerability: Implications for successful adaptation to extreme stress. *American Journal of Psychiatry, 161*(2), 195–216.

Copeland, J. L., Consitt, L. A., & Tremblay, M. S. (2002). Hormonal response to endurance and resistance exercise in female aged 19-69 years. *The e Journal of Gerontology. Series A, Biological Sciences and Medical Sciences, 57*(4), B158–B165. doi: 10.1093/Gerona/57.4.B158

Costanzo, E. S., Sood, A. K., & Lutgendorf, S. K. (2011). Biobehavioural influences on cancer progression. *Immunology and Allergy Clinics of North America, 31*, 109–132. PubMedCentralPubMedGoogle Scholar

Cumming, E (1968). New thoughts on the theory of disengagement. *International Journal of Psychiatry, 6*, 53–67.

Daugherty, C. K., Fitchett, G., Murphy, P. E., Peterman, A. H., Banik, D. M., Hlubocky, F., & Tartaro, J. (2005). Trusting God and medicine: Spirituality in advanced cancer patients volunteering for clinical trials of experimental agents. *Psycho-Oncology: Journal of the Psychological, Social and Behavioral Dimensions of Cancer, 14*(2), 135–146.

Davidson, R. (2000). *Anxiety, depression and emotions*. New York: Oxford University Press.

deKloet, E. R., Joels, M., & Holsboer, F. (2005). Stress and the brain: From adaptation to disease. *Nature Reviews Neuroscience, 6*(6), 463–475.

DeNisco, S. (2011). Exploring the relationship between resilience and diabetes outcomes in African Americans. *Journal of the American Academy of Nurse Practitioners, 23*(11), 602–610.

Devi, D., & Bagga, A. (1997). Health status of older women of Manipur. *Indian Journal Gerontology, 7*, 27–42.

Feder, A., Nestler, E. J., & Charney, D. S. (2009). Psychobiology and molecular genetics of resilience. *Nature Reviews Neuroscience, 10*(6), 446–457.

Garmezy, N. (1971). Vulnerability research and the issues of primary prevention. *American Journal of Orthopsychiartry, 41*(1), 101–116.

Gotay, C. C., Isaacs, P., & Pagano, I. (2004). Quality of life in patients who survive a dire prognosis compared to control cancer survivors. *Psycho-Oncology: Journal of the Psychological, Social and Behavioral Dimensions of Cancer, 13*(12), 882–892.

Hariharan, M. (1990). *Invulnerable children: Some studies on disadvantaged children's competence and coping style* (Unpublished doctoral thesis). Utkal University, Orissa, India.

Hariharan, M., Karimi, M., & Kishore, M. T. (2014). Resilience in persons with physical disabilities: Role of perceived environment and emotional intelligence. *Journal of the Indian Academy of Applied Psychology, 40*(1), 96–101.

Hariharan, M., & Rana, S. (2016). Conceptual complexity of resilience: Synergy approach to measurement. In: U. Kumar (Ed.), *The Routledge international handbook of psychosocial resilience* (pp. 101–118). New York: Routledge.

Havighurst, R. J. (1961). The nature and values of meaningful free-time activity. In R. W. Kleemeier (Ed.), *Aging and Leisure* (309–344). New York: Oxford University Press.

Helgeson, V. S. (1992). Moderators of the relation between perceived control and adjustment to chronic illness. *Journal of Personality and Social Psychology, 63*(4), 656.

Jamuna, D. (1988). Role activity and general adjustment of middle aged and older women. *Journal of Psychological Researches, 32*, 37–40.

Jamuna, D. (1994). Psychological and social correlates of successful aging among elderly Indian women. *Institute of Journal of Gerontology, 8*, 29–36.

Jamuna, D., & Ramamurti, P. V. (2000a). Burnout among caregivers of disabled elderly: Effect of intervention. *Psychological Studies, 45*, 150–155.

Jamuna, D., & Ramamurti, P.V. (2000b). Psychological correlates of long lived individuals. Project report submitted to the university Grants Commission (UGC) New Delhi.

Jamuna, D., & Ramamurti, P. V. (2001). *An investigation of psychological factors including quality of life of very senior citizens from rural and urban areas of Andhra Pradesh*. New-Delhi: Indian Council of Social Science Research.

Johnston-Brooks, C. H., Lewis, M. A., & Garg, S. (2002). Self-efficacy impacts self-care and HbA1c in young adults with Type I diabetes. *Psychosomatic Medicine, 64*(1), 43–51.

Kapur, M. (2013). Resilience and competence in childhood. In: G. Misra (Ed.), *History of science, philosophy and culture in Indian civilization*, Volume XIII, Part 3, Psychology and psychoanalysis (pp. 255–267). New Delhi: Munshiram Manoharlal Publishers Pvt. Ltd.

Keyes, C. L. M. (2004). Risk and resilience in human development: An introduction. *Research in Human Development, 1*(4), 223–227.

Kobasa, S. (1982). Hardiness and health: A prospective study. *Journal of Personality and Social Psychology, 42*, 168–177.

Kohli, N., & Dalal, A. K. (1998). Culture as a factor in casual understanding of illness: A study of cancer patients. *Psychology and Developing Societies, 10*(2), 115–129.

Kumar, R. (2002). Self and intersubjectivity in autism: Directions in research. *Asia Pacific Disability Rehabilitation Journal, 14*, 95–104.

Kumar, V. (1998). Perspectives on activities and aging in the world: physical activity and old persons in India. *Journal of Ageing and Physical Activity, 6*, 205–206.

Lalnuntluangi, R., Chelli, K., & Padhy, M. (2017). Self-efficacy, outcome expectancy and self-management of type 2 diabetes patients. *Indian Journal of Health & Wellbeing, 8*(9), 1040–1043.

Leder, D. (1996). Spiritual community in later life: A modest proposal. *Journal of Ageing Studies, 10*, 103–116.

Leventhal, R. C. (1997). Aging consumers and their effects on the marketplace. *Journal of Consumer Marketing, 14*(4), 276–281.

Leventhal, T. (2003). Moving to opportunity: An experimental study of neighborhood effects on mental health. *American Journal of Public Health, 93*, 1576–1582.

Lisha, S. (2012). *Factors of resilience among physically disabled-an interpretative phenomenological analysis* (M. Phil. Dissertation). Bharathiar University, Coimbatore.

Luther, S. S. (1990). Vulnerability and resilience: A study of high-risk adolescents. *Child Development, 62*, 600–616.

Luther, S.S., Doernberger, C. H., & Zigler, E. (1993). Resilience is not a unidimensional construct: Insights from a prospective study on inner-city adolescents. *Development and Psychopathology, 5*, 730–717.

Ma, L. C., Chang, H. J., Liu, Y. M., Hsieh, H. L., Lo, L., Lin, M. Y., & Lu, K. C. (2013). The relationship between health-promoting behaviors and resilience in patients with chronic kidney disease. *Scientific World Journal*, 2013, 124973.

Masten, A. S. (2001). Ordinary magic: Resilience processes in development. *American Psychologist*, *56*(3), 227.

Masten, A. S. (2007). Resilience in developing systems: Progress and promise as the fourth wave rises. *Development and Psychopathology*, *19*(3), 921–930.

Masten, A., Best, K., & Garmezy, N. (1990). Resilience and development: Contributions from the study of children who overcome adversity. *Development Psychopathology*, *2*, 425–444.

Masten, A. S. (1994). Resilience in individual development: Successful adaptation despite risk and adversity. In: M. C. Wang and E. W. Gordon (Eds.), *Educational resilience in inner city America: Challenges and prospects* (pp. 3–25). Hillsdale, NJ: Erlbaum.

Mattison, J. A., Lave, M. A., Roth, G. S., & Ingram, D. K. (2003). Calorie restriction in rhesus monkeys. *Experimental Gerontology*, *38*(1–2), 35–46.

Morgan, C. A., 3rd, Southwick, S., Hazlett, G., Rasmusson, A., Hoyt, G., Zimolo, Z., & Charney, D. S. (2004). Relationships among plasma dehydroepiandrosteronesulfate and cortisol levels, symptoms of dissociation, and objective performance in humans exposed to acute stress. *Archives of General Psychiatry*, *61*(8), 819–825.

Morille, M., Passirani, C., Vonarbourg, A., Clavreul, A., & Benoit, J. P. (2008). Progress in developing cationic vectors for non-viral systemic gene therapy against cancer. *Biomaterials*, *29*(24–25), 3477–3496.

Moser, D., & Dracup, K. (1995). Psychosocial recovery from a cardiac event: The influence of perceived control. *Heart & Lung, The Journal of Critical Care*, *24*, 273–280.

Narayanan, A. (2015). Predictors of resilience among adolescents of low socio-economic states in India. *International Review of Psychiatry*, *23*(3), 204–217. doi: 10.3109/09540261.2015.1066763

Narváez, J., Bianchi, M. M., Santo, P., de la Fuente, D., Ríos-Rodriguez, V., Bolao, F., ... & Nolla, J. M. (2010). Pancreatitis, panniculitis, and polyarthritis. *Seminars in Arthritis and Rheumatism*, *39*(5), 417–423.

Orbuch, T. L., Parry, C., Chesler, M., Fritz, J., & Repetto, P. (2005). Parent-child relationships and quality of life: Resilience among childhood cancer survivors. *Family Relations*, *54*(2), 171–183.

Padhy, M., Chottai, P., & Lalnutluangi, R. (2017). Wellbeing of patients with type 2 diabetes: Role of self-efficacy and outcome expectancy. *International Journal of Social and Allied Research*, *6*(1), 9–16.

Pakenham, K. I., & Cox, S. (2009). The dimensional structure of benefit finding in multiple sclerosis and relations with positive and negative adjustment: A longitudinal study. *Psychology and Health*, *24*(4), 373–393.

Parry, C. (2003). Embracing uncertainty: An exploration of the experiences of childhood cancer survivors. *Qualitative Health Research*, *13*, 227–246.

Parry, C., & Chesler, M. A. (2005). Thematic evidence of psychosocial thriving in childhood cancer survivors. *Qualitative Health Research*, *15*(8), 1055–1073.

Perna, L., Mielck, A., Lacruz, M. E., Emeny, R. T., von EisenhartRothe, A., Meisinger, C., & Ladwig, K. H. (2015). The association between resilience and diabetic neuropathy by socioeconomic position: Cross-sectional findings from the KORA-Age study. *Journal of Health Psychology*, *20*(9), 1222–1228.

Prakash, V., Archana (2017). Role of genetics and temperament in resilience. In: U. Kumar (Ed.), *Handbook of psychosocial resilience* (pp. 75–87). London and New York: Routledge Intervention.

Priti, Yadava, A., & Sharma, N. R. (2012). Identification of charater strengths associated with health maintenance and prognosis. In: A. Yadava, D. Hooda and N. R. Sharma (Eds.), *Biopsychosocial issues in positive health* (pp. 171–183). New Delhi: Global Vision Publishing House.

Prochaska, J. O., & DiClemente, C. C. (1982). Transtheoretical therapy: Toward a more integrative model of change. *Psychotherapy: Theory, Research & Practice*, *19*(3), 276–288. doi: 10.1037/h0088437

Rajan, A. M., & John, R. (2016). Resilience and impact of children's intellectual disability on Indian parents. *Journal of Intellectual Disabilities*, *21*(4), doi: 10.1177/1744629516654588.

Rajendran, A. (2019). Development and validation of resilience tool (Unpublished Doctoral Thesis). University of Hyderabad.

Rajendran, A., Hariharan, M., & Rao, C. R. (2019). A holistic approach to measuring resilience: Development and initial validation of resilience test battery. *International Journal of Humanities and Social Science Studies*, *4*(3), 52–64. doi: 10.29032/ijihsss.v6.i3.2019.52-64

Ramamurti, P. V. (1987). Empirically derived constituents for a happy ageing. In: K. Subbarao and V. Prabhakar (Eds.), *Aging: A multi factorial discussion* (pp. 13–118). Hyderabad: Association of Gerontology India (AGI).

Ramamurti, P. V. (1989). Old age as a stress: Strategies for its management. *Proceedings of the Workshop on Awareness, Welfare and Productive Utilisation of Elderly Component of Human Population*, ChinmayaSeva Trust, Rewa, October.

Ramamurti, P. V. (2003). Empowering the older persons in India. *Research and Developmental Journal* (Help age India), *9*, 16–21.

Ramamurti, P. V., & Jamuna, D. (2010). Geropsychology in India. *Psychology in India*, *3*, 185–253.

Rao, A. P. (2000). Kind of supports requires in different kinds of elderly. *Paper presented at the Asia-Sub Regional Seminar for Social Security for Elderly*. Social Security Association of India, New Delhi.

Richardson, G. E. (2002). The metatheory of resilience and resiliency. *Journal of Clinical Psychology*, *58*(3), 307–321.

Robinson-Smith, G., Johnston, M. V., & Allen, J. (2000). Self-care self-efficacy, quality of life, and depression after stroke. *Archives of Physical Medicine and Rehabilitation*, *81*(4), 460–464.

Robottom, B. J., Gruber-Baldini, A. L., Anderson, K. E., Reich, S. G., Fishman, P. S., Weiner, W. J., & Shulman, L. M. (2012). What determines resilience in patients with Parkinson's disease? *Parkinsonism & Related Disorders*, *18*(2), 174–177.

Rogers, R. W. (1975). A protection motivation theory of fear appeals and attitude change. *The Journal of Psychology*, *91*(1), 93–114.

Rutter, M. (1987). Psychosocial resilience and protective mechanisms. *American Journal of Orthopsychiatry*, *57*(3), 316–331.

Sachdev, P. (1998). Schizophrenia-like psychosis and epilepsy: The status of the association. *American Journal of Psychiatry*, *155*(3), 325–336.

Saraf, S., Singh, T. B., & Khuvana, S. (2013). Cervical cancer survivors: Meaning in life. *Psychological Studies*, *58*, 144–152.

Savita, V., & Darshan, S. (1999). Factors affecting health of aged. *Ageing and Society: The Indian Journal Gerontology*, *9*, 21–37.

Schwarzer, R. (1999). Self-regulatory processes in the adoption and maintenance of health behaviors. *Journal of Health Psychology*, *4*(2), 115–127.

Sharma, A. (Ed.). (1994). *Religion and women*. New York: SUNY Press.

Sharma, S., & Misra, G. (2010). Health psychology: Progress and challenges. In: G. Mishra (Ed.), *Psychology in India* (Vol. 3, pp. 265–316). India: Pearson Education.

Shi, Y., Sears, L. E., Coberley, C. R., & Pope, J. E. (2013). The association between modifiable well-being risks and productivity: A longitudinal study in pooled employer sample. *Journal of Occupational and Environmental Medicine*, *55*(4), 353–364.

Singh, R. R. (1993). Welfare system and psycho-social support for the aged. *Proceedings of National Seminar on Aging Scenario in India by 2001 A.D. Help Age India and Age Care India*, New-Delhi.

Sinha, S. P. (1999). Role of social support in alleviating residential crowding stress among elderly. *Indian Journal of Gerontology*, *13*, 105–110.

Smith, B. W., & Zautra, A. J. (2008). Vulnerability and resilience in women with arthritis: Test of a two-factor model. *Journal of Consulting and Clinical Psychology*, *76*(5), 799.

Soma Sundaram, R.O., & Devamani, K. A. (2016). A comparative study on resilience, perceived social support and hopelessness among cancer patients treated with curative and palliative care. *Indian Journal of Palliative Care*, *22*(2), 135–140.

Subramanyan, K. (1989). *Perception of community support in relation to adjustment and roles among aged*0. University of Calicut, Calicut.

Sullivan, M. D., LaCroix, A. Z., Russo, J., & Katon, W. J. (1998). Self-efficacy and self-reported functional status in coronary heart disease: A six-month prospective study. *Psychosomatic Medicine*, *60*(4), 473–478.

Symister, P., & Friend, R. (2003). The influence of social support and problematic support on optimism and depression in chronic illness: A prospective study evaluating self-esteem as a mediator. *Health Psychology, 22*(2), 123.

Taylor, N. (2019). The science of wellbeing: Where neuroscience Ayurveda and yoga meet, Health Ayurveda and Natural Remedies. Yogainternational.com/articles/view/the science_of_well-being_where_ neuroscience_ayurveda_and_yoga_meet. Retrieved on 19.9.2019

Thomas, M., Hariharan, M., & Rana, S. (2016). Psychological distress as predictor of adherence and prognosis among patients undergoing coronary artery bypass grafting. *Journal of the Indian Academy of Applied Psychology, 42*(1), 161.

Umadevi, A. (1991). *Study of disability in old age and perception of social supports* (Master's Dissertation). Sri Venkateswara University, Tirupati.

Ungar, M. (2013). The impact of youth-adult relationship on resilience. *International Journal of Child, Youth and Family Studies, 3*, 328–336.

Upadhyay, S. (2002). *Influence of optimism, future orientation and detachment on health inn deprivational environment* (Unpublished doctoral dissertation). D.D.U. Gorakhpur University, Gorakhpur.

Weinstein, N. D., Rothman, A. J., & Sutton, S. R. (1998). Stage theories of health behaviour: Conceptual and methodological issues. *Health Psychology, 17*(3), 290.

Werner, E., & Smith, R. S. (1982). Vulnerable but invincible: A longitudinal study of children and youth. New York: Adams, Bannister and Cox.

Wright, L. J., Zautra, A. J., & Going, S. (2008). Adaptation to early knee osteoarthritis: The role of risk, resilience, and disease severity on pain and physical functioning. *Annals of Behavioral Medicine, 36*(1), 70–80.

Wright, M. O. D., Masten, A. S., & Narayan, A. J. (2013). Resilience processes in development: Four waves of research on positive adaptation in the context of adversity. In: S. Goldstein, & R. B. Brooks (Eds.), *Handbook of resilience in children* (pp. 15–37). Boston, MA: Springer.

Yi, J. P., Vitaliano, P. P., Smith, R. E., Yi, J. C., & Weinger, K. (2008). The role of resilience on psychological adjustment and physical health in patients with diabetes. *British Journal of Health Psychology, 13*(2), 311–325.

11 Pain and Its Psychosocial Correlates

The following is the experience of different people travelling in the same train that met with a ghastly accident in the darkness of a night.

Ashwin, a 37-year-old officer from a government department, suddenly experienced the bang that threw him out of his berth. He remembers hitting against a hard surface and fell on his back. He was conscious. After what appeared to him as a long wait, some people came and tried to help him out. He screamed in pain when they tried to move him out because he experienced excruciating pain in his back. He was moved to a vehicle in a stretcher, and driven to the hospital. The following day, he was told that he had a fracture in his hip and needed surgery. The pain he experienced in his back brought tears into his eyes though he was put on strong pain killers.

Vipasha, a 52-year-old woman travelling in the same train who was in the lower berth, suddenly woke up when she hit against the berth opposite hers. She remained in the same compartment, which escaped the bad impact. She first tried to locate her two children who were found to be safe. They clung to each other and were relieved to see that they were safe. Vipasha, however, felt a pain in her chest and found it difficult to breathe. But, she gathered herself and with the help of someone in the compartment was helped to get down from the train along with her children. Later, the three were moved to the hospital by the rescue team. Vipasha was diagnosed with hairline fracture in her ribs, which the doctors said will have to heal on their own and she may have to live with it and that they are not considered harmful.

Rakesh, the 13-year-old boy, was travelling in the same train along with his parents. Their compartment was the one that took the worst impact. All the three were trapped in the compartment partially crushed. Rakesh's left leg was trapped under something heavy. He could not move out. He could see his father about 5 m away from him. He started calling out for his dad, but there was no response. Rakesh could hear the feeble voice of his mother calling his name for a while, and then, there was silence. He started crying out for help. There were few other voices doing the same. There was no response. It seemed like an eternity before Rakesh was woken up by someone patting on his shoulder. The heavy thing from his leg was removed, and he was moved to the hospital. He was told that he had very mild injuries and that he would be discharged after few hours of being under observation. Rakesh asked the hospital authorities about his parents. They said they would let him know. The following day, he was taken to his mother who just underwent amputation of her leg. Rakesh was taken to the mortuary to identify his father's body. The row of dead bodies in the mortuary, the wailing of relatives, the smell of the place, the disfigured bodies… Rakesh had to encounter all these all alone as his mother was still in ICU. It took about two days before Rakesh's uncle could reach there.

Ashwin who had a hip fracture suffered from acute pain. The rib fracture for Vipasha gave her a chronic pain; Rakesh's mother who underwent amputation had acute pain, and lived with the trauma of losing a limb. Rakesh had only mild physical injury and pain but the trauma he

DOI: 10.4324/9781003438908-11

experienced robbed the smile in his face, changed his original bubbly personality. He would wake up from his sleep often with a flash of the same experience when he lied immobile in the crushed compartment of the train calling out for his father, hearing the mother's faint voice, then identifying his father's body in the mortuary. Though Rakesh suffered no physical pain, the trauma that he experienced continued for several years.

Thus, when we talk of the pain, we cannot limit ourselves to the physical pain though physical pain and the intervention for it continues to occupy the nucleus of pain management programmes.

What Is Pain?

Way back in 1979, the International Association of the Study of Pain (IASP) adopted the definition of pain given by the subcommittee on Taxonomy. They defined pain as "An unpleasant sensory and emotional experience associated with actual or potential tissue damage, or described in terms of such damage". In 2018, the IASP formed a 14-member, multinational Presidential Task Force, which after deliberations and consultation for two years came up with a revision of the definition. The revised version defined pain as "An unpleasant sensory and emotional experience associated with, or resembling that associated with, actual or potential tissue damage" (Raja et al., 2020). The earlier definition's focus was on the tissue damage, while the revised definition extended it to what resembles or is associated with tissue damage. What is important to note is that both the definitions endorsed the significance of emotional experience in pain. The revised definition has extended the definition of pain beyond nociception. Nociception refers to the process of neural activities that encodes and processes noxious stimuli (Loeser & Treede, 2008). It is initiated by the signal given to the central nervous system triggered by a stimulation of specialized sensory receptors called nociceptors located in peripheral nervous system. The nociceptors are triggered to action by noxious stimulus of three types within the target tissue, viz. thermal (temperature), mechanical (stretch and strain) and chemical (e.g. pH change due to local inflammatory process). Nociception is in fact a mechanism that protects the organism by triggering physiological and behavioural response that helps in preventing one from further damage of tissues. This happens because by experiencing or perceiving the pain, the activity of the organism is suspended or withdrawn so that further damage of the tissue is prevented. Thus, the experience of pain is in fact a positive phenomenon that is protective in nature.

Types of Pain

Pain is a subjective experience. Hence, there is likely to be as many types of pain as the existence of human beings. Even from the medical perspective, there are various types of pain. We will discuss here the four most common types of pain.

Acute Pain

This is something that ranges in its duration from few minutes to six months. It refers to the pain severe in nature and serves as a warning to the body, which can be the onset or presence of a disease, injury or an event in natural physiological process (such as labour pains before child birth, angina pain preceding a cardiac attack, abdominal pain indicating an infected appendix). Acute pain is also caused by surgical wounds, fractured bones, bruises due to cuts and burns, and dental problems. There is always an underlying cause behind the pain. Once the cause is identified and treated, the pain also fades away. However, in certain cases where the pain persists, it may even turn out into a chronic pain requiring continuous medical care and management. Examples of such instances are pain experienced in sciatica, arthritis etc.

Chronic Pain

Chronic pain lasts for more than six months. The intensity of the pain may range from mild to severe. The duration may run into years. The frequency ranges depending on the nature and condition of the disease, and many other psychosocial factors. The typical examples of chronic pain are back ache, neck pain, pain in the toes or fingers, and pain in the limbs or joints. Very often, these pains are the manifestations of existing health conditions such as diabetes, arthritis, gout, spondylitis. Unlike the acute pain, the patients suffering from chronic pain need to cope with it almost life-long by adopting effective pain management technics.

Neuropathic Pain

Neuropathic pain is caused by a damage to the nerve or part of the nervous system. The pain experience is described as stabbing, shooting, sharp or burning sensation. It is also common to experience a tingling sensation, electric shock etc. Some of the known causes for neuropathic pain are diabetes, cancer, stroke, multiple sclerosis, amputation of a limb, alcoholism, radiation or chemotherapy. The other causes can be vitamin B deficiency, carpal tunnel syndrome, thyroid problems, arthritis in the spine and facial nerve problem. It is estimated that about 30% of all nerve pain are traced back to diabetes. One common symptom of neuropathic pain is its spontaneous onset with no trigger stimulation. Sometimes, non-painful stimuli such as coming in contact with hot or cold sensation, gentle brush against the skin may induce this pain. The onset of the pain being spontaneous, one is likely to be caught unawares with the pain. This has several psychosocial implications.

Nociceptive Pain

Nociceptive pain is the most common caused by potentially harmful stimuli to body in the form of damage to the cells detected by the nociceptors located in the body. This happens due to minor and major accidents such as a hit, rub, fall, scrape, sprain or twist. The cell damage may be in the skin, muscle, tendon, ligament, bone or joints.

Nociceptive pain is of three types, viz. somatic, visceral and radicular. Somatic pain refers to the pain that is usually localized and stimulated by movements. This is experienced when the pain receptors in the tissues, skin, muscle or bone are triggered into action. Examples of somatic pain are headaches and cuts. Visceral pain refers to the pain originating from any of the visceral organs. Visceral organs are the soft interior organs of the body such as lungs, heart, and organs in the gastrointestinal system, excretory system and reproductive system. There are several characteristic features of the visceral pain. It originates in the middle of the body but felt in other areas. It is a vague pain with difficulty in locating it because the pain is rather diffused. The cause of such diffusion is because the pain receptors in visceral organs are not closely packed or evenly distributed. Hence, the location is difficult to trace. Visceral pain is described in different ways. Sometimes, it is described as dull pain, other times as gnawing, twisting, colicky, deep or pressure experience. Visceral pain typically involves the autonomic nervous system. Hence, the clinical presentation includes a host of symptoms such as sweating, palpitations, change in blood pressure, nausea and vomiting. In addition, there is also change in affect state with symptoms of anxiety and panic. The description is vague and subjective.

Radicular pain refers to the pain that radiates. The pain originates in the nerve roots of the spinal cord. Such pain radiates from the back, hip and into the legs through the spine sometimes culminating in the numbness, tingling or weakness in the leg muscles. It is experienced when there is irritation in the nerve ends in the spinal cord because of the compression or inflammation. The radicular pain is classified, depending on the location of the compression of the nerve along the spine. The location can be one of the three, viz. cervical (neck), thoracic (upper middle back) or lumbar (low back).

Theories of Pain

In the process of understanding and explaining the phenomenon of pain, biologists, medical professionals, physicists and psychologists postulated their own theories. Thus, it helped in the evolution of better theories in understanding pain. In fact, the theories of pain can be traced back to several centuries. These theories are explained in brief so as to track the trajectory in understanding the evolutionary path of unravelling the process involved in the experience of pain.

Dualistic Theory

Pain was first perceived as a punishment of God for the evil mankind indulged in. However, this did not deter the inquiry into the experience of pain. When the dualistic theory that perceived body and mind as two mutually exclusive entities was in in prevalence, pain was construed as a harm directed at the physical or psychological plane. However, the two were understood as two mutually exclusive processes without any scope for generating a synthesized experience. Descartes added that suffering is related to the soul. He further identified that pineal gland constitutes the soul of the pain. This indicated that the brain played the role of moderator in experiencing the pain. Descartes advocated that the pain perception of pain existed in the brain. Independently, he also described pain as a sensory transduction that is carried through the nerves to the brain. He never postulated any connectivity between the sensory transduction and perception of pain in the brain. He theorized comparing the body to a machine where the pain is a disturbance that travelled through the nerves to the destination of brain. One great change brought by this theory is to shift the perception of pain from spiritual to physical domain. Once it is construed as a physical phenomenon, it opens the possibility of locating the nerve fibres, treating them for relief or cure. Thus, due credit may be ascribed to Descartes for bringing the first major shift in conceptualizing pain.

Intensive Theory

The nucleus of this theory is the process of summation in experiencing pain. This theory has been postulated at different times in the history. The initial conceptualization was by Plato who stated that pain is not a unique sensory experience. He conceived it as an emotion that resulted when the individual experienced a stimulus that is stronger than normal. This is an extension of Aristotle's concept of pain, which is the consequence of excessive stimulation originating from touch. Several years later in 1859, Bernhard Naunyn conducted an experiment on patients of syphilis with degenerating dorsal columns. These patients were administered tactile stimuli of very low intensity, which is below the threshold of tactile perception. When such low-intensity tactile stimulation was repeated from 60 to 600 times, the patients reported to have rapidly developed what they termed as unbearable pain. The same results were produced with stimulus variations such as electrical stimuli. Naunyn concluded that some process of summation must be taking place for elevating the subthreshold stimuli to unbearable pain. Based on these experiments, Arthur Goldscheider postulated that repeated subthreshold stimulations or subthreshold hypersensitive stimulation culminates in severe pain. In this neurophysiological model, he is also specified that the in the grey matter of the spinal cord that the increased sensory stimuli would converge and summate. Thus, it is the repetition of the stimuli though at a subthreshold level resulted in intense pain because of the summation process.

Specificity Theory

Max von Frey, a psychophysicist based on his experimental observations, advocated the four kinds of sensory spots, viz. pressure, cold, warmth and pain. He inferred the presence of specific receptive structures and special afferent ending of pain.

Specificity theory advocates that pain is a sensation independent of touch and other similar senses (Bonica, 1990). Just as the vision and auditory sensations have their independent mechanisms, pain has its own sensory process. Charles Sherrington came with the observation that pain cannot be construed as an independent sense because it can be evoked by different stimuli such as mechanical, chemical and thermal unlike the other sensations, which had their stimuli defined. He elaborated the theory with his further logic that the common feature among the three stimuli causing pain is the damage to the tissue. He proposed that any stimuli that are capable of causing the tissue damage be labelled as 'noxious'. From here, he coined the word 'nociception' that originated from the Latin verb 'nocere' meaning 'to harm'. The selective afferent nerves carrying the message of tissue damage were named as nociceptors.

According to the specificity theory, the independent sensation of pain has its specialized sensory receptors called nociceptors. The nerve endings of nociceptors are so tuned to respond to the damage to the tissues and trigger signals and carry the message through the pathways along the nervous system until they reach the target pain centres in the brain. These signals are processed in the pain centres so that the experience of pain is produced.

Aspect Theory

Strong (1895) discussed the aspect theory. This theory refers to pain and pleasure. According to this, pain is defined as the highest form of displeasure experienced as the tactile or thermal sensation. He proposed that pain is a combination of experience of a noxious stimulation and the psychic reaction of displeasure elicited by the sensation. Explaining with reference to the stages of evolution, he stated that heat was the first sensation. Only after that the sensation of pain came. In the process of evolution, sensations were the nervous system's modifications. Thus, pain was just limited to a sensation. Only later in the process of evolution, when ego developed, the sensation expanded to the emotion of displeasure. The major contribution of Strong's theory is the recognition of the associated negative affect with the noxious stimulation in the experience of pain.

Pattern Theory

Nafe (1929) came up with the quantitative theory of feeling. He set aside the earlier theories that advocated the summation of sensation or specialized nerves for specific sensations. He theorized that there are no specific nerve fibres carrying specific sensory messages. Different sensations are experienced because of a particular pattern of neural firing. The encoding of spatial and temporal profile of firing of peripheral nerves results in the experience of the specific type and intensity of sensation. There are no special receptors of pain. The same receptors carry messages of touch and pain. The difference in pain or non-painful sensation is based on the pattern of signals carried by peripheral nerves. Pain is felt with certain patterns of neural activity of high level as a result of intense stimulus. It does not depend on the location of the stimulus. For example, being hit hard on the back results in pain, while caressing or rubbing the same spot does not cause pain. Thus, it is the temporal and spatial patterns of nerve impulses that result in pain experience than the specific types of nerves. In a way, this theory opened the gates for the gate control theory of pain.

Gate Control Theory

Gate control theory of pain was proposed by Melzack and Walls (1965). It is originated when they identified the gaps in pattern theory and specificity theory. Pattern theory proposed that the sensation of pain is the result of a particular pattern of high neural activity. Specificity theory identified the nociceptors as the special pain fibres. Mezack and Walls discussed the shortcomings of these two theories and tried to fill the gaps in these two landmark theories of the era. They came up with a model that explained these two apparently opposing theories. At the outset, they accepted the presence of nociceptors and touch fibres. According to them, these two fibres form synapse.

According to this model, when there is stimulation on the skin, the primary afferent nerves carry the message of sensation and transmit the same to three regions in the spinal cord: (1) cells within the substantia gelatinosa in dorsal horn, (2) fibres in the dorsal column and (3) a group of cells called transmission cells located in the dorsal horn. Substantia gelatinosa located in the dorsal horn constitutes the gate to the spinal cord. The small nerves with narrow diameter carry the pain stimulation, while the large nerves with wider diameters carry the stimulation of touch and pressure. Both the types of fibres carry information to two areas of the dorsal horn. The sensory information from primary afferent nerves will have to pass through this gate to reach the transmission cells in the spinal cord before the message reaching the brain. The experience of pain is the result of a complex interaction between the three components in the spinal cord. However, the pain information passes through to brain only when the 'gate' opens. There are some conditions for the 'gate' to open and close.

1. Stronger the noxious stimulus, more the activity in the small fibres intensifying the stimulus. When the intensity of the stimulus on the skin reaches certain level, the 'gate' opens and allows the signal to pass through, transmitted to brain. It is processed in the brain for the individual to feel the pain. Small fibre activity tends to impede the inhibitory interneurons that have the power to close the 'gate'. Hence, the 'gate' is open allowing the transmission of pain impulses to pass through the transmission cells and reach the brain.
2. When the activity in wide diameter fibres that carry harmless stimuli such as touch or rub is high, the 'gate' tends to close for the fibre carrying the impulses of noxious stimuli because they excite the inhibitory neurons. This explains why we tend to treat pain by applying pressure or massage at the spot of pain and get relief.
3. Melzack and Walls suggested that in addition to substantia gelatinosa, there existed another control mechanism located in the cortical region. Recent research (Garland, 2012) postulated that these cortical control centres play a role in the individual experiencing pain as a result of cognitive and emotional factors. A person in negative state of mind has a 'gate' that tends to open more often so that the pain impulses pass through resulting in the individual experiencing pain from a stimulus that is otherwise perceived as normal. Further research suggested the relationship between lifestyle and pain experience. Certain unhealthy lifestyle seems to result in opening the 'gate' leading to experience of pain disproportionate to the stimulus (Nijs et al., 2020; Senba & Kami, 2017).

It can be summarized that the 'gate opens when

1 The noxious stimulus is intense
2 When the individual's emotional state is negative
3 When the individual's cognition is focused on the pain located

The 'gate' is closed when the individual is

1 Relaxed and contented
2 Is engaged in activity and exercise
3 Takes interest in life and is optimistic

Mezack and Walls are the first theorists whose model gave due significance to psychosocial factors in the experience of pain. Counterstimulation techniques such as massaging for pain relief are well explained by this model. Distraction techniques such as applying ointments with strong smell and tingling sensation to skin in pain location also fall into the logic of this model.

Is Pain a Biomedical or Biopsychosocial Phenomenon?

The biomedical model of pain construes pain as a physical/physiological phenomenon that involves the cells in the skin, muscles, nerves, ligaments, bones and so on. The focus is on nociception. The treatment approach concentrates on the relief through medication surgery or physiotherapy that works on the principle of counterstimulation, distraction or repair of the damaged cells.

Pain is not just a physiological phenomenon. It elicits emotions. For example, it is not uncommon to see people crying in pain. It is also not uncommon to see people in constant pain slowly getting into depressive state. There are a number of cases where people took the extreme step of taking their lives unable to cope with the pain. Conceptualizing, expressing, treating and coping with the pain have a number of associated psychological and sociocultural factors, which cannot be ignored in the process of diagnosis, treatment and management of pain. Hence, it is in the best interest of the patients that pain should be approached from biopsychosocial perspective.

Psychological and Social Factors of Pain

The very definition of pain includes the emotional component making the experience psychophysiological. The psychological factors in pain include cognition, emotion and behaviour. Apart from the psychological factors, pain also involves certain major sociocultural factors that guide the expression of emotion and the pain relief-seeking behaviour. Figure 11.1 summarizes the psychological and sociocultural factors associated with pain. Though the figure depicts the process in a sequence for the sake of better explanation, the cognitive, affective and behavioural factors are interconnected and have their inherent link with sociocultural factors at various levels.

Figure 11.1 explains that the once the message of nociceptive stimulus passes through the 'gate' and reaches the brain, the individual's attention is drawn to the pain stimulus. This process happens so fast that the focus of attention appears to be instantaneous. The attention is immediately followed by interpretation of the pain stimulus. This is where cognitive mediation happens. With the help of some past experience and inputs from the sociocultural factors, the

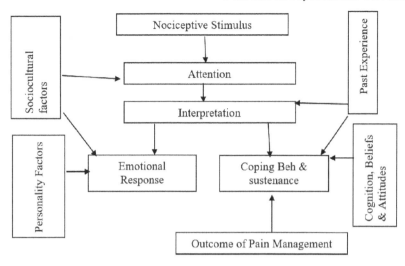

Figure 11.1 Psychosocial Factors of Pain.

individual interprets the pain. For example, a person from the rural area having experience in the agricultural field walking in the garden on a rainy day suddenly feels a piercing pain on a spot near the ankle will immediately pay attention to the spot and realize it as a snake bite at once. This interpretation comes because of his past experience and the inputs from the sociocultural set-up where snake bite during the monsoon is common. However, the same situation for an urban dweller on a visit to the village, though will draw the attention, will fail to help with the correct interpretation. The person from urban area may interpret it as an injury due to thorn or a sharp stone. The emotions and the subsequent behaviour depend significantly on the interpretation. The person from rural area might take immediate action for the pain and the cause, while the urban dweller may ignore it as a minor injury until the poison starts acting on him. The interpretation of the pain simultaneously leads to two responses—the emotional reaction and the coping behavioural response. The emotional expression is majorly determined by the sociocultural factors and the personality of the individual. The coping behaviour is determined by the individual's past experience and health cognition, beliefs and attitudes. The villager who realizes that he had a snake bite may immediately shout for help, and show panic reaction because of the knowledge that the snakes in the area are highly poisonous. He may feel relieved when someone brings a hen and makes it suck the blood from the wound created at the spot. This is because of the cultural practice where the immediate first aid to snake bite is to tightly tie up the place above the snake bite and make the hen suck the blood so that the poison is prevented from getting into blood circulation and the poison already in the blood is sucked out. The urban dweller may not show any emotion because of the interpretation of the wound as a thorn or stone hit injury that is minor and he has no cognition about the snakes and snake bites of the region. He would panic later when the poison starts having its impact on him because of not having any clue about the cause of the pain. Once he knows that it was a snake bite, he may not be comfortable with the first aid using the hen but may insist on being taken to the hospital to be administered the antidote for snake bite because of his cognition and beliefs about the snake bites. Thus, the cognition, affect and behaviour as associates of pain are closely interrelated and are linked to the past experience, personality factors and sociocultural factors of the individual in pain. We will now examine each of the basic psychological factors involved in pain.

Attention

Attention to pain should be considered a boon. Because attention, though, is a process controlled by the brain, the psychological function of attention is to motivate one to act. The attention is very spontaneous and automatic. The attention to pain functions as a warning that one should stop the activity one is engaged in. This prevents further damage to the tissue and harm to the individual. For example, when one is walking on a terrain with an upward slope and suddenly feels a severe pain in the chest, the attention to the pain helps the person to continue the walk. In case the pain is related to the cardiac system, stopping the walk/climb prevents the heart from taking further pressure and thus staking further damage.

On many occasions, it is intriguing to observe that the pain (such as chronic muscular pain) over which one has very little control gets a lot of attention but does not attend to the one that is a real warning signal (such as a deep cut in an accident) and engage in helping the other family member from slipping into unconscious state. This happens because of the release of a hormone called endorphin, which is normally released during pleasurable activities and eustress. They help in relieving pain and continue the action, which in normal conditions of injury is difficult to carry out.

Sometimes, a seemingly small injury results in intense pain. The cause for this is vigilance. Vigilance refers to an abnormally high attention on signals of pain. When there is intense focus on the pain signals, the pain experienced appears magnified (Leeuw et al., 2007). This phenomenon highlights the close connection between the cognition and emotion related to pain (Linton, 2005; Villemure & Bushnell, 2002). This factor underscores the subjectivity involved in pain perception. The subjectivity is related to the attention one pays to the pain. A common phenomenon observed among the children is that when they have a fall and see the bruise in their body, they start crying. When their attention is diverted to something else, they stop crying. But again the minute they start looking at their bruise, they resume crying. This is a factor related to attention, pain experience and emotion. This phenomenon making the pain experience and expression subjective is a challenge to objective assessment of pain. Patients with chronic pain who are not engaged in activities complain of more pain than those who engage themselves and keep busy. This factor of pain strongly supports the advocacy for psychosocial approach to pain than a biomedical approach.

Interpretation

Interpretation of the pain is done through cognitive mediation. Cognition in interpreting pain is influenced by learning through past experience, sociocultural factors. In turn, it is the interpretation of the pain that triggers emotions and motivates the individual's pain-relief behaviour. It may be appropriate to state that there is mutuality between emotion and pain interpretation. The interpretation of the pain is likely to be very negative when one's affect state is that of depression or anxiety, while it will be interpreted not so negatively when one is in positive affect state. The influence of cognition and sociocultural factors on interpretation is well evidenced in case of the inevitable menstrual pain among the woman folk. Some understand it as a natural biological process and go about taking the pain as a natural phenomenon, or find remedies in case the noxious stimulus is high. Others who interpret it as pathological, or curse on the womanhood tend to catastrophize the pain and as a consequence experience a negative affect throughout the process repeated in every cycle. One more factor that influences the interpretation of pain is the expectation of consequences. For example, there is always a difference in interpretation of labour pain and cancer pain with the intensity of pain being constant. This is because the cognition, emotions and expectations are poles apart for the two. Cognitive and emotional factors explain as to why sometimes a mild pressure is construed as severe pain, while a real severe pain is perceived as tolerable.

Cognition, Beliefs and Attitudes

Past experience helps in developing some schema. For example, experiencing a pain in the abdomen may indicate that it is likely to be colic pain that one had the previous year. Sometimes, the existing schema may also play a significant role in misleading the interpretation. For example, a middle-aged person who feels uneasy and an undefined pain in the chest may pass it as the symptom of acidity and gas due to his existing schema, while the symptoms actually relate to cardiac-related pain.

Certain beliefs and attitudes about pain have an influence in the interpretation and experience of it. Certain beliefs and attitudes have been found to contribute to development of persistent pain (Main, Foster, & Buchbinder, 2010). The belief that pain is a threat and if not responded with rest would harm results in the individual stopping the activity altogether that results in persistent pain. For example, a patient with spondylitis guided by the belief to rest because of pain instead of exercising as per the physician's advice may end up having persistent pain than any relief.

The beliefs and attitudes also contribute to expectations, which in turn may be crucial in triggering motivation to act in a particular way. If the expectations are supported by health literacy and inputs from the medical professional, the subsequent behaviour and affect state are positive. In case the expectations are based on the wrong beliefs, it may result in unsuitable behaviour and negative affect state. For example, if a patient with a pain due to ligament tear in the ankle equates the pain with one's cousin who had pain due to sprained ankle and expects to get relieved of the pain in three to four days will be disappointed as the pain relief in ligament tear takes much longer compared to that of a sprain. As a result, the patient may feel the treatment not effective and seek second opinion or go for alternative medicine. Setting the right expectations in the patient constitutes a part of biopsychosocial approach. The patients undergoing Coronary Artery Bypass Grafting (CABG) who were exposed to a biopsychosocial intervention that included the post-operative pain expectation were found to recover faster compared to their counterparts in the control group (Savio & Hariharan, 2020)

This proves the close connection between the cognition, affect and behaviour.

Emotions

Pain is not an isolated physical phenomenon. The most significant aspect of pain is the associated emotions. The emotions associated with pain are fear, anger, guilt, anxiety, depression and distress. The more intense are the emotions, the higher is the perceived severity of the pain and longer is the healing process. The same intensity of stimulus may create different intensities of pain when emotions vary. A patient of chronic arthritis pain may experience tolerable pain and move about with routine activities when in a joyous mood. But on another occasion when the day started with an argument with a family member, and the negative mood continued, the same intensity of noxious stimulus is experienced as a severe pain by the person. Several aspects explain the reason. One of the reasons is the physiological changes that happen within the body due to stress. There is a drop or an increase in skin temperature depending on the location (e.g. the temperature in finger tips drops, while in males, there is an increase in the temperature in cheeks), muscular tone changes to becoming rigid, blood flow into the vessels increases, breathing gets shallow, to mention a few. Some of these changes such as tightening of muscles or breathing shallowly worsen the pain further. The stress level increases with the worsening of pain, thus creating a vicious circle.

The interconnection between pain and emotions also may have a neurological explanation. In human brain, the areas processing sensory, emotional and cognitive information have profound interconnections. Research findings indicate that people persistent pain also manifest symptoms of anxiety disorder than those without pain (Peters, 2015). The most prominent manifestation of anxiety noticed in patients with pain is negative thoughts with 'what if' apprehensions that take the shape of worry (Barlow, 2004).

Depression is yet another affect state closely associated with chronic pain. With depression, the pain intensity felt is high. The potent risk of disability is also a factor that triggers the mutually contributing association between pain and depression. Depression may not be diagnosed as clinical depression in many pain patients. Yet, the presence of depression lowers the prognosis in chronic pain patients. One of the reasons could be the striking characteristic of inertia in chronic pain patients. The inertia prevents them from following the physical activities, which are detrimental. Further, isolating one from socializing or cognitive activities results in more focus on the pain. The more the attention, the worse the experience of pain. The same is true about anxiety.

Sociocultural Factors in Pain

While physiological factors of pain are obvious and endorsed, psychological aspects have to be emphasized for a deliberate focus so that the approach to pain is optimized. However, very often the sociocultural aspects of pain fail to get the attention they deserve. Pain has a huge cultural loading. Hence, it is necessary to understand the sociocultural dimensions related to pain, particularly in contemporary times when medical tourism is a common phenomenon and encouraged. While the nociception and pain are universal experiences, the expression associated with pain has wide cultural variations. The expression of emotion and the overt reactions are behaviours learned appropriate to one's culture. The culture-appropriate behaviour is learned and assimilated because of the reinforcement factor of reward and punishment of culture-appropriate behaviour.

It is very difficult to standardize 'the normal pain response' because of its wide variations. Expression of pain can be classified into extroversion and introversion types (Mohan, 2011). Extroversion of pain is explicit, catches the attention and hence is likely to receive immediate help. The introversion type of pain prompts the victim to limit the expression to covert level, and hence, the intervention is likely to get delayed. Another argument is that the extroversion sometimes may get discounted as exaggeration or attention-seeking behaviour. Thus, it is a challenge to standardize and objectivize the measurement of pain, which is bound to be coloured with lot of subjectivity due to individual differences in pain threshold levels and the cultural factors related to endurance. The only way is to understand the cultural norms and be sensitive to it in assessing the pain. Mohan (2010) reported a qualitative difference in expression of pain across nations spread over three continents. According to him, pain expression among Indian patients is loud, African patients irrespective of loud or silent are found to be attention-seeking, while Dutch patients manifest silent expression. According to the author, the variation in expression is the outcome of child-rearing process in the culture.

Though the common belief is that women, who are biologically predisposed to endure the menstrual and labour pain, endure more pain, the research evidence is contrary. Women are found to be more sensitive but less enduring of pain (Wise et al., 2002).

In view of the wide variations among the gender, age and cultures, the merit lies in assessing pain with all its subjectivity. The report and rating given by the patient need to be taken at face value and assessed by the interventionists.

Coping Behaviour

Nociceptive stimulus is a deviation from norm, and the experience of pain places the wellbeing at stake. The associated emotion is negative. None of these contribute to the homeostatic state or biopsychological equilibrium. Hence, the normal response to pain experience is a pain-relieving behaviour. This is what is coping with the pain or pain management steps. In case of pain due to an accident and injury to the body, the immediate natural course of action is to seek first aid and relief from pain. In case of chronic pain, the natural course of action is to seek medical advice for effective pain management that may involve invasive procedures, medication, physiotherapy, diet management and stress management. The patient takes up these measures with an expectation of pain relief. In case the expectation is total relief from pain at once, the patient is likely to be disappointed and frustrated. Since the outcome is not within the expected time and extent, the patient sees an absence of reward for the effort. Hence, it may be difficult to sustain the pain management behaviour. On the contrary, if the health communication from the treating doctor sets realistic outcome and the patient works on the pain relief measures with realistic expectations and experiences relief as a result of following medical advice on medication, exercise and diet, he/she is likely to sustain the adherence behaviour and cope effectively with the pain. Thus, the sustenance of coping with pain is a function of the outcome of the coping behaviour. This is nothing but the simple application of operant conditioning.

Psychosocial Interventions in Pain Management

At the outset, it has to be mentioned that the psychosocial interventions are not the primary but constitute supplementary to the invasive or medical management so as to optimize the outcome of treatment. Psychosocial interventions are normally beneficial in managing chronic pain. The major psychosocial factors contributing to pain perception and experience are as follows: (1) attention, (2) cognition, (3) affect and (4) behaviour. Guided by these, the intervention plan should also address these psychological dimensions. The research has proved that the higher the attention to the pain stimulus, the higher will be the trauma. Secondly, the pre-existing schema and beliefs about the pain and its consequences influence the pain. Thirdly, the negative affect state magnifies the pain experience. Finally, the coping with pain and its outcome contributes to pain management substantially. The major psychosocial interventions work on the following broad principles:

1. Use distraction techniques so that the patient's attention is off the pain spot
2. Help the patient have a strong cognitive base about the pain
3. Create and sustain positive affect in the patient
4. Ensure sound adherence to pain management behaviour

Distraction Techniques

External applications: Distracting the patient can be achieved in many ways. The balms, ointments and massages with aromatic or material with strong smell accomplish this goal. The balms, spray or ointments applied on the pain spot of the skin generate not only an olfactory sensation, but some of them also change the temperature in the applied part of the skin. All these work as good attention distractors.

Cognitive distractors: Patients with chronic pain need to have good cognitive engagement. In the absence of it, the attention automatically gets focused on the pain, thus increasing the perception of severity of pain. Developing a hobby, engaging in reading, spiritual practices or engaging in religious rituals helps the patients occupied in meaningfully busy schedule. This prevents the attention from getting focused on the pain. Engaging oneself in harmless light physical activities also functions as cognitive distractor. A general observation of senior citizens suggests that those who occupy their time in reading, solving puzzles, hobbies such as gardening, painting or knitting and those who show interest in learning new skills are the ones who have less complaints about the pain than those who have a lot of leisure time.

Socializing: Socializing and active participation in community activities physically or intellectually is a good attention distractor. Further, it also helps in sustaining a positive affect of a sense of satisfaction. Altruistic activities keep the attention on the problems of the others; thus, the focus is diverted from one's pain perception. Further, the positive feedback about one's actions helps in distracting the focus from the negativity of pain. Engaging in interpersonal interactions within and outside the family attracts the attention on a number of issues and topics rather than thinking and feeling the chronic pain. In affiliation-oriented cultures like Indian society, increasing the social network is one sure method of distracting the chronic patient's attention from pain.

Creating Cognitive Base

The theories of health behaviour converge on one point, which states that the health behaviour has a strong influence of health cognition. Pain is no exception in this. Understanding pain in terms of the cause, duration, frequency, precipitating actions and its prognosis in the realistic way helps the patient cope with it better. A prospective mother going through the labour pain has the knowledge that it would end soon and the outcome of having the baby in her arms is a pleasant experience to look forward to. Hence, the labour pain limits her anxiety. Otherwise, the intense pain it causes should have caused extreme panic in all mothers making them incapable of recovering to attend to the babies. If all patients of pain are made aware of the nature and outcome of their pain, the knowledge factor may work positively in managing their pain. Majority of pain patients panic because of the phenomenon called 'fear of the unknown' when they don't understand the cause and nature of the pain. For example, if one is to have a sudden shooting pain in the throat, one tends to panic because of the unknown cause. On the contrary, if one slowly develops the throat pain that gets intense gradually over the day, one has scope to detect that the cause of the pain is the ice cream party the previous night in a windy weather. This would not create so much anxiety. Thus, knowledge is a great cognitive component that feeds to one's emotions. Lack of knowledge or incomplete knowledge invokes negative emotions. This is applicable to the pain experience too. A patient of chronic pain such as arthritis should have complete knowledge that one can minimize the pain with medication and other lifestyle changes but cannot expect a quick cure. This helps in creating a mental readiness though it may sometimes take a little time. The second cognitive factor relates to apprising the patient on the lifestyle factor and one's own role in minimizing the pain. This enhances the self-efficacy in the patient and thereby adherence behaviour. Wrong knowledge, false beliefs and fallacious inferences based on wrong examples or models, superstitions originating from irrational thoughts or information may prove disastrous for pain patients. This may lead to negative emotions and catastrophizing the pain and worsening of the illness. The treatment approach should include appropriate psychoeducation and provide scope for clarifying doubts in the patient. This calls for a sound health communication system that can be one-to-one or group sessions. Explaining the pathology involved in the muscular/skeletal/nervous system if explained with diagrams followed by how the medication or lifestyle changes address these issues would help in laying a sound foundation of knowledge about one's condition and the rationale behind lifestyle changes. This in turn contributes to enhance adherence behaviour.

Maintaining Positive Affect

Pain is associated with negative affect. Fear, anxiety, apprehension, anger, guilt, depression and distress are some of the negative affect states associated with pain. This association has both neurological and psychological explanations. Continuous attention on pain enhances the negative affect and negative thoughts, thus creating a vicious circle. Applying the principle of classical conditioning, it may be stated that since the pain and negative affect are associated, if we try to induce positive affect, then the substitution of affect state will result in reducing the pain. Some of the therapeutic interventions help in keeping away the negative affect away and replacing them with positive affect.

THOUGHT SUBSTITUTION

Repeated negative thoughts, to a great extent, generate negative affect. One way to control the negative affect is to handle the negative thoughts. Thought substitution is a method where one examines the value of the thought in terms of contributing to wellbeing. Then, try to identify a contrary positive thought to substitute it. In case a positive thought is difficult, then a neutral thought may be identified to substitute the negative. For example, if a patient with sciatica is found to be engaged with the thought that the pain is going to incapacitate and end up in making one physically disabled, the possible steps are as follows: (1) help encourage the patient to examine if this extreme thought is rational, (2) assess if such thoughts are useful and contribute to good feelings, (3) help the patient to identify the facts that the intensity of the pain varies and the flare-ups are the experiences that cause the negative thoughts, (4) help the patient identify the measures that are useful in subsiding the pain and the factors precipitating it, (5) evolve substitute thoughts about the initiatives that contribute to preventing precipitations and minimizing the pain when there is a flare-up and (6)help the patient substitute the catastrophizing thoughts with the small remedial or preventive behaviours that are successful in managing the pain. Thought substitution helps in reinstating hope in the patients, which is positive. Alternative methods are to distract the thoughts by reminiscing some positive past experiences and create a positive affect in self. The patient may be assigned some simple task of writing or narrating a pleasant experience in life. Narrate the funny situation one was caught in. This helps in replacing the repetitive negative thoughts with that of positive, thereby mellowing down the pain perception.

RELAXATION TECHNIQUES

There are a number of standardized relaxation techniques to ameliorate the anxiety and stress. Jacobson's Progressive Muscular Relaxation (JPMR), Guided Imagery, *Yoga nidra, Pranayama* and variant breathing exercises are a few to mention.

JPMR is a relaxation technique where the patient follows the instructions of the psychologist and alternates between tensing and relaxing every muscle. This contrast between tightening and relaxing the muscles helps in enhancing the experience of relaxation. The process also involves relaxing every muscle and experiencing the weight of the body at the end when every part of the body totally relaxes by lying loose. The patient is allowed to remain in this relaxed state for a while before the instructor guides him/her to open the eyes and gradually feel the environment. One needs to use the discretion in administering this technique of relaxation on patients suffering from pain since this involves tightening of the muscles. This technique may not suit post-operative patients, those with pain due to injuries and patients with severe muscular pain or pain due to bone degeneration. It is advisable to administer JPMR after clearance from the treating doctors of patients in pain.

Guided Imagery is a safe technique with patients with any type of pain. In Guided Imagery, the patient is instructed to visualize being in a pleasant physical environment such as a beach, garden, hill station. The instructor describes the place and surroundings when the patient has to live the experience of the imagery described. For example when the instructor narrates "you are now walking barefoot slowly on the lawns of the garden. You feel the moist tender grass under the feet, as the slow soothing wind carrying the fragrance of the jasmine flowers brush against your arms, face and head", the patient lives the situation with all the sensory inputs. Guided Imagery has the potential to generate the pleasant experience and clear the neural pathways. Pain cannot coexist with the pleasant sensations. Further, the impact of the pleasant experience and relaxed state lingers and helps in maintaining a positive affect state, which helps in lowering the pain perception.

Yoga nidra is a relaxation technique of Indian origin that has been practised by spiritual seekers for centuries. This technique combines the principles of JPMR and Guided Imagery. The technique involves instructions that make the patient conscious of different parts of the body, relax each part. It carries the patient through visualizing, and imageries of sensory experiences that are polar opposites, such as visualizing a huge elephant standing followed by the visualization of a small cat, experiencing a bright light followed by the pitch darkness. These sensory polar opposites are similar to muscular tension and relaxation in JPMR. The purpose of this is explained to carry the function of neural pathways. The patient is made to resolve not to fall asleep during the practice of *yoga nidra*. Towards the end, the patient is put to total relaxation through instructions to relax each muscle, feel the lightness of the body and enjoy the state.

Pranayama is an ancient Indian method of regulating the breath that results in relaxation. The method requires the follower to use one's thumb and ring finger and follow the steps described below:

1. One has to first close the left nostril with the ring finger and breathe in slowly and steadily until the lungs are filled.
2. Release the left nostril and close the right nostril with the thumb and release the air through the left nostril until the lungs are emptied.
3. In the second half, continue to keep the right nostril closed, breathe in through the left nostril.
4. Release the right nostril, and close the left with the ring finger and release the air slowly and steadily through the right nostril.

This completes one round. Repeat the process. The principle behind *Pranayama* is that the activation of sympathetic system results in disturbing the breathing, which becomes fast and shallow. This conditioned association between anxiety and breathing is disrupted by *pranayama*, which makes the breathing steady and normal. Along with this, the blood pressure and galvanic skin response also change to normal. These changes in the physiological system work on the psychological process, and the individual's affect state is no more negative.

DISTRACTION AND DESENSITIZATION

Eye Movement Desensitization and Reprocessing (EMDR) is a therapeutic process aimed at treating pain effectively (Grant & Threlfo, 2002). The ground on which EMDR stands is that pain is found to become chronic due to maladaptive measures in processing the emotions, which need to be handled effectively. This method is found to be useful in desensitizing and processing the emotional distress. The use of this therapy is gradually gaining popularity, particularly with chronic patients manifesting anxiety, stress and psychological comorbidity. Randomized control clinical trials are in vogue to prove the safety and efficacy of this method in various pain treatments.

EMDR gained popularity in treating the patients with post-traumatic stress disorder (PTSD). Chronic pain involves changes in the brain and nervous system similar to the situation of PTSD. Hence, EMDR may be effective in chronic pain also. In this therapy, the patient is asked to focus on memories related to pain, or the pain experienced currently or on the pain and stress apprehended in future. Once this is done, the patient is asked to indulge in these memories; the therapist moves his/her finger back and forth rapidly following a rhythm within the visual field of the patient. The finger is kept approximately at a distance of one foot from the patient's face. This is repeated for 24 cycles at the rate of one cycle per second (Jena, 2008). After one set of 24 cycles, the patient is instructed to blank out of the focus of pain and take a deep breath. The principle behind is that while the patient is focusing on the pain, he/she is distracted. This distraction weakens the vividness of the memory and associated emotions, thus resulting in desensitization of the associated thoughts and emotions triggered along with the pain.

Adherence Behaviour

Pain management calls for changes in lifestyle. In case of chronic pain, the medical advice may include regular physical exercises despite discomfort or mild pain. Further, the patient may be advised to follow restrictions in diet, which may not suit one's personal choice. Avoiding socialization, confining to bed, isolating oneself, brooding and indulgence in thinking and talking about the pain may get into one's habit, which may have to be changed. Adherence behaviour thus involves unlearning of the old habits and replacing them with the new learned behaviour. In order to achieve this, the patient should be able to visualize the new behaviour attractive with a positive reinforcement value, and the old behaviour should lose its reward value if any. This requires appropriate counselling from a professional health psychologist. To invoke and strengthen health adherence behaviour, the counselling should aim at cognitive restructuring and invoking motivation, and work on reinforcements within the family and social environment. This calls for individual sessions with the patient, support group formation involving a set of patients experiencing chronic pain of similar kind, and family counselling that orients the family members how to identify the reinforcers in the natural setting and how to utilize the same in strengthening the adherence behaviour in the patient.

In view of all the factors discussed, it can be concluded that for optimizing the prognosis in treating pain, the approach should necessarily be biopsychosocial. The psychosocial factors should be integrated right from the time of assessment and continue as a follow-up too. The pain medicine is thus a multidisciplinary branch than in control of pure medical management.

References

Barlow, D. H. (2004). *Anxiety and its disorders: The nature and treatment of anxiety and panic*. New York: Guilford Press.
Bonica, J. J. (1990). History of pain concepts and therapies. In: J. J. Bonica (Ed.), *The management of pain* (2nd ed., pp. 2–17). London: Lea & Febiger.

Garland, E. L. (2012). Pain processing in the human nervous system: A selective review of nociceptive and biobehavioral pathways. *Primary Care: Clinics in Office Practice, 39*(3), 561–571.

Grant, M., & Threlfo, C. (2002). EMDR in the treatment of chronic pain. *Journal of Clinical Psychology, 58*(12), 1505–1520. doi: 10.1002/jclp.10101

Jena, S. P. K. (2008). *Behaviour therapy: Techniques, research and applications.* New Delhi: SAGE Publications India.

Leeuw, M., Goossens, M. E., Linton, S. J., Crombez, G., Boersma, K., & Vlaeyen, J. W. (2007). The fear-avoidance model of musculoskeletal pain: Current state of scientific evidence. *Journal of Behavioral Medicine, 30,* 77–94.

Linton, S. J. (2005). *Understanding pain for better clinical practice: A psychological perspective.* Edinburgh: Elsevier.

Loeser, J. D., & Treede, R. D. (2008). The Kyoto protocol of IASP basic pain terminology. *PAIN®, 137*(3), 473–477. doi: 10.1016/j.pain.2008.04.025

Main, C. J., Foster, N., & Buchbinder, R. (2010). How important are back pain beliefs and expectations for satisfactory recovery from back pain? *Best Practice & Research Clinical Rheumatology, 24*(2), 205–217.

Melzack, R., Wall, P. D. (1965). Pain mechanisms: A new theory. *Science, 150*(3699), 971–979. doi: 10.1126/science.150.3699.971. PMID: 5320816.

Mohan, H. (2010). Cultural markers in expression of pain and trauma. In: M. Hariharan, G. Padmaja & M. Padhy (Eds.), *Trauma and pain: Biopsychosocial perspectives* (pp. 71–78). New Delhi: Global Vision Publishers.

Nafe, J. P. (1929). A quantitative theory of feeling. *The Journal of General Psychology, 2*(2–3), 199–211. doi: 10.1080/00221309.1929.9918059

Nijs, J., D'Hondt, E., Clarys, P., Deliens, T., Polli, A., Malfliet, A., ... & Ickmans, K. (2020). Lifestyle and chronic pain across the lifespan: an inconvenient truth? *Pm&r, 12*(4), 410–419.

Peters, M. L. (2015). Emotional and cognitive influences on pain experience. *Modern Trends in Pharmacopsychiatry, 30,* 138–152. doi: 10.1159/000435938

Raja, S. N., Carr, D. B., Cohen, M., Finnerup, N. B., Flor, H., Gibson, S., ... & Vader, K. (2020). The revised international association for the study of pain definition of pain: Concepts, challenges, and compromises. *Pain, 161*(9), 1976–1982. doi: 10.1097/j.pain.0000000000001939

Savio, M. T., & Hariharan, M. (2020). Impact of psychosocial intervention on prognosis of cardiac surgery patients. *Health Psychology Research, 8*(3), 139–146. doi:10.4081/hpr.2020.8887

Senba, E., & Kami, K. (2017). A new aspect of chronic pain as a lifestyle-related disease. *Neurobiology of Pain, 1,* 6–15.

Strong, C. A. (1895). The psychology of pain. *Psychological Review, 2*(4), 329–347. doi: 10.1037/h0075245

Villemure, C., & Bushnell, M. C. (2002). Cognitive modulation of pain: How do attention and emotion influence pain processing? *Pain, 95*(3), 195–199.

Wise, E. A., Price, D. D., Myers, C. D., Heft, M. W., & Robinson, M. E. (2002). Gender role expectations of pain: Relationship to experimental pain perception. *Pain, 96*(3), 335–342.

Index

Note: **Bold** page numbers refer to tables; *italic* page numbers refer to figures.

abducens nerve 200
abnormal sleep *(aswabhavika)* 68
Abraído-Lanza, A. F. 420
accessory muscles 217
accessory nerve 200
Accredited Social Health Activists (ASHA) 75
Acharya Charaka 17
acid-alkaline balance (pH) 227
Acquired Deficiency Syndrome (AIDS) 91–92
acquired habits: alcohol consumption 98–104; health risk behaviour as 93–104; smoking behaviour 93–98; tobacco consumption 98
action self-efficacy 151, 152, *152*
active-passive model 378–379
activities of daily living (ADL) 359
acute kidney failure 107
acute pain 437–438
adaptation 328–329
Ader, R. 12, 268
adherence behaviour 451
Adler, N. E. 8
adrenal gland 202, 204, 206
adrenal medulla 206
adrenocorticotrophin-releasing hormone (ACTH) 206
aether 2
affect state 11, 31, 50, 57; factors related to 113; negative 63, 68, 113; positive 60, 68
afferent neurons (sensory neurons) 189
Affleck, G. 415
Agarwal, A. 383
Agarwal, M. 414, 415
ageing 254; and cardiomyopathy 299; and health resilience 422–424; productive 424
Ahankara (Ego) 34
Ahn, J. 123
Ajzen, I. 132
Alabaster, E. 156
Albarracin, D. 134
alcohol consumption 98–104, *100*; consequences 104–105; digestive system 106; family support 113–114; health risks of 109–110; immune system 107–108; impact on cardiovascular system 106; impact on nervous system 105–106; kidneys 107; and liver 106–107; long-term effects 105; mental health 108; onset and progression of drinking behaviour 99–100; onset of 100–101; and pancreas 106–107; problem drinking and alcoholism 101–104; progression in drinking 101; psychosocial repercussions 108–109; reproductive system 107; short-term effects 104–105; skeletal system 107; standards 99; vision 108
alcoholic fatty liver disease 106
alcoholism 101–104; early alcoholic 102; late alcoholic 103–104; mild alcoholic 102; pre-alcoholism 102; stages 102–104, *103*
aldosterone 227
Alhassan, A. A. 111
allostasis 247–248
allostatic load theory 247–248
Alzheimer's disease 308, 375
American Medical Association (AMA) 8
American Psychological Association (APA) 1, 8, 13
American Psychosomatic Society 10
amine hormones 204
Amrutanjan (a pain balm) 364
Anand, J. 414
Ananda (bliss) 31–32
Andrew, A. 38, 334, 339, 426
angina (chest pain) 295
angina pectoris 297
Annalakshmi, N. 422
Anthony, E. J. 403–405
anthropogenic stress 259–260
antigens 234
antiseptics 6
Antoni, M. H. 317
Antonovsky, A. 404

454 Index

Apgar test 70
Aquinas, St. Thomas 5
Arango-Lasprilla, J. C. 376
Arifin, W. N. 146
Aristotle 2
Arjunan, I. 372
aroma therapy 19
arteriosclerosis (hardening of the arteries) 295
Artha (monitory returns) 34
arthritis: and health resilience 419–420; rheumatoid 270, 311–312
'asanas' (set postures of the physical body) 36
Asatmendriyartha Samyoga 34–35
Asclepius 1
Asha, D. 22, 23
Ashtanga Hridayam Sangraha 17
Ashtanga Yoga 36
aspect theory 440
asthma 302–303
aswasthata 34; *Asatmendriyartha Samyoga* 34–35; *Kala* 35; *Prajnaparadha* 35; reasons/sources of 34–35
Atharva Veda 17
'atma' (self) 17
atrioventricular valves 210
Attention Deficit Hyperactive Disease (ADHD) 19
attention to pain 444
Au, A. 376
Austin, D. 65
autoimmune diseases 270
autonomous orientation 163
autonomy, defined 161
Avsar, U. 364
Awasthi, P. 330, 343
axon 187
Ayurveda: approach to health 17–18; *Atharva Veda* 17; and biopsychosocial model of health 32, 35; on exercise 61; and Health Psychology 16–20; healthy eating 56–57, 58; healthy sleep 67–69; *Nada Yoga* 19; panchabhootas 32–33; prescribed lifestyle in 36; specialized branches 18; treatment procedure in 19; tridoshas 32–33
Ayurveda 428
Ayush (Ayurved, Yoga, Unani, Siddha and Homeopathy) 20

Badger, T. 366
Bandura, A. 146
Banerjee, A. 389
Banhato, E. F. C. 320
Barker, C. 271
basal ganglia 196
Basal Metabolic Rate (BMR) 61
Basic Psychological Needs Theory (BPNT) 163
Baum, A. 240
Bäuml, J. 340

BCG vaccine 74
Beck, A. T. 11
Becker, M. H. 120, 121
Beck's Depression Inventory (BDI) 319
Beecher, H. K: 'the Powerful Placebo' 10
behaviour: defined 49; goal of 49; health 50–51; health protective 51–52; immunization 72–74; positive health 49–77
behavioural change 345–346
behavioural control: and achievement motivation 136; and self-efficacy 136–137
behavioural deviation: from healthy practices 81–93; unhealthy diet 82–87; unhealthy sexual behaviour 90–93; unhealthy sleep behaviour 87–90
behavioural intention 132
behavioural interventions 343, 345
Behavioural Neuroscience 12
behaviour modification programme 296
Behaviour Repertory Appraisal 130
benefit-finding 418, 420, *420*, 421, 425
Bencrjee, S. P. 424
Bennett, P. 22, 156
Benyamini, Y. 23
Best, K. 404
Bethell, C. D. 428
Bharadwaja 17
Bhatia, U. 101
Bhattacharjee, M. 360
Bhava Prakasa 17
Bhui, K. 258
Biglu, M. H. 383
biochemical and physiological changes in the body 241
biofeedback 12
biofeedback interventions 348–349
biomedical model 24–28, *25*; vs. biopsychosocial model 31–32; cause of disease 24–25; significant aspects of 26
biopsychosocial model of health 28–32, *30*; and Ayurveda 32, 35; vs. biomedical model 31–32; treatment process 31
bipolar neurons 188
Biswas, U. N. 342
Blalock, S. J. 150
blastocyte 232
Blaxter, M. 23
Block, G. 55
blood pressure (BP) 226–227, 294–295
blood vessels 210–211
Bockow, T. B. 321
body: biochemical and physiological changes in 241; defence system 238
Body Mass Index (BMI) 301
bone marrow 235
brain: basal ganglia 196; cerebellum 198; cerebrum 194; diencephalon 196;

forebrain 194; frontal lobe 195; hindbrain 198; hypothalamus 196–197, *197*; limbic system 196; major anatomical map of 193–199; metencephalon 198; midbrain 197; myelencephalon medulla oblongata 198; natural protection to 191, *192*; occipital lobe 195; parietal lobes 195; periaqueductal grey matter 197–198; pons 198; red nucleus 197; reticular formation 197; spinal cord 198–199, *199*; substantia nigra 197; tectum 197; tegmentum 197; temporal lobe 195; thalamus 196, *197*
Brayne, C. 422
breasts 230–231
breathing and the control centre 217
breathing mechanism—pressure relationship 217–218
Brihadaranyaka Upanishad 22
British Journal of Health Psychology 13
Broadbent, E. 316
bronchi 216
Brown, R. G. 376
Buckworth, J. 173
Buddhi (Intelligence) 34
Buhse, M. 359
Burles, F. 67
burnout *see* physician burnout
Butalid, L. 380
bypass surgery 296

Cabeza, R. 428
Cai, Y. 92
Cain, C. J. 360
cancer: caregivers of, patients 372, 376; and health resilience 418–419
Cangemi, E. 255
Cannon, W. B. 8, 13, 244
Cao, X. 427
Caplin, D. A. 361
cardiac cycle 213
cardiac functioning 212–213
cardiomyopathy 298–299
cardiovascular diseases (CVDs) 66, 294–301; and alcohol 106; angina pectoris 297; cardiomyopathy 298–299; congestive heart failure (CHF) 298; coronary artery disease (CAD)/coronary heart disease (CHD) 295–296; and health resilience 414–416; hypertension 294–295; myocardial infarction 297–298; and stress 270–271; stroke/cerebrovascular accident 300–301; varicose veins 299–300
cardiovascular system 209–214; atrioventricular valves 210; blood vessels 210–211; cardiac cycle 213; cardiac functioning 212–213; chambers of the heart 210; coronary arteries 211–212; electrical system of the heart 213–214; endocardium 210; epicardium 210; heart 209–210; heart valves 210; heart walls 210; myocardium 210; pulmonary veins 211; semilunar valves 210
caregivers: assessment 370; burden 359, 363–364; of cancer patients 372, 376; care providers 377–378; case studies 355–357; cognitive behavioural therapy 375–376; crisis 358; doctor-patient communication 379–395; doctor-patient relationship 378–379; emotional health 362–367; impact of patient care on 359–360; impact on physical health 361–362; interventions for psychological distress 372–374; multitasking of *368*; nature 358–359; negative impact 361; overview 354–355; patient care 357–358; perspective 357–358; positive impacts 360–361; primary 358; psychoeducation 370–372; psychology of 355–357; psychosocial interventions for 369; relationship between patient and *366*; responsibilities 359; secondary 358; social life 367–369
care providers 377–378
Catalano, D. 255
catastrophizing 336
causality orientation 166
Causality Orientation Theory (COT) 163–164; autonomous orientation 163; controlled orientation 164; impersonal orientation 164
Cauter, E. Van 66
cell body/soma 187
cell-mediated immunity 236
central nervous system (CNS) 191
cerebellum 198
cerebral embolism 300
cerebral haemorrhage 300–301
cerebral thrombosis 300
cerebrospinal fluid (CSF) 193, 318
cerebrum 194
chambers of the heart 210
Chan, K. Y. 373
Chandra, S. 383
Chang, C. S. 383
Charaka 56, **56,** 61, 68
Charaka Samhita 17
Charney, D. S. 411
Chelli, K. 330, 417
chemical balance 227
chemical stress 259
Chesler, M. A. 419
childhood stress 280–282, *282*; behavioural indicators of 283–284; diagnostic methods and tools 284; interventions for 284; preventive steps 284; remedial measures 284–285

456   *Index*

Chipidza, F. E. 377
Chivukula, U. 38, 330, 334, 341
Chottai, P. 417
Christian, B. 361
chronic condition 317
chronic diseases 290–291; and health resilience 413–414
chronic glomerulonephritis 305–306
chronic illnesses: behavioural change 345–346; biopsychosocial impact of **326**; cardiovascular diseases 294–301; cognitive therapy 338–345; defined 290–291; endocrine system and related diseases 303–305; gastrointestinal diseases 309–311; immune system and related diseases 311–312; methods to handle obstructions 347–349; nervous system and diseases 306–309; and physiological systems 292–294; principles of psychological therapy 335–338; psychosocial intervention to *333*; pulmonary diseases 301–303; renal diseases 305–306; reproductive system and diseases 312–331; and therapeutic interventions 332–334
chronic kidney disease (CKD) 107, 371, 372, 421
Chronic Obstructive Pulmonary Disease (COPD) 303, 319
chronic pain 362, 438–439
Chrousos, G. P. 247
cirrhosis of liver 106
Clark, D. M. 271
climate stress 259
Clinical Health Psychology 14
clinical intervention 426
Cobb, S. 50
cognitive appraisal 241, *251,* 251–252
cognitive base 448–449
cognitive behavioural therapy (CBT) 296, 375–376
cognitive distortions 335–337; interventions to 337–338
cognitive distractors 448
Cognitive Evaluation Theory (CET) 159–161; intrinsic motivation 160–161; types of motivation 159–160, *160*
cognitive factors: health risk behaviour 112
cognitive interventions 338
cognitive schemas 335–337
cognitive therapy (CT) 11, 338–345; assumption 338; behavioural interventions 343; doctor-patient communication 338–339; group interventions 339–340; motivational and behavioural intervention 345; new behaviour 343–344; positive affect and thought induction 342; prompting and fading 344–345; psychoeducation 340–342; response shaping 344; social support 342–343; stimulus shaping 344; systematic desensitization 345

Cohen, N. 12, 268
Colón, R. M. 420
colour therapy 19
Community Health Psychology 14
community-level interventions 427–428
comorbid psychological condition 42–43
competence, defined 161
concepts 119
conditioning experiment 5, *5*
confrontive coping 329–330
congestive heart failure (CHF) 298
consciousness raising 143
contemporary physiological model: allostatic load theory 247–248
contingency management 144
Continuous Ambulatory Peritoneal Dialysis (CAPD) 364
controlled orientation 164
conversion hysteria 6
coping (behaviour) 320–321; adaptation 328–329; with chronic illness 327, 329–331; confrontive 329–330; distancing 331; god/religion/faith 331; pain 447; positive reappraisal 330–331; seeking social support 330
coping appraisal 128
coronary arteries 211–212
Coronary Artery Bypass Grafting (CABG) 28, 296, 337, 445; *see also* bypass surgery
coronary artery disease (CAD)/coronary heart disease (CHD) 295–296; aetiology 295; biomedical intervention 296; psychosocial interventions 296; symptoms 296; treatment 296
coronary heart diseases (CHDs) 37, 66
corticotrophin-releasing hormone (CRH) 41
Costanzo, E. S. 418
Costlow, C. 66
counterconditioning 145
Coutinho, R. A. 124
Covinsky, K. E. 368
Cox, S. 421
Coyne, J. C. 250
Crabtree, B. F. 383
Craik, R. 38
crisis caregiver 358
Critical Health Psychology 14
Crohn's disease (CD) 310
Cronk, N. J. 98
cystic fibrosis (CF) 301–302, *302*

daily hassles 264
Dalal, A. K. 27, 31, 382, 414
Dalal, P. M. 360
Dalton, K. 312

Darwin, Charles 5
Daugherty, C. K. 418
Davidson, R. 412
Davison, S. N. 329
DeBord, K. 280
Deci, E. L. 160, 166–167
decisional balance 145
dehydroepiandrosterone (DHEA) 411–412
delayed hypersensitivity T cells 236
demands on self 240
dementia 308; *see also* Alzheimer's disease
dendrites 187
DeNisco, S. 417
De Ridder, D. 329
Descartes, Rene 4
desensitization 451
Devamani, K. A. 418
De Wit, J. B. 124
Dhanwantri 17
Dharma (social responsibilities) 34
dhyana (meditation) 36
diabetes mellitus (DM) 304–305; and health resilience 416–418; type 1 305, 416; type 2 305, 416
dichotomous thinking 336
DiClemente, C. C. 138, 141, 143, 146
diencephalon 196
diet 55; unhealthy 82–87
difficulty in initiating and maintaining behaviour 346
digestive system 219–224; alcohol consumption 106; functions of liver 223; large intestine 221–223; liver 223; mouth 219; oesophagus 220; small intestine 221; stomach 220–221
'*Dinacharya*' (daily routine) 36
Dinh, K. T. 97
Dinos, S. 258
direct association 317, 318
disabilities: and health resilience 421–422
Disability-Adjusted Life Years (DALY) 365
discrepancy 348
diseases: biomedical model 26–27; defined 27; lifestyle **41**, 41–44; psychological factors as antecedents of 37; screening for detecting 71–72
distancing 331
distraction techniques 447–448, 451
doctor-patient communication 338–339, 379–395; causes of physician burnout 392; impact of 380; impact of burnout 392–393; impact on doctors 387–389; impact on doctor's satisfaction 384–385; impact on health and wellbeing 380–382; impact on patient satisfaction 382–384; onset and progress of physician burnout 390–392; patient care 387–389

doctor-patient relationship 377, 378; active-passive model 378–379; guidance—cooperation model 379; impact on health outcome variables 385; models of 378–379; mutual participation model 379; negative impact 386–387; reciprocal 378
doctor's satisfaction 384–385
doshas 17–19, 33–34
Doswell, Braxter, Cha and Kim 134
DPT vaccine 74
Dracup, K. 415
dramatic relief 143
dualistic theory 439
Duda, J. L. 167

East India Company 19
eating behaviour 55, 85, *85*
economic poverty 368
Edmunds, J. 167
efferent neurons (motor neurons) 189
ego 119
Ehde, D. M. 321
electrical system of the heart 213–214
emotional empathy 67
emotional health 362–365
emotions: negative 317, 363, 427; pain 445–446; positive 362–363
empathy 347
endocardium 210
endocrine system and related diseases 203–209, 303–305; control centre of 204–208; diabetes mellitus (DM) 304–305; thyroid gland 304
endometrium 230
endorphin 60
End Stage Renal Disease (ESRD) 364
energetic stress 260
Engedashet, E. 93
Engel, George 13, 28–30
Engel, J. M. 321
environmental reevaluation 143
environmental stress 258
epicardium 210
epilepsy 307
Eppright, D. R. 130
ergonomic stress 260–261
Erikssen, G. 59
errors in immune system and autoimmune diseases 270
European Health Psychology Society 13
exercise: impact on immune system 59–60; impact on mental health 60–61; inadequacy 58–59; motivations for 63; physical 58
explanatory style and stress 277
external applications 447–448
external regulation 162

extrinsic goals 164
Eye Movement Desensitization and Reprocessing (EMDR) 451

facial nerve 200
fading 344–345
fallopian tube 230
Family Caregiver Cancer Education Programme (FCCEP) 372
family intervention 426
family support 113–114
fear of novelty 346
Feder, A. 411
female reproductive system 229–232; breasts 230–231; fallopian tube 230; ovaries 229; uterine cycle 231–232; uterus 230; vagina 230; vulva 230
Fencing, Alexander 8
Ferrara, M. 67
fight-or-flight response 244–245
Fishbein, M. I. 132
5-hydroxyindoleacetic acid (5-HIAA) 318
Fleshner, M. 269
Flocke, S. A. 383
Folkman, S. 252
forebrain 194
Fortner, M. 66
Fredrickson, B. L. 342
Freud, Sigmund 6, 7, 13, 119; *Studies on Hysteria* 6
Frey, Max von 440
Friedman, D. S. 382
Friedman, H. S. 8
Friedman, M. 10, 37, 271
Friend, R. 421
frontal lobe 195
functionalism 6

Galant-Miecznikowska, M. 258
Galen, Claudius 2–4
galvanic skin response (GSR) 349
gamma-aminobutyric acid (GABA) 104
Gandhi, Mahatma 429
Garmezy, N. 403–404
gastrointestinal diseases 309–311; Inflammatory Bowel Diseases (IBD) 310; Irritable Bowel Syndrome (IBS) 311; Peptic Ulcer Disease (PUD) 310–311
gastrointestinal system: and stress 272–273
Gastrooesophageal Reflux Disease (GERD) 273
gate control theory 441–442
Gawali, K. 360
Geenen, R. 329
General Adaptation Syndrome (GAS) 9, 245–247, *246*; alarm reaction 245; criticism 246–247; stage of exhaustion 246; stage of resistance 246
General Health Questionnaire (GHQ-28) 376

Gillin, J. C. 66
Given, B. 359, 376
Given, C. W. 359
Glanz, K. 120
Global Youth Tobacco Survey (GYTS) 96
glossopharyngeal nerves 200
glucocorticoid receptor (GR) 413
glucocorticoids 206
Goal Contents Theory (GCT) 164
goals: extrinsic 164; intrinsic 164; life 166
Gochman, D. S. 50
god/religion/faith 331
Going, S. 420
Gold, P. W. 247
Goldscheider, Arthur 440
gonadocorticoids 206
gonads 206
Gonzalez, A. B. 371
Gopinath, D. 372
Gotay, C. C. 418
Gras, M. J. 124
Grave's disease 304
Greene, R. 312
Grindley, E. J. 131
group interventions 339–340
Grunfeld, E. 363
Guadagni, V. 67
guidance—cooperation model 379
Guided Imagery 310, 342, 349, 394, 449–450
Guier, C. 420
Gururaj, G. 85, 96
Guten, S. 51, **52**
gutkha 98

Haas, J. S. 384
Hajar 1
Haley, W. E. 360
Hanigan, D. 23
hardiness 276–277, 403, 404, 425
Hariharan, M. 22, 23, 38, 258, 265, 280, 319, 330, 334, 385, 406, 422, 426
Hariharan-Rajendran Synergy Model of 406–407, *409*; adversity 407; outcome indicators 407–409; protective and promoting factors 407; resistance 407
Harris, D. M. 51, **52**
Haste, H. 55
Havens, B. 323
Havighurst, R. J. 422
Haygarth, J. 10
headache 308–309; migraine 309; primary 308–309; secondary 309; tension-type/muscle contraction 309
healing process 19
healing through sound 19
health 22; Ayurveda approach to 17–18; defined 10, 24; direct impact of stress on 266; indirect impact of stress on 266–267;

models of 24–32; practices in West 1; promotion 39–40; *purusharthas* 34; status of the individual 30; as understood by people 22–24
Health Action Process Approach (HAPA) 151–158, 413; application 156; criticisms 156; description 151–153; HAPA mechanism explained 153–155, *155*; intentions 151; outcome expectancies 151; planning 152–153; principles of 155–156; research on 157; risk perception 151; self-efficacy 151–152, *152*; self-monitoring/action control 153; two phases in **153**
health behaviour 50–51; defined 50; and lifestyle 50–51; model of self-determination theory explained in context of 165–166
Health Behaviour Model 413
Health Belief Model (HBM) 11, 120–126, *122*; application 123–124; genesis 120–121; limitations 124–125
health care professionals *see* care providers
health protective behaviour 51–52
Health Psychology 36–38; 4th–6th century BCE 1–2; 18th and 19th century 5–9; 20th century 9–15; aims and scope of 38–40; application 39–40; and Ayurveda 16–20; change in lifestyle 40–41; emergence of 1; framework of 44–46, *45*; in India 15–16; interventional studies of 12; need for 40–44; relevance of *46*; scope of 44–46; theorizing 38–39
health resilience 402–430; and ageing 422–424; and arthritis 419–420; and cancer 418–419; and cardiovascular disease 414–416; and chronic diseases 413–414, 425; clinical intervention 426; community-level interventions 427–428; concept of 403; in context of health 410–411; and dehydroepiandrosterone (DHEA) 411–412; and diabetes mellitus 416–418; and disabilities 421–422; family intervention 426; genetic influence on 412–413; Hariharan-Rajendran Synergy Model of 406, *409*; HPA activation 411; impacting factors 409–410; Indian perspective of intervention 428–429; interventions in educational institutions 427; interventions to 424–426; meta-theory of 405; and neurobiological response 412; and other chronic diseases 421; phenomenon of 404; physiology of 411–413; positive factors 413; as process 404–406; research 403–404; and resiliency 403–404; resilient woman 402–403; theories 413
health risk behaviour 80–115, **81**; as acquired habits 93–104; behavioural deviation from healthy practices 81–93; categories 81; cognitive factors 112; defined 80; maintaining 112; motivational factors 113
health screening behaviour 69
healthy eating 56–57, *58*; seasonal considerations for **57**
heart 209–210; chambers of 210; electrical system of 213–214; valves 210; walls 210
Helgeson, V. S. 415
helper T cells 237
Herzlich, C. 24
hindbrain 198
hippocampus 412
Hippocrates 2–4
Hochbaum, G. M. 123
Hoek, A. V. D. 124
Hollender, M. H. 378
Holmen, H. 146
Holmes, T. H. 248, 264
Holsboer, F. 411, 413
homeostasis 9, 247–248
Hospital Anxiety and Depression Scale (HADS) 319
HPA activation 411
H pylori bacteria 311
Huang, F. 92
Huang, H. 92
Huchting, K. 138
'human chronic gonadotrophin' (HCG) 232
Human Immunodeficiency Virus (HIV) 91–92; prevalence in India **91**; prevalence in world **91**
human physiology: cardiovascular system 209–214; digestive system 219–224; endocrine system 203–209; immune system 233–238; nervous system 186–203; renal system 224–227; reproductive system 228–233; respiratory system 214–219
human vulnerability to microbes 234–235
humoral immunity 237
humoural theory 2–3
Hunt, J. B. 130
hypertension 291, 294–295; aetiology of 294; prevention of 295; primary/essential 294; secondary 294; symptoms 295; treatment for 295
hyperthyroidism (overactive thyroid) 304
hypoglossal nerve 200
hypothalamic-pituitary-adrenal (HPA) 318
hypothalamic-pituitary-adrenal (HPA) axis response system 242–244, *244*
hypothalamus 196–197, *197*
hypothyroidism (underactive thyroid) 304

Ian, B. 315
Iaria, G. 67
identification, regulation through 162

illness: behaviour 321; biomedical model 26–27; cognition 315–316; cure 39; defined 27; management behaviour 291; prevention 40, 52–53, *53*; psychosocial aspects of 38; status of the individual 30; stress and 266–270, 320–321
immune system 233–238; alcohol consumption 107–108; and autoimmune diseases 270; errors in 270; exercise impact on 59–60; functions *237*; human vulnerability to microbes 234–235; operation of the body's defence system 238; stress and 267–269, *268*; white blood cells (WBC) or leucocytes 235–237
immune system and related diseases 311–312; pancreatitis 312; rheumatoid arthritis 311–312
immunization: behaviour 72–74; behaviour through patient education 75; drive in rural India 74; rates and socioeconomic status 73
impersonal orientation 164
India: Ayurveda (*see* Ayurveda); Health Psychology in 15–16; HIV prevalence in **91**; immunization drive in rural 74; obesity 85; top causes of death in **81**; University of Hyderabad 15
Indian independence 429
Indian perspective of intervention 428–429
Indian perspective of resilience intervention 428–429
Indian Space Research Organisation (ISRO) 427
indirect association 317, 318–320
'*Indriya*' (sense organs) 17
Inflammatory Bowel Disease (IBD) 273, 310
inner sound 19
instrumental activities of daily living (IADL) 359
insulin-dependent diabetes mellitus (IDDM) 305; *see also* type 1 diabetes
integrated regulation 162–163
intensive care units (ICU) 334
intensive theory 439–440
intercostal muscles 217
intermediate emotional state 130
internal stress: external sources 255; family environment 255; social environment 255–256; work content 257; work context 257–258; work environment 256–257
International Association of Applied Psychology (IAAP) 13
International Association of the Study of Pain (IASP) 437
International Society for Health Psychology Research (ISHPR) 13
Internet addiction 110–112
interneurons (association neurons) 189
interpretation of pain 444–445

interventions: behavioural 343, 345; biofeedback 348–349; for caregiver 369; for chronic illness management 334; clinical 426; to cognitive distortions 337–338; community-level 427–428; in educational institutions 427; family 426; to foster resilience 424–426; to health resilience 424–426; Indian perspective of 428–429; motivational 345; in pain management 447–451; positive thought 342; for psychological distress 372–374; psychosocial 447–451
intrinsic goals 164
intrinsic motivation 160–161
introjected regulation 162
Irritable Bowel Syndrome (IBS) 273, 311
Irwin, M. 66
ischaemia (reduced blood supply) 295
ischaemic stroke 300

Jackson, K. M. 104
Jacobson's Progressive Muscular Relaxation (JPMR) 449
James, William 6, 13
James-Lange theory of emotion 6
Jamuna, D. 424
Janis, I. L. 10
Japanese Health Psychology 13
Jay, G. M. 23
Jeihooni 124
Jekauc, D. 59
Jensen, M. P. 321
Jhangri, G. S. 329
Joels, M. 411, 413
John, R. 422
Johnston-Brooks, C. H. 416
de Jongh, B. 258
Journal of Health Communication 13
Journal of Health Psychology 13
Journal of Indian Health Psychology 13
Journal of Occupational Health Psychology 13
Jutras, S. 23
'juxtaglomerular cells' 226

Kala 35
Kala parinama 35
Kama (sensual enjoyments) 34, 56
Kanbay, Y. 97
Kanner, A. D. 250
kapha 17
Kapha dosha 61
Kapur, S. 428
Karadoğan, D. 97
Karimi, M. 422
Kashyapa 17
Kasl, S. V. 50
Katon, W. 319

Kayachikitsa (internal medicine) 17
Keller, M. 104
Kerlinger, R. 119
Key, T. J. 55
kidneys 224–225; acid-alkaline balance (pH) 227; alcohol consumption 107; blood pressure 226–227; chemical balance 227; glomeruli (filtering system) 305; microscopic parts in 225–227; osmolarity 227
killer T cells 236
Kim, H. S. 123
Kim, Y. 146
Kimmel, S. R. 73
Kirby, T. E. 173
Kishore, M. T. 319, 422
Kleinman, A. 27
deKloet, E. R. 411, 413
Knott, K. 38
Knowlden, A. P. 62
knowledge intervention 339–341; impact of *341*
Kobasa, S. 276, 404
Kohli, N. 414
Kopparty, S. 367
Krause, N. M. 23
Kroenke, K. 319
Kuan, G. 146
Kueh, Y. C. 146
Kuijer, R. 329
Kumar, B. S. 98
Kumar, G. A. 93
Kumar, R. 424
Kwon, O. Y. 376

labelling/mislabelling 337
laboratory experiments 265
LaBrie, J. W. 138
Lac, A. 138
Lalnuntluangi, R. 330, 417
Langade, D. 390
Lange, Carl 6
large intestine 221–223
Larsen, P. D. 291
larynx 216
Lawton, M. P. 361
Lazarus, R. S. 10, 127, 250, 252
Leder, D. 424
Lee, A. Y. 137
Leproult, R. 66
Leventhal, E. A. 23, 127, 318
Leventhal, H. 23, 177, 291, 315, 318
Leventhal, H. O. R. 315, 318
Li, S. 92
life events 263–264
life goals 166
lifestyle: change in 40–41; defined 50; diseases **41**, 41–44, 332; and health behaviour 50–51; risk 43–44

light sleep 88
limbic system 196
Lin, E. H. 319
Lin, L. 65
lipid hormones 204
Lisha, S. 421
Liu, K. T. 146
liver 223; and alcohol consumption 106–107; functions of 223
Lleras, A. 111
locus of control (LoC) 274–275, *275*
López, M. A. 62
Losada, A. 376
loss of control 324–325
loss of dignity and stigma 325–326
lungs 216; protection for 216–217
lymphatic system 235
lymphocytes 236

Ma, L. C. 421
Mackinnon, N. 101
Madaan, V. 60
Madhava Nidanam 17
Magliano, L. 365
magnification/minimization 337
Maier, S. F. 269
maintenance self-efficacy 151, 152, *152*
major anatomical map of the brain 193–199
male reproductive system 229; penis 229; prostate gland 229
malnutrition: India 85; unhealthy diet 83, **84**
Manas (thoughts) 34
Manning, M. R. 276
Manser, T. 393
mantra (prayer) 19, 22, 428
Markland, D. 166
Martines, G. F. 255
Martinsen, E. W. 60
Mason, J. W. 246–247
massage, and sleep 69
Masten, A. 404, 406
Matarazzo, J. D. 51
McClintick, J. 66
McEwen, B. S. 247, 248
measles 74
measuring stress 262–263
Meier, L. L. 393
melatonin 88
Melzack, R. 10, 441, 442
memory T cells 236
meninges 192
menopause 231–232
mental health: alcohol consumption 108; exercise impact on 60–61; and sleep 67; smoking behaviour 96
metencephalon 198
Metgud, R. 98

462 *Index*

Miaskowski, C. 362
microbes: human vulnerability to 234–235
microscopic parts in kidney 225–227
midbrain 197
Middendorp, H. van 329
Migliorini, R. 259
Mignot, E. 65
migraine headache 309
Miller, Janis 13
Miller, Neal 12
Miller, W. L. 383
mind-body dualism 2, *4*
mind-reading 336
mineralocorticoids 206
mini-theories 164–165
Mishra, R. C. 330, 343
Misra, G. 414
Moattar, M. 124
models: defined 119; of stress 241; *vs.* theory/ies 119
Mohammadnezhad, M. 383
Mohan, H. 446
Mok, W. K. 137
Moksha (liberation) 34
Moksnes, U. K. 280
Monico, N. 106
Monteiro, S. R. 22, 23
Moore, M. R. 321
Morille, M. 418
Moser, D. 415
Mossey, J. M. 38
motivation: intrinsic 160–161; types of 159–160, *160*
motivational factors: health risk behaviour 113
motivational interventions 345
motivational interviewing 296, 347–348
mouth 219
multipolar neuron 188
Murphy, N. A. 361
Murthy, N. S. 372
Murugesh, C. J. 98
muscular function 217
Mutran, E. 38
mutual participation model 379
myelencephalon medulla oblongata 198
myocardial infarction 297–298
myocardium 210, 295

Nada Yoga 19
Nadkarni, A. 101
Nafe, J. P. 440
Naik, S. 98
Nandinee, D. 341
Narayanan, A. 428
NarishaktiPuraskar 402
Narváez, J. 420
Nasypany, A. M. 131

National Family Health Survey (NFHS-4) 99
National Opinion Research Centre 360
natural disaster 258
natural protection to brain 191, *192*
natural sleep *(swabhavika)* 68
Naunyn, Bernhard 439
negative emotional state 241
negative emotions 317, 363, 427
Nehru, Jawaharlal 429
Neighbors, M. 294
nervous system 186–203; alcohol consumption impact on 105–106; axon 187; cell body/soma 187; central nervous system (CNS) 191; cerebrospinal fluid (CSF) 193; dendrites 187; major anatomical map of the brain 193–199; meninges 192; natural protection to brain 191, *192*; neural communication as function of neuron 189–191; neurons 187; peripheral nervous system (PNS) 199–201; reflex arc 189; somatic nervous system 201–202; structure of a neuron 187, *188*; support for neurons 189; sympathetic nervous system 202; terminal buttons 187; types of neurons 188–189
nervous system and diseases 306–309; dementia 308; epilepsy 307; headache 308–309; Parkinson's disease 307; spinal cord injury 307–308
Nestler, E. J. 411
neural communication as function of neuron 189–191
neurobiological response 412
neurogenesis 60
neurons 187; afferent 189; bipolar 188; efferent 189; interneurons 189; multipolar 188; neural communication as function of 189–191; structure of 187, *188*; support for 189; types of 188–189; unipolar 188–189
neuropathic pain 438
Nicholson, N. R. 323–324
'*Nidra*' (sleep) *see* sleep
Niermann, C. 59
Nishkamakarma (doing with no expectation of reward) 362
No, J. K. 123
nociceptive pain 438–439
non-communicable diseases (NCDs) 19, 41; exercise inadequacy 58–59; and sleep 66–67
non–insulin-dependent diabetes mellitus (NIDDM) 305; *see also* Type 2 diabetes
Non-Rapid Eye Movement (NREM) sleep 88
Normandeau, S. 23
normative beliefs 133
Northouse, L. L. 370
nose 215

Novoa, S. O. 371
Ntoumanis, N. 167

obesity: India 85; prevalence among adults **82**; unhealthy diet 82–85
Obradovich, N. 259
observational learning/modelling 169
occipital lobe 195
Occupational Health Psychology 14
oculomotor nerve 200
oesophagus 220
oestrogen 206–207
Ogden, J. 121
olfactory nerve 200
Önal, Ö. 97
Onstad, L. E. 97
operant conditioning 75–76
operation of the body's defence system 238
optic nerve 200
optimum stress level (OSL) 261–262, *262*
Orbuch, T. L. 418
'Ordered Protection Motivation Schema' (OPM) 130
Organismic Integration Theory (OIT) 161–163; external regulation 162; integrated regulation 162–163; introjected regulation 162; regulation through identification 162
orientation: autonomous 163; causality 166; controlled 164; impersonal 164
osmolarity 227
O'Toole, M. S. 376
ovarian cycle 231
ovaries 229
overgeneralization 336–337

paan masala 98
Paba, D. P. 62
Pace, P. 255
Padhy, M. 330, 334, 385, 417
Padiri, R. A. 330
Padmaja, G. 366–367
pain 436–451; acute 437–438; attention to 444; biomedical model of 442–451; biopsychosocial phenomenon 442–451; chronic 438–439; cognition, beliefs and attitudes 445; coping behaviour 447; defined 437; emotions 445–446; interpretation of 444–445; neuropathic 438; nociceptive 438–439; psychological and social factors of 442–447; psychosocial factors of *443*; psychosocial interventions in 447–451; radicular 439; sociocultural factors in 446–447; somatic 438; theories of 439–442; types of 437; visceral 438
Pakenham, K. I. 421
panchabhootas 32–33
panchamahabhootas 17, *33*

Panchatantra 428
pancreas 207; and alcohol consumption 106–107
pancreatitis 107, 312
Panova, T. 111
parathyroid glands 207–208
parietal lobes 195
Parkinson's disease 307, 375, 421
Parry, C. 419
Parsons, T. 10
Pasacreta, J. V. 372
Pasteur, Louis 6, *7*, 8
pasteurization 6
Patel, Sardar 429
patient and caregiver relationship *366*
patient care 39, 357–358, 387–389; impact on caregiver 359–360
Patient Health Questionnaire 9 (PHQ 9) 319
patient satisfaction 382–384
pattern theory 440–441
Patterson, B. 55
Paulus, M. P. 259
Pavlov, Ivan 5, 13
Payaprom, Y. 156
Pearson, S. D. 377
Peltzer, K. 319
Pengpid, S. 319
penicillin 8
Peptic Ulcer Disease (PUD) 310–311
peptide hormones 204
perceived behavioural control 136–137
perceived susceptibility 120
periaqueductal grey matter 197–198
perimetrium 230
peripheral nervous system (PNS) 199–201
Perna, L. 423
Pertaub, D. P. 271
Peterson, A. V. 97
Petrie, K. J. 316
Petty, F. D. 60
phagocytes 235–236
pharynx 216
physical ambience, and sleep 68
physical environment: and stress 258
physical exercise 58
physical health 361–362
physician burnout: causes of 392; coping with 394; handling at individual level 393–394; impact of 392; impact on health care system 393; impact on patients 393; intervention at institutional level 394–395; intervention at policy level 395; interventions for 393; onset and progress of 390–392, *391*; symptoms 389, 390
physiological measures of stress: biochemical analysis 263; electrical and mechanical equipment 263; psychological scales 263–266

physiological systems 292–294
Piasecki, T. M. 98
Pienyu, R. 334
pineal gland 207–208
pitta 17, 34
pituitary gland 204–205
placebo effect 10
planful problem solving 330
polio 74
pons 198
positive affect 342, 449
positive emotions 362–363
positive health behaviour 49–77; body weight and sleep duration 65–66; diet 55; exercise 58–61; factors influencing 75–76; health protective behaviour 51–52; health screening behaviour 69; healthy eating 56–57, *58*; illness prevention 52–53, *53*; immunization behaviour 72–74; mental health and sleep 67; NCDs and sleep 66–67; physical exercise 58; primary prevention 53–54; secondary prevention 54; sleep and immune function 66; sleep behaviour 64–65, **65**; tertiary prevention 54–55; *Yoga asana* 62–63
positive reappraisal 330–331
positive stress 283
positive thought intervention 342
positive thoughts 342
post-traumatic stress disorder (PTSD) 392, 451
'the Powerful Placebo' (Beecher) 10
powerlessness 324–325
pragmatism 6
Prajnaparadha 35
Prakash, V. 412
Prakruti 35
'*pranayama*' (breathing exercises) 36, 450
Prasad, K. 258
prasannatmendriyamanah 17
Precaution Adoption Process Model (PAPM) 148–150, *149*
premenstrual syndrome (PMS)/premenstrual dysphoric disorder (PMDD) 312–331; adaptation 328–329; aetiology 313, *313*; affect state 317; biopsychosocial symptoms of *314*; chronic condition and negative emotions 317; chronic illness 313–315; coping 329–331; coping with chronic illness 327; described 312–313; direct association 317, 318; illness cognition 315–316; illness-stress relationship 320–321; indirect association 317, 318–320; loss of control 324–325; loss of dignity and stigma 325–326; powerlessness 324–325; psychological factors 313–315; social isolation 323–324; symptom perception 316–317; symptoms 313; treatment 313, *314*; uncertainty 321–323; vulnerability 325–326
prevalence 390
prevalence of depression and anxiety **319**
prevention of social isolation 324
preventive behaviour 53
primary appraisal 252
primary caregivers 358
primary/essential hypertension 294
primary headache 308–309
primary prevention 53–54
principles of psychological therapy 335–338
Priya, N. K. 98
problem drinking 101–104
process of filtration 226
Prochaska, J. O. 138, 141, 143, 146
progesterone 207
Programme for Affective and Cognitive Education (PACE) 341–342
prompting 344–345
prostate-specific antigen (PSA) 371
protection motivation 128
Protection Motivation Theory (PMT) 413; application 130–131; description 127–130, *128–129*; limitations 131; overview 127
psychoeducation 296, 340–342, 370–372
psychological interventions 296, 373, 374
psychological therapy: cognitive interventions 338; cognitive schemas and distortions 335–337; interventions to cognitive distortions 337–338; principles of 335–338
Psychology, Health and Medicine 13
Psychology and Health: An International Review 13
psychology of caregiver 355–357
psychoneuroimmunology 270
psychosocial care 38
psychosocial interventions for caregiver 369
psychosocial intervention to chronic illness *333*
psychosocial moderators of stress 274–285; behavioural indicators of stress in children 283–284; causes of 277; childhood stress 280–282; explanatory style and stress 277; hardiness 276–277; impact of a negative event 277; interventions for childhood stress 284; locus of control (LoC) 274–275, *275*; outcome of a negative event 277–279; positive stress 283; self-efficacy 276; stakes-effort balance & stress 279, *279*; tolerable stress 283; toxic stress 283
Psychosomatic Medicine 9–10
puberty 228, 230
Public Health Psychology 14
pulmonary diseases 301–303; asthma 302–303; Chronic Obstructive Pulmonary Disease (COPD) 303; cystic fibrosis (CF) 301–302
pulmonary veins 211
purusharthas 34

quasi-experiments in natural setting 265–266
Quiñonez, N. 62

radicular pain 439
Radley, A. 26
Raeke, L. H. 377
Ragitha, R. 422
Rahe, R. H. 248, 264
Rahwan, I. 259
Raina, P. 361
Rajan, A. M. 422
Rajas (royal) 33–34
Rajendran, A. 408, 409
Rajeski, W. J. 60
Rakhshani, A. 63
Ramamurti, P. V. 424
Rana, S. 38, 330, 334, 406
Rao, C. R. 22, 23, 409
Rapid Eye Movement (REM) sleep 88
Rashmi, P. 98
Rath, R. 280
Ray, M. L. 129
recovery self-efficacy 151, 152, *152*
red nucleus 197
reductionist theory of mind 2
reflex arc 189
regulation: external 162; integrated 162–163; introjected 162; through identification 162
Reiner, M. 59
reinforcements 169
relatedness: defined 164
Relationship Motivation Theory (RMT) 164–166; model of self-determination theory explained in the context of health behaviour 165–166; model that integrates all the mini-theories 164–165
relaxation techniques 12, 449–450
renal diseases 305–306; chronic glomerulonephritis 305–306; renal failure 306
renal failure 306
renal system 224–227; kidneys 224–225; microscopic parts in kidney 225–227; process of filtration 226; structure of renal system 224–225; ureters 225; urethra 226; urinary bladder 225–226
reproductive system 228–233; alcohol consumption 107; female reproductive system 229–232; male reproductive system 229; reproduction and preparation for the body 232; and stress 273–274
reproductive system and diseases 312–331; premenstrual syndrome (PMS)/premenstrual dysphoric disorder (PMDD) 312–331
research evidence 322
resilience *see* health resilience

Resilience Test Battery 409
resiliency 403–404
resistance 347
resistance to change 346
respiratory cycle 217
respiratory system 214–219; breathing and the control centre 217; breathing mechanism—pressure relationship 217–218; bronchi 216; larynx 216; lungs 216; nose 215; pharynx 216; protection for lungs 216–217; and stress 271–274; trachea 216; voluntary control over breath 218
response shaping 344
reticular formation 197
rheumatoid arthritis 311–312, 419–420
Richardson, G. E. 405–407, 412
Rimer, B. K. 120
Rippetoe, P. A. 129
'Ritucharya' (seasonal diet) 36
Rivera, J. V. 371
Robinson-Smith, G. 416
Robottom, B. J. 421
Rogers, R. W. 127, 129
Rosenman, R. H. 10, 37, 271
Rosenstock, I. M. 120–121
Rothman, A. J. 148
Ruland, C. M. 362
Ryan, R. M. 160, 166–167

Sachdev, P. 424
'Sadvritta' (social behaviour) 36
Sandman, P. M. 150
Sapkal, Sindhu (Sindhu Tai) 402–403
Saraf, S. 418
Sarafino, E. P. 52, 54
Sarason, I. G. 97
Satish, L. 62
Sattva (truth/reality) 33–34
'Satya' (the purest form) 17
Schaefer, C. 250
Schwarzer, R. 151, 156
screening: for detecting disease 71–72; for health risk 69–71
scrotum 229
Sebastian, N. M. 384
Secker, D. L. 376
secondary appraisal 252
secondary caregivers 358
secondary headache 309
secondary hypertension 294
secondary prevention 54
seeking social support 330
Seema, N. N. 334
selective abstraction 336
Self-Determination Theory (SDT) 158–168; application 166–167; Basic Psychological

466 Index

Needs Theory (BPNT) 163; causality orientation 166; Causality Orientation Theory (COT) 163–164; Cognitive Evaluation Theory (CET) 159–161; Goal Contents Theory (GCT) 164; health care climate *165,* 165–166; life goals 166; Organismic Integration Theory (OIT) 161–163; Relationship Motivation Theory (RMT) 164–166; subtheories of 159–166
self-efficacy 113, 121, 136, 145–146, 169, 276, 347–348, 413, 416–417, *417,* 420; action 151, 152, *152;* beliefs of 171; maintenance 151, 152, *152;* recovery 151, 152, *152*
self-image: and smoking behaviour 97–98
self-liberation 144
self-management 325
self-reevaluation 144
self-regulation 346
Self-Regulation Model (SRM) 174–178, 413; application 177; basic constructs 175; description 175–177, *176;* illness representation 175
Selye, H. 9, 13, 245–247
semilunar valves 210
sense of coherence (SoC) 403–404, 418, 425
sexually transmitted infections (STI) 92
shaping: response 344; stimulus 344; use of 343–344
'*Sharira*' (the body) 17
Sharma, A. 60, 424
Sharma, M. 62
Sharma, S. 414
Sharngdhara Samhita 17
Shastri, Lal Bahadur 429
Shellman, J. 323
Shen, X. 92
Sherman, W. M. 173
Sherrington, Charles 440
Shetty, H. 389
Shukla, A. 69
skeletal system: alcohol consumption 107
Slater, M. 271
sleep: behaviour 64–65, **65**; duration, and body weight 65–66; healthy, and Ayurveda 67–69; hygiene 89–90; and immune function 66; and mental health 67; and NCDs 66–67; stages of 88
sleep-debt condition 66
sleep posture 69
sleep-recovery period 66
slow wave sleep (SWS) 88
small intestine 221
Smith, B. W. 420
Smith, R. S. 403
smoking behaviour 93–98; antecedents to smoking 96; cancer 95; cardiovascular system 93–94; circulatory system 94; contributing factors 96–97; and fertility 96; mental health 96; respiratory system 94–95; and self-image 97–98; synergistic effects of smoke 94
social cognition process 143
Social Cognitive Theory (SCT) 168–174, 413; application 173; explanation of the theory in general context 169–170; limitations 173; observational learning/modelling 169; outcome expectations 169; personal factors 170; reinforcements 169; self-efficacy 169; social environmental factors 170; theory explained in the context of health behaviour 170–172, *172*
social facilitation and barriers 346
social isolation 323–324
socializing 448
social learning or modelling 76
social liberation 144
social media addiction 110–112
Social Readjustment Rating Scale (SRRS) 248, **249,** 250, 264
social support 113, 330, 342–343
Socrates 2
Soma Sundaram, R.O. 418
somatic nervous system 201–202
somatic pain 438
sources of stress 254, *256*
specificity theory 440
Spiegel, K. 66
spinal cord 198–199, *199*
spinal cord injury 307–308
spleen 235
Srimad Bhagavad Gita 331
Srinadh, B. 334
Srivastava, A. 414
stakes-effort balance & stress 279, *279*
standard physical exercise training 296
Stansfeld, S. 258
Stellar, E. 247
Stenberg, U. 362, 363
Stewart, M. 381
stimulus control 145
stimulus shaping 344
stomach 220–221
Strecher, V. J. 121
stress 240–245; anthropogenic 259–260; biochemical and physiological changes in the body 241; and cardiovascular disorders 270–271; chemical 259; climate 259; cognitive appraisal 241; daily hassles 264; defined 240; demands on self 240; energetic 260; environmental 258; ergonomic 260–261; fight-or-flight response 244–245; and gastrointestinal system 272–273;

hypothalamic-pituitary-adrenal (HPA) axis response system 242–244, *244*; and illness 266–270; and immune system 267–269, *268*; laboratory experiments 265; life events 263–264; limited resources 240–241; measuring 262–263; and medicophysiological models 242; models of 241; negative emotional state 241; positive 283; psychosocial moderators of 274–285; quasi-experiments in natural setting 265–266; and reproductive system 273–274; and respiratory system 271–274; as response 242; sources of 254, *256*; as a stimulus 248–250; Sympathetic Adrenomedullary Response System (SAM) 242, *243*; tolerable 283; toxic 283
stress management training 296
stroke/cerebrovascular accident 300–301; *see also* ischaemic stroke
Strong, C. A. 440
Studies on Hysteria (Freud) 6
Subar, A. 55
Subramanyan, K. 413
substantia nigra 197
Suchman, A. L. 384
Sugai, D. Y. 381
Sullivan, M. D. 415
Sunitha, S. 85, 96
suppressor T cells 237
susceptibility: defined 120; perceived 120
Sushruta 61
Sushruta Samhita 17
Sutton, S. R. 148
Svastha 17
Swain, S. 258, 330, 334, 381
swastha 31, 34
Symister, P. 421
Sympathetic Adrenomedullary Response System (SAM) 242, *243*
sympathetic nervous system 202
symptom perception 316–317
systematic desensitization 345
system theory 29
Szasz, T. S. 378

Taheri, S. 65
Tak, A. 98
Tamas 33–34
Tannehill-Jones, R. 294
Tanner Jr. J. F. 130
Tantipong, H. 156
Taylor, N. 428
Taylor, S. E. 50, 93
tectum 197
tegmentum 197
temporal lobe 195
tension-type/muscle contraction headache 309

terminal buttons 187
tertiary prevention 54–55
Tesfaye, G. 93
testes 229
testosterone 207
thalamus 196, *197*
theory/ies: defined 119; of health behavioural change **179–182**; *vs.* model 119; of pain 439–442; usefulness of 120
Theory of Planned Behaviour (TPB) 135–138, *137*; application 137–138; behavioural control and achievement motivation 136; behavioural control and locus of control 136; behavioural control and self-efficacy 136–137; description 135; limitations 138; perceived behavioural control 136
Theory of Reasoned Action (TRA) 132–134, *133*; application 134; limitations 134; overview 132–133
therapeutic interventions 332–334; baseline assessment 334; for chronic illness management 334
Thomas, M. 38, 334, 341
Thomas, S. 334
thought substitution 449
threat appraisal 128
thymus 235
thyroid gland 206, 304; *see also* hyperthyroidism (overactive thyroid); hypothyroidism (underactive thyroid)
tobacco consumption 98
Tobin, V. J. 166
tolerable stress 283
Tornay, E. 372
toxic stress 283
trachea 216
transactional theory of stress 250–266; anthropogenic stress 259–260; chemical stress 259; climate stress 259; energetic stress 260; ergonomic stress 260–261; external sources 255; family environment 255; internal sources 254–258; measuring stress 262–263; natural disaster 258; optimum stress level (OSL) 261–262, *262*; physical environment 258; physiological measure 263–266; primary appraisal 252; secondary appraisal 252; social environment 255–256; sources of stress 254, *256*; work content 257; work context 257–258; work environment 256–257
transmission cells 441
Transtheoretical Model (TTM) 138–148, *139,* 413; applications 146; limitations 146–147; stages of *140,* 141–146; stages of change 139
tridoshas 32–33, 35; and *trigunas* 33–36

trigeminal nerve 200
trigunas: Rajas (*see Rajas* (royal)); *Sattva* (*see Sattva* (truth/reality)); *Tamas* (*see Tamas*); and *tridoshas* 33–36
trochlear nerve 200
Trovato, F. M. 255
Trovato, G. M. 255
tuberculosis 74
type 1 diabetes 305, 416
type 2 diabetes 290–291, 305, 416
type A personality 37

ulcerative colitis (UC) 310
Unani 19
uncertainty 321–323, *323*
Ungar, M. 426
unhealthy diet 82–87; adolescence 86; adulthood 86–87; childhood 86; elderly 87
unhealthy sexual behaviour 90–93; knowledge deficiency 92; trigger to 92–93
unhealthy sleep behaviour 87–90; habits that interfere with sleep 88–89; sleep hygiene 89–90; stages of sleep 88
unipolar neurons 188–189
Upadhyay, S. 414
ureters 225
urethra 226
urinary bladder 225–226
uterine cycle 231–232
uterus 230

vagina 230
vagus nerve 200
VaidyoNaraayanoHarih 377
Vaillant, G. E. 104
Vairale, J. 360
varicose veins 299–300
vata 17
Velásquez, A. M. 62
Verma, A. 32
Verma, S. K. 32
vestibulocochlear nerve 200
visceral pain 438
vision: alcohol consumption 108
Viswanath, K. 120
voluntary control over breath 218
vulnerability 325–326
vulva 230
vyayama 61

Walker, C. 325
Wall, P. D. 10, 441, 442
Wallace, L. S. 173
Walters, J. R. 259
Wang, D. 427
Ward, P. 383
Warshaw, G. 290
Watkins, L. R. 269
Weinstein, N. D. 148, 150
Welp, A. 393
Werner, E. 403
Wernicke-Korsakoff Syndrome 105
Wernicke's disease (WD) 105–106
West, R. 97
Western psychology 19
Westman, J. C. 259
White, J. 66
white blood cells (WBC) or leucocytes 235–237
Wicks, M. N. 360
Wiggers, L. C. 124
Wilkie, W. L. 129
Williams, G. C. 166–167
Williams, R. F. 276
Wilson, I. B. 382
Wins, I. 23
Wolfe, D. M. 276
Woll, A. 59
Worku, A. 93
World Health Organization (WHO) 291, 409–410, 413; on alcohol consumption 99; definition of health 10, 24; population-wide screening tests criteria 71; on smoking behaviour 93
World War II 8
wound healing 269
Wright, L. J. 420

Xu, G. 92

Yan, Y. 131
Yang, C. 427
Yi, J. P. 416
Yoga 428
Yoga asana 62–63
yoga nidra 450
Young, P. C. 361
Young, T. 65

Zautra, A. J. 420
Zizzi, S. J. 131